Springer Series in Statistics

Advisors:
P. Bickel, P. Diggle, S. Fienberg, U. Gather,
I. Olkin, S. Zeger

Springer Series in Statistics

Andersen/Borgan/Gill/Keiding: Statistical Models Based on Counting Processes.
Atkinson/Riani: Robust Diagnostic Regression Analysis.
Atkinson/Riani/Cerioli: Exploring Multivariate Data with the Forward Search.
Berger: Statistical Decision Theory and Bayesian Analysis, 2nd edition.
Borg/Groenen: Modern Multidimensional Scaling: Theory and Applications.
Brockwell/Davis: Time Series: Theory and Methods, 2nd edition.
Bucklew: Introduction to Rare Event Simulation.
Chan/Tong: Chaos: A Statistical Perspective.
Chen/Shao/Ibrahim: Monte Carlo Methods in Bayesian Computation.
Coles: An Introduction to Statistical Modeling of Extreme Values.
David/Edwards: Annotated Readings in the History of Statistics.
Devroye/Lugosi: Combinatorial Methods in Density Estimation.
Efromovich: Nonparametric Curve Estimation: Methods, Theory, and Applications.
Eggermont/LaRiccia: Maximum Penalized Likelihood Estimation, Volume I: Density Estimation.
Fahrmeir/Tutz: Multivariate Statistical Modelling Based on Generalized Linear Models, 2nd edition.
Fan/Yao: Nonlinear Time Series: Nonparametric and Parametric Methods.
Farebrother: Fitting Linear Relationships: A History of the Calculus of Observations 1750-1900.
Federer: Statistical Design and Analysis for Intercropping Experiments, Volume I: Two Crops.
Federer: Statistical Design and Analysis for Intercropping Experiments, Volume II: Three or More Crops.
Ghosh/Ramamoorthi: Bayesian Nonparametrics.
Glaz/Naus/Wallenstein: Scan Statistics.
Good: Permutation Tests: A Practical Guide to Resampling Methods for Testing Hypotheses, 2nd edition.
Good: Permutation Tests: Parametric and Bootstrap Tests of Hypotheses, 3rd edition.
Gouriéroux: ARCH Models and Financial Applications.
Gu: Smoothing Spline ANOVA Models.
Györfi/Kohler/Krzyżak/ Walk: A Distribution-Free Theory of Nonparametric Regression.
Haberman: Advanced Statistics, Volume I: Description of Populations.
Hall: The Bootstrap and Edgeworth Expansion.
Härdle: Smoothing Techniques: With Implementation in S.
Harrell: Regression Modeling Strategies: With Applications to Linear Models, Logistic Regression, and Survival Analysis.
Hart: Nonparametric Smoothing and Lack-of-Fit Tests.
Hastie/Tibshirani/Friedman: The Elements of Statistical Learning: Data Mining, Inference, and Prediction.
Hedayat/Sloane/Stufken: Orthogonal Arrays: Theory and Applications.
Heyde: Quasi-Likelihood and its Application: A General Approach to Optimal Parameter Estimation.

(continued after index)

Geert Molenberghs
Geert Verbeke

Models for Discrete Longitudinal Data

With 61 Figures

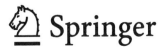

Geert Molenberghs
Center for Statistics
Universiteit Hasselt
Agoralaan 1
B-3590 Diepenbeek
Belgium
Geert.Molenberghs@uhasselt.be

Geert Verbeke
Biostatistical Centre
K.U. Leuven
Kapucijnenvoer 35
B-3000 Leuven
Belgium
Geert.Verbeke@med.kuleuven.be

Library of Congress Control Number: 2005923258

ISBN-10: 0-387-25144-8   Printed on acid-free paper.
ISBN-13: 978-0387-25144-8

© 2005 Springer Science+Business Media, Inc.
All rights reserved. This work may not be translated or copied in whole or in part without the written permission of the publisher (Springer Science+Business Media, Inc., 233 Spring Sreet., New York, NY 10013, USA), except for brief excerpts in connection with reviews or scholarly analysis. Use in connection with any form of information storage and retrieval, electronic adaptation, computer software, or by similar or dissimilar methodology now known or hereafter developed is forbidden.
The use in this publication of trade names, trademarks, service marks, and similar terms, even if they are not identified as such, is not to be taken as an expression of opinion as to whether or not they are subject to proprietary rights.

Printed in the United States of America.   (MVY)

9 8 7 6 5 4 3 2 1

springeronline.com

To Conny, An, and Jasper

To Godewina, Lien, Noor, and Aart

Preface

The linear mixed model has become the main parametric tool for the analysis of continuous longitudinal data. Verbeke and Molenberghs (2000) devoted an entire text to the model, a number of its extensions, and how to deal with incompletely observed longitudinal profiles. The model can be fitted in a wide variety of commercially available software packages, such as the SAS procedure MIXED, the SPlus function lme, the MLwiN package, etc. Although the model can be interpreted as a natural hierarchical extension of linear regression and analysis of variance, it is our experience from courses, scientific collaboration, and statistical consultancy that the model remains surrounded with non-trivial issues such as the difference between a hierarchical and a marginal interpretation, complexities arising with inference for variance components, assessing goodness-of-fit, the effect of (mis-)specifying the random-effects distribution, etc.

Our courses, consultancy, and research in the area of longitudinal data analysis have included the non-Gaussian setting as well, including binary, ordinal repeated measures, as well as counts measured repeatedly over time. Our experience has been that the issues in this field are a multiple of those in the continuous case, predominantly due to the lack of an unambiguous counterpart of the multivariate normal distribution. Almost all models exhibit a certain amount of non-linearity. Even when attention is restricted to the special non-linear models of the generalized linear type, important differences between the classes of marginal, conditional, and subject-specific models arise. Within each of these, subfamilies can be identified within which, in turn, many different models can be placed. Different problems may call for different solutions and hence different modeling strategies.

In addition, due to computational complexity, many models require the use of approximate numeric methods, each one with its advantages and disadvantages. The issues are further compounded when planned measurement sequences are incompletely observed and strategies to deal with such incompleteness may depend in important ways on the inferential framework within which a particular model is framed. Fortunately, a variety of standard statistical software tools is now available to handle, possibly incomplete, non-Gaussian repeated measures, including the SAS procedures GENMOD, GLIMMIX, NLMIXED, MI, and MIANALYZE.

Verbeke and Molenberghs (2000) have not dealt with the non-Gaussian case, and we aim to fill this gap with the current text. Regular and short courses have helped shape our thinking regarding the selection of material and the emphasis to put on various model families, models, and inferential aspects. We mention in particular the regular courses on Correlated and Multivariate Data in the Master of Science in Applied Statistics Programme of the Limburgs Universitair Centrum, the Longitudinal Data Analysis and Advanced Modeling Techniques courses of the Master of Science in Biostatistics Programme of the Limburgs Universitair Centrum, and the Repeated Measures course in the International Study Programme in Statistics of the Katholieke Universiteit Leuven. We further learned a lot from teaching short courses to audiences with various backgrounds at numerous locations in Europe, North and South America, the Caribbean, Australia, and Asia.

Just as with Verbeke and Molenberghs (2000), we hope this book will be of value to a wide audience, including applied statisticians and biomedical researchers, particularly in the biopharmaceutical industry, medical and public health research organizations, contract research organizations, and academic departments. The majority of the chapters are explanatory rather than research oriented, although some chapters contain advanced material. A perspective is given in Chapter 1. Practice is emphasized rather than mathematical rigor. In this respect, guidance and advice on practical issues are important focuses of the text, and numerous extensively analyzed examples are included, many running across several chapters.

Virtually all of the statistical analyses were performed using SAS procedures such as MIXED, GENMOD, GLIMMIX, NLMIXED, MI, and MIANALYZE, as well as the SAS macro GLIMMIX. Almost all analyses were done using the SAS Version 9.1. The GLIMMIX procedure used here is experimental. Nevertheless, both the methodological development and the analysis of the case studies are presented in a software-independent fashion. Illustration of how to use SAS for the various model strategies is concentrated in a small number of chapters and sections, and the text can be read without any problem if these software excursions are ignored. Selected programs, macros, output, and publicly available datasets can be found at Springer-Verlag's URL: `www.springer-ny.com`, as well as at the authors' web site.

Geert Molenberghs (Diepenbeek) and Geert Verbeke (Leuven)

Acknowledgments

This text has benefited from the help of a large number of people. A lot of the more advanced chapters are based on joint research with many colleagues, as well as with current and past doctoral students. We gratefully acknowledge the support of these co-authors: Marc Aerts (Limburgs Universitair Centrum), Ariel Alonso (Limburgs Universitair Centrum), Caroline Beunckens (Limburgs Universitair Centrum), Larry Brant (National Institute of Aging and The Johns Hopkins University, Baltimore), Luc Bijnens (Johnson & Johnson Pharmaceutical Research and Development, Beerse), Tomasz Burzykowski (Limburgs Universitair Centrum), Marc Buyse (International Institute for Drug Development, Brussels), Raymond J. Carroll (Texas A& M University, College Station), Paul Catalano (Harvard School of Public Health, Boston), José Cortiñas Abrahantes (Limburgs Universitair Centrum), Linda Danielson (UCB, Braine-l'Alleud), Paul De Boeck (Katholieke Universiteit Leuven), Steffen Fieuws (Katholieke Universiteit Leuven), Krista Fisher-Lapp (Tartu University), Helena Geys (Johnson & Johnson Pharmaceutical Research and Development, Beerse), Els Goetghebeur (Universiteit Gent), Niel Hens (Limburgs Universitair Centrum), Ivy Jansen (Limburgs Universitair Centrum), Michael G. Kenward (London School of Hygiene and Tropical Medicine), Emmanuel Lesaffre (Katholieke Universiteit Leuven), Stuart Lipsitz (Medical University of South Carolina, Charleston), Craig Mallinckrodt (Eli Lilly and Company, Indianapolis), Bart Michiels (Janssen Research Foundation, Beerse), Christopher Morrell (National Institute of Aging and Loyola College, Baltimore), Meredith Regan (Harvard School of Public Health, Boston), Didier Renard (Eli Lilly and Company, Mont-Saint-Guibert),

Louise Ryan (Harvard School of Public Health, Boston), Jan Serroyen (Limburgs Universitair Centrum), Bart Spiessens (Glaxo Smith Kline Belgium), Herbert Thijs (Limburgs Universitair Centrum), Fabián Tibaldi (Eli Lilly and Company, Mont-Saint-Guibert), Tony Vangeneugden (Virco-Tibotec, Mechelen), Kristel Van Steen (Harvard School of Public Health, Boston), and Paige Williams (Harvard School of Public Health, Boston).

Several people have helped us with the computational side of the models presented. We mention in particular Caroline Beunckens, Steffen Fieuws, and Oliver Schabenberger (SAS Institute, Cary, North Carolina).

We gratefully acknowledge support from Research Project Fonds voor Wetenschappelijk Onderzoek Vlaanderen G.0002.98, "Sensitivity Analysis for Incomplete Data"; NATO Collaborative Research Grant CRG950648, "Statistical Research for Environmental Risk Assessment"; Onderzoeksfonds K.U.Leuven grant PDM/96/105, and Belgian IUAP/PAI network "Statistical Techniques and Modeling for Complex Substantive Questions with Complex Data."

The feedback we received from our regular and short course audiences has been invaluable. We are grateful for such interactions in Australia (Cairns, Coolangatta), Belgium (Beerse, Braine-l'Alleud, Brussels, Diepenbeek, Gent, Leuven, Wavre), Brasil (Piracicaba), Canada (Toronto), Cuba (La Habana, Varadero), Finland (Turku), France (Marseille, Toulouse, Vannes), Germany (Freiburg, Heidelberg), Ireland (Dublin), Spain (Barcelona, Pamplona, Santiago de Compostela), and the United States of America (Ann Arbor, Arlington, Atlanta, New York City, Rockville, San Francisco, Tampa, Washington, DC).

As always, it has been a pleasure to work with John Kimmel at Springer and his colleagues from the production department, in particular C. Curioli and M. Koy.

We apologize to our wives, daughters, and sons for the time not spent with them during the preparation of this book, and we are very grateful for their understanding. The preparation of this book has been a period of close collaboration and stimulating exchange, of which we will keep good memories.

Geert and Geert
Kessel-Lo and Herent, Belgium, February 2005

Contents

Preface   vii

Acknowledgments   ix

I Introductory Material   1

1 Introduction   3

2 Motivating Studies   7
  2.1   Introduction   7
  2.2   The Analgesic Trial   8
  2.3   The Toenail Data   8
  2.4   The Fluvoxamine Trial 12
  2.5   The Epilepsy Data 14
  2.6   The Project on Preterm and Small for Gestational
        Age Infants (POPS) Study   14
  2.7   National Toxicology Program Data   17
        2.7.1   Ethylene Glycol 18
        2.7.2   Di(2-ethylhexyl)Phthalate 18
        2.7.3   Diethylene Glycol Dimethyl Ether 22
  2.8   The Sports Injuries Trial 23
  2.9   Age Related Macular Degeneration Trial   24

3 Generalized Linear Models — 27
- 3.1 Introduction — 27
- 3.2 The Exponential Family — 27
- 3.3 The Generalized Linear Model (GLM) — 28
- 3.4 Examples — 29
  - 3.4.1 The Linear Regression Model for Continuous Data — 29
  - 3.4.2 Logistic and Probit Regression for Binary Data — 29
  - 3.4.3 Poisson Regression for Counts — 29
- 3.5 Maximum Likelihood Estimation and Inference — 30
- 3.6 Logistic Regression for the Toenail Data — 31
- 3.7 Poisson Regression for the Epilepsy Data — 32

4 Linear Mixed Models for Gaussian Longitudinal Data — 35
- 4.1 Introduction — 35
- 4.2 Marginal Multivariate Model — 36
- 4.3 The Linear Mixed Model — 36
- 4.4 Estimation and Inference for the Marginal Model — 39
- 4.5 Inference for the Random Effects — 41

5 Model Families — 45
- 5.1 Introduction — 45
- 5.2 The Gaussian Case — 46
- 5.3 Model Families in General — 47
  - 5.3.1 Marginal Models — 48
  - 5.3.2 Conditional Models — 49
  - 5.3.3 Subject-specific Models — 50
- 5.4 Inferential Paradigms — 52

II Marginal Models — 53

6 The Strength of Marginal Models — 55
- 6.1 Introduction — 55
- 6.2 Marginal Models in Contingency Tables — 56
  - 6.2.1 Multivariate Logistic Models — 57
  - 6.2.2 Goodman's Local Association Models — 58
  - 6.2.3 Dale's Marginal Models — 59
  - 6.2.4 A General Class of Models — 61
- 6.3 British Occupational Status Study — 62
- 6.4 The Caithness Data — 62
- 6.5 Analysis of the Fluvoxamine Trial — 64
- 6.6 Extensions — 68
  - 6.6.1 Covariates — 69

		6.6.2 Three-way Contingency Tables	72
	6.7	Relation to Latent Continuous Densities	79
	6.8	Conclusions and Perspective	80

7 Likelihood-based Marginal Models   83

	7.1	Notation	84
	7.2	The Bahadur Model	86
		7.2.1 A General Bahadur Model Formulation	86
		7.2.2 The Bahadur Model for Clustered Data	88
		7.2.3 Analysis of the NTP Data	90
		7.2.4 Analysis of the Fluvoxamine Trial	92
	7.3	A General Framework for Fully Specified Marginal Models	93
		7.3.1 Univariate Link Functions	94
		7.3.2 Higher-order Link Functions	94
	7.4	Maximum Likelihood Estimation	99
	7.5	An Influenza Study	99
		7.5.1 The Cross-over Study	100
		7.5.2 The Longitudinal Study	101
	7.6	The Multivariate Probit Model	102
		7.6.1 Probit Models	103
		7.6.2 Tetrachoric and Polychoric Correlation	104
		7.6.3 The Univariate Probit Model	105
		7.6.4 The Bivariate Probit Model	106
		7.6.5 Ordered Categorical Outcomes	110
		7.6.6 The Multivariate Probit Model	112
	7.7	The Dale Model	113
		7.7.1 Two Binary Responses	113
		7.7.2 The Bivariate Dale Model	115
		7.7.3 Some Properties of the Bivariate Dale Model	117
		7.7.4 The Multivariate Plackett Distribution	117
		7.7.5 The Multivariate Dale Model	117
		7.7.6 Maximum Likelihood Estimation	119
		7.7.7 The BIRNH Study	119
	7.8	Hybrid Marginal-conditional Specification	122
		7.8.1 A Mixed Marginal-conditional Model	123
		7.8.2 Categorical Outcomes	126
	7.9	A Cross-over Trial: An Example in Primary Dysmenorrhoea	127
		7.9.1 Analyzing Cross-over Data	128
		7.9.2 Analysis of the Primary Dysmenorrhoea Data	130
	7.10	Multivariate Analysis of the POPS Data	131
	7.11	Longitudinal Analysis of the Fluvoxamine Study	134
	7.12	Appendix: Maximum Likelihood Estimation	136

		7.12.1 Score Equations and Maximization	136
		7.12.2 Newton-Raphson Algorithm with Cumulative Counts	139
		7.12.3 Determining the Joint Probabilities	140
	7.13	Appendix: The Multivariate Plackett Distribution	142
	7.14	Appendix: Maximum Likelihood Estimation for the Dale Model	147

8 Generalized Estimating Equations — 151
- 8.1 Introduction . . . 151
- 8.2 Standard GEE Theory . . . 153
- 8.3 Alternative GEE Methods . . . 161
- 8.4 Prentice's GEE Method . . . 162
- 8.5 Second-order Generalized Estimating Equations (GEE2) . . . 164
- 8.6 GEE with Odds Ratios and Alternating Logistic Regression . . . 165
- 8.7 GEE2 Based on a Hybrid Marginal-conditional Model . . 168
- 8.8 A Method Based on Linearization . . . 169
- 8.9 Analysis of the NTP Data . . . 170
- 8.10 The Heatshock Study . . . 174
- 8.11 The Sports Injuries Trial . . . 181
  - 8.11.1 Longitudinal Analysis . . . 181
  - 8.11.2 A Bivariate Longitudinal Analysis . . . 186

9 Pseudo-Likelihood — 189
- 9.1 Introduction . . . 189
- 9.2 Pseudo-Likelihood: Definition and Asymptotic Properties . . . 190
  - 9.2.1 Definition . . . 190
  - 9.2.2 Consistency and Asymptotic Normality . . . 191
- 9.3 Pseudo-Likelihood Inference . . . 192
  - 9.3.1 Wald Statistic . . . 193
  - 9.3.2 Pseudo-Score Statistics . . . 193
  - 9.3.3 Pseudo-Likelihood Ratio Statistics . . . 194
- 9.4 Marginal Pseudo-Likelihood . . . 195
  - 9.4.1 Definition of Marginal Pseudo-Likelihood . . . 195
  - 9.4.2 A Generalized Linear Model Representation . . . 198
- 9.5 Comparison with Generalized Estimating Equations . . . 199
- 9.6 Analysis of NTP Data . . . 200

10 Fitting Marginal Models with SAS — 203
- 10.1 Introduction . . . 203
- 10.2 The Toenail Data . . . 203

10.3	GEE1 with Correlations	204
	10.3.1 The SAS Program	205
	10.3.2 The SAS Output	206
10.4	Alternating Logistic Regressions	212
10.5	A Method Based on Linearization	215
	10.5.1 The SAS Program for the GLIMMIX Macro	215
	10.5.2 The SAS Output from the GLIMMIX Macro	216
	10.5.3 The Program for the SAS Procedure GLIMMIX	218
	10.5.4 Output from the GLIMMIX Procedure	218
10.6	Programs for the NTP Data	219
10.7	Alternative Software Tools	221

III Conditional Models   223

11 Conditional Models   225

11.1	Introduction	225
11.2	Conditional Models	226
	11.2.1 A Pure Multivariate Setting	227
	11.2.2 A Single Repeated Outcome	229
	11.2.3 Repeated Multivariate Outcomes	230
11.3	Marginal *versus* Conditional Models	233
11.4	Analysis of the NTP Data	234
11.5	Transition Models	236
	11.5.1 Analysis of the Toenail Data	238
	11.5.2 Fitting Transition Models in SAS	240

12 Pseudo-Likehood   243

12.1	Introduction	243
12.2	Pseudo-Likelihood for a Single Repeated Binary Outcome	244
12.3	Pseudo-Likelihood for a Multivariate Repeated Binary Outcome	245
12.4	Analysis of the NTP Data	246
	12.4.1 Parameter Estimation	247
	12.4.2 Inference and Model Selection	249

IV Subject-specific Models   255

13 From Subject-specific to Random-effects Models   257

13.1	Introduction	257
13.2	General Model Formulation	257
13.3	Three Ways to Handle Subject-specific Parameters	258

13.3.1	Treated as Fixed Unknown Parameters	258
13.3.2	Conditional Inference	258
13.3.3	Random-effects Approach	259
13.4	Random-effects Models: Special Cases	260
13.4.1	The Linear Mixed Model	260
13.4.2	The Beta-binomial Model	260
13.4.3	The Probit-normal Model	262
13.4.4	The Generalized Linear Mixed Model	262
13.4.5	The Hierarchical Generalized Linear Model	263

14 The Generalized Linear Mixed Model (GLMM)   265
14.1 Introduction 265
14.2 Model Formulation and Approaches to Estimation 265
    14.2.1 Model Formulation 265
    14.2.2 Bayesian Approach to Model Fitting 266
    14.2.3 Maximum Likelihood Estimation 266
    14.2.4 Empirical Bayes Estimation 268
14.3 Estimation: Approximation of the Integrand 268
14.4 Estimation: Approximation of the Data 269
    14.4.1 Penalized Quasi-Likelihood (PQL) 270
    14.4.2 Marginal Quasi-Likelihood (MQL) 270
    14.4.3 Discussion and Extensions 271
14.5 Estimation: Approximation of the Integral 273
    14.5.1 Gaussian Quadrature 274
    14.5.2 Adaptive Gaussian Quadrature 275
14.6 Inference in Generalized Linear Mixed Models 276
14.7 Analyzing the NTP Data 277
14.8 Analyzing the Toenail Data 278

15 Fitting Generalized Linear Mixed Models with SAS   281
15.1 Introduction 281
15.2 The GLIMMIX Procedure for Quasi-Likelihood 282
    15.2.1 The SAS Program 283
    15.2.2 The SAS Output 284
15.3 The GLIMMIX Macro for Quasi-Likelihood 287
    15.3.1 The SAS Program 288
    15.3.2 Selected SAS Output 289
15.4 The NLMIXED Procedure for Numerical Quadrature . . 290
    15.4.1 The SAS Program 290
    15.4.2 The SAS Output 293
15.5 Alternative Software Tools 296

16 Marginal *versus* Random-effects Models   297
16.1 Introduction 297

	16.2	Example: The Toenail Data	297
	16.3	Parameter Interpretation	298
	16.4	Toenail Data: Marginal *versus* Mixed Models	301
	16.5	Analysis of the NTP Data	304

V Case Studies and Extensions   307

17 The Analgesic Trial   309
   17.1 Introduction 309
   17.2 Marginal Analyses of the Analgesic Trial 310
   17.3 Random-effects Analyses of the Analgesic Trial 314
   17.4 Comparing Marginal and Random-effects Analyses .. 317
   17.5 Programs for the Analgesic Trial 318
       17.5.1 Marginal Models with SAS 318
       17.5.2 Random-effects Models with SAS 320
       17.5.3 MIXOR 321
       17.5.4 MLwiN 323

18 Ordinal Data   325
   18.1 Regression Models for Ordinal Data 326
       18.1.1 The Fluvoxamine Trial 328
   18.2 Marginal Models for Repeated Ordinal Data 329
   18.3 Random-effects Models for Repeated Ordinal Data .. 331
   18.4 Ordinal Analysis of the Analgesic Trial 332
   18.5 Programs for the Analgesic Trial 334

19 The Epilepsy Data   337
   19.1 Introduction 337
   19.2 A Marginal GEE Analysis 337
   19.3 A Generalized Linear Mixed Model 340
   19.4 Marginalizing the Mixed Model 342

20 Non-linear Models   347
   20.1 Introduction 347
   20.2 Univariate Non-linear Models 349
   20.3 The Indomethacin Study: Non-hierarchical Analysis .. 351
   20.4 Non-linear Models for Longitudinal Data 355
   20.5 Non-linear Mixed Models 357
   20.6 The Orange Tree Data 358
   20.7 Pharmacokinetic and Pharmacodynamic Models 360
       20.7.1 Hierarchical Analysis of the Indomethacin Study 361
       20.7.2 Pharmacokinetic Modeling and the Theophylline Data 363

	20.7.3 Pharmacodynamic Data	367
20.8	The Songbird Data	368
	20.8.1 Introduction	368
	20.8.2 A Non-linear Mixed-effects Model	370
	20.8.3 Analysis of SI at RA	371
	20.8.4 Model Strategies for HVC	372
	20.8.5 Analysis of SI at HVC	374
20.9	Discrete Outcomes	376
	20.9.1 Analysis of the NTP Data	377
20.10	Hypothesis Testing and Non-linear Models	379
20.11	Flexible Functions	379
	20.11.1 Random Smoothing Splines	381
	20.11.2 Analysis of the Analgesic Trial	383
20.12	Using SAS for Non-linear Mixed-effects Models	384
	20.12.1 SAS Program for the Orange Tree Data Analysis	384
	20.12.2 SAS Programs for the Indomethacin Analyses	385
	20.12.3 SAS Programs for the Theophylline Analyses	386
	20.12.4 SAS Program for the Songbird Data	387
	20.12.5 SAS Program for the NTP Data	388
	20.12.6 SAS Program for the Random Smoothing Spline Model	388

21 Pseudo-Likelihood for a Hierarchical Model — 393
21.1	Introduction	393
21.2	Pseudo-Likelihood Estimation	394
21.3	Two Binary Endpoints	397
21.4	A Meta-analysis of Trials in Schizophrenic Subjects	401
21.5	Concluding Remarks	403

22 Random-effects Models with Serial Correlation — 405
22.1	Introduction	405
22.2	A Multilevel Probit Model with Autocorrelation	406
22.3	Parameter Estimation for the Multilevel Probit Model	408
22.4	A Generalized Linear Mixed Model with Autocorrelation	410
22.5	A Meta-analysis of Trials in Schizophrenic Subjects	412
22.6	SAS Code for Random-effects Models with Autocorrelation	415
22.7	Concluding Remarks	417

23 Non-Gaussian Random Effects — 419
| 23.1 | Introduction | 419 |

23.2		The Heterogeneity Model	421
23.3		Estimation and Inference	423
23.4		Empirical Bayes Estimation and Classification	427
23.5		The Verbal Aggression Data	428
23.6		Concluding Remarks	435

24 Joint Continuous and Discrete Responses   437

24.1		Introduction	437
24.2		A Continuous and a Binary Endpoint	439
	24.2.1	A Probit-normal Formulation	439
	24.2.2	A Plackett-Dale Formulation	441
	24.2.3	A Generalized Linear Mixed Model Formulation	442
24.3		Hierarchical Joint Models	445
	24.3.1	Two-stage Analysis	445
	24.3.2	Fully Hierarchical Modeling	446
24.4		Age Related Macular Degeneration Trial	448
	24.4.1	Bivariate Marginal Analyses	448
	24.4.2	Bivariate Random-effects Analyses	452
	24.4.3	Hierarchical Analyses	453
24.5		Joint Models in SAS	455
24.6		Concluding Remarks	464

25 High-dimensional Joint Models   467

25.1		Introduction	467
25.2		Joint Mixed Model	469
25.3		Model Fitting and Inference	471
	25.3.1	Pairwise Fitting	471
	25.3.2	Inference for Ψ	472
	25.3.3	Combining Information: Inference for Ψ^*	473
25.4		A Study in Psycho-Cognitive Functioning	473

VI   Missing Data   479

26 Missing Data Concepts   481

26.1		Introduction	481
26.2		A Formal Taxonomy	482
	26.2.1	Missing Data Frameworks	484
	26.2.2	Missing Data Mechanisms	485
	26.2.3	Ignorability	487

27 Simple Methods, Direct Likelihood, and WGEE   489

27.1		Introduction	489
27.2		Longitudinal Analysis or Not?	490

27.3	Simple Methods	491
27.4	Bias in LOCF, CC, and Ignorable Likelihood	495
27.5	Weighted Generalized Estimating Equations	498
27.6	The Depression Trial	499
	27.6.1 The Data	499
	27.6.2 Marginal Models	501
	27.6.3 Random-effects Models	502
27.7	Age Related Macular Degeneration Trial	503
27.8	The Analgesic Trial	507

28 Multiple Imputation and the EM Algorithm — 511

28.1	Introduction	511
28.2	Multiple Imputation	511
	28.2.1 Theoretical Justification	512
	28.2.2 Pooling Information	513
	28.2.3 Hypothesis Testing	514
	28.2.4 Efficiency	514
	28.2.5 Imputation Mechanisms	515
28.3	The Expectation-Maximization Algorithm	516
	28.3.1 The Algorithm	517
	28.3.2 Missing Information	518
	28.3.3 Rate of Convergence	519
	28.3.4 EM Acceleration	520
	28.3.5 Calculation of Precision Estimates	520
	28.3.6 A Simple Illustration	521
28.4	Which Method to Use?	526
28.5	Age Related Macular Degeneration Study	527
28.6	Concluding Remarks	529

29 Selection Models — 531

29.1	Introduction	531
29.2	An MNAR Dale Model	532
	29.2.1 Likelihood Function	533
	29.2.2 Maximization Using the EM Algorithm	535
	29.2.3 Analysis of the Fluvoxamine Data	537
29.3	A Model for Non-monotone Missingness	543
	29.3.1 Analysis of the Fluvoxamine Data	546
29.4	Concluding Remarks	552

30 Pattern-mixture Models — 555

30.1	Introduction	555
30.2	Pattern-mixture Modeling Approach	556
30.3	Identifying Restriction Strategies	557
	30.3.1 How to Use Restrictions?	560

30.4	A Unifying Framework for Selection and Pattern-mixture Models		561
30.5	Selection Models *versus* Pattern-mixture Models		563
	30.5.1	Selection Models	564
	30.5.2	Pattern-mixture Models	565
	30.5.3	Identifying Restrictions	566
	30.5.4	Precision Estimation with Pattern-mixture Models	566
30.6	Analysis of the Fluvoxamine Data		567
	30.6.1	Selection Modeling	568
	30.6.2	Pattern-mixture Modeling	569
	30.6.3	Comparison	572
30.7	Concluding Remarks		572

31 Sensitivity Analysis 575

31.1	Introduction		575
31.2	Sensitivity Analysis for Selection Models		576
31.3	A Local Influence Approach for Ordinal Data with Dropout		578
	31.3.1	General Principles	578
	31.3.2	Analysis of the Fluvoxamine Data	581
31.4	A Local Influence Approach for Incomplete Binary Data		585
	31.4.1	General Principles	585
	31.4.2	Analysis of the Fluvoxamine Data	586
31.5	Interval of Ignorance		590
	31.5.1	General Principle	591
	31.5.2	Sensitivity Parameter Approach	593
	31.5.3	Models for Monotone Patterns and a Bernoulli Experiment	594
	31.5.4	Analysis of the Fluvoxamine Data	599
31.6	Sensitivity Analysis and Pattern-mixture Models		604
31.7	Concluding Remarks		605

32 Incomplete Data and SAS 607

32.1	Introduction		607
32.2	Complete Case Analysis		607
32.3	Last Observation Carried Forward		609
32.4	Direct Likelihood		611
32.5	Weighted Estimating Equations (WGEE)		613
32.6	Multiple Imputation		618
	32.6.1	The MI Procedure for the Imputation Task	618
	32.6.2	The Analysis Task	624
	32.6.3	The Inference Task	629

	32.6.4	The MI Procedure to Create Monotone Missingness	633
32.7		The EM Algorithm	633
32.8		MNAR Models and Sensitivity Analysis Tools	635

References   **637**

Index   **671**

Part I

Introductory Material

1
Introduction

In contemporary quantitative research, the collection of *correlated data* is very common. In agreement with Verbeke and Molenberghs (2000), we use this term in a generic sense and understand it to encompass such structures as multivariate observations, clustered data, repeated measurements, longitudinal data, and spatially correlated data.

In a multivariate study (Seber 1984, Krzanowski 1988, Johnson and Wichern 1992), a number of different characteristics are measured on the same unit. This occurs, for example, when three test scores are recorded on each child enrolled in a study (Section 2.6). If the same characteristic is measures several times, perhaps under varying experimental condition, then we are confronted with repeated measures. When the same characteristic is measured repeatedly over time, and time itself is, at least in part, a subject of scientific investigation, we refer to *longitudinal data*. A related setting, obtained by replacing the time dimension by one or more spatial dimensions, yields so-called *spatial data* (Cressie 1991). All of these correlated designs are based on a hierarchy in the data. Other hierarchies are found in classical agricultural designs, in sociological experiments (e.g., pupils within classes, within schools, within districts, ...).

Longitudinal or otherwise hierarchical data are made up, by definition, of more than one source of variability. Continuous longitudinal data are often analyzed by means of the general linear mixed-effects model (Verbeke and Molenberghs 2000), which encompasses three sources of variability: (1) subject-specific effects, (2) serial correlation, resulting from additional autoregressive effects in the data, and (3) measurement error. Autoregressive models are commonly used in the time-series and spatial literatures

(Ripley 1981, Diggle 1983, Cressie 1991), whereas subject or unit-specific effects are commonly used in variance component models (Searle, Casella, and McCulloch 1992). The fact that longitudinal data exhibit replication 'in two directions,' subjects on the one hand and repeated measurements within subject collected over time on the other hand, with in addition the specific structure imposed by the uni-directional time dimension, makes them rich in structure.

A key characteristic of correlated data is the type of outcome. For a univariate continuous outcome, linear or, more parametrically, Gaussian models, are often appropriate. The structure of the covariates further distinguishes between such subfamilies as linear regression and analysis of variance, but the choice of the broader family is defined by the outcome. Univariate categorical outcomes are analyzed using loglinear models, logistic regression, probit regression, etc., with Poisson regression reserved for the analysis of univariate count data. Of course, all of these can be framed within the generalized linear model family (McCullagh and Nelder 1989), but the normal distribution, underlying parametric linear regression, is a somewhat special member of this family, and linear regression is special among the various forms of regression, primarily and simply due to the normality and linearity of the model.

In longitudinal settings, each individual has a *vector* Y of responses with a natural (time) ordering among the components. This leads to several, generally nonequivalent, extensions of univariate models. In a *marginal model*, marginal distributions are used to describe the outcome vector Y, given a set X of predictor variables. The correlation among the components of Y can then be captured either by adopting a fully parametric approach or by modeling a limited number of lower-order moments only. Alternatively, in a *random-effects model*, the predictor variables X are supplemented with a vector b of subject-specific effects, conditional upon which the components of Y are often assumed to be independent. This does not preclude that more elaborate models are possible if residual dependence is detected. Finally, a *conditional model* describes the distribution of the components of Y, conditional on X but also conditional on (a subset of) the other components of Y. In a longitudinal context, a particular relevant class of conditional models describes a component of Y given the ones recorded earlier in time, the so-called *autoregressive* or *transition models*.

This taxonomy allows us to indicate an important distinction between Gaussian and non-Gaussian repeated measures. In the Gaussian case, the linear mixed model is widely accepted as the unifying framework for a variety of correlated settings, including but not limited to repeated measures, longitudinal data, correlated data, and hierarchical data. In addition, it plays a prominent role in the area of spatial statistics. The model encompasses subject-specific and autoregressive effects at the same time. Furthermore, this general hierarchical model marginalizes in a straightforward way to a multivariate normal model with directly interpretable mean and covariance parameters.

These results are entirely based on powerful but unique properties of the normal distribution, including that both the conditional and marginal distributions of a multivariate normal distribution are again normal. Virtually nothing of this carries over to the non-Gaussian case, as there is no natural analog to the multivariate normal distribution for, say, repeated binary or ordinal data, or longitudinally measured counts. As a consequence, each of the three model families (marginal, subject-specific, and conditional) stands to a large extent on its own and no straightforward transfers are possible. Although models for longitudinally measured non-Gaussian outcomes are typically based on two important building blocks, being the linear mixed model on the one hand and generalized linear models on the other hand, there are additional choices to be made as to precisely how these two will be combined and, importantly, within which of the three model families the resulting model will be framed. Depending on the choices made, one may end up with, for example, generalized estimating equations or with the generalized linear mixed-effects model.

Specific challenges arise when the longitudinally measured profiles are incomplete. Missing data already received a lot of attention in Verbeke and Molenberghs (2000), and it is treated in detail here as well, as various modeling approaches, often within a different inferential framework, require specific measures to correctly deal with incompleteness.

The book is divided into six parts. The first part presents the key motivating studies (Chapter 2) as well as brief reviews of the two major building blocks mentioned earlier: generalized linear models in Chapter 3 and the linear mixed-effects model in Chapter 4. The introductory part ends with a chapter detailing the three model families within which models for non-Gaussian repeated measures can be framed (Chapter 5). All of the material in this part is easily accessible, also for the less technically interested reader. Even though the title of the book contains the word 'longitudinal,' many of the examples are of a more general nature, including clustered and multivariate data. Although longitudinal examples form the backbone of the methodological developments and illustrations alike, we aim to show the methodology is more broadly applicable.

The second, third, and fourth part zoom in on marginal, conditional, and subject-specific models, respectively. Turning to marginal models first, Chapter 6 provides a gentle introduction to the concept of marginal models, confining attention for the better part to bivariate outcomes and contingency-table settings. Chapter 7 gives a broad overview of likelihood-based marginal models, illustrating both use and computational complexity. This naturally leads to the need for likelihood alternatives, such as generalized estimating equations (Chapter 8) and pseudo-likelihood (Chapter 9). The final Chapter 10 reviews the use of SAS for fitting marginal models.

The third part, on conditional models, is rather brief, with a general overview in Chapter 11 and the use of pseudo-likelihood in this context in Chapter 12.

The fourth part on subject-specific models starts off with a perspective on the various ways to deal with subject-specific effects (Chapter 13), and then puts a lot of emphasis on the specific but versatile class constituted by the generalized linear mixed model (GLMM) in Chapter 14. In analogy with Chapter 10, Chapter 15 illustrates how SAS can be used to fit GLMMs. Chapter 16 discusses the similarities, differences, and connections between marginal and random-effects models.

The fifth part is devoted to a number of case studies and extensions. An overview of the various model strategies, using a case study, is presented in Chapter 18. Chapters 18 and 19 are devoted to the specific cases of ordinal outcomes and counts, respectively. Extensions to non-linear models, for both Gaussian and non-Gaussian outcomes, are presented in Chapter 20. A pseudo-likelihood approach to hierarchical data is given in Chapter 21, and the model presented here is extended further to encompass serial correlation in Chapter 22. Whereas the GLMM assumes random effects to follow a normal distribution, an approach with non-Gaussian random effects is discussed in Chapter 23. Chapter 24 introduces models for multivariate outcomes of a combined Gaussian and discrete nature and, in fact, for any combination of outcome types. The specifically challenging case of high-dimensional multivariate repeated measures is considered in Chapter 25.

The sixth and last part is devoted to incomplete data. General concepts are introduced in Chapter 26. Simple methods and the so-called direct likelihood and weighted generalized estimating equations methods are studied in Chapter 27. Chapter 28 studies two specific approaches, the expectation-maximization algorithm and multiple imputation. Chapters 29 and 30 are devoted to two important model families for incomplete longitudinal data, selection models, and pattern-mixture models. When data are incomplete, a number of model assumptions made cannot be verified using the observed data only, and hence sensitivity analysis (Chapter 31) may be very appropriate. In the final chapter of this part, it is shown how progress can be made with the analysis of incomplete longitudinal data, using SAS procedures, supplemented with a number of macros.

2
Motivating Studies

2.1 Introduction

In this chapter, we present a number of studies that motivate this work and/or are used repeatedly throughout the text. Upon going through the book, the reader will find more examples. These are either used once or at least confined to one or a few chapters. A single-arm clinical trial conducted in patients with chronic pain, the analgesic trial, is introduced in Section 2.2. Section 2.3 is devoted to a two-armed clinical trial in patients treated for toenail infection. The fluvoxamine study, a post-marketing study conducted in psychiatric patients, is introduced in Section 2.4. A controlled clinical trial, conducted in patients suffering from epileptic seizures, is presented in Section 2.5. All studies introduced thus far are longitudinal in nature. Section 2.6 discusses the Project on Preterm and Small for Gestational Age Infants study (POPS), an epidemiologic study in which interest lies in a multivariate outcome. A key clustered data example from the developmental toxicology area, conducted under the U.S. National Toxicology Program (NTP), is presented in Section 2.7. Section 2.8 introduces the sports injuries trial, studying two longitudinal post-operative outcomes. Finally, Section 2.9 is devoted to the Age Related Macular Degeneration Study (ARMD), an ophthalmologic clinical trial in which both a continuous as well as a categorical longitudinally measured outcome is of interest.

2.2 The Analgesic Trial

These data come from a single-arm clinical trial in 395 patients who are given analgesic treatment for pain caused by chronic nonmalignant disease. Treatment was to be administered for 12 months and assessed by means of a 'Global Satisfaction Assessment' (GSA) scale, rated on a five-point scale:

$$\text{GSA} = \begin{cases} 1 & : \quad \text{very good,} \\ 2 & : \quad \text{good,} \\ 3 & : \quad \text{indifferent,} \\ 4 & : \quad \text{bad,} \\ 5 & : \quad \text{very bad.} \end{cases} \quad (2.1)$$

Many of our analyses will focus on a dichotomized version, defined in (17.1), but Chapter 18 will consider the ordinal version of the outcome. Apart from the outcome of interest, a number of covariates are available, such as age, sex, weight, duration of pain in years prior to the start of the study, type of pain, physical functioning, psychiatric condition, respiratory problems, etc.

GSA was rated by each person four times during the trial, at months 3, 6, 9, and 12. An overview of the frequencies per follow up time is given in Table 2.1. Inspecting Table 2.1 reveals that the total per column is variable. This is due to missingness. At three months, 10 subjects lack a measure, with these numbers being 93, 168, and 172 at subsequent times. Not only monotone missingness or dropout occurs, there are also subjects with intermittent values.

An overview of the extent of missingness is shown in Table 2.2. Note that only around 40% of the subjects have complete data. The dropout sequences amount to roughly another 40%, with close to 20% of the patterns showing intermittent missingness. This example underscores that a satisfactory longitudinal analysis will oftentimes have to address the missing data problem.

2.3 The Toenail Data

The data introduced in this section were obtained from a randomized, double-blind, parallel group, multicenter study for the comparison of two oral treatments (in what follows coded as A and B) for toenail dermatophyte onychomycosis (TDO), described in full detail by De Backer *et al* (1996). TDO is a common toenail infection, difficult to treat, affecting more than 2 out of 100 persons (Roberts 1992). Antifungal compounds, classically used for treatment of TDO, need to be taken until the whole nail has grown out healthy. The development of new compounds, however,

TABLE 2.1. *Analgesic Trial. Absolute and relative frequencies of the five GSA categories for each of the four follow up times.*

GSA	Month 3		Month 6		Month 9		Month 12	
1	55	14.3%	38	12.6%	40	17.6%	30	13.5%
2	112	29.1%	84	27.8%	67	29.5%	66	29.6%
3	151	39.2%	115	38.1%	76	33.5%	97	43.5%
4	52	13.5%	51	16.9%	33	14.5%	27	12.1%
5	15	3.9%	14	4.6%	11	4.9%	3	1.4%
Tot	385		302		227		223	

TABLE 2.2. *Analgesic Trial. Overview of missingness patterns and the frequencies with which they occur. 'O' indicates observed and 'M' indicates missing.*

Measurement occasion					
Month 3	Month 6	Month 9	Month 12	Number	%
Completers					
O	O	O	O	163	41.2
Dropouts					
O	O	O	M	51	12.91
O	O	M	M	51	12.91
O	M	M	M	63	15.95
Non-monotone missingness					
O	O	M	O	30	7.59
O	M	O	O	7	1.77
O	M	O	M	2	0.51
O	M	M	O	18	4.56
M	O	O	O	2	0.51
M	O	O	M	1	0.25
M	O	M	O	1	0.25
M	O	M	M	3	0.76

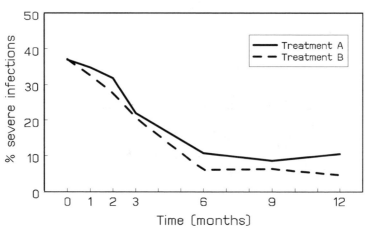

FIGURE 2.1. *Toenail Data. Evolution of the percentage of severe toenail infections in the two treatment groups separately.*

has reduced the treatment duration to 3 months. The aim of the present study was to compare the efficacy and safety of 12 weeks of continuous therapy with treatment A or with treatment B.

In total, 2×189 patients were randomized, distributed over 36 centers. Subjects were followed during 12 weeks (3 months) of treatment and followed further, up to a total of 48 weeks (12 months). Measurements were taken at baseline, every month during treatment, and every 3 months afterwards, resulting in a maximum of 7 measurements per subject. At the first occasion, the treating physician indicates one of the affected toenails as the target nail, the nail which will be followed over time. We will restrict our analyses to only those patients for which the target nail was one of the two big toenails. This reduces our sample under consideration to 146 and 148 subjects, in group A and group B, respectively.

One of the responses of interest was the unaffected nail length, measured from the nail bed to the infected part of the nail, which is always at the free end of the nail, expressed in mm. This outcome has been studied extensively in Verbeke and Molenberghs (2000). Another important outcome in this study was the severity of the infection, coded as 0 (not severe) or 1 (severe). The question of interest was whether the percentage of severe infections decreased over time, and whether that evolution was different for the two treatment groups. A summary of the number of patients in the study at each time-point, and the number of patients with severe infections is given in Table 2.3. A graphical representation is given in Figure 2.1.

Due to a variety of reasons, the outcome has been measured at all 7 scheduled time points, for only 224 (76%) out of the 298 participants. Table 2.4 summarizes the number of available repeated measurements per

TABLE 2.3. *Toenail Data. Number and percentage of patients (N) with severe toenail infection, for each treatment arm separately.*

	Group A			Group B		
	# Severe	N	%	# Severe	N	%
Baseline	54	146	37.0%	55	148	37.2%
1 month	49	141	34.7%	48	147	32.6%
2 months	44	138	31.9%	40	145	27.6%
3 months	29	132	22.0%	29	140	20.7%
6 months	14	130	10.8%	8	133	6.0%
9 months	10	117	8.5%	8	127	6.3%
12 months	14	133	10.5%	6	131	4.6%

TABLE 2.4. *Toenail Data. Number of available repeated measurements per subject, for each treatment arm separately.*

	Group A		Group B	
# Obs.	N	%	N	%
1	4	2.74%	1	0.68%
2	2	1.37%	1	0.68%
3	4	2.74%	3	2.03%
4	2	1.37%	4	2.70%
5	2	1.37%	8	5.41%
6	25	17.12%	14	9.46%
7	107	73.29%	117	79.05%
Total:	146	100%	148	100%

subject, for both treatment groups separately. We see that the occurrence of missingness is similar in both treatment groups.

2.4 The Fluvoxamine Trial

Accumulated experience with fluvoxamine, a serotonin reuptake inhibitor, in controlled clinical trials has shown it to be as effective as conventional antidepressant drugs and more effective than placebo in the treatment of depression (Burton 1991). However, many patients who suffer from depression have concomitant morbidity with conditions such as obsessive-compulsive disorder, anxiety disorders and, to some extent, panic disorders. In most trials, patients with comorbidity are excluded, and therefore, it is of interest to gather evidence as to the importance of such factors, with a view on improved diagnosis and treatment. The general aim of this study was to determine the profile of fluvoxamine in ambulatory clinical psychiatric practice.

A total of 315 patients were enrolled with one or more of the following diagnoses: depression, obsessive, compulsive disorder, and panic disorder. Several covariates were recorded, such as gender and initial severity on a 5-point ordinal scale, where severity increases with category. After recruitment of the patient in the study, he or she was investigated at four visits (weeks 2, 4, 8, and 12). On the basis of about twenty psychiatric symptoms, the therapeutic effect and the side-effects were scored at each visit in an ordinal manner. Side effect is coded as (1) = no; (2) = not interfering with functionality of patient; (3) = interfering significantly with functionality of patient; (4) = the side-effect surpasses the therapeutic effect. Similarly, the effect of therapy is recorded on a four-point ordinal scale: (1) no improvement over baseline or worsening; (2) minimal improvement (not changing functionality); (3) moderate improvement (partial disappearance of symptoms); and (4) important improvement (almost disappearance of symptoms). Thus, a side effect occurs if new symptoms occur while there is therapeutic effect if old symptoms disappear. These data were used, among others, by Molenberghs and Lesaffre (1994), Molenberghs, Kenward, and Lesaffre (1997), and Lapp, Molenberghs, and Lesaffre (1998), Van Steen et al (2001), and Jansen et al (2003).

Table 2.5 gives the absolute and relative frequencies over the four categories of side effects and therapeutic effect for each of the four follow-up times. Because there are 315 subjects enrolled in the trial, it is clear that at the four times there are 16, 46, 72, and 89 subjects missing, respectively. The missing data patterns, common to both outcomes, are represented in Table 2.6. Note that a much larger fraction is fully observed than in, for example, the analgesic trial (Section 2.2). Among the incomplete sequences, dropout is much more common than intermittent missingness, the latter

TABLE 2.5. *Fluvoxamine Trial. Absolute and relative frequencies of the four side effects and therapeutic effect categories for each of the four follow-up times.*

	Week 2		Week 4		Week 8		Week 12	
			Side effects					
0	128	42.8%	144	52.5%	156	64.2%	148	65.5%
1	128	42.8%	103	38.3%	79	32.5%	71	31.4%
2	28	9.4%	17	6.3%	6	2.5%	7	3.1%
3	15	5.2%	5	1.9%	2	0.8%	0	0.0%
			Therapeutic effects					
0	19	6.4%	64	23.8%	110	45.3%	135	59.7%
1	95	31.8%	114	42.4%	93	38.3%	62	27.4%
2	102	34.1%	62	23.1%	30	12.4%	19	8.4%
3	83	27.8%	29	10.8%	10	4.1%	10	4.4%
Tot	299		269		243		226	

TABLE 2.6. *Fluvoxamine Trial. Overview of missingness patterns and the frequencies with which they occur. 'O' indicates observed and 'M' indicates missing.*

Measurement occasion					
Month 3	Month 6	Month 9	Month 12	Number	%
		Completers			
O	O	O	O	224	71.11
		Dropouts			
O	O	O	M	18	5.71
O	O	M	M	26	8.25
O	M	M	M	31	9.84
M	M	M	M	14	4.44
		Non-monotone missingness			
M	O	O	O	1	0.32
M	M	M	O	1	0.32

14   2. Motivating Studies

type confined to two sequences only. Observe that, unlike in Table 2.2, there are subjects, 14 in total without any follow-up measurements. This group of subjects is still an integral part of the trial, as they contain baseline information, including covariate information and baseline assessment of severity of the mental illness.

2.5   The Epilepsy Data

The data considered here are obtained from a randomized, double-blind, parallel group multi-center study for the comparison of placebo with a new anti-epileptic drug (AED), in combination with one or two other AED's. The study is described in full detail in Faught *et al* (1996). The randomization of epilepsy patients took place after a 12-week baseline period that served as a stabilization period for the use of AED's, and during which the number of seizures were counted. After that period, 45 patients were assigned to the placebo group, 44 to the active (new) treatment group. Patients were then measured weekly. Patients were followed (double-blind) during 16 weeks, after which they were entered into a long-term open-extension study. Some patients were followed for up to 27 weeks. The outcome of interest is the number of epileptic seizures experienced during the last week, i.e., since the last time the outcome was measured. The key research question is whether or not the additional new treatment reduces the number of epileptic seizures. As a summary of the data, Figure 2.2 shows a frequency plot, over all visits, over both treatment groups. We observe a very skewed distribution, with largest observed value equal to 73 seizures in one week time. Average and median evolutions are shown in Figure 2.3. The unstable behavior can be explained by the presence of extreme values, but is also the result of the fact that very little observations are available at some of the time-points, especially past week 20. This is also reflected in Table 2.7, which shows the number of measurements at a selection of time-points. Note the serious drop in number of measurements past the end of the actual double-blind period, i.e., past week 16.

2.6   The Project on Preterm and Small for Gestational Age Infants (POPS) Study

The Project On Preterm and Small-for-gestational age infants (POPS) collected information on 1338 infants born in The Netherlands in 1983 and having gestational age less than 32 weeks and/or birthweight less than 1500 g (Verloove *et al* 1988). In total, 133 clinics were involved. The study population represents 94% of the births in that year with similar gestational age and birthweight characteristics. Prenatal, perinatal, and postnatal in-

2.6 The Project on Preterm and Small for Gestational Age Infants (POPS) Study

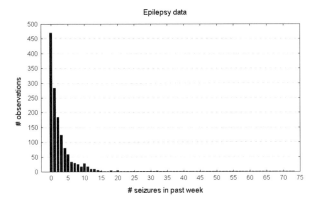

FIGURE 2.2. *Epilepsy Data. Frequency plot, over all visits, over both treatment groups.*

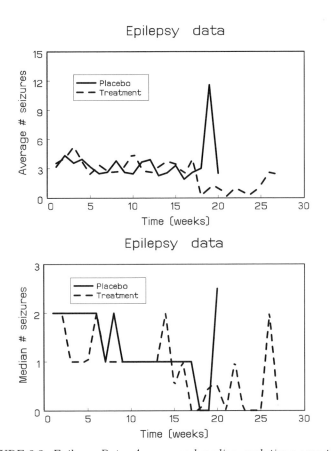

FIGURE 2.3. *Epilepsy Data. Average and median evolutions over time.*

TABLE 2.7. *Epilepsy Data. Number of measurements available at a selection of time-points, for both treatment groups separately.*

	# Observations		
Week	Placebo	Treatment	Total
1	45	44	89
5	42	42	84
10	41	40	81
15	40	38	78
16	40	37	77
17	18	17	35
20	2	8	10
27	0	3	3

formation as well as two year follow-up data were collected. Furthermore, the data base contains information on the delivery and specific details of the infant. After two years the child was reexamined. Lesaffre and Molenberghs (1991) and Molenberghs and Lesaffre (1994) studied the relationship between three ability scores measured at the age of two and risk factors measured at delivery. All ability scores were recorded in a dichotomous manner. They were available for 799 children. The first score ($ABIL_1$) checks whether the child can pile three bricks, $ABIL_1 = 1$ corresponds to 'no,' whereas $ABIL_1 = 2$ to 'yes.' The second score ($ABIL_2$) measures whether the physical movements of the child are natural, $ABIL_2 = 1$(no) and $ABIL_2 = 2$(yes). Although $ABIL_2$ is a purely physical ability score, $ABIL_1$ is a combination of physical and mental qualities. The third ability score, $ABIL_3$, expresses whether or not the child is able to put a ball in a box if he or she is asked to do so. The problem is to determine the risk factors for low performance at the three tests. Further it is of interest to compare the predicted probabilities taking into account the relationship between the responses to those calculated under the assumption of independent responses.

The defining variables of the POPS study, birth weight and gestational age, are shown graphically in Figure 2.4. It is clear from the figure that at least one of these needs to be low to be enrolled into the study.

The three ability scores are tabulated in Table 2.8. Of the 1338 subjects, 818 (61.1%) have all three ability scores observed, and 471 (35.2%) have none of them. Only 49 (3.7%) have partial information. The latter is not unexpected, since two years lapsed between enrollment and the assessment of the ability scores.

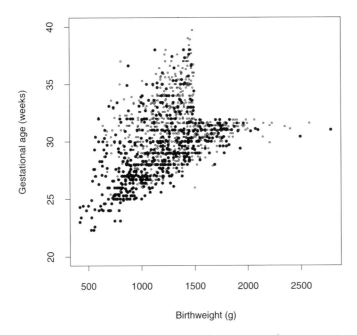

FIGURE 2.4. *POPS Study. The open circles correspond to zero outcomes.*

TABLE 2.8. *POPS Study. Frequency table of the three binary ability scores. Missing values are represented by M.*

		ABIL$_3$		
ABIL$_1$	ABIL$_2$	0	1	M
0	0	685	20	19
0	1	30	5	2
0	M	1	0	1
0	0	25	11	1
0	1	10	32	0
0	M	0	0	0
0	0	5	0	15
0	1	0	2	2
0	M	1	0	471

2.7 National Toxicology Program Data

The developmental toxicity studies introduced in this section are conducted at the Research Triangle Institute, which is under contract to the National

18   2. Motivating Studies

Toxicology Program of the United States (NTP data). These studies investigate the effects in mice of five chemicals: ethylene glycol (Price et al 1985), diethylene glycol dimethyl ether (Price et al 1987), and di(2-ethylhexyl)phthalate (Tyl et al 1988).

2.7.1 Ethylene Glycol

Ethylene glycol (EG) is also called 1,2-ethanediol and can be represented by the chemical formula $HOCH_2CH_2OH$. It is a high-volume industrial chemical with many applications. EG is used as an antifreeze in cooling and heating systems, as one of the components of hydraulic brake fluids, as an ingredient of electrolytic condensers, and as a solvent in the paint and plastics industries. Furthermore, EG is employed in the formulation of several types of inks, as a softening agent for cellophane, and as a stabilizer for soybean foam used to extinguish oil and gasoline fires. Also, one uses EG in the synthesis of various chemical products, such as plasticizers, synthetic fibers, and waxes (Windholz 1983).

EG may represent little hazard to human health in normal industrial handling, except possibly when used as an aerosol or at elevated temperatures. EG at ambient temperatures has a low vapor pressure and is not very irritating to the eyes or skin. However, accidental or intentional ingestion of antifreeze products, of which approximately 95% is EG, is toxic and may result in death (Rowe 1963, Price et al 1985).

Price et al (1985) describe a study in which timed-pregnant CD-1 mice were dosed by gavage with EG in distilled water. Dosing occurred during the period of organogenesis and structural development of the foetuses (gestational days 8 through 15). The doses selected for the study were 0, 750, 1500, or 3000 mg/kg/day. Table 2.9 shows, for each dose group and for all five NTP toxic agents, the number of dams containing at least one implant, the number of dams having at least one viable fetus, the number of live foetuses, the mean litter size, and the percentage of malformation for three different classes: external malformations, visceral malformations, and skeletal malformations. While for EG, skeletal malformations are substantial in the highest dose group, external and visceral malformations show only slight dose effects. The distribution of the number of implants is given in Table 2.10 for each of these five chemicals.

Figures 2.5 and 2.6 show for each of these studies and for each dose group the observed and averaged malformation rates in mice.

2.7.2 Di(2-ethylhexyl)Phthalate

Di(2-ethylhexyl)phthalate (DEHP) is also called octoil, dioctyl phthalate, or 1,2-benzenedicarboxylic acid bis(2-ethylhexyl) ester. It can be represented by $C_{24}H_{38}O_4$. DEHP is used in vacuum pumps (Windholz 1983).

2.7 National Toxicology Program Data 19

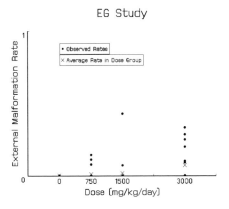

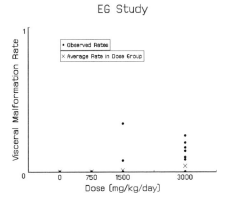

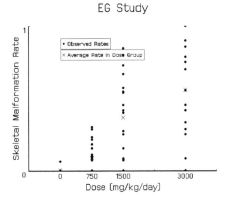

FIGURE 2.5. *NTP Data. EG Study in Mice. Observed and averaged malformation rates.*

2. Motivating Studies

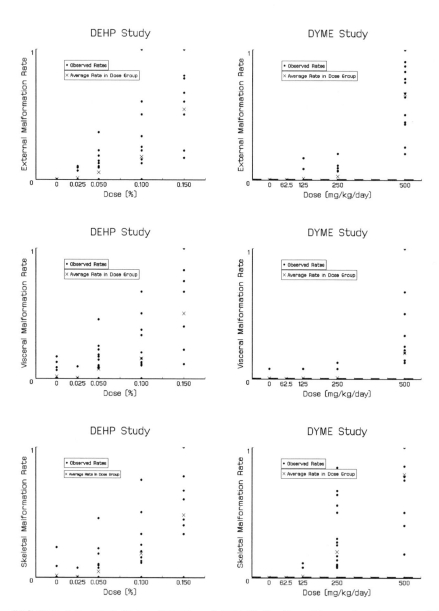

FIGURE 2.6. *NTP Data. DEHP and DYME Studies. Observed and averaged malformation rates.*

TABLE 2.9. *NTP Data. Summary data by study in mice. The dose is in mg/kg/day.*

Exposure	Dose	# Dams, ≥ 1 Impl.	# Dams, ≥ 1 Viab.	Live	Litter Size (mean)	Malformations Ext.	Malformations Visc.	Malformations Skel.
EG	0	25	25	297	11.9	0.0	0.0	0.3
	750	24	24	276	11.5	1.1	0.0	8.7
	1500	23	22	229	10.4	1.7	0.9	36.7
	3000	23	23	226	9.8	7.1	4.0	55.8
DEHP	0	30	30	330	13.2	0.0	1.5	1.2
	44	26	26	288	11.1	1.0	0.4	0.4
	91	26	26	277	10.7	5.4	7.2	4.3
	191	24	17	137	8.1	17.5	15.3	18.3
	292	25	9	50	5.6	54.0	50.0	48.0
DYME	0	21	21	282	13.4	0.0	0.0	0.0
	62.5	20	20	225	11.3	0.0	0.0	0.0
	125	24	24	290	12.1	1.0	0.0	1.0
	250	23	23	261	11.3	2.7	0.1	20.0
	500	22	22	141	6.1	66.0	19.9	79.4

Furthermore, this ester as well as other phthalic acid esters are used extensively as plasticizers for numerous plastic devices made of polyvinyl chloride. DEHP provides the finished plastic products with desirable flexibility and clarity (Shiota, Chou, and Nishimura 1980).

It has been well documented that small quantities of phthalic acid esters may leak out of polyvinyl chloride plastic containers in the presence of food, milk, blood, or various solvents. Due to their ubiquitous distribution and presence in human and animal tissues, considerable concern has developed as to the possible toxic effects of the phthalic acid esters (e.g., Autian 1973).

In particular, the developmental toxicity study described by Tyl *et al* (1988) has attracted much interest in the toxicity of DEHP. The doses selected for the study were 0, 0.025, 0.05, 0.1, and 0.15%, corresponding to a DEHP consumption of 0, 44, 91, 191, and 292 mg/kg/day, respectively. Females were observed daily during treatment, but no maternal deaths or distinctive clinical signs were observed. The dams were sacrificed, slightly prior to normal delivery, and the status of uterine implantation sites recorded. A total of 1082 live foetuses were dissected from the uterus, anesthetized, and examined for external, visceral, and skeletal malformations.

TABLE 2.10. *NTP Data. Frequency distribution of the number of implants.*

Number of implants	EG	DEHP	DYME
1	0	1	0
2	0	1	0
3	1	0	1
4	0	2	1
5	1	0	0
6	0	2	0
7	2	0	2
8	1	4	2
9	8	5	2
10	4	7	7
11	8	18	10
12	19	21	15
13	16	26	27
14	11	21	19
15	16	10	9
16	6	8	10
17	1	2	5
18	0	2	0
19	1	1	0
	95	131	110

Table 2.9 suggests clear dose-related trends in the malformation rates. The average litter size (number of viable animals) decreases with increased levels of exposure to DEHP, a finding that is attributable to the dose-related increase in fetal deaths.

2.7.3 *Diethylene Glycol Dimethyl Ether*

Other names for diethylene glycol dimethyl ether (DYME) are diglyme and bis(2-methoxyethyl) ether. DYME has as its chemical formula

$$CH_3O(CH_2)_2O(CH_2)_2OCH_3$$

(Windholz 1983). It is a component of industrial solvents. These are widely used in the manufacture of protective coatings such as lacquers, metal coatings, baking enamels, etc. (NIOSH 1983). Although to date, several at-

TABLE 2.11. *Sports Injuries Trial. Cross-classification of awakeness measurements at 10 and 20 minutes, on a four-point ordinal scale.*

Score at 10 mins	Score at 20 mins			
	0	1	2	3
0	42	119	6	0
1	0	68	31	3
2	0	0	3	2
3	0	0	0	2

tempts have proven inadequate to evaluate the potential of glycol ethers to produce human reproductive toxicity, structurally related compounds have been identified as reproductive toxicants in several mammalian species, producing (1) testicular toxicity and (2) embryotoxicity.

Price *et al* (1987) describe a study in which timed-pregnant mice were dosed with DYME throughout major organogenesis (gestational days 8 through 15). The doses selected for the study were 0, 62.5, 125, 250 and 500 mg/kg/day. Table 2.9 summarizes the data.

2.8 The Sports Injuries Trial

These data come from a randomized, parallel group, double-blind trial in men comparing the effect of an active treatment to placebo on post-operative shivering and per-operative hemodynamics. The primary responses of interest were severity of post-operative shivering measured from the end of anesthesia every 5 minutes during 30 minutes as none (0), mild (1), moderate (2), or severe (3), and effect of treatment on overall consciousness assessed from the end of anesthesia at 10, 20, 30, 45, 60, 90, and 120 minutes as impossible to awake (0), difficult to awake (1), easy to awake (2), and awake, eyes open (3). One hundred forty patients were assigned to each treatment group.

Since this trial occurred in a very short time period, there is very little missing data. There was one patient who had no response information for either variable, so this patient is excluded from all analyses. There were also 3 patients with some missing information on shivering or overall consciousness, leaving 138 patients with complete information.

One interesting feature of these data is that there are structural zeros in the awake variables. A patient could never become less awake over time, thus the cross-tabulation of the score over time contains zeros in the lower left corner. Data from 10 and 20 minutes are presented in Table 2.11. The zero in the upper right hand corner (0 at 10 minutes and 3 at 20 minutes)

TABLE 2.12. *Sports Injuries Trial. Cross-classification of four dichotomized shivering measurements (at 5, 10, 15, and 20 minutes).*

(5 mins, 10 mins)	(15 mins, 20 mins)			
	(0,0)	(0,1)	(1,0)	(1,1)
	Placebo arm			
(0,0)	37	11	8	16
(0,1)	6	2	6	23
(1,0)	1	0	0	1
(1,1)	2	0	4	21
	Treatment arm			
(0,0)	59	10	4	9
(0,1)	10	1	11	22
(1,0)	0	0	0	0
(1,1)	1	0	2	10

is a sampling zero because it is possible for a patient to go from being completely asleep to awake with eyes open, but rather unlikely. On the other hand, the zeros in the lower left hand corner of the table are all structural zeros because once a patient reached a certain level of consciousness, he could never return to a lower level. The longitudinal nature of the data is seen in Table 2.12, where the cross-classification of four dichotomized shivering measures, at 5, 10, 15, and 20 minutes, is shown.

2.9 Age Related Macular Degeneration Trial

These data arise from a randomized multi-centric clinical trial comparing an experimental treatment (interferon-α) to a corresponding placebo in the treatment of patients with age-related macular degeneration. Throughout the analyses done, we focus on the comparison between placebo and the highest dose (6 million units daily) of interferon-α (Z), but the full results of this trial have been reported elsewhere (Pharmacological Therapy for Macular Degeneration Study Group 1997). Patients with macular degeneration progressively lose vision. In the trial, the patients' visual acuity was assessed at different time points (4 weeks, 12 weeks, 24 weeks, and 52 weeks) through their ability to read lines of letters on standardized vision charts. These charts display lines of 5 letters of decreasing size, which the patient must read from top (largest letters) to bottom (smallest letters). Each line with at least 4 letters correctly read is called one 'line of vision.'

TABLE 2.13. *Age Related Macular Degeneration Trial. Loss of at least 3 lines of vision at 1 year according to loss of at least 2 lines of vision at 6 months and according to randomized treatment group (placebo versus interferon-α).*

	12 months			
	Placebo		Active	
6 months	0	1	0	1
No event (0)	56	9	31	9
Event (1)	8	30	9	38

TABLE 2.14. *Age Related Macular Degeneration Trial. Mean (standard error) of visual acuity at baseline, at 6 months and at 1 year according to randomized treatment group (placebo versus interferon-α).*

Time point	Placebo	Active	Total
Baseline	55.3 (1.4)	54.6 (1.3)	55.0 (1.0)
6 months	49.3 (1.8)	45.5 (1.8)	47.5 (1.3)
1 year	44.4 (1.8)	39.1 (1.9)	42.0 (1.3)

The patient's visual acuity is the total number of letters correctly read. The primary endpoint of the trial was the loss of at least 3 lines of vision at 1 year, compared to their baseline performance (a binary endpoint). The secondary endpoint of the trial was the visual acuity at 1 year (treated as a continuous endpoint). Buyse and Molenberghs (1998) examined whether the patient's performance at 6 months could be used as a surrogate for their performance at 1 year with respect to the effect of interferon-α. They looked at whether the loss of 2 lines of vision at 6 months could be used as a surrogate for the loss of at least 3 lines of vision at 1 year (Table 2.13). They also looked at whether visual acuity at 6 months could be used as a surrogate for visual acuity at 1 year.

Table 2.14 shows the visual acuity (mean and standard error) by treatment group at baseline, at 6 months, and at 1 year. Visual acuity can be measured in several ways. First, one can record the number of letters read. Alternatively, dichotomized versions (at least 3 lines of vision lost, or at least 3 lines of vision lost) can be used as well. Therefore, these data will be useful to illustrate methods for the joint modeling of continuous and binary outcomes, with or without taking the longitudinal nature into account. In addition, though there are 190 subjects with both month 6 and month 12 measurements available, the total number of longitudinal profiles is 240, but only for 188 of these have the four follow-up measurements been made.

3
Generalized Linear Models

3.1 Introduction

Most models that have been proposed in the statistical literature for the analysis of discrete repeated measurements can be considered extensions of generalized linear models (McCullagh and Nelder 1989) to the context of correlated observations. In this chapter, these models will be introduced, inference will be briefly discussed, and several frequently used specific cases will be given special attention.

3.2 The Exponential Family

A random variable Y follows a distribution that belongs to the exponential family if the density is of the form

$$f(y) \equiv f(y|\theta, \phi) = \exp\left\{\phi^{-1}[y\theta - \psi(\theta)] + c(y, \phi)\right\} \qquad (3.1)$$

for a specific set of unknown parameters θ and ϕ, and for known functions $\psi(\cdot)$ and $c(\cdot, \cdot)$. Often, θ and ϕ are termed 'natural parameter' (or 'canonical parameter') and 'scale parameter,' respectively.

The first two moments can easily be derived as follows. Starting from the property $\int f(y|\theta, \phi)dy = 1$ and taking the first- and second-order derivatives from both sides of the equation, we get that

$$\begin{cases} \int [y - \psi'(\theta)] \, f(y|\theta,\phi) \, dy = 0, \\ \int \{\phi^{-1}[y - \psi'(\theta)]^2 - \psi''(\theta)\} \, f(y|\theta,\phi) \, dy = 0, \end{cases}$$

from which it directly follows that the average $\mu = \mathrm{E}(Y)$ equals $\psi'(\theta)$ and the variance $\sigma^2 = \mathrm{Var}(Y)$ is given by $\phi\psi''(\theta)$. An important implication is that, in general, the mean and variance are related through $\sigma^2 = \phi\psi''[\psi'^{-1}(\mu)] = \phi v(\mu)$ for an appropriate function $v(\mu)$, called the variance function.

In some of the models that will be discussed in this book, a quasi-likelihood perspective is taken. Although the above relation between the mean and the variance immediately follows from the density (3.1), one sometimes starts from specifying a mean and a variance function,

$$\begin{aligned} \mathrm{E}(Y) &= \mu, \\ \mathrm{Var}(Y) &= \phi v(\mu). \end{aligned}$$

The variance function $v(\mu)$ can be chosen in accordance with a particular member of the exponential family. If not, then parameters cannot be estimated using maximum likelihood principles. Instead, a set of estimating equations needs to be specified, the solution of which is referred to as the quasi-likelihood estimates. Examples of this approach will be given in Chapter 8.

3.3 The Generalized Linear Model (GLM)

In a regression context, where one wishes to explain variability between outcome values based on measured covariate values, the model needs to incorporate covariates. This leads to so-called generalized linear models. Let $Y_1, \ldots, Y_N$ be a set of independent outcomes, and let $\boldsymbol{x}_1, \ldots, \boldsymbol{x}_N$ represent the corresponding p-dimensional vectors of covariate values. It is assumed that all Y_i have densities $f(y_i|\theta_i, \phi)$ which belong to the exponential family, but a different natural parameter θ_i is allowed per observation. Specification of the generalized linear model is completed by modeling the means μ_i as functions of the covariate values. More specifically, it is assumed that

$$\mu_i = h(\eta_i) = h(\boldsymbol{x_i}'\boldsymbol{\beta}),$$

for a known function $h(\cdot)$, and with $\boldsymbol{\beta}$ a vector of p fixed unknown regression coefficients. Usually, $h^{-1}(\cdot)$ is called the link function. In most applications, the so-called natural link function is used, i.e., $h(\cdot) = \psi'(\cdot)$, which is equivalent to assuming $\theta_i = \boldsymbol{x_i}'\boldsymbol{\beta}$. Hence, it is assumed that the natural parameter satisfies a linear regression model.

3.4 Examples

3.4.1 The Linear Regression Model for Continuous Data

Let Y be normally distributed with mean μ and variance σ^2. The density can be written as

$$f(y) = \exp\left\{\frac{1}{\sigma^2}\left(y\mu - \frac{\mu^2}{2}\right) + \left(\frac{\ln(2\pi\sigma^2)}{2} - \frac{y^2}{2\sigma^2}\right)\right\},$$

which implies that the normal distribution belongs to the exponential family, with natural parameter θ equal to μ, scale parameter ϕ equal to σ^2, and variance function $v(\mu) = 1$. Hence, the normal distribution is very particular in the sense that there is no mean-variance relation, as will be shown to be present for other exponential family distributions. The natural link function equals the identity function, leading to the classical linear regression model $Y_i \sim N(\mu_i, \sigma^2)$ with $\mu_i = \boldsymbol{x_i}'\boldsymbol{\beta}$.

3.4.2 Logistic and Probit Regression for Binary Data

Let Y be Bernoulli distributed with success probability $P(Y = 1) = \pi$. The density can be written as

$$f(y) = \exp\left\{y\ln\left(\frac{\pi}{1-\pi}\right) + \ln(1-\pi)\right\},$$

which implies that the Bernoulli distribution belongs to the exonential family, with natural parameter θ equal to the logit, i.e., $\ln[\pi/(1-\pi)]$, of π, scale parameter $\phi = 1$, with mean $\mu = \pi$ and with variance function $v(\pi) = \pi(1-\pi)$. The natural link function is the logit link, leading to the classical logistic regression model $Y_i \sim \text{Bernoulli}(\pi_i)$ with $\ln[\pi_i/(1-\pi_i)] = \boldsymbol{x_i}'\boldsymbol{\beta}$ or equivalently

$$\pi_i = \frac{\exp(\boldsymbol{x_i}'\boldsymbol{\beta})}{[1 + \exp(\boldsymbol{x_i}'\boldsymbol{\beta})]}.$$

Sometimes, the logit link function is replaced by the probit link, which is the inverse of the standard normal distribution function, Φ^{-1}. It has been repeatedly shown (Agresti 1990) that the logit and probit link functions behave very similarly, in the sense that for probabilities other than extreme ones (say, outside of the interval $[0.2; 0.8]$) logistic and probit regression provide approximately the same parameter estimates, up to a scaling factor equal to $\pi/\sqrt{3}$, the ratio of the standard deviations of a logistic and a standard normal variable.

3.4.3 Poisson Regression for Counts

Let Y be Poisson distributed with mean λ. The density can be written as

$$f(y) = \exp\{y\ln\lambda - \lambda - \ln y!\},$$

from which it follows that the Poisson distribution belongs to the exponential family, with natural parameter θ equal to $\ln \lambda$, scale parameter $\phi = 1$, and variance function $v(\lambda) = \lambda$. The logarithm is the natural link function, leading to the classical Poisson regression model $Y_i \sim \text{Poisson}(\lambda_i)$, with $\ln \lambda_i = \boldsymbol{x}_i' \boldsymbol{\beta}$.

3.5 Maximum Likelihood Estimation and Inference

Estimation of the regression parameters in $\boldsymbol{\beta}$ is usually done using maximum likelihood (ML) estimation. Assuming independence of the observations, the log-likelihood is given by

$$\ell(\boldsymbol{\beta}, \phi) = \frac{1}{\phi} \sum_{i=1}^{N} [y_i \theta_i - \psi(\theta_i)] + \sum_i c(y_i, \phi).$$

The score equations obtained from equating the first-order derivatives of the log-likelihood to zero take the form

$$S(\boldsymbol{\beta}) = \sum_i \frac{\partial \theta_i}{\partial \boldsymbol{\beta}} [y_i - \psi'(\theta_i)] = 0.$$

Because $\mu_i = \psi'(\theta_i)$ and $v_i = v(\mu_i) = \psi''(\theta_i)$, we have that

$$\frac{\partial \mu_i}{\partial \boldsymbol{\beta}} = \psi''(\theta_i) \frac{\partial \theta_i}{\partial \boldsymbol{\beta}} = v_i \frac{\partial \theta_i}{\partial \boldsymbol{\beta}}$$

which implies the following score equations:

$$S(\boldsymbol{\beta}) = \sum_i \frac{\partial \mu_i}{\partial \boldsymbol{\beta}} v_i^{-1} (y_i - \mu_i) = 0.$$

In general, these score equations need to be solved iteratively, using numerical algorithms such as iteratively (re-)weighted least squares, Newton-Raphson, or Fisher scoring.

Once the ML estimates have been obtained, classical inference based on asymptotic likelihood theory becomes available, including Wald-type tests, likelihood ratio tests, and score tests, all asymptotically equivalent.

In some cases, such as in the logistic regression model, ϕ is a known constant. In other examples, such as the linear normal model, estimation of ϕ may be required to estimate the standard errors of the elements in $\boldsymbol{\beta}$. Because $\text{Var}(Y_i) = \phi v_i$, an obvious estimate for ϕ is given by

$$\widehat{\phi} = \frac{1}{N-p} \sum_i (y_i - \widehat{\mu}_i)^2 / v_i(\widehat{\mu}_i).$$

TABLE 3.1. *Toenail Data. Logistic regression, ignoring the association structure. Parameter estimates, associated standard errors, and inferences for the parameters in model (3.2).*

Parameter	Estimate	s.e.	p-value
β_0	-0.5571	0.1090	<0.0001
β_1	0.0240	0.1565	0.8780
β_2	-0.1769	0.0246	<0.0001
β_3	-0.0783	0.0394	0.0470

For example, under the normal model, this would yield

$$\widehat{\sigma}^2 = \frac{1}{N-p} \sum_i (y_i - x_i'\widehat{\beta})^2,$$

which is the mean squared error used in linear regression models to estimate the residual variance.

We refer to McCullagh and Nelder (1989) and to Agresti (1990) for more details on estimation and inference in the GLM's.

3.6 Logistic Regression for the Toenail Data

As an example of logistic regression, we analyze the toenail data introduced in Section 2.3, ignoring the correlation structure due to the repeated measurements within subjects. This would be correct if measurements at different time points would also be taken on different subjects. In Section 10.3, the results obtained here will be used as starting values in the fitting of more complicated models that do account for the association structure. Let Y_i be the binary outcome indicating severity of the toenail infection, for the ith observation. A logistic model will be assumed, with linear time trends, for both treatment groups separately. More specifically, the model is given by

$$Y_i \sim \text{Bernoulli}(\pi_i),$$
$$\text{logit}(\pi_i) = \beta_0 + \beta_1 T_i + \beta_2 t_i + \beta_3 T_i t_i, \tag{3.2}$$

in which T_i is the treatment indicator for this observation, and t_i is the time-point at which the observation was taken. The results are shown in Table 3.1. The maximized log-likelihood value equals -905.91 and could be used in likelihood ratio tests for the validity of simpler models. Note the significant interaction ($p = 0.0470$) suggesting different trends in the two treatment groups.

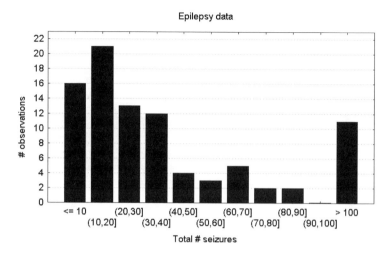

FIGURE 3.1. *Epilepsy Study. Frequency plot of the post-randomization total number of epileptic seizures, over both treatment groups.*

3.7 Poisson Regression for the Epilepsy Data

As an example of Poisson regression, we analyze the epilepsy data introduced in Section 2.5. Our response of interest will be the total number of seizures a patient has experienced during the study, after randomization took place. We want to test for a treatment effect on number of seizures, correcting for the average number of seizures during the 12-week baseline phase, prior to the treatment. Let Y_i be the total number of seizures for subject i. A histogram of the observed values is given in Figure 3.1. Note that this histogram does not correct for the fact that the subjects have not been followed for an equal number of weeks. Let n_i be the number of weeks subject i has been followed; we will correct for the differences in follow-up time by assuming that

$$Y_i \sim \text{Poisson}(\lambda_i),$$
$$\ln(\lambda_i/n_i) = \beta_0 + \beta_1 \text{Baseline}_i + \beta_2 T_i, \tag{3.3}$$

in which T_i is the treatment indicator and where Baseline_i is the baseline seizure rate. Note that model (3.3) is equivalent to

$$\ln(\lambda_i) = \ln(n_i) + \beta_0 + \beta_1 \text{Baseline}_i + \beta_2 T_i \tag{3.4}$$

which is a traditional Poisson model with constant term $\ln(n_i)$ added to the linear predictor. This term is often called an 'offset'.

The results are shown in Table 3.2. The maximized log-likelihood equals 14837.31. Note the highly significant positive effect of the baseline rate.

3.7 Poisson Regression for the Epilepsy Data

TABLE 3.2. *Epilepsy Study. Poisson regression for the total number of epileptic seizures. Parameter estimates, associated standard errors, and inferences for the parameters in model (3.4).*

Parameter	Estimate	S.e.	p-value
β_0	0.8710	0.0218	<0.0001
β_1	0.0172	0.0002	<0.0001
β_2	-0.4987	0.0341	<0.0001

Further, correcting for baseline rate, the treatment significantly reduces the average weekly number of epileptic seizures ($p < 0.0001$).

4
Linear Mixed Models for Gaussian Longitudinal Data

4.1 Introduction

Although this book focuses on models for repeated categorical data, it is helpful to first consider some key topics in the analysis of continuous longitudinal data, where most parametric models are based on underlying normality assumptions. Two general extensions of the univariate linear regression models to repeated measures can be distinguished. First, a multivariate model can be formulated, in which each component is modeled using a univariate linear regression model, and with the association structure directly modeled through a marginal covariance matrix. Second, a random-effects approach can be followed. In the next sections, these two model families will be discussed in turn. We will compare both approaches, and we will summarize how estimation and inference proceeds.

Ideas will be illustrated in the simple context of a response Y measured repeatedly on a homogeneous set of subjects i, $i = 1, \ldots, N$, and where it is believed that Y evolves linearly over time. This can immediately be generalized to more complex settings with non-linear trends and/or to models in which covariates are included to model the believe that trends may depend on subject-specific covariates.

4.2 Marginal Multivariate Model

Let Y_{ij} be the jth measurement available for the ith subject or cluster, $i = 1, \ldots, N$, $j = 1, \ldots, n_i$. Further, $\boldsymbol{Y}_i = (Y_{i1}, \ldots, Y_{in_i})'$ is the n_i-dimensional vector with all observations available for subject i. Assuming an average linear trend for Y as a function of time, a multivariate regression model can be obtained by assuming that the elements Y_{ij} in $\boldsymbol{Y}_i$ satisfy $Y_{ij} = \beta_0 + \beta_1 t_{ij} + \varepsilon_{ij}$, with the assumption that the error components ε_{ij} are normally distributed with mean zero. In vector notation, we get $\boldsymbol{Y}_i = X_i \boldsymbol{\beta} + \boldsymbol{\varepsilon}_i$ for an appropriate design matrix X_i, with $\boldsymbol{\beta}' = (\beta_0, \beta_1)$ and with $\boldsymbol{\varepsilon}'_i = (\varepsilon_{i1}, \varepsilon_{i2}, \ldots, \varepsilon_{in_i})$. The model is completed by specifying an appropriate covariance matrix V_i for $\boldsymbol{\varepsilon}_i$, leading to the multivariate model

$$\boldsymbol{Y}_i \sim N(X_i \boldsymbol{\beta}, V_i). \tag{4.1}$$

Let I_{n_i} denote the identity matrix of dimension n_i, then we have that $V_i = \sigma^2 I_{n_i}$ corresponds to the univariate linear regression model, assuming all repeated measurements Y_{ij} to be independent, i.e., ignoring the fact that repeated measures within subjects may be (highly) correlated. In the case of balanced data, i.e., when a fixed number n of measurements is taken for all subjects, and when measurements are taken at fixed timepoints $t_1, \ldots, t_n$, a useful covariance model is $V_i = V$, where V is a general (unstructured) $n \times n$ positive definite covariance matrix. This yields the classical mulivariate regression model (Seber 1984, Chapter 8).

Depending on the context and the actual data at hand, other choices may be appropriate. For example, a first-order autoregressive model assumes that the covariance between two measurements Y_{ij} and Y_{ik} from the same subject i is of the form $\sigma^2 \rho^{|t_{ij} - t_{ik}|}$ for unknown parameters σ^2 and ρ. Another example is compound symmetry, which assumes the covariance to be of the form $\sigma^2 + \gamma \delta_{jk}$ for unknown parameters σ^2 and $\gamma > -\sigma^2$, and where δ_{jk} equals one for $j = k$ and zero otherwise. These are examples of homogeneous covariance structures since they assume the variance of all Y_{ij} to be equal. Heterogeneous versions can be formulated as well (Verbeke and Molenberghs 2000).

4.3 The Linear Mixed Model

The random-effects approach toward extending the univariate linear regression model to longitudinal settings is based on the assumption that, for every subject, the response can be modeled by a linear regression model, but with subject-specific regression coefficients. Continuing our simple example, suppose that the individual trajectories of the response Y are of the type as shown in Figure 4.1. Obviously, a linear regression model with intercept and linear time effect seems plausible to describe the data of

4.3 The Linear Mixed Model

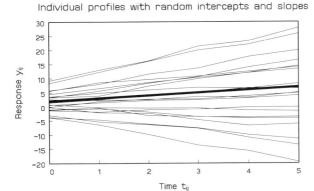

FIGURE 4.1. *Hypothetical example of continuous longitudinal data that can be well described by a linear mixed model with random intercepts and random slopes. The thin lines represent the observed subject-specific evolutions. The bold line represents the population-averaged evolution.*

each person separately. However, different persons tend to have different intercepts and different slopes. One can therefore assume that the outcome Y_{ij}, measured at time t_{ij} satisfies $Y_{ij} = \widetilde{\beta}_{i0} + \widetilde{\beta}_{i1} t_{ij} + \varepsilon_{ij}$. As before, $\varepsilon_i = (\varepsilon_{i1}, \varepsilon_{i2}, \ldots, \varepsilon_{in_i})'$ is assumed to be normally distributed with mean vector zero, and some covariance matrix which we now denote by Σ_i.

Because subjects are randomly sampled from a population of subjects, it is natural to assume that the subject-specific regression coefficients $\widetilde{\boldsymbol{\beta}}_i = (\widetilde{\beta}_{i0}, \widetilde{\beta}_{i1})'$ are randomly sampled from a population of regression coefficients. It is customary to assume the $\widetilde{\boldsymbol{\beta}}_i$ to be (multivariate) normal, but extensions can be formulated (Verbeke and Lesaffre 1996, Magder and Zeger 1996). Assuming $\widetilde{\boldsymbol{\beta}}_i$ to be bivariate normal with mean $(\beta_0, \beta_1)'$ and 2×2 covariance matrix D we can reformulate the model as

$$Y_{ij} = (\beta_0 + b_{i0}) + (\beta_1 + b_{i1}) t_{pi} + \varepsilon_{ij}, \qquad (4.2)$$

with $\widetilde{\beta}_{i0} = \beta_0 + b_{i0}$ and $\widetilde{\beta}_{i1} = \beta_1 + b_{i1}$, and the new random effects $\boldsymbol{b}_i = (b_{i0}, b_{i1})'$ are now normal with mean zero and covariance D. The population-averaged profile is linear, with intercept β_0 and slope β_1, and is represented by the bold line in Figure 4.1.

The above model is a special case of the general linear mixed model which assumes that the vector $\boldsymbol{Y}_i$ of repeated measurements for the ith subject satisfies

$$\boldsymbol{Y}_i | \boldsymbol{b}_i \sim N(X_i \boldsymbol{\beta} + Z_i \boldsymbol{b}_i, \Sigma_i) \qquad (4.3)$$
$$\boldsymbol{b}_i \sim N(\boldsymbol{0}, D), \qquad (4.4)$$

for $n_i \times p$ and $n_i \times q$ known design matrices X_i and Z_i, for a p-dimensional vector $\boldsymbol{\beta}$ of unknown regression coefficients, for a q-dimensional vector $\boldsymbol{b}_i$

of subject-specific regression coefficients assumed to be sampled from the q-dimensional normal distribution with mean zero and covariance D, and with Σ_i a covariance matrix parameterized through a set of unknown parameters. The components in $\boldsymbol{\beta}$ are called 'fixed effects,' the components in $\boldsymbol{b}_i$ are called 'random effects.' The fact that the model contains fixed as well as random effects motivates the term 'mixed models.'

Unless the model is fitted in a Bayesian framework (Gelman et al 1995), estimation and inference are based on the marginal distribution for the response vector $\boldsymbol{Y}_i$. Let $f_i(\boldsymbol{y}_i|\boldsymbol{b}_i)$ and $f(\boldsymbol{b}_i)$ be the density functions corresponding to (4.3) and (4.4), respectively, the marginal density function of $\boldsymbol{Y}_i$ is

$$f_i(\boldsymbol{y}_i) = \int f_i(\boldsymbol{y}_i|\boldsymbol{b}_i)\, f(\boldsymbol{b}_i)\, d\boldsymbol{b}_i,$$

which can easily be shown to be the density function of an n_i-dimensional normal distribution with mean vector $X_i\boldsymbol{\beta}$ and with covariance matrix $V_i = Z_i D Z_i' + \Sigma_i$. Note that the linear mixed model implies a marginal model of the form (4.1), but with a very specific parametric form for the marginal covariance matrix V_i, easily allowing highly unbalanced data. In this respect, the linear mixed model can be interpreted as a procedure to obtain flexible multivariate marginal models. As was already shown in our earlier example, the fixed effects describe the population-averaged evolution.

Because the mixed model is defined through the distributions $f_i(\boldsymbol{y}_i|\boldsymbol{b}_i)$ and $f(\boldsymbol{b}_i)$, this will be called the hierarchical formulation of the linear mixed model. The corresponding marginal normal distribution with mean $X_i\boldsymbol{\beta}$ and covariance $V_i = Z_i D Z_i' + \Sigma_i$ is called the marginal formulation of the model. Note that, although the marginal model naturally follows from the hierarchical one, both these models are not equivalent. Indeed, different random-effects models can produce the same marginal model. To see this, consider the case where every subject is measured twice ($n_i = 2$). First, assume that the random-effects structure is confined to a random intercept (b_i is scalar), and the residual error structure $\Sigma_i = \Sigma = \text{diag}(\sigma_1^2, \sigma_2^2)$ (Model I). The resulting marginal covariance matrix is

$$V = \begin{pmatrix} 1 \\ 1 \end{pmatrix} (d) \begin{pmatrix} 1 & 1 \end{pmatrix} + \begin{pmatrix} \sigma_1^2 & 0 \\ 0 & \sigma_2^2 \end{pmatrix} = \begin{pmatrix} d + \sigma_1^2 & d \\ d & d + \sigma_2^2 \end{pmatrix}. \quad (4.5)$$

Second, consider the random effects to consist of a random intercept and a random slope ($\boldsymbol{b}_i = (b_{0i}, b_{1i})'$), mutually uncorrelated, with residual error structure $\Sigma_i = \Sigma = \sigma^2 I_2$ (Model II). The resulting covariance matrix now equals

$$V = \begin{pmatrix} 1 & 0 \\ 1 & 1 \end{pmatrix} \begin{pmatrix} d_1 & 0 \\ 0 & d_2 \end{pmatrix} \begin{pmatrix} 1 & 1 \\ 0 & 1 \end{pmatrix} + \begin{pmatrix} \sigma^2 & 0 \\ 0 & \sigma^2 \end{pmatrix}$$

$$= \begin{pmatrix} d_1 + \sigma^2 & d_1 \\ d_1 & d_1 + d_2 + \sigma^2 \end{pmatrix}. \quad (4.6)$$

Obviously, the parametric models (4.5) and (4.6) for the marginal covariance are equivalent: $d_1 = d$, $d_2 = \sigma_2^2 - \sigma_1^2$, and $\sigma^2 = \sigma_1^2$. Thus, (at least) two different hierarchical models can produce the same marginal model, illustrating that a good fit of the marginal model should not be seen as equally strong evidence for any of the mixed models. Arguably, a satisfactory treatment of the random-effects model is only possible within a Bayesian context.

In addition, it is important to see that there are even marginal models that are not implied by a mixed model. The simplest example is found by considering the marginal model with compound symmetric covariance structure (Section 4.2). If the within-subject correlation is positive ($\gamma \geq 0$), this model could have been implied by a mixed model with random intercepts b_i that are normally distributed with mean 0 and variance γ, and with uncorrelated error components with common variance σ^2. However, if the within-cluster correlation is negative ($\gamma < 0$), the resulting marginal model cannot be implied by an appropriate random-effects model. This would be the case, for example, in a context of competition such as when littermates compete for the same food resources.

4.4 Estimation and Inference for the Marginal Model

As indicated earlier, the fitting of a linear mixed model is usually based on the marginal model that, for subject i, is multivariate normal with mean $X_i\beta$ and covariance $V_i(\alpha) = Z_i D Z_i' + \Sigma_i$, hereby explicitly denoting that V_i depends on an unknown vector α of parameters in the covariance matrices D and Σ_i. The parameters in α are usually called 'variance components.' The classical approach to estimation and inference is based on maximum likelihood (ML). Assuming independence across subjects, the likelihood takes the form

$$L_{\mathrm{ML}}(\boldsymbol{\theta}) = \prod_{i=1}^{N} \left\{ (2\pi)^{-n_i/2} |V_i(\boldsymbol{\alpha})|^{-\frac{1}{2}} \right.$$
$$\left. \times \exp\left[-\frac{1}{2} (\boldsymbol{Y}_i - X_i\boldsymbol{\beta})' V_i^{-1}(\boldsymbol{\alpha}) (\boldsymbol{Y}_i - X_i\boldsymbol{\beta}) \right] \right\}. \quad (4.7)$$

Estimation of $\boldsymbol{\theta}' = (\boldsymbol{\beta}', \boldsymbol{\alpha}')$ requires joint maximization of (4.7) with respect to all elements in $\boldsymbol{\theta}$. In general, no analytic solutions are available, calling for numerical optimization routines.

Conditionally on $\boldsymbol{\alpha}$, the maximum likelihood estimator (MLE) of $\boldsymbol{\beta}$ is given by (Laird and Ware 1982):

$$\widehat{\boldsymbol{\beta}}(\boldsymbol{\alpha}) = \left(\sum_{i=1}^{N} X_i' W_i X_i \right)^{-1} \sum_{i=1}^{N} X_i' W_i Y_i, \qquad (4.8)$$

where W_i equals V_i^{-1}. In practice, $\boldsymbol{\alpha}$ is not known and can be replaced by its MLE $\widehat{\boldsymbol{\alpha}}$. However, one often also uses the so-called restricted maximum likelihood (REML) estimator for $\boldsymbol{\alpha}$ (Harville 1974), which allows to estimate $\boldsymbol{\alpha}$ without having to estimate the fixed effects in $\boldsymbol{\beta}$ first. It is known from simpler models, such as linear regression models, that, while classical ML estimators are biased downwards, this is not the case for the REML estimators (Verbeke and Molenberghs 2000, Section 5.3).

When it comes to inference, in practice, the fixed effects in $\boldsymbol{\beta}$ are often of primary interest, as they describe the average evolution in the population. Conditionally on $\boldsymbol{\alpha}$, the maximum likelihood (ML) estimate for $\boldsymbol{\beta}$ is given by (4.8), which is normally distributed with mean

$$E\left[\widehat{\boldsymbol{\beta}}(\boldsymbol{\alpha})\right] = \left(\sum_{i=1}^{N} X_i' W_i X_i \right)^{-1} \sum_{i=1}^{N} X_i' W_i E\left[Y_i\right] = \boldsymbol{\beta}, \qquad (4.9)$$

and covariance

$$\begin{aligned}
\text{Var}\left[\widehat{\boldsymbol{\beta}}(\boldsymbol{\alpha})\right] &= \left(\sum_{i=1}^{N} X_i' W_i X_i \right)^{-1} \\
&\quad \times \left(\sum_{i=1}^{N} X_i' W_i \text{Var}\left[Y_i\right] W_i X_i \right) \\
&\quad \times \left(\sum_{i=1}^{N} X_i' W_i X_i \right)^{-1} \qquad (4.10) \\
&= \left(\sum_{i=1}^{N} X_i' W_i X_i \right)^{-1}, \qquad (4.11)
\end{aligned}$$

provided that the mean and covariance were correctly specified in our model, i.e., provided that $E(Y_i) = X_i \boldsymbol{\beta}$ and $\text{Var}(Y_i) = V_i = Z_i D Z_i' + \Sigma_i$. Approximate Wald-type tests for components in $\boldsymbol{\beta}$ can now easily be obtained.

Note however, that these Wald tests are based on standard errors obtained from replacing $\boldsymbol{\alpha}$ in (4.11) by its ML or REML estimate and therefore underestimate the true variability in $\widehat{\boldsymbol{\beta}}$ because they do not take into account the variability introduced by estimating $\boldsymbol{\alpha}$. Therefore, the classical normal or chi-squared reference distributions are often replaced by t or F-distributions, with the same numerator degrees of freedom as the original chi-squared distribution. The denominator degrees of freedom need to be estimated from the data. This is often based on so-called Satterthwaite-type approximations (Satterthwaite 1941), and is only fully developed for the case of linear mixed models. We refer to Verbeke and Molenberghs (2000, Section 6.2) for more information on this aspect. In most longitudinal applications, different persons contribute independent information, which results in numbers of denominator degrees of freedom which are typically large enough, whatever estimation method is used, to lead to very similar p-values. Only for very small samples in terms of independent replicates, or when mixed models would be used with crossed random effects (random effects for persons as well as for items) different estimation methods for degrees of freedom may lead to severe differences in the resulting p-values.

Note also that the standard errors based on (4.11) are valid, only if the mean and covariance were correctly specified, while the only condition for $\widehat{\beta}$ to be unbiased is that the mean is correctly specified. Because in practice, it is often difficult to assess correct specification of the covariance structure, one often prefers standard errors to be based on (4.10), rather than (4.11), but with Var(Y_i) estimated by $(y_i - X_i\widehat{\beta})(y_i - X_i\widehat{\beta})'$ rather than $\widehat{V}_i$. The so-called robust or empirical standard errors are consistent, as long as the mean is correctly specified. This procedure is a special case of the theory on generalized estimating equations (GEE), introduced by Liang and Zeger (1986) which will be applied in Chapter 8 in the context of discrete outcomes.

When interest is also in inference for some of the variance components in α, classical asymptotic Wald, likelihood ratio, and score tests can be used. However, due to restrictions on the parameter spaces, some hypotheses of interest may be on the boundary of the parameter space, implying that classical testing procedures are no longer valid. In some special but important cases, analytic results are available on how to correctly test such hypotheses. We herefore refer to Stram and Lee (1994, 1995) for results on the likelihood ratio test, and to Verbeke and Molenberghs (2003) for results on the score test. A detailed discussion on inference for the marginal linear mixed model can be found in Verbeke and Molenberghs (2000, Chapter 6).

4.5 Inference for the Random Effects

Although in practice, one is usually primarily interested in estimating the parameters in the marginal model, it is often useful to calculate estimates for the random effects b_i as well, as they reflect how much the subject-specific profiles deviate from the overall average profile. Such estimates can then be interpreted as residuals which may be helpful for detecting special profiles (i.e., outlying individuals) or groups of individuals evolving differently over time. Also, estimates for the random effects are needed whenever interest is in prediction of subject-specific evolutions. Obviously, it is then no longer sufficient to assume that the data can be described well by the marginal model $N(X_i\beta, V_i)$. Instead, one has to explicitly assume that the hierarchical model specification (4.3) and (4.4) is appropriate. Because random effects represent a natural heterogeneity between the subjects, this assumption will often be justified for data where the between-subjects variability is large in comparison to the within-subject variability.

Because the subject-specific parameters b_i are assumed random, it is most natural to estimate them using Bayesian techniques (Box and Tiao 1992, Gelman *et al* 1995). Conditional on b_i, Y_i follows a multivariate normal distribution with mean vector $X_i\beta + Z_i b_i$ and with covariance matrix Σ_i. In combination with the distributional assumptions for b_i, one can easily derive (Smith 1973, Lindley and Smith 1972) that, conditionally on $Y_i = y_i$, b_i follows a multivariate normal posterior distribution with mean $\widehat{b}_i(\theta) = DZ_i'V_i^{-1}(\alpha)(y_i - X_i\beta)$, which is used in practice as an estimator for b_i. Its covariance estimator is equal to

$$\text{var}(\widehat{b}_i(\theta))$$
$$= DZ_i' \left\{ V_i^{-1} - V_i^{-1} X_i \left(\sum_{i=1}^{N} X_i' V_i^{-1} X_i \right)^{-1} X_i' V_i^{-1} \right\} Z_i D. \quad (4.12)$$

Note that (4.12) underestimates the variability in $\widehat{b}_i(\theta) - b_i$ since it ignores the variation of b_i. Therefore, inference for b_i is usually based on

$$\text{var}[\widehat{b}_i(\theta) - b_i] = D - \text{var}[\widehat{b}_i(\theta)] \quad (4.13)$$

as an estimator for the variation in $\widehat{b}_i(\theta) - b_i$ (Laird and Ware 1982).

So far, all calculations were performed conditionally upon the vector θ of parameters in the marginal model. In practice, the unknown parameters β and α in $\widehat{b}_i(\theta)$, (4.12), and (4.13) are replaced by their maximum or restricted maximum likelihood estimates. The resulting estimates for the random effects are called "Empirical Bayes" (EB) estimates, which we will denote by $\widehat{b}_i$. Note that (4.12) and (4.13) then underestimate the true variability in the obtained estimate $\widehat{b}_i$ because they do not take into account the variability introduced by replacing the unknown parameter θ by its estimate. Similarly as for the fixed effects, inference is therefore often based on approximate t-tests or F-tests, rather than on traditional Wald tests.

It immediately follows from (4.13) that for any linear combination λb_i of the random effects, $\text{var}(\lambda'\widehat{b}_i) \leq \text{var}(\lambda'b_i)$, indicating that the EB estimates show less variability than actually present in the random-effects population. This phenomenon is usually referred to as shrinkage (Carlin and Louis 1996, Strenio, Weisberg, and Bryk 1983). The shrinkage is also seen in the prediction $\widehat{\boldsymbol{y}}_i \equiv X_i\widehat{\boldsymbol{\beta}}+Z_i\widehat{\boldsymbol{b}}_i$ of the ith profile, which can be rewritten as $\widehat{\boldsymbol{y}}_i = \Sigma_i V_i^{-1} X_i\widehat{\boldsymbol{\beta}}+[I_{n_i}-\Sigma_i V_i^{-1}]\boldsymbol{y}_i$. Note that $\widehat{\boldsymbol{y}}_i$ can be interpreted as a weighted average of the population-averaged profile $X_i\widehat{\boldsymbol{\beta}}$ and the observed data $\boldsymbol{y}_i$, with weights $\Sigma_i V_i^{-1}$ and $I_{n_i} - \Sigma_i V_i^{-1}$, respectively. The "numerator" of $\Sigma_i V_i^{-1}$ is the residual covariance matrix Σ_i and the "denominator" is the overall covariance matrix V_i. Hence, severe shrinkage is to be expected when the residual variability is large in comparison to the between-subject variability (modeled by the random effects), whereas little shrinkage will occur if the opposite is true.

In practice, one often uses histograms and scatter plots of components of $\widehat{\boldsymbol{b}}_i$ for diagnostic purposes, such as the detection of outliers, which are subjects who seem to evolve differently from the other subjects in the data set. Examples and more details on the use of EB estimates can be found in Verbeke and Molenberghs (2000, Chapter 7) or in DeGruttola, Lange, and Dafni (1991) and Waternaux, Laird, and Ware (1989). It should be emphasized that the EB estimates cannot be used to check the underlying normality assumption about the random effects. Verbeke and Lesaffre (1996) have shown that, in some cases with severe deviations from normality, the normality assumption forces the EB estimates to look like a normal distribution. They propose to use more general random-effects distributions, such as mixtures of normals. In Chapter 23, we will use related ideas in the context of models for non-continuous responses.

5
Model Families

5.1 Introduction

In Chapter 4, we reviewed how the linear mixed model can be a versatile model for the analysis of continuous longitudinal data, based on Gaussian assumptions. A full account is given in Verbeke and Molenberghs (2000). The linear mixed model enjoys a lot of properties, to a large extent based on linearity features and properties of the multivariate normal distribution. Therefore, although some of its features can be extended and modified to model longitudinal data of a non-Gaussian type, thereby using ideas from generalized linear models (Chapter 3), one has to be aware of important differences. For example, in Sections 4.3 and 4.5, the connection between a fully hierarchical specification of the linear mixed model and the marginal model derived thereof was reviewed. In fact, the connection is so natural and easy that one often needs to be reminded of important differences between the marginal and hierarchical model. One such difference is the different view one should adopt on negative variance components, depending on whether a marginal or a hierarchical point of view is taken.

Such straightforward connections do not exist in the non-Gaussian case. It is therefore important to carefully distinguish between modeling families when dealing with models for non-normally distributed outcomes. Section 5.2 will review the key model families in the Gaussian case, and Section 5.3 presents the equivalent but different concepts in the general situation. Parts II–IV will provide a detailed treatment for each of the families in turn.

5.2 The Gaussian Case

In Chapter 4, we have reviewed the linear mixed model for longitudinal data. As stated before, in Sections 4.3 and 4.5 we referred to the difference between a marginal and a hierarchical (random-effects) interpretation of such a model. From a general perspective, marginal and random-effects models are two important sub-families of models for repeated measures. Several authors, such as Diggle, Liang, and Zeger (1994), Diggle et al (2002), and Aerts et al (2002), distinguish between three families. Let us first formalize these for Gaussian outcomes or, more generally, for models with a linear mean structure. This will then provide a useful basis for developing the equivalent families in general (Section 5.3).

A marginal model is characterized by a marginal mean function of the form

$$E(Y_{ij}|\boldsymbol{x}_{ij}) = \boldsymbol{x}'_{ij}\boldsymbol{\beta}, \qquad (5.1)$$

where $\boldsymbol{x}_{ij}$ is a vector of covariates for subject i at occasion j and $\boldsymbol{\beta}$ is a vector of regression parameters. It is clear that we refer to the model as marginal, even though the mean is expressed conditional upon the vector of covariates. Here and throughout most of this book, dependence on covariates is taken for granted, and sometimes suppressed from notation.

In a random-effects model we focus on the expectation, additionally conditioning upon a random-effects vector $\boldsymbol{b}_i$:

$$E(Y_{ij}|\boldsymbol{b}_i, \boldsymbol{x}_{ij}) = \boldsymbol{x}'_{ij}\boldsymbol{\beta} + \boldsymbol{z}'_{ij}\boldsymbol{b}_i. \qquad (5.2)$$

Finally, a third family of models conditions a particular outcome on the other responses or a subset thereof. In particular, a simple first-order stationary transition model focuses on expectations of the form

$$E(Y_{ij}|Y_{i,j-1}, \ldots, Y_{i1}, \boldsymbol{x}_{ij}) = \boldsymbol{x}'_{ij}\boldsymbol{\beta} + \alpha Y_{i,j-1}. \qquad (5.3)$$

Alternatively, one might condition upon all outcomes except the one being modeled:

$$E(Y_{ij}|Y_{ik,k \neq j}, \boldsymbol{x}_{ij}) = \boldsymbol{x}'_{ij}\boldsymbol{\beta} + \overline{\boldsymbol{Y}}'_{ij}\boldsymbol{\alpha}, \qquad (5.4)$$

where $\overline{\boldsymbol{Y}}_{ij}$ represents $\boldsymbol{Y}_i$ with the jth component omitted.

As shown by Verbeke and Molenberghs (2000) and reviewed in Chapter 4, random-effects models imply a simple marginal model in the linear mixed model case. This is due to the elegant properties of the multivariate normal distribution. In particular, expectation (5.1) follows from (5.2) by either (a) marginalizing over the random effects or (b) by conditioning on the random-effects vector $\boldsymbol{b}_i = \boldsymbol{0}$. Hence, the fixed-effects parameters $\boldsymbol{\beta}$ have a marginal and a hierarchical model interpretation at the same time. Finally, certain auto-regressive models in which later-time residuals are expressed in terms of earlier ones lead to particular instances of the general linear mixed effects model as well, and hence have a marginal function of the form (5.1).

Although each of the three model families exist in general, there is no close connection between them when outcomes are of a non-Gaussian type, such as binary, categorical, or discrete. We will consider each of the model families in turn and point to some relevant issues.

5.3 Model Families in General

Within the linear mixed model, both the random-effects structure and the serial correlation process are devices to capture association within units and accommodate within the model. In the general, non-Gaussian setting, there are several ways to handle such association and, unlike in the linear mixed model case, choices may be mutually exclusive. This is partly due to the lack of a discrete analogue to the multivariate normal distribution. Building upon the taxonomy of Section 5.2, and in line with Fahrmeir and Tutz (1994, 2001) and Diggle *et al* (2002), we also distinguish between

- *marginal models,* in which responses are modeled marginalized over all other responses; the association structure is then typically captured using a set of association parameters, such as correlations, odds ratios, etc.;

- *conditionally specified models,* in which any response within the sequence of repeated measures is modeled conditional upon (subsets of) the other outcomes (this could be the set of all past measurements or a subset thereof, in transition models);

- *subject-specific models,* in which the responses are assumed independent, given a collection of subject-specific parameters.

Broadly, one can treat the subject-specific effects as either fixed effects or as random effects. A third alternative consists of conditioning upon the subject-specific effects, a principle well-known in the context of matched case-control studies, where conditional logistic regression is a frequently used technique (Breslow and Day 1987, Agresti 2002). The fixed-effects approach is subject to severe criticisms, as it leaves several sources of variability unaccounted for and, to worsen matters, the number of fixed-effects parameters increases with sample size, jeopardizing consistency of such approaches.

The answer to the question as to which model family is to be preferred depends principally upon the research question(s) to be answered. In conditionally specified models the expectation of the response at a given occasion is modeled in terms of the responses at the other occasions, as well as on covariates. In marginal models, the covariates are directly related to the marginal expectations. Subject-specific models differ from the two previous models by the inclusion of parameters that are specific to the subject or unit of independent replication. Which *method* is used to fit the model should also depend on the assumptions the investigator is willing to make. A pragmatic but unavoidable restriction comes from the availability of computational algorithms. If one is willing to fully specify the joint model, maximum likelihood methods can be adopted. Yet, if only a partial description in terms of marginal or conditional probabilities is given, one has to rely on non-likelihood methods such as generalized estimating equations (Chapter 8), alternating logistic regressions (Section 8.6), or pseudo-likelihood methods (Chapter 9).

5.3.1 Marginal Models

In marginal or population-averaged models, the parameters characterize the marginal expectation (e.g., the marginal probability of success at a given point in time when the response is binary) of a subset of the outcomes, without conditioning on other outcomes. Part II is devoted to marginal models.

Bahadur (1961) proposed a marginal model, accounting for the association via marginal correlations. This model has also been studied by Cox (1972), Kupper and Haseman (1978), and Altham (1978). The general formulation of the Bahadur model requires the specification of a number of parameters, exponential in the number of repeated measures, indicating that this type of model may be prohibitive if the number of repeated measures per subject is relatively large, unless considerable simplification is done. Such simplification occurs, for example, when exchangeability can be assumed, in the sense that the expectation at every occasion is the same and all association parameters of a certain order are the same. Moreover, one may want to set all association parameters from a certain order onwards equal to zero. However, whereas such assumptions could be plausible for settings such as clustered data, they may be less plausible for repeated measures over time. In addition, whether or not restrictions are applied, the parameter space of the Bahadur model is typically of a peculiar shape, with large regions of parameter combinations not leading to a valid model. A general study of this phenomenon is given in Declerck, Aerts, and Molenberghs (1998).

Molenberghs and Lesaffre (1994) and Lang and Agresti (1994) have proposed models that parameterize the association in terms of marginal odds ratios. Dale (1986) defined the bivariate global odds ratio model, based on a bivariate Plackett distribution (Plackett 1965). Molenberghs and Lesaffre (1994, 1999) extended this model to multivariate ordinal outcomes. They generalize the bivariate Plackett distribution to establish the multivariate cell probabilities. Their 1994 method involves solving polynomials of high degree and computing the derivatives thereof, whereas in 1999 generalized linear models theory is exploited, together with the use of an appropriately adapted iterative proportional fitting algorithm. Lang and Agresti (1994) exploit the equivalence between direct modeling and imposing restrictions on the multinomial probabilities, using undetermined Lagrange multipliers. Alternatively, the cell probabilities can be fitted using a Newton iteration scheme, as suggested by Glonek and McCullagh (1995). Further marginal models include the correlated binomial models of Altham (1978) and the double binomial model of Efron (1986). A discussion of likelihood-based marginal approaches is offered in Chapter 7.

However, even though a variety of flexible models exist, maximum likelihood can be unattractive due to excessive computational requirements, especially when high dimensional vectors of correlated data arise, as alluded to in the context of the Bahadur model. As a consequence, alternative methods have been in demand. Liang and Zeger (1986) proposed so-called *generalized estimating equations* (GEE), which only require the correct specification of the univariate marginal distributions provided one is willing to adopt "working" assumptions about the association structure (Chapter 8). An alternative to this approach is given by so-called *alternating logistic regressions* (ALR, Carey, Zeger, and Diggle 1993) (Section 8.6). le Cessie and van Houwelingen (1994) suggested to approximate the true likelihood by means of a pseudo-likelihood (PL) function that is easier to evaluate and to maximize (Chapters 9). Both GEE and PL yield consistent and asymptotically normal estimators, with an empirically corrected variance estimator, often referred to as the sandwich estimator. However, GEE is typically geared toward marginal models, whereas PL can be used with both marginal (le Cessie and Van Houwelingen 1994, Geys, Molenberghs, and Lipsitz 1998) and conditional models (Geys, Molenberghs, and Ryan 1997, 1999). Ample detail can be found in Aerts *et al* (2002).

5.3.2 Conditional Models

In a conditional model the parameters describe a feature (expectation, probability, odds, logit, ...) of (a set of) responses, given values for the other responses (Cox 1972). The best known example is undoubtedly the log-linear model. Rosner (1984) described a conditional logistic model. Due to the popularity of marginal models, especially generalized estimating equations, and random-effects models for repeated measures, conditional models have received relatively little attention within this context. Diggle *et al* (2002, pp. 142–144) criticized the conditional approach because the interpretation of a fixed effect parameter (e.g., time evolution or treatment effect) of one response is conditional on other responses for the same subject, outcomes of other subjects, and the number of repeated measures. Not only may such parameters make answering the substantive question difficult, they are also ill founded when the number of measurements per subject is not constant.

In spite of these criticisms, conditional models have enjoyed some popularity in a number of areas, such as multivariate analysis, in particular with applications in the social sciences. Perhaps the most important reasons for this popularity is the mathematical convenience of, for example, the log-linear model. Indeed, it belongs to the exponential family, with all due advantages for model fitting, given that efficient algorithms exist, based on matching observed and expected values of sufficient statistics (Agresti 2002). In addition, the parameter space is rectangular, implying that all combinations of the parameter vector lead to a valid model formulation. However, these advantages come at the cost of difficulty with parameter interpretation.

For these reasons, conditional models are not the central focus of this book. Nevertheless, they are discussed in some detail in Chapter 11. Special attention is devoted to transition models, useful in a longitudinal context. Even though a large class of conditional models are relatively easy to fit, in a number of cases, especially with long sequences of measurements, the evaluation of the normalizing constant can become prohibitive. In such a case, pseudo-likelihood can come to the rescue. The use of pseudo-likelihood in a conditional setting is discussed in Chapter 12.

5.3.3 Subject-specific Models

Subject-specific models are differentiated from marginal or population-averaged models by the inclusion of parameters specific to the subject. Unlike for correlated Gaussian responses, the parameters of a subject-specific and of population-averaged models for non-Gaussian data describe different types of effects of the covariates on the expectations (Neuhaus 1992). For example, when responses are binary, the effect of covariates on the response probabilities is conditional upon the level of the subject-specific effect. This means that a unit change in the covariate translates to an appropriate change in probability, keeping the level of the subject-specific effect fixed. They are useful if one is interested in within-subject changes (Neuhaus, Kalbfleisch, and Hauck 1991). In a marginal model, such a difference in covariate translates into a difference of the response probability, marginal over the subject-specific effects. Not only are there interpretational differences between both families but when comparing parameter estimates across families, one often observes substantial differences. The key reason is that they estimate different "true" parameters. It is fair to say this issue is surrounded with a lot of confusion. It is treated in detail in Chapters 16.

Sometimes, the term 'subject-specific approach' is equated to 'random-effects approach.' This is not entirely adequate as subject-specific parameters can be dealt with in essentially three ways: (1) as fixed effects, (2) as random-effects, and (3) by conditioning upon them. These three ways to deal with subject-specific parameters are studied in detail in Chapter 13.

The first approach is seemingly simplest but in many cases flawed because the number of parameters then increases with a rate proportional to the sample size, thereby invalidating most standard inferential results. The second approach is very popular. There are several routes to introduce randomness into the model parameters. Stiratelli, Laird, and Ware (1984) assume the parameter vector to be normally distributed. This idea has been carried further in the work on so-called *generalized linear mixed models* (Breslow and Clayton 1993), which is closely related to linear and non-linear mixed models. It implies that the random effects operate linearly at the level of the linear predictor. For binary data, for example, this would be at the logit scale. Alternatively, Skellam (1948) introduced the beta-binomial model, in which the adverse event probability of any member of a particular cluster comes from a beta distribution. Hence, this model can also be viewed as a random effects model. The difference with the previous one is that the random effects operate at the probability scale. The third approach is well-known in epidemiology, more precisely in the context of matched case-control studies. In particular, conditional logistic regression is then often considered (Breslow and Day 1987). In general, with so-called conditional likelihood methods, one conditions on the sufficient statistics for the subject-specific effects (Ten Have, Landis, and Weaver 1995, Conaway 1989). The various approaches to introducing subject-specific effects are considered in Chapter 13.

It is implicit in the treatment here that the models will be fitted to data using maximum likelihood, or using related or derived estimation methods. The presence of subject-specific parameters, in conjunction with the non-linear aspects of the model (e.g., the link functions), poses computational difficulties, and a variety of approximate likelihood maximization techniques have been proposed. Thus, before discussing inferential tools in Section 14.6, numerical approximation methods are reviewed in Sections 14.3, 14.4, and 14.5. Because different numerical approximations may lead to sometimes substantially different parameters, careful attention needs to be paid to the various software tools available and to the approximations on which they are based (Chapters 15). Alternatively, a fully Bayesian treatment could be envisaged (Carlin and Louis 1996). This is outside of the scope of this book.

Specific models for specific contexts have been developed. For example, Foulley and Gianola (1996) and Jaffrézic, Robert-Granié, and Foulley (1999) developed mixed-effects threshold models for ordered categorical data, allowing for heteroscedasticity, with emphasis on genetic applications.

5.4 Inferential Paradigms

Throughout this chapter, we have made informal connections between the three model families and inferential paradigms. Strictly speaking, selecting an inferential tool differs from selecting the model family. However, some inferential methods naturally go together with a model family. Because in all three model families maximum likelihood is possible, at least in some subset of cases, they all call for approximations and alternatives. Within the marginal families such tools as generalized estimating equations and alternating logistic regressions have been proposed. In all cases, pseudo-likelihood can be envisaged. Using ideas from quasi-likelihood methodology (McCullagh and Nelder 1989) or employing numerical quadrature strategies, a number of variations to the likelihood theme have been devised for the random-effects family. Also, conditional likelihood ideas have been in use for a number of decades in the context of conditional logistic regression.

Part II

Marginal Models

6
The Strength of Marginal Models

6.1 Introduction

In the past century, a vast part of the literature devoted to multivariate categorical data focused on describing the association structure between two or more variables. Eminent early references are Yule and Kendall (1950) and Goodman (1969, 1979, 1981a, 1981b, 1985).

Recently, the focus in multivariate categorical data has somewhat shifted to regression models, intended mainly for the analysis of longitudinal data. It is fair to say that the gap between classical contingency table and categorical data analysis on the one hand and categorical longitudinal data on the other hand is less wide than the corresponding gap for Gaussian data, where multivariate and longitudinal methods have their own focus and flavor. As a consequence, not only classically used models such as log-linear models (Cox 1972, Agresti 2002) ought to be considered, but also marginal models can be of great use. Perhaps it is not sufficiently recognized that these models provide a versatile basis, not only for regressing multiple outcomes on predictor variables, as will be done in Chapter 7, but also to study the association between two (or more) categorical variables. In other words, they can be used for the *analysis of association*. To this end, it is necessary to construct more complex association structures than are often needed for longitudinal applications. For this purpose, one can borrow flexible association structures as used in more conventional models, such as the ones described in Goodman (1981a).

In Section 6.2, we first sketch the so-called multivariate logistic models (McCullagh and Nelder 1989, Glonek and McCullagh 1995). Then we review the classical row-column (RC) association models (Goodman 1981a) and the marginal association model (Dale 1986, Molenberghs and Lesaffre 1994). It is indicated that both families can be seen as specific multivariate logistic models. This naturally leads to the observation that, within the multivariate logistic models family, very general association models can be constructed. Sections 6.3 and 6.4 present two simple but illustrative examples: the British occupational study and the Caithness data.

The fluvoxamine trial, introduced in Section 2.4, is analyzed in Section 6.5. These data are rich in the sense that two important outcomes, therapeutic effect and side effects, measured on 4-point ordinal scales, are measured repeatedly over time, and both continuous and discrete covariates are measured. Here, we first restrict attention to two-way contingency tables, and then, in Section 6.6, two extensions are presented, the first one to contingency tables in the presence of a categorical covariate, the second one to three-way tables. Both of these extensions will be put within a general framework in Chapter 7. In Section 6.7, we sketch how the association models can be embedded in families of models, arising as discretizations of continuous distributions.

6.2 Marginal Models in Contingency Tables

We first introduce the notation, needed for this chapter. A general notational framework is given in Section 7.1. The notation here is somewhat different from the notation used in the purely longitudinal chapters but allows us to efficiently deal with the contingency table nature of the data in this chapter. Suppose a contingency table arises from cross-classifying N subjects with respect to two categorical variables Y_1 and Y_2, having I and J levels respectively. It is convenient to introduce both ordinary multinomial cell counts

$$Z^*_{ijr} = \begin{cases} 1 & \text{if } Y_{1r} = i \text{ and } Y_{2r} = j, \\ 0 & \text{otherwise.} \end{cases}$$

as well as their cumulative counterparts

$$Z_{ijr} = \begin{cases} 1 & \text{if } Y_{1r} \leq i \text{ and } Y_{2r} \leq j, \\ 0 & \text{otherwise,} \end{cases} \tag{6.1}$$

with a subscript r denoting the rth subject. The corresponding probabilities are defined by $\mu^*_{ij} = \text{pr}(Z^*_{ijr} = 1)$ and $\mu_{ij} = \text{pr}(Z_{ijr} = 1)$. This notation will be used to describe the association models. Should the probabilities depend on the subject (for example, through the introduction of covariate information), then a subscript r will be added (μ^*_{ijr} and μ_{ijr}). We will first introduce a general framework, largely due to McCullagh and Nelder (1989) and Glonek and McCullagh (1995). Then, the RC family of models (Goodman 1981a) and the Dale (1986) model are shown to fit within this framework, conditional on a slight generalization in the RC case. Finally, it is indicated how the modeling framework can be used to combine useful aspects of both subclasses to yield a very wide and versatile class, which, in addition, allows extension to covariates as well as to higher order tables.

6.2.1 Multivariate Logistic Models

McCullagh and Nelder (1989) defined a useful class of generalized linear models, by writing the vector link function in terms of the joint probabilities in the following way:

$$\boldsymbol{\eta} = C' \ln(L\boldsymbol{\mu}^*), \quad (6.2)$$

where $\boldsymbol{\mu}^*$ is the vector of joint probabilities, formed by stacking the μ_{ij}^*. The matrix L consists solely of zeros and ones, such that $L\boldsymbol{\mu}^*$ contains the probabilities necessary to construct the required link functions. Then, contrasts of log-probabilities are equated to a vector of linear predictors $\boldsymbol{\eta}$ using the contrast matrix C. Contrasts of log-probabilities encompass many commonly used links for both marginal probabilities and associations. Within this model formulation, the marginal means can be modeled via, e.g., baseline category logits, adjacent category logits, continuation-ratio logits, or cumulative logits. The association can be described in terms of, e.g., local or global cross-ratios. This means that this formulation applies to binary, ordinal, and nominal data. When cumulative logits and/or global cross-ratios are used, the model can be expressed directly in terms of the cumulative probabilities μ_{ij}, such that (6.2) becomes $\boldsymbol{\eta} = C' \ln(L\boldsymbol{\mu})$. In this case, L may contain other elements than merely zeros and ones. Alternatively, the connection between μ_{ij} and μ_{ij}^* ($\boldsymbol{\mu} = B\boldsymbol{\mu}^*$, for some constant matrix B) can be absorbed into the matrix L as well. As counterexamples, modeling the marginal distribution via, e.g., the probit or the complementary log-log link is excluded from (6.2). One usually requires that $\boldsymbol{\mu}^*$ and $\boldsymbol{\eta}$ are in 1-to-1 relationship. Model (6.2) is called the *multivariate logistic transform* by Glonek and McCullagh (1995). They illustrate its use for both marginal and conditional regression models, as well as for mixed marginal-conditional parameterizations. A general and flexible class of marginal logistic models of the form (6.2) was studied by Lang and Agresti (1994), who allow a many-to-one relationship between $\boldsymbol{\mu}^*$ and $\boldsymbol{\eta}$ because they do not require that the (higher order) associations are modeled explicitly. Examples will be given in the next two sections.

In the spirit of generalized *linear* modeling (Chapter 3), McCullagh and Nelder (1989) completed (6.2) by

$$\boldsymbol{\eta} = X\boldsymbol{\xi}, \quad (6.3)$$

i.e., by adopting a vector of linear predictors. Here, X is a known design and/or covariate matrix and $\boldsymbol{\xi}$ is a vector of parameters of direct interest. Glonek and McCullagh (1995) call the resulting family *multivariate logistic regression models*.

When not only regression aspects are of scientific interest, but focus is placed on the association structure as well, it is useful to generalize the vector of linear predictors (6.3) to the potentially non-linear class

$$\boldsymbol{\eta} = C' \ln(L\boldsymbol{\mu}^*) = \boldsymbol{g}(\boldsymbol{\xi}), \tag{6.4}$$

where $\boldsymbol{g}(\boldsymbol{\xi})$ is a known vector-valued function.

6.2.2 Goodman's Local Association Models

Goodman (1981a) defines association models in terms of log local cross-ratios for $I \times J$ tables. These log cross-ratios are given by

$$\ln \theta_{ij}^* = \ln \left(\frac{\text{pr}(Y_1 = i, Y_2 = j)\text{pr}(Y_1 = i+1, Y_2 = j+1)}{\text{pr}(Y_1 = i, Y_2 = j+1)\text{pr}(Y_1 = i+1, Y_2 = j)} \right)$$

$$= \ln \frac{\mu_{ij}^* \mu_{i+1,j+1}^*}{\mu_{i,j+1}^* \mu_{i+1,j}^*},$$

with $i = 1, \ldots, I-1$ and $j = 1, \ldots, J-1$. They naturally follow from the following closed form model for the joint cell probabilities:

$$\mu_{ij}^* = \alpha_i \beta_j e^{\phi \lambda_i \nu_j}, \tag{6.5}$$

($i = 1, \ldots, I; j = 1, \ldots, J$). Here, α_i and β_j are main effect parameters while λ_i, ν_j and ϕ describe the association structure. Indeed, the local cross-ratios are $\ln \theta_{ij}^* = \phi(\lambda_i - \lambda_{i+1})(\nu_j - \nu_{j+1})$. Identifiability constraints have to be imposed on the parameters in (6.5). This model is also called the row-column model (RC model).

Note that this model is not fully marginal in nature since the marginal probabilities or transformations thereof do not easily follow from the model parameters. In fact, the model has a close connection to log-linear models, which are conditional in nature. In this sense, it bridges the gap between the models treated here and those in Part III.

Model (6.5) can be seen as a member of (6.4) by setting L and C equal to the identity matrix: $\boldsymbol{\eta} = \ln \boldsymbol{\mu}^* = \boldsymbol{g}(\boldsymbol{\xi})$, with $\boldsymbol{g}(\boldsymbol{\xi})$ defined by

$$g_{ij}(\boldsymbol{\xi}) = \ln \alpha_i + \ln \beta_j + \phi \lambda_i \nu_j. \tag{6.6}$$

Due to its third term, the predictor function (6.6) is non-linear. Note that (6.6) is a mixture of main effect and association parameters. By setting C equal to the identity matrix, the concept of *contrasts* of log-probabilities is not maintained and thus (6.4) is slightly extended.

6.2 Marginal Models in Contingency Tables

An alternative association parameterization is additive in the log cross-ratios: $\ln\theta^*_{ij} = \delta_{1i} + \delta_{2j}$. This model is induced by the following expression for the cell probabilities:

$$\mu^*_{ij} = \alpha_i \beta_j \gamma_{1i}^j \gamma_{2j}^i. \tag{6.7}$$

For this parameterization (6.6) changes to

$$g_{ij}(\boldsymbol{\xi}) = \ln\alpha_i + \ln\beta_j + j\ln\gamma_{1i} + i\ln\gamma_{2j}. \tag{6.8}$$

Note that this predictor is of the linear type in $\ln\alpha_i$, etc. Fitting algorithms for (6.5) and (6.7) can be found in Goodman (1981a).

Goodman (1981a) generalizes model (6.5) to:

$$\mu^*_{ij} = \alpha_i \beta_j \exp\left(\sum_{k=1}^{4} \phi_k \lambda_{ki} \nu_{kj}\right), \tag{6.9}$$

where λ_{1i} and λ_{3i} are linear functions of the index i and ν_{1j} and ν_{2j} are linear in j. The others are allowed to be non-linear. He shows that the log cross-ratios can be written as

$$\ln\theta^*_{ij} = \eta + \eta_i^I + \eta_j^J + \zeta_i^I \zeta_j^J. \tag{6.10}$$

This model allows the inclusion of additive effects on the association. Goodman calls it the R+C+RC model.

Although the above models provide an elegant description of the association in contingency tables, a disadvantage of the RC family is the cumbersome form they induce for the marginal distributions. The model presented next is built marginally.

6.2.3 Dale's Marginal Models

Dale (1986) and Molenberghs and Lesaffre (1994, 1999) define a marginal model for ordinal data in terms of marginal cumulative logits and global cross-ratios. We will describe it here for the purpose of our contingency table type data setting, and defer a fully general, longitudinal introduction to Chapter 7. The cumulative logits

$$\eta_{1i} = \text{logit}[\text{pr}(Y_1 \leq i)] = \ln(\mu_{iJ}) - \ln(1 - \mu_{iJ}), \tag{6.11}$$
$$\eta_{2j} = \text{logit}[\text{pr}(Y_2 \leq j)] = \ln(\mu_{Ij}) - \ln(1 - \mu_{Ij}), \tag{6.12}$$

$(i = 1, \ldots, I-1; j = 1, \ldots, J-1)$, and the global cross-ratios

$$\ln\psi_{ij} = \ln\left(\frac{\text{pr}(Y_1 \leq i, Y_2 \leq j)\text{pr}(Y_1 > i, Y_2 > j)}{\text{pr}(Y_1 \leq i, Y_2 > j)\text{pr}(Y_1 > i, Y_2 \leq j)}\right)$$

$$= \ln\frac{\mu_{ij}(1 - \mu_{Ij} - \mu_{iJ} + \mu_{ij})}{(\mu_{iJ} - \mu_{ij})(\mu_{Ij} - \mu_{ij})} \tag{6.13}$$

6. The Strength of Marginal Models

define the joint probabilities.

It is clear from (6.11), (6.12), and (6.13) that this model is a member of (6.2). For the special case of binary data ($I = J = 2$), (6.2) becomes

$$\begin{pmatrix} \eta_1 \\ \eta_2 \\ \eta_3 \end{pmatrix} = \begin{pmatrix} 0 & 0 & 0 & 0 & 1 & -1 & 0 & 0 \\ 0 & 0 & 0 & 0 & 0 & 0 & 1 & -1 \\ 1 & -1 & -1 & 1 & 0 & 0 & 0 & 0 \end{pmatrix} \times$$

$$\times \ln \begin{pmatrix} 1 & 0 & 0 & 0 \\ 0 & 1 & 0 & 0 \\ 0 & 0 & 1 & 0 \\ 0 & 0 & 0 & 1 \\ 1 & 1 & 0 & 0 \\ 0 & 0 & 1 & 1 \\ 1 & 0 & 1 & 0 \\ 0 & 1 & 0 & 1 \end{pmatrix} \begin{pmatrix} \mu_{11}^* \\ \mu_{12}^* \\ \mu_{21}^* \\ \mu_{22}^* \end{pmatrix},$$

where the model is written in terms of the cell probabilities μ_{jk}^*. Because

$$\begin{pmatrix} \mu_{11}^* \\ \mu_{12}^* \\ \mu_{21}^* \\ \mu_{22}^* \end{pmatrix} = \begin{pmatrix} 1 & 0 & 0 & 0 \\ -1 & 1 & 0 & 0 \\ -1 & 0 & 1 & 0 \\ 1 & -1 & -1 & 1 \end{pmatrix} \begin{pmatrix} \mu_{11} \\ \mu_{12} \\ \mu_{21} \\ \mu_{22} \end{pmatrix},$$

an expression in terms of the cumulative probabilities μ_{jk} is immediate. Should it be thought reasonable, then local cross-ratios:

$$\ln \psi_{ij}^* = \ln \frac{\mu_{ij}^*(1 - \mu_{i+1,j}^* - \mu_{i,j+1}^* + \mu_{ij}^*)}{(\mu_{i,j+1}^* - \mu_{ij}^*)(\mu_{i+1,j}^* - \mu_{ij}^*)} \tag{6.14}$$

can be used instead. For the particular case of binary variables, both types of cross-ratios coincide.

For the association (6.13), we will pay particular attention to

$$\ln \psi_{ij} = \phi + \rho_{1i} + \rho_{2j} + \sigma_{1i}\sigma_{2j}, \tag{6.15}$$

including a constant association parameter, row and column effects, and interactions between rows and columns, respectively. This model is identified, e.g., by imposing $\rho_{1I} = \rho_{2J} = \sigma_{1I} = \sigma_{2J} = 0$ and $\sigma_{11} = 1$. Due to the fourth term of (6.15) this parameterization is a member of the non-linear family (6.4). It is very similar in structure to the local cross-ratios of the R+Ċ+RC model (6.10). Of course, model (6.15) is only one of many possibilities, since there is a whole spectrum of possible models between independence and constant association on the one hand and a saturated association model on the other hand. When the number of categories increases, it becomes more crucial to look for parsimonious association models in order to reduce the number of parameters in the model. To this end, the more flexible class (6.4) might be preferable over (6.3).

Model fitting proceeds, e.g., via Newton-Raphson or Fisher scoring techniques. Details, for the general case, can be found in Section 7.7.6. To do so, the cumulative cell probabilities need to be computed. First, note that $\mu_{IJ} = 1$. Then, μ_{iJ} and μ_{Ij} follow from η_{1i} and η_{2j}, i.e., (6.11) and (6.12) are solved for μ_{iJ} and μ_{Ij}. The other counts follow from

$$\mu_{ij} = \begin{cases} \frac{1+[\mu_{iJ}+\mu_{Ij}](\psi_{ij}-1)-S_{ij}}{2(\psi_{ij}-1)} & \text{if } \psi_{ij} \neq 1, \\ \mu_{iJ}\mu_{Ij} & \text{otherwise,} \end{cases} \quad (6.16)$$

where

$$S_{ij} = \sqrt{[1+(\psi_{ij}-1)(\mu_{iJ}+\mu_{Ij})]^2 + 4\psi_{ij}(1-\psi_{ij})\mu_{iJ}\mu_{Ij}}.$$

Molenberghs and Lesaffre (1994, 1999) show how to extend this class of models to more than two variables. They also indicate how to adopt other association measures, such as marginal correlations, which corresponds to the Bahadur (1961) model. Molenberghs (1994) and Lesaffre, Verbeke, and Molenberghs (1994) provide details on maximum likelihood estimation for the two-way and higher order versions of the model. See also Section 7.7.

6.2.4 A General Class of Models

The models described in Sections 6.2.2 and 6.2.3 differ in two respects:

1. The association in the RC model is in terms of local cross-ratios, while the Dale model is based on global cross-ratios. This difference is not essential, as we argued that local cross-ratios can be incorporated into the marginal model without problem.

2. The marginal probabilities of the RC model are complex functions of the model parameters, whereas the Dale model is expressed directly in terms of the marginal logits.

However, upon generalizing (6.4) slightly, both models are seen as subclasses of this flexible family. For both models, linear and non-linear predictors are possible. Indeed, for the RC family, (6.8) is linear whereas (6.6) is non-linear. For the Dale model, (6.15) is non-linear, but if the fourth term is dropped, it becomes a linear predictor.

The advantage of this result is that completely general models can be constructed, combining and extending interesting aspects of both the RC

TABLE 6.1. *British Occupational Study. Cross-classification of male sample according to each subject's occupational status category and his father's occupational category, using seven status categories*

Father's status	\multicolumn{7}{c}{Subject's status}						
	1	2	3	4	5	6	7
1	50	19	26	8	18	6	2
2	16	40	34	18	31	8	3
3	12	35	65	66	123	23	21
4	11	20	58	110	223	64	32
5	14	36	114	185	714	258	189
6	0	6	19	40	179	143	71
7	0	3	14	32	141	91	106

and the Dale model. For example, a genuine marginal model can be constructed, with an association function of the RC type. Depending on the data problem, one can opt for local or for global cross-ratios. Arguably, local cross-ratios are suitable for nominal variables, whereas global cross-ratios are a natural choice for cross-classified ordinal variables.

6.3 British Occupational Status Study

We re-analyze the data presented in Goodman (1979). Subjects are cross-classified, according to their occupational status and their father's occupational status, using seven ordered categories. The data are presented in Table 6.1

Standard RC and Dale models, fitted to Table 6.1, are presented in Table 6.2. The Dale model with row effects, column effects, and interactions, provides a good fit, based on a deviance χ^2 approach. This means that no model of the form (6.3) fits the data and that the full non-linear version (6.15) is necessary to achieve an acceptable fit. No RC model, not even the R+C+RC model, fits the data well.

6.4 The Caithness Data

Goodman (1981a) studied association models for two-way contingency tables with ordered categories. The cross-classification of eye color and hair color of 5387 children is reproduced in Table 6.3.

Goodman treated these responses as ordinal that, although sensible, might be open to discussion. We combine marginal probabilities, one set

TABLE 6.2. *British Occupational Study. Deviance χ^2 goodness-of-fit statistics for Dale and RC models, fitted to the data in Table 6.1. The models with an acceptable fit (p > 0.05) are indicated by an asterisk.*

	Dale		RC	
Description	df	χ^2	df	χ^2
Independence	36	897.52	36	897.52
Constant association	35	207.23	35	98.19
Row effects only	30	105.23	30	87.14
Column effects only	30	100.69	30	80.74
Row and column effects	25	42.94	25	75.59
Row, column, interactions	16	*20.11	16	38.09
Saturated model	0	0.00	0	0.00

TABLE 6.3. *Caithness Data. Eye color and hair color of 5387 children in Caithness (Goodman 1981a).*

Eye color	Hair color				
	Fair	Red	Medium	Dark	Black
Blue	326	38	241	110	3
Light	688	116	584	188	4
Medium	343	84	909	412	26
Dark	98	48	403	681	85

for each variable, with local odds ratios to describe the association. We consider two models. The first one (8 parameters) assumes a constant local odds ratio. The simpler model which assumes independence between both responses has been shown by Goodman to provide a poor fit and will not be considered here. The second, saturated, model allows an unstructured 3×4 table of local odds ratios. The marginal probabilities for *both* models are $(0.13, 0.29, 0.33, 0.25)$ for eye color and $(0.27, 0.05, 0.40, 0.26, 0.02)$ for hair color. The common local odds ratio for the first model equals 1.50. The deviance is 131.10 on 11 degrees of freedom, rejecting the constant (or uniform) association model. Note that Goodman's *conditional* model for uniform association exhibited a much poorer deviance of 265.03 on 11 degrees of freedom. The 12 local odds ratios, organized as an association

TABLE 6.4. *Fluvoxamine Trial. Cross-classification of initial severity and side effect at the second occasion. In parentheses, the fitted values for the independence model are shown.*

	Side 2			
Severity	1	2	3	4
1	1	0	1	0
	(0.86)	(0.86)	(0.18)	(0.10)
2	21	28	5	5
	(25.29)	(25.29)	(5.42)	(3.01)
3	62	62	15	7
	(62.57)	(62.57)	(13.41)	(7.45)
4	41	31	6	2
	(34.29)	(34.29)	(7.35)	(4.08)
5	1	5	0	1
	(3.00)	(3.00)	(0.64)	(0.36)

table, are:

	1/2	2/3	3/4	4/5
1/2	1.45	0.79	0.71	0.78
2/3	1.45	2.15	1.41	2.97
3/4	2.00	0.78	3.73	1.98

Although there is some fluctuation in the association structure, it is very hard to pinpoint a clear trend. This is typically much harder for multivariate data than for genuinely longitudinal data where, for example, exchangeable (constant) or exponentially decaying structures are commonly encountered.

6.5 Analysis of the Fluvoxamine Trial

Let us consider the fluvoxamine trial, presented in Section 2.4. Further analyses will be given in various sections of Chapter 7, as well as in the missing data Chapters 29, 30, and 31.

Because the focus here is on marginal models for contingency tables coming from repeated categorical data, we select four two-way classifications from the fluvoxamine study. We will first consider a cross-classification of side effects and initial severity (Table 6.4). Then, we cross-classify the

6.5 Analysis of the Fluvoxamine Trial

TABLE 6.5. *Fluvoxamine Trial. Cross-Classification of therapeutic effect at the second and third Occasion. In parentheses, the fitted values: the first entry corresponds to the constant association Dale model, while the second entry stands for the row and column local association model.*

	Ther. 3			
Ther. 2	1	2	3	4
1	13	2	0	0
	(11.64)	(2.87)	(0.49)	(0.15)
	(13.06)	(1.87)	(0.06)	(0.01)
2	37	40	8	4
	(40.46)	(39.77)	(5.50)	(1.39)
	(34.98)	(44.28)	(7.55)	(2.20)
3	13	58	18	4
	(10.09)	(53.94)	(23.38)	(4.77)
	(15.65)	(52.42)	(18.49)	(6.45)
4	1	13	36	21
	(2.68)	(16.71)	(32.52)	(21.64)
	(0.32)	(14.44)	(35.91)	(20.34)

measurements on therapeutic effect at visits 2 and 3 in Table 6.5. A similar table is constructed for side effects (Table 6.6). Finally, we consider a cross-classification of side effects and therapeutic effect, recorded at visit 2 (Table 6.7). Note that the total of Table 6.7 (299) is higher than the total of Table 6.4 (294), as there are 5 subjects with information on therapeutic and side effects, but without initial severity measurement. These tables cover different settings: a cross-classification of an outcome and a baseline variable, the same outcome at subsequent measurement times and a "cross-sectional" picture, composed of two variables measured simultaneously. Table 6.8 shows the data from Table 6.7, split by sex category.

Let us now analyze these data. Table 6.9 summarizes the deviance χ^2 goodness-of-fit statistics for the models fitted to Tables 6.4–6.8.

Table 6.4 shows a complete lack of association. As a consequence, the independence model is accepted for both the Dale and the RC model. Of course, the deviance for the independence model in both families is exactly the same. Initial severity measures symptoms present at baseline, whereas side effects measures symptoms induced by the therapy. Thus the independence model implies that incidence and intensity of side effects do not depend on the initial conditions. Note that for Tables 6.4–6.8 the R+C+RC

TABLE 6.6. *Fluvoxamine Trial. Cross-classification of side effects at the second and third occasion. In parentheses, the fitted values: the first entry corresponds to the row and column effects Dale model, while the second entry corresponds to model (6.7).*

	Side 3			
Side 2	1	2	3	4
1	105	14	0	0
	(104.98)	(13.84)	(0.16)	(0.00)
	(105.01)	(13.98)	(0.01)	(0.00)
2	34	80	7	1
	(33.88)	(80.46)	(7.27)	(0.27)
	(33.63)	(79.96)	(8.20)	(0.22)
3	2	7	10	2
	(2.09)	(7.02)	(8.76)	(2.91)
	(2.71)	(7.14)	(7.58)	(3.57)
4	3	1	0	2
	(3.14)	(1.01)	(0.00)	(2.21)
	(2.65)	(0.92)	(1.21)	(1.22)

model is overparameterized and thus coincides with the saturated model, whence it is not included in Table 6.9.

For Table 6.5, we find a strong association main effect with the Dale model. The constant global cross-ratio is very high: $\widehat{\psi} = \widehat{\psi}_{ij} = \exp(2.52) = 12.43$. Note that this model corresponds to an underlying Plackett (1965) distribution, as such a distribution is characterized by a constant global cross-ratio. The fit improves by 7.68 on 2 degrees of freedom if we add a row effect. This model deserves our preference. For the RC family, there is certainly a strong constant association effect, but the fit is not acceptable at that point. A fully satisfactory fit is provided by the row and column association model.

There is also a clear global association main effect in Table 6.6. Including this parameter improves the fit of the model dramatically, although adding both row and column effects provides a better fit. Associations are shown in Table 6.10. Some of the observed cross-ratios are infinite, due to zero cells in the contingency table. All but one associations are high to extremely high. High associations in the upper right corner are explained by the fact that side effects over time are of course highly correlated, but also tend to go down, and only rarely go up, showing that the drug has a beneficial effect. It is remarkable that no RC model fits the data well, as can be learned

TABLE 6.7. *Fluvoxamine Trial. Cross-classification of side effects and therapeutic effect at the second occasion. In parentheses, the fitted values are shown. The first model is the global association column effects model. The second global cross-ratio model includes row and column effects, as well as interactions. The third set of fitted values corresponds to the RC model (row and column effects).*

		Therapeutic 2			
Side 2		1	2	3	4
	1	8	40	40	40
		(7.46)	(38.32)	(44.19)	(38.11)
		(8.10)	(39.58)	(40.41)	(39.50)
		(8.91)	(38.18)	(41.85)	(39.05)
	2	7	45	51	25
		(9.73)	(45.60)	(43.33)	(29.09)
		(6.61)	(46.37)	(49.46)	(25.49)
		(6.33)	(46.92)	(48.99)	(25.75)
	3	2	9	8	9
		(1.37)	(7.82)	(10.39)	(8.52)
		(2.22)	(7.49)	(9.66)	(8.64)
		(2.02)	(8.12)	(8.95)	(8.91)
	4	2	1	3	9
		(0.32)	(2.15)	(4.45)	(8.15)
		(2.24)	(1.30)	(2.52)	(8.95)
		(1.74)	(1.77)	(2.20)	(9.29)

from Table 6.9. In conclusion, a marginal model such as the Dale model fits the data better than a model from the RC family. Should one choose to remain within the RC family, then a model of a more elaborate nature, such as the ones discussed in Section 6.7, might be needed. Note, again, that the R+C+RC model is no alternative, as it is overparameterized. Fitting related model (6.7) to Table 6.7 yields an acceptable fit: $\chi^2 = 6.33$ on 4 degrees of freedom ($p = 0.1760$).

Both Tables 6.5 and 6.6 are cross-classifications of an ordinal variable, recorded at two subsequent measurement times. In both cases, a parsimonious global association model explains the data well. It seems to be much harder to fit these data with local association models.

For Table 6.7, the row effects model is the most parsimonious one that provides an acceptable fit. One might argue that it is careful to retain the model adding column effects and interactions as well. Therefore, fitted frequencies for both models are shown in Table 6.7. Table 6.11 shows the global cross-ratios for the data of Table 6.7, together with the pre-

TABLE 6.8. *Fluvoxamine Trial. Cross-classification of side effects and therapeutic effect at the second occasion, split by sex.*

	Therapeutic 2			
Side 2	1	2	3	4
Male subjects				
1	4	18	12	16
2	0	9	19	9
3	0	4	3	4
4	0	1	1	5
Female subjects				
1	4	22	28	24
2	7	36	32	16
3	2	5	5	5
4	2	0	2	4

dicted values under both models. We observe two patterns in Table 6.11. First, the association increases along the main diagonal. This means that the association between the variables $I(\text{SIDE2} \leq 1)$ and $I(\text{THER2} \leq 1)$ is smaller than the association between the variables $I(\text{SIDE2} \leq 3)$ and $I(\text{THER2} \leq 3)$. Here, $I(\cdot)$ is an indicator function. Also, the association becomes "negative" (i.e., smaller than 1 on the cross-ratio scale) for pairs such as $I(\text{SIDE2} \leq 3)$ and $I(\text{THER2} \leq 1)$. The RC models, fitted to this table, suggest the selection of the row and column effects model. The fitted model is also presented in Table 6.7. All RC models are based on model (6.5).

In conclusion, the Dale model yields a non-linear association model for Tables 6.1 and 6.7, through the interaction terms in (6.15), which is a very natural association model as it is a Dale model analogue of Goodman's R+C+RC model, of which the cross-ratios are given by (6.10). For Tables 6.4–6.6, simpler association models, including at most row and/or column effects, but no interactions, are found to be acceptable. The models of RC type fitted to these data tend to be of a more complex nature, arguably because they model the association through local cross-ratios even though the data are ordered categorical.

6.6 Extensions

As mentioned earlier, the fluvoxamine study recorded more than two outcomes and further there is covariate information available. We consider

TABLE 6.9. *Fluvoxamine Trial. Deviance χ^2 goodness-of-fit statistics for Dale and RC models, fitted to Tables 6.4–6.8 (models with an acceptable fit are indicated by an asterisk).*

Description	Table 6.4 df	χ^2	Table 6.5 df	χ^2	Table 6.6 df	χ^2	Table 6.7 df	χ^2
			Dale models					
Independence	12	*14.20	9	141.95	9	158.15	9	17.12
Constant association	11	*11.71	8	*11.48	8	18.27	8	17.12
Row effects only	8	*8.34	6	*3.80	6	14.49	6	*9.78
Column effects only	9	*11.37	6	*10.26	6	*12.29	6	16.74
Row and column effects	6	*8.03	4	*1.29	4	*2.05	4	*9.31
Row, column, interactions	2	*0.22	1	*0.31	1	*0.35	1	*0.94
Saturated model	0	0.00	0	0.00	0	0.00	0	0.00
			RC models					
Independence	12	*14.20	9	141.95	9	158.15	9	17.12
Constant association	11	*12.04	8	19.46	8	48.66	8	16.71
Row effects only	8	*8.21	6	12.90	6	18.84	6	*11.69
Column effects only	9	*11.88	6	14.35	6	45.12	6	15.14
Row and column effects	6	*2.22	4	*5.16	4	10.48	4	*1.44
Saturated model	0	0.00	0	0.00	0	0.00	0	0.00

in turn two ways of extending the models described so far, while still remaining within the contingency table framework. First, in Section 6.6.1, we discuss the inclusion of a dichotomous covariates in marginal association models, followed by a generalization to three-way tables (Section 6.6.2). These extensions are members of the class (6.4). Completely general covariates, as well as multi-way tables and fully longitudinal models are the subject of Chapter 7.

6.6.1 Covariates

The marginal Dale model presented here is flexible in incorporating covariate effects. Their influence on the marginal means and on the association can be described in separate ways. For example, age could be found to influence the marginal response functions, while the association could be seen to change with sex. We will exemplify the possibilities that are brought about by this feature using two covariates. First, the data presented in Table 6.7 are split into two sex groups (Table 6.8). Second, we will add the effect

TABLE 6.10. *Fluvoxamine Trial. Global cross ratios for the classification of side effects at time 2 versus time 3 (Data in Table 6.6).*

Side 2	Side 3		
	1	2	3
	Observed		
1	21.15	$+\infty$	$+\infty$
2	6.00	31.37	41.74
3	1.17	6.05	43.17
	Row and column effects		
1	21.07	116.88	760.06
2	5.70	31.65	205.37
3	1.20	6.67	43.26

of the continuous covariate age on the responses and on the association between responses.

Let us consider sex first. Selected models, fitted to these data, are presented in Table 6.12. Obviously the marginal regressions are independent of sex, but we do find a sex effect in the association. If we add row effects (but no column effects), the fit is satisfactory ($p = 0.12$). The association structure of this model is:

$$\ln \psi_{ijr} = 1.64 - 0.88 \text{sex}_r - 1.24 I(i=1) - 0.56 I(i=2),$$

where ψ_{ijr} is the global cross-ratio, depending on subject r through their sex, and $I(.)$ is the indicator function. The association is stronger for males than for females ($p = 0.0402$).

Even though Table 6.8 contains four sampling zeros, no convergence problems are encountered and all parameters lie in the interior of their space. The Dale likelihood attains its maximum in the interior of the parameter space under very mild conditions, a feature shared with univariate ordinal logistic regression, which it generalizes. First, there must not be a complete separation in the covariate space between response groups. A similar condition was derived for the multigroup logistic model by Albert and Lesaffre (1986). Second, even with zero cell counts, models can be constructed for which the MLE lies in the interior of the space. For example, in a 3×3 table with cells $(1,1)$, $(1,3)$, $(2,2)$, $(3,1)$, and $(3,3)$ equal to zero (with the other cells non-zero), a model with global cross-ratio dependent on row and column classification, yields finite estimates. We can easily include such continuous covariates as age. For 296 subjects out of 299 recorded in Table 6.7, age (in years) is recorded. Age ranges from 16

TABLE 6.11. *Fluvoxamine Trial. Global cross ratios for the classification of side effects versus therapeutic effect (both at the second occasion).*

	Therapeutic 2		
Side 2	1	2	3
	Observed		
1	0.97	0.95	0.74
2	0.61	1.33	2.12
3	0.41	2.57	4.26
	Column effects only		
1	0.86	0.86	0.86
2	1.77	1.77	1.77
3	3.24	3.24	3.24
	Row, column, interaction		
1	0.92	0.86	0.80
2	0.55	1.55	1.92
3	0.37	2.17	4.00

to 75 years, with a mean of 42.2 years (median is 40.5 years). There are 97 distinct age by sex combinations, which yields an average of about 3 subjects per distinct 4×4 table! Thus, we have a generalization of a purely contingency table analysis to multivariate ordinal regression. Obviously, a saturated model is not meaningful here, as the number of covariate levels (and hence the number of cells) increases with the sample size. Derivation of formal goodness-of-fit tools, such as appropriate residuals, requires further research. The most complex model we will consider, contains sex and age effects in both the marginal mean and in the association and lets the association further depend on row and column classification. Clearly, this model could be extended (for example, by means of higher order effects of age and interactions between sex and age). Table 6.13 reports on a backward selection performed to simplify the model. In the final model, the marginal logits are simplified such that only SIDE2 depends on age. The association is independent of the column classification. Although sex and age could be omitted from the association when comparing Models 4 and 5 with 3 (numbers referring to Table 6.13), or 6 with 4 and 5, a direct comparison of Model 6 (no covariate influence on association) with Model 3 (both age and sex influence the association) is significant at the 5% level. Therefore, we prefer Model 3. The cumulative logits (6.11) and (6.12) for

72   6. The Strength of Marginal Models

TABLE 6.12. *Fluvoxamine Trial. Deviance χ^2 goodness-of-fit statistics for Dale models, fitted to Table 6.8 (distinguishing between sex groups). Models with an acceptable fit ($p > 0.05$) are indicated by an asterisk.*

Marginal model	Association model	df	χ^2
No sex effect	Constant	23	39.32
No sex effect	Sex, row	20	*27.76
No sex effect	Sex, row, column	18	*27.30
Sex effect	Constant	21	36.80
Sex effect	Sex effect	20	31.74
Sex effect	Sex, row, column	16	*25.53
Saturated	Saturated	0	0.00

subject r are

$$\eta_{1ir} = 0.54I(i=1) + 2.63I(i=2) + 3.75I(i=3) - 0.019\text{age}_r,$$
$$\eta_{2jr} = -2.69I(j=1) - 0.47I(j=2) + 0.95I(j=3),$$

and the association structure is

$$\ln\psi_{ijr} = 2.94 - 0.80\text{sex}_r - 0.028\text{age}_r - 1.44I(i=1) - 0.63I(i=2).$$

The logit for side effects decreases with age, implying, e.g., that the probability of category 1 (no side effects) decreases and the probability of category 4 (highest level of side effects) increases with age. The association is stronger for males than for females (consistent with Table 6.12) and decreases with age.

6.6.2   Three-way Contingency Tables

Molenberghs and Lesaffre (1994) extended the Dale model, originally constructed for two response variables, to arbitrary dimensions. This implies that the model is suitable to analyze multi-way contingency tables. Computational details can be found in Molenberghs and Lesaffre (1994). We apply the general method technique on the fluvoxamine data set, more specifically to a cross-classification of therapeutic effect at visits 2, 3, and 4. The data are presented as a $4 \times 4 \times 4$ contingency table (Tables 6.14–6.17). There are 242 patients with measurements on all three outcomes.

Let the variables Y_1, Y_2, and Y_3 have I, J, and K levels, respectively, and define cumulative three-way probabilities μ_{ijk} ($i = 1, \ldots, I; j = 1, \ldots, J; k = 1, \ldots, K$), similar to the definition in Section 6.2.

The model extends as follows. Apart from three sets of marginal parameters, one for each measurement time:

$$\eta_{1i} = \text{logit}[\text{pr}(Y_1 \leq i)] = \ln(\mu_{iJK}) - \ln(1 - \mu_{iJK}), \quad (6.17)$$

6.6 Extensions

TABLE 6.13. *Fluvoxamine Trial. Backward selection for Dale models, fitted to Table 6.8 (including sex and age). The number of model parameters (Par), the deviance (Dev) of the model are reported. For each model comparison, the reference model (Vs), and the corresponding χ^2 statistic and p-value are reported. ('R' stands for row effects and 'C' stands for column effects.)*

Nr	Side 2	Ther. 2	Association	Par	Dev	Vs	df	χ^2	p
1	Sex, age	Sex, age	Sex, age, R, C	17	1372.5				
2	Age	—	Sex, age, R, C	14	1375.0	1	3	2.52	0.472
3	Age	—	Sex, age, R	12	1375.5	2	2	0.50	0.779
4	Age	—	Age, R	11	1379.0	3	1	3.47	0.063
5	Age	—	Sex, R	11	1379.0	3	1	3.49	0.062
6	Age	—	R	10	1382.7	4	1	3.66	0.056
6	Age	—	R	10	1382.7	3	2	7.13	0.028

$$\eta_{2j} = \text{logit}[\text{pr}(Y_2 \leq j)] = \ln(\mu_{IjK}) - \ln(1 - \mu_{IjK}), \quad (6.18)$$

$$\eta_{3k} = \text{logit}[\text{pr}(Y_3 \leq k)] = \ln(\mu_{IJk}) - \ln(1 - \mu_{IJk}), \quad (6.19)$$

($i = 1, \ldots, I - 1; j = 1, \ldots, J - 1; k = 1, \ldots, K - 1$), there are also three sets of pairwise association parameters:

$$\ln \psi_{12,ij} = \ln \frac{\mu_{ijK}(1 - \mu_{IjK} - \mu_{iJK} + \mu_{ijK})}{(\mu_{iJK} - \mu_{ijK})(\mu_{IjK} - \mu_{ijK})}, \quad (6.20)$$

$$\ln \psi_{13,ik} = \ln \frac{\mu_{iJk}(1 - \mu_{IJk} - \mu_{iJK} + \mu_{iJk})}{(\mu_{iJK} - \mu_{iJk})(\mu_{IJk} - \mu_{iJk})}, \quad (6.21)$$

$$\ln \psi_{23,jk} = \ln \frac{\mu_{Ijk}(1 - \mu_{IJk} - \mu_{IjK} + \mu_{Ijk})}{(\mu_{IJk} - \mu_{Ijk})(\mu_{IjK} - \mu_{Ijk})}, \quad (6.22)$$

together with a set of three-way associations (generalized cross-ratios):

$$\ln \psi_{123,ijk} =$$

$$\ln \left[\frac{\mu_{ijk}(\mu_{iJK} - \mu_{ijK} - \mu_{iJk} + \mu_{ijk})}{(\mu_{ijK} - \mu_{ijk})(\mu_{iJk} - \mu_{ijk})} \right.$$

$$\times \frac{(\mu_{IjK} - \mu_{ijK} - \mu_{Ijk} + \mu_{ijk})}{(\mu_{Ijk} - \mu_{ijk})}$$

$$\left. \times \frac{(\mu_{IJk} - \mu_{iJk} - \mu_{Ijk} + \mu_{ijk})}{(1 - \mu_{iJK} - \mu_{IjK} - \mu_{IJk} + \mu_{ijK} + \mu_{iJk} + \mu_{Ijk} - \mu_{ijk})} \right]. (6.23)$$

Clearly, the link functions (6.17)–(6.23) are all expressed in terms of contrasts of log-probabilities and hence fit in (6.2). Molenberghs and Lesaffre

TABLE 6.14. *Fluvoxamine Trial. Cross-classification of therapeutic effect at the second, third, and fourth occasion. In parentheses, the fitted values. The first entry corresponds to Model 1, the second entry corresponds to Model 2, the third entry corresponds to the generalized RC model. Part I.*

Side 2	Side 3	Side 4 1	2	3	4
1	1	11	1	0	0
		(10.18)	(1.19)	(0.10)	(0.02)
		(13.75)	(2.07)	(0.18)	(0.05)
		(10.99)	(0.48)	(0.00)	(0.00)
	2	0	1	1	0
		(0.60)	(1.46)	(0.30)	(0.06)
		(0.89)	(1.88)	(0.40)	(0.10)
		(1.16)	(0.97)	(0.02)	(0.00)
	3	0	0	0	0
		(0.05)	(0.18)	(0.15)	(0.06)
		(0.08)	(0.21)	(0.13)	(0.05)
		(0.05)	(0.15)	(0.07)	(0.01)
	4	0	0	0	0
		(0.01)	(0.03)	(0.04)	(0.02)
		(0.02)	(0.05)	(0.04)	(0.02)
		(0.01)	(0.02)	(0.03)	(0.03)

(1994, 1999) describe ways to determine the joint probabilities μ_{ijk} from the links and to compute maximum likelihood estimates. Indeed, the key issue in a marginal model of this type is the construction of the joint probabilities. The univariate marginal probabilities μ_{iJK}, μ_{IjK}, and μ_{IJk} are easily determined from inverting (6.17)–(6.19), just as with (6.11) and (6.12). The pairwise marginal probabilities μ_{ijK}, μ_{iJk}, and μ_{Ijk}, can be written in analogy with (6.16), as links (6.20)–(6.22) have the same form as (6.13). Determining the third order cumulative probabilities μ_{ijk} is more difficult and details are given in Chapter 7, in particular in Sections 7.3 and 7.7.

To illustrate the model, let us analyze the three therapeutic effect measurements. Model 1 assumes the marginal logits (6.17)–(6.19) are independent of covariate effects, yielding 9 marginal parameters. Each of the association parameters ψ in (6.20)–(6.23) is assumed independent of covariate effects as well as of the category indicators i, j, and k, yielding three pairwise and one three-way association parameters. This brings the

TABLE 6.15. *Fluvoxamine Trial. Cross-classification of therapeutic effect at the second, third, and fourth occasion. In parentheses, the fitted values. The first entry corresponds to Model 1, the second entry corresponds to Model 2, the third entry corresponds to the generalized RC model. Part II.*

		Side 4			
Side 2	Side 3	1	2	3	4
2	1	33	2	0	0
		(36.27)	(2.92)	(0.33)	(0.08)
		(30.39)	(3.18)	(0.35)	(0.09)
		(32.34)	(2.76)	(0.00)	(0.00)
	2	13	23	2	0
		(13.80)	(18.28)	(2.14)	(0.39)
		(13.03)	(16.81)	(2.19)	(0.46)
		(16.88)	(17.72)	(0.73)	(0.00)
	3	1	2	3	0
		(0.47)	(1.84)	(1.87)	(0.62)
		(0.44)	(1.31)	(1.05)	(0.40)
		(1.48)	(4.48)	(2.39)	(0.24)
	4	0	1	1	1
		(0.10)	(0.30)	(0.34)	(0.21)
		(0.10)	(0.29)	(0.22)	(0.11)
		(0.20)	(0.83)	(0.99)	(0.95)

total number of parameters to 13. Marginal parameter estimates (standard errors in parentheses) are

$\hat{\eta}_{11} = -2.76(0.27)$ $\hat{\eta}_{21} = -1.04(0.14)$ $\hat{\eta}_{31} = -0.21(0.13)$
$\hat{\eta}_{12} = -0.45(0.13)$ $\hat{\eta}_{22} = 0.75(0.13)$ $\hat{\eta}_{32} = 1.58(0.17)$
$\hat{\eta}_{13} = 1.00(0.15)$ $\hat{\eta}_{23} = 2.40(0.22)$ $\hat{\eta}_{33} = 3.12(0.32)$.

The constant global cross-ratios are $\hat{\psi}_{12} = \hat{\psi}_{12,ij} = \exp(2.58) = 13.18(3.08)$ for the first and the second outcome, $\hat{\psi}_{13} = \hat{\psi}_{13,ik} = \exp(1.38) = 3.99(0.89)$ for the first and the third outcome, and $\hat{\psi}_{23} = \hat{\psi}_{23,jk} = \exp(3.08) = 21.76(5.74)$ for the second and the third outcome. The three-way interaction, $\hat{\psi}_{123} = \hat{\psi}_{123,ijk} = \exp(0.18) = 1.19(0.66)$, is not significantly different from 1. Fitted frequencies are given in Tables 6.14–6.17.

The overall deviance goodness-of-fit statistic is 37.13 on 50 degrees of freedom ($p = 0.9115$). Inspecting standardized residuals, 62 out of 64 are

76   6. The Strength of Marginal Models

TABLE 6.16. *Fluvoxamine Trial. Cross-classification of therapeutic effect at the second, third, and fourth occasion. In parentheses, the fitted values. The first entry corresponds to Model 1, the second entry corresponds to Model 2, the third entry corresponds to the generalized RC model. Part III.*

		Side 4			
Side 2	Side 3	1	2	3	4
3	1	12	1	0	0
		(8.39)	(1.04)	(0.16)	(0.04)
		(7.41)	(1.12)	(0.17)	(0.05)
		(12.59)	(1.70)	(0.00)	(0.00)
	2	25	25	1	1
		(22.86)	(24.33)	(1.45)	(0.27)
		(24.97)	(28.79)	(2.09)	(0.38)
		(19.74)	(24.31)	(1.48)	(0.00)
	3	1	8	5	1
		(1.15)	(10.76)	(7.30)	(1.56)
		(1.33)	(9.96)	(6.61)	(1.64)
		(2.75)	(8.61)	(4.98)	(0.63)
	4	0	3	0	0
		(0.22)	(0.83)	(1.16)	(0.97)
		(0.30)	(1.05)	(1.02)	(0.71)
		(0.43)	(1.78)	(2.07)	(1.91)

less than 2 in absolute value, the remaining ones being 2.24 and 2.39. Thus, model fit is acceptable, but one might want to simplify the model further. We will in turn simplify the marginal and association structures. First, the three sets of logits reveal an increase over time, suggesting an improving response to therapy. A simpler model would assume: $\eta_{1i} = \alpha_i$, $\eta_{2j} = \alpha_j + \pi_2$, and $\eta_{3k} = \alpha_k + \pi_3$ $(i,j,k = 1,2,3)$. We interpret α_1, α_2, and α_3 as cut-off points at the first occasion and π_2 and π_3 as "proportional" shift parameters at occasions 2 and 3 respectively. Second, one might argue that the association between outcomes is mainly a function of the time lag between the outcomes, but not so much of the measurement times themselves. This is supported by the fact that $\ln \psi_{12}$ and $\ln \psi_{23}$ are roughly the same (given their standard errors of about 0.24), with $\ln \psi_{13}$ approximately half of the other association. Should one grant belief to this assumption, then an association model of the form $\gamma = \ln \psi_{12} = 2 \ln \psi_{13} = \ln \psi_{23}$ might be considered. The multiplier 0.5 for $\ln \psi_{13}$ is suggested by the data and has

TABLE 6.17. *Fluvoxamine Trial. Cross-classification of therapeutic effect at the second, third, and fourth occasion. In parentheses, the fitted values. The first entry corresponds to Model 1, the second entry corresponds to Model 2, the third entry corresponds to the generalized RC model. Part IV.*

			Side 4		
Side 2	Side 3	1	2	3	4
4	1	1	0	0	0
		(1.96)	(0.42)	(0.07)	(0.02)
		(1.42)	(0.36)	(0.06)	(0.02)
		(0.08)	(0.05)	(0.00)	(0.00)
	2	5	6	0	0
		(8.87)	(5.58)	(0.46)	(0.11)
		(8.16)	(5.55)	(0.44)	(0.11)
		(5.50)	(11.75)	(2.70)	(0.03)
	3	7	18	9	1
		(3.07)	(19.88)	(7.74)	(0.99)
		(3.26)	(19.69)	(6.67)	(0.97)
		(3.82)	(13.39)	(10.15)	(2.78)
	4	0	2	8	6
		(0.51)	(3.13)	(7.48)	(4.78)
		(0.68)	(4.42)	(7.84)	(4.45)
		(0.98)	(3.98)	(4.37)	(3.41)

limited empirical or theoretical support. Alternatively, one could estimate this parameter from the data. Third, the three-way interaction can be set to zero. There are six parameters in total.

Parameter estimates (standard errors) for this model are estimated to be $\hat{\alpha}_1 = -2.41(0.17)$, $\hat{\alpha}_2 = -0.52$ (0.12), $\hat{\alpha}_3 = 1.02(0.14)$ for the cut-off points, with time shifts $\hat{\pi}_2 = 1.32(0.11)$ for the second period and $\hat{\pi}_3 = 2.17(0.16)$ for the third period. The single association parameter is equal to $\hat{\gamma} = 2.81(0.17)$, resulting in $\hat{\psi}_{12} = \hat{\psi}_{23} = 16.56(2.77)$ and $\hat{\psi}_{13} = \sqrt{16.56} = 4.07(0.34)$. Fitted frequencies are given in Table 6.14–6.17. This model has a deviance of 43.67 on 57 degrees of freedom ($p = 0.9029$), and again only two standardized residuals are larger than 2 (being 2.07 and 2.70), showing that there is some support in the data for the assumed model. Finally, comparing Models 1 and 2, yields a deviance of 6.54 on 7 degrees of freedom ($p = 0.4782$), indicating that the first and more complex model is not necessary.

A similar model is obtained from the analysis of side effects at times 2, 3, and 4. Analyzing initial severity, side effects at time 2, and therapeutic effect at time 2, yields a satisfactory model with only constant association. No details on these models are included. These results are promising because they support the thesis that for a range of ordinal data applications, parsimonious marginal global cross-ratio models are sufficient to describe the data.

In case nominal data are to be analyzed, then the model can be adapted to cell probabilities μ_{ijk}^*. This would mean that (6.17)–(6.23) have to be changed in the spirit of (6.14). In particular, the global cross-ratios might have to be replaced by their local counterparts.

In addition to the extensions studied sofar, it is possible to extend the RC model to more than two dimensions. One option is to generalize Model (6.5) by defining

$$\mu_{ijk}^* = \alpha_i \beta_j \gamma_k e^{\phi \lambda_i \nu_j \omega_k} \tag{6.24}$$

with obvious notation. Of course, the marginal pairwise local odds ratio for a pair (i,j) has a very complicated form and (6.5) is not a submodel of (6.24) in the sense that the interpretation of the parameters will change in passing from a bivariate to a trivariate model. The conditional pairwise odds ratio on the other hand is $\ln \theta_{ij|k}^* = \phi \omega_k (\lambda_i - \lambda_{i+1})(\nu_j - \nu_{j+1})$, where ω_k can be considered an adjustment for the category conditioned upon. The three-way odds ratio is similar in structure to the two-way odds ratio of the bivariate model (6.5).

Fitting Model (6.24) to the trivariate therapeutic data of Tables 6.14–6.17 yields a deviance of 67.96 on 47 degrees of freedom ($p = 0.0243$), indicating that the fit is not satisfactory. Fitted frequencies are displayed in Table 6.14–6.17. One could consider more elaborate alternatives, such as trivariate versions of the R+C+RC model (9.9). However, as indicated earlier, for this kind of data, the marginal model defined in terms of cumulative probabilities seems to be more promising, as it yields very parsimonious descriptions of the association structure.

An alternative fashion to extend (6.5) would start from three pairwise marginal RC models:

$$\mu_{ij+}^* = \alpha_i^{(12)} \beta_j^{(12)} e^{\phi^{(12)} \lambda_i^{(12)} \nu_j^{(12)}}, \tag{6.25}$$

$$\mu_{i+k}^* = \alpha_i^{(13)} \gamma_k^{(13)} e^{\phi^{(13)} \lambda_i^{(13)} \tau_k^{(13)}}, \tag{6.26}$$

$$\mu_{+jk}^* = \beta_j^{(23)} \gamma_k^{(23)} e^{\phi^{(23)} \nu_j^{(23)} \tau_k^{(23)}}, \tag{6.27}$$

$(i = 1, \ldots, I; j = 1, \ldots, J; k = 1, \ldots, K)$. For (6.25)–(6.27) to define a valid probability mass function μ_{ijk}^*, complicated restrictions must be satisfied: summing (6.25) over j and (6.26) over k yields I restrictions:

$$\alpha_i^{(12)} \sum_{j=1}^{J} \beta_j^{(12)} e^{\phi^{(12)} \lambda_i^{(12)} \nu_j^{(12)}} = \alpha_i^{(13)} \sum_{k=1}^{K} \gamma_k^{(13)} e^{\phi^{(13)} \lambda_i^{(13)} \tau_k^{(13)}},$$

($i=1,\ldots,I$), with similarly J and K restrictions for the other two marginals.

6.7 Relation to Latent Continuous Densities

Several publications are devoted to the comparison of local and global association models. Important references are Goodman (1981b), Mardia (1970), Dale (1984), and Becker (1989). An argument, often used to claim superiority of local over global association models, is the close relationship between Goodman's UM model and discretizations of the bivariate normal distribution (Goodman 1981b, Becker 1989). Also, their close connection with log-linear modeling is brought forward.

Holland and Wang (1987) introduced the *local dependence function* (LDF) of a bivariate continuous density function f as an analog to the local cross-ratios for contingency tables (Yule and Kendall 1950). The probability of a rectangular cell around (x,y) with edges dx and dy is approximated by $f(x,y)dxdy$. For cells around (x,y), (x,v), (u,y) and (u,v), the log local cross-ratio is given by

$$\theta(x,y;u,v) = \ln\left[\frac{f(x,y)f(u,v)}{f(x,v)f(u,y)}\right].$$

The *local dependence function* (LDF) at (x,y) is defined as

$$\gamma_f(x,y) = \lim_{dx\to 0, dy\to 0}\frac{\theta(x,y;x+dx,y+dy)}{dx\,dy} = \frac{\partial^2}{\partial x \partial y}\ln f(x,y). \quad (6.28)$$

Holland and Wang (1987) show that a bivariate density is characterized by its LDF and its two marginal densities. Further, a bivariate normal is characterized by a constant LDF and two normal marginal densities. Precise statements and proofs are found in Holland and Wang (1987).

The LDF of a normal density with correlation ρ is equal to $\phi = \rho/(1-\rho^2)$. Exactly this quantity, together with appropriately chosen scores α_i, β_j, λ_i and ν_j, are used by Becker (1989) to approximate the discretized normal by (6.5). Note that a special version of the RC model, i.e., the UM model, implies a constant local cross-ratio. It can be observed from Wang (1987), who provides an alternative way of computing normal probabilities, that the local association model introduced by (6.5) and the bivariate normal naturally go together. This explains why the local association models fit far better the discretized normal than do global cross-ratio models. In general, local association models correspond to bivariate densities via the LDF.

An analogous relationship holds between the Dale model and the Plackett distribution (Plackett 1965, Mardia 1970). If the global cross-ratio is constant (or in particular zero) throughout a contingency table, then it corresponds to a bivariate Plackett distribution (constant "Yulean association"). This was the case for the global association models, selected in the case of Tables 6.4 and 6.5.

However, we observed that model construction is restricted to neither a constant local association, nor a constant global association. Within family (6.4), one can even consider non-linear association models. In particular, we considered various types of row and column effects, together with interactions. This suggests that the normal distribution and the Plackett distribution are not the only ones of interest as continuous distributions, underlying a contingency table. Different forms for the local and global cross-ratios correspond to different distributions.

The correspondence between contingency tables and distribution functions in the Dale model case is very easy. The definition of the distribution is found by the continuous version of (6.16), of which the explicit form is straightforward. A continuous version of (6.15) would include linear (and quadratic) terms in x and y, together with an interaction term.

Let us again turn attention to Goodman's R+C+RC model (6.9). To construct a continuous density having a similar association structure, we first select a local dependence function of the form

$$\gamma(\boldsymbol{\phi}; x, y) = \phi_1 + \phi_2 f_2(x) + \phi_3 g_3(y) + \phi_4 f_4(x) g_4(y), \qquad (6.29)$$

where f_k and g_k are integrable functions. Molenberghs and Lesaffre (1999) show how the corresponding density can be approximated. The RC model is found by setting all terms, except those with subscript 4, equal to zero.

The models, fitted to Table 6.1, can be seen as extensions of both an underlying normal and an underlying Plackett distribution. The choice between different models should not be made on the ground of potential classes of underlying densities, but on the shape (structure) of associations. Figure 6.1 presents local and global cross-ratios found from the fitted values of both the RC+R+C model and the global cross-ratio model with row and column effects, as well as interactions. Obviously, there is little pattern in the local cross-ratios, whereas the global cross-ratios show a clear tendency: all associations are high, with an increase if the dichotomy is constructed closer to the categories with low labels, being highest between the variables I(Father's status ≤ 1) and I(Child's status ≤ 1). This implies that social mobility increases with increasing category. There is also slight evidence that the association surface is symmetric, which would then correspond to a global cross-ratio distribution with symmetric global cross-ratio function, such as a symmetric second-degree polynomial.

6.8 Conclusions and Perspective

In this chapter, we presented association models for cross-classified data that belong to the unified multivariate logistic framework, described by

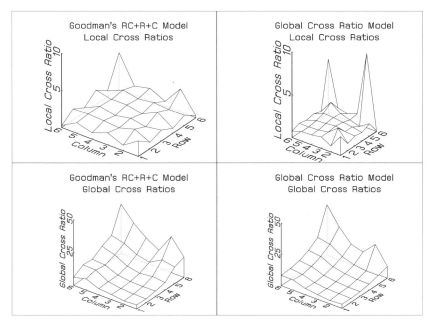

FIGURE 6.1. *Fluvoxamine Trial. Local and global cross-ratios, found from fitting the RC+R+C model and the global cross-ratio model.*

McCullagh and Nelder (1989) and Glonek and McCullagh (1995). This family provides a versatile way of exploring the association structure of cross-classified data. It encompasses both local and global measures of association, with emphasis on cross-ratios (odds ratios), as log cross-ratios can be written as contrasts of log-probabilities. Both fully marginal models, such as the Dale model and its multivariate extensions, as models with a conditional flavor, such as Goodman's (1981a) RC model, are members of this family. Further, linear as well as non-linear link functions (e.g., involving interactions between row and column effects) fit within this family.

We argue that, in spite of the close connection between an RC model and an underlying normal density and the absence of this connection with a fully marginal model, this last category of models provides a flexible toolkit to explore the association structure of cross-classified data, whether of nominal or of ordinal type. We infer from the examples that they often yield parsimonious descriptions of the association structure. Further, marginal association models are easily extended to marginal regression models to include covariate effects. Extensions to multi-way tables are possible, both with the RC as well as with the marginal family.

Both Dale (1984) and Anscombe (1981) suggest the use of global cross-ratios as soon as the outcomes are recorded as ordinal variables. We have shown that this choice is supported by a very good fit for this kind of model to a range of applications. Further, we claim that the global cross-ratio can lead to interesting interpretations of the association structure itself, which we think is an often neglected aspect of data analysis.

An argument, in favor of RC models, is their computational simplicity. However, with the current state of high quality statistical software, fitting marginal global association models poses no problems.

The Dale model, being a marginal model, is a member of a wider class of marginal models encompassing, for example, the probit model, and allowing for the analysis of multivariate and longitudinal data, with or without covariates, and with measurements sequences of length longer than two. This is the topic of the next chapter.

7
Likelihood-based Marginal Models

In Section 5.3.1, a general overview of marginal models is presented. Specific versions, largely focused on contingency tables, were presented in Chapter 6. In this chapter, we contemplate the fully general situation. We focus on fully specified probabilistic models, in contrast to specifying a few low-order moments only, such as in generalized estimating equations (GEE). Although undoubtedly complicating both the theory and the computations, there are at least two situations in which this route is the preferred one. First, the scientific question may require careful modeling of the association structure, in addition to the univariate response function. Second, one may be interested in the joint probability of a number of events (e.g., what is the probability of side effects occurring at two subsequent measurement occasions). In such a case, the association structure is not of direct interest, but is still indirectly needed to calculate such joint, or union, probabilities. An additional reason is that, such models as the Bahadur model (Section 7.2) or the global odds ratio model (the Dale model, Section 7.7) are the underlying basis for non-likelihood methods discussed later. For example, standard GEE, such as introduced by Liang and Zeger (1986) and studied in Chapter 8, is based on Bahadur's probabilistic model, while the version proposed by Lipsitz, Laird, and Harrington (1991) can be seen as rooted in the Dale model.

We begin by presenting the Bahadur model (Section 7.2). It has a relatively simple genesis, but at the same time suffer from severe drawbacks. Section 7.3 presents a general framework, encompassing a wide class of marginal models, while details on maximum likelihood estimation are given in Section 7.4. The ideas developed in Sections 7.3 and 7.4 are exemplified, using an influenza study, in Section 7.5. Two specific families, the multivariate probit model (Section 7.6) and the multivariate Dale model, or global odds ratio model (Section 7.7) are presented next. Section 7.8 presents a hybrid model, combining marginal and conditional model specifications. Three case studies, a cross-over trial in primary dysmenorrhoea (Section 7.9), the multivariate POPS study (Section 7.10, introduced in Section 2.6), and the longitudinal fluvoxamine trial (Section 7.11) are presented.

7.1 Notation

In Chapter 4, we indicated, for each individual, subject, or experimental unit $i = 1, \ldots, N$ in a study, a series of measurements by $\boldsymbol{Y}_i = (Y_{i1}, \ldots, Y_{n_i})'$, along with covariate information, usually grouped into a matrix X_i. We will refer to this convention as the *regression notation*.

When data are non-Gaussian in nature, this notation can sometimes be used without too much modification, such as in the later chapters in this part (e.g., on generalized estimating equations in Chapter 8), or in Part IV on subject-specific models. On the other hand, note that in Chapter 6 we merely needed indices to indicate cells in a contingency table. For example, (i, j) in a two-way contingency table refers to row i and column j. In each such cell, *a number of* subjects are grouped. When a two-way contingency table is further split over levels of, say, a dichotomous covariate, such as in Section 6.6.1, one often merely adds an additional index. This is similar to the conventions in analysis of variance and in contrast to linear regression.

In the present chapter, we need a hybrid system. On the one hand, the focus is on (longer) sequences of measurements, together with sets of covariates that can be continuous, categorical, or a mixture of these. In later chapters, it will be sufficient to use the regression-type notation, sketched at the start of this section. However, here we will need to describe not just marginal, univariate regressions, also the association structure needs to be modeled. This brings us close to a contingency table setting. When we have, for example, one covariate with two levels and five repeated binary measures, we can view the data as consisting of two 2^5 contingency tables. But the same view can be adopted when we have covariates with more levels, and even when some or all of the covariates are continuous. For continuous covariates, measured with high accuracy, there may be one or at most a few study subjects corresponding to it. Rather than being a problem, it is merely a way of conveniently framing both genuine contingency table settings and categorical data regression settings into a single, contingency table notational convention.

Thus, in this chapter, we will let $r = 1, \ldots, N$ indicate the covariate or design levels, each containing N_r subjects. For example, when there is one covariate with two levels, $N = 2$ and the total sample size is $N_1 + N_2$.

When the covariate is continuous and such that there is only one subject per covariate level, then each $N_r = 1$ and the total sample size is N. The consequence of our choice is that, for the time being, we need an additional index i for subjects within design lvels.

The outcome for subject i at the rth level (group) is a series of measurements Y_{rij} ($j = 1, \ldots, n_r$). In case there are subjects sharing covariates, but with a different number of repeated measurements taken, then these should be split over several design levels, implying that r defines unique combinations of covariate levels and numbers of repeated measurements. An additional notational element is that our outcome Y_{rij} can be binary (usually taking the values 0 and 1), but also categorical, ordered, or unordered. We then need additional notation and assume that in such case variable Y_{rij} can take on c_j distinct (possibly ordered) values. Without loss of generality, denote them by $1, \ldots, c_j$. In examples of a multivariate nature, the measurement sequence usually is equally long for all subjects, i.e., $n_r \equiv n$ but the number c_j of categories per outcome can be variable. In longitudinal settings, the number of measurements could also be different from subject to subject, but when the same outcome is measured repeatedly over time, one typically sees that $c_j \equiv c$. The more elaborate notation will be referred to as the *contingency table notation*.

In the specific case of categorical data with more than two, possibly ordered, categories, it is useful to make use of some additional notation. All information about the responses on the units in the rth group is contained in a cross-classification of the outcomes Y_{rij} into a $c_1 \times \ldots \times c_{n_r}$ dimensional contingency table with cell counts

$$Z_r^*(\boldsymbol{k}) \equiv Z_r^*(k_1, \ldots, k_{n_r}), \qquad (7.1)$$

where cell $\boldsymbol{k} = (k_1, \ldots, k_{n_r})$ corresponds to the subjects with $Y_{rij} = k_j$, for $j = 1, \ldots, n_r$.

Along with the outcomes, a vector of explanatory variables x_{rj} is recorded. The covariate vector is allowed to change over time. It can include continuous and discrete variables. Available covariate information, along with other relevant design features, are incorporated in a design matrix X_r.

In harmony with the possibility to use cumulative measures for ordinal data, we construct the table of cumulative counts:

$$Z_r(\boldsymbol{k}) = \sum_{\boldsymbol{\ell} \leq \boldsymbol{k}} Z_r^*(\boldsymbol{\ell}). \qquad (7.2)$$

Thus, $Z_r(\boldsymbol{k})$, where $\boldsymbol{k} = (k_1, \ldots, k_{n_r})$, is just the number of individuals in group r whose observed response vector is $\boldsymbol{k}$, and likewise for $Z_r(\boldsymbol{k})^*$. The corresponding probabilities are

$$\mu_r^*(\boldsymbol{k}) = P(\boldsymbol{Y}_{ri} = \boldsymbol{k} | X_r, \boldsymbol{\beta}) \qquad (7.3)$$

and $\mu_r(\mathbf{k}) = P(\mathbf{Y}_{ri} \leq \mathbf{k}|X_r, \boldsymbol{\beta})$. Let $\mathbf{Z}_r$ be the vector of all cumulative cell counts with $\boldsymbol{\mu}_r$ the corresponding vector of probabilities. Note that $Z_r(c_1,\ldots,c_{n_r}) = n_r$ and $\mu_r(c_1,\ldots,c_{n_r}) = 1$. Therefore, omitting these two entries from $\mathbf{Z}_r$ and $\boldsymbol{\mu}_r$, respectively, yields non-redundant sets. $\mathbf{Z}_r^*$ and $\boldsymbol{\mu}_r^*$ are defined similarly, and simple matrix equalities

$$\boldsymbol{\mu}_r^* = B_r \boldsymbol{\mu}_r, \qquad \mathbf{Z}_r^* = B_r \mathbf{Z}_r \qquad (7.4)$$

hold. As an example, consider a bivariate binary outcome vector, with probabilities $\boldsymbol{\mu}_r^* = (\mu_{11}^*, \mu_{12}^*, \mu_{21}^*, \mu_{22}^*)$ and a similar ordering for $\boldsymbol{\mu}_r$. The matrix B_r is found by

$$B_r^{-1} = \begin{pmatrix} 1 & 0 & 0 & 0 \\ 1 & 1 & 0 & 0 \\ 1 & 0 & 1 & 0 \\ 1 & 1 & 1 & 1 \end{pmatrix}.$$

The marginal counts are given by all counts for which all but one index are equal to their maximal value: $Z_{rjk} \equiv Z_r(c_1,\ldots,c_{j-1}, k, c_{j+1},\ldots,c_{n_r})$. Bivariate cell counts, i.e., cell counts of a cross-classification of a pair of outcomes, follow from setting all but two indices k_s equal to c_s. Therefore, this description very naturally combines univariate, bivariate, and multivariate information. The ordering needed to stack the multi-indexed counts and probabilities into a vector will be assumed fixed. Several orderings of both $\mathbf{Z}_r$ and $\boldsymbol{\mu}_r$ are possible. A natural choice is the lexicographic ordering, but this has the disadvantage of dispersing the univariate marginal counts and means over the entire vector. Therefore, we will typically group the elements by dimensionality first.

7.2 The Bahadur Model

7.2.1 A General Bahadur Model Formulation

Bahadur (1961) introduced this model, with its elegant closed form, but with a number of computational problems surrounding it, stemming from the complicated and highly restrictive form of its parameter space. The model is conceived for binary data and can be introduced using the simpler regression notation, outlined in Section 7.1. Thus, let the binary response Y_{ij} indicate whether or not measurement j on subject i exhibits the event under investigation.

Assume the marginal distribution of Y_{ij} to be Bernoulli with

$$E(Y_{ij}) = P(Y_{ij} = 1) \equiv \pi_{ij}.$$

7.2 The Bahadur Model

This expectation can be taken conditional upon covariates X_i. For simplicity, they are suppressed from notation. To start describing the association, the pairwise probability

$$P(Y_{ij_1} = 1, Y_{ij_2} = 1) = E(Y_{ij_1} Y_{ij_2}) \equiv \pi_{ij_1 j_2}$$

needs to be characterized. This "success probability" of two measurements taken in the same subject can be modeled in terms of the two marginal probabilities π_{ij_1} and π_{ij_2}, as well as an association parameter, this being the marginal correlation coefficient in Bahadur's model.

The marginal correlation coefficient assumes the form

$$\text{Corr}(Y_{ij_1}, Y_{ij_2}) \equiv \rho_{ij_1 j_2} = \frac{\pi_{ij_1 j_2} - \pi_{ij_1} \pi_{ij_2}}{[\pi_{ij_1}(1 - \pi_{ij_2})\pi_{ij_2}(1 - \pi_{ij_2})]^{1/2}}. \quad (7.5)$$

In terms of this association parameter, the joint probability $\pi_{ij_1 j_2}$ can then be written as

$$\pi_{ij_1 j_2} = \pi_{ij_1} \pi_{ij_2} + \rho_{ij_1 j_2} [\pi_{ij_1}(1 - \pi_{ij_1})\pi_{ij_2}(1 - \pi_{ij_2})]^{1/2}. \quad (7.6)$$

Hence, given the marginal correlation coefficient $\rho_{ij_1 j_2}$ and the univariate probabilities π_{ij_1} and π_{ij_2}, the pairwise probability $\pi_{ij_1 j_2}$ can be calculated with ease.

The first and second moments of the distribution have now been specified. However, a likelihood-based approach requires the complete representation of the joint probabilities of the vector of binary responses in each unit. The full joint distribution $f(y)$ of $Y_i = (Y_{i1}, \ldots, Y_{in_i})'$ is multinomial with a 2^{n_i} probability vector. Bahadur used, apart from the conventional two-way correlation coefficient, third- and higher- order correlation coefficients to completely specify the joint distribution. To this end, let

$$\varepsilon_{ij} = \frac{Y_{ij} - \pi_{ij}}{\sqrt{\pi_{ij}(1 - \pi_{ij})}} \quad \text{and} \quad e_{ij} = \frac{y_{ij} - \pi_{ij}}{\sqrt{\pi_{ij}(1 - \pi_{ij})}}, \quad (7.7)$$

where y_{ij} is an actual value of the binary response variable Y_{ij}. Further, let

$$\begin{aligned}
\rho_{ij_1 j_2} &= E(\varepsilon_{ij_1} \varepsilon_{ij_2}), \\
\rho_{ij_1 j_2 j_3} &= E(\varepsilon_{ij_1} \varepsilon_{ij_2} \varepsilon_{ij_3}), \\
&\vdots, \\
\rho_{i12\ldots n_i} &= E(\varepsilon_{i1} \varepsilon_{i2} \ldots \varepsilon_{in_i}).
\end{aligned} \quad (7.8)$$

Then, the general Bahadur model can be represented by the expression $f(\mathbf{y}_i) = f_1(\mathbf{y}_i) c(\mathbf{y}_i)$, where

$$f_1(\mathbf{y}_i) = \prod_{j=1}^{n_i} \pi_{ij}^{y_{ij}} (1 - \pi_{ij})^{1 - y_{ij}}$$

and

$$c(\boldsymbol{y}_i) = 1 + \sum_{j_1<j_2} \rho_{ij_1j_2} e_{ij_1} e_{ij_2} + \sum_{j_1<j_2<j_3} \rho_{ij_1j_2j_3} e_{ij_1} e_{ij_2} e_{ij_3}$$
$$+ \ldots + \rho_{i12\ldots n_i} e_{i1} e_{i2} \ldots e_{in_i}.$$

Thus, the probability mass function is the product of the independence model $f_1(\boldsymbol{y}_i)$ and the correction factor $c(\boldsymbol{y}_i)$. One view-point is to consider the factor $c(\boldsymbol{y}_i)$ as a model for overdispersion.

7.2.2 The Bahadur Model for Clustered Data

To enhance understanding, let us consider the Bahadur model for the case of exchangeably clustered data. This version of the model was of use for Aerts et al (2002) who studied models for clustered data arising in an environmental context.

When the focus is on the special case of clustered data, this assumes on the one hand that each measurement within a unit (individual, family, litter, cluster,...) has the same response probability, i.e., $\pi_{ij} = \pi_i$. On the other hand, it usually implies that within a litter, the associations of a particular order are constant, i.e., $\rho_{ij_1j_2} = \rho_{i(2)}$ for $j_1 < j_2$, $\rho_{ij_1j_2j_3} = \rho_{i(3)}$ for $j_1 < j_2 < j_3,\ldots$, $\rho_{i12\ldots n_i} = \rho_{i(n_i)}$, with $i = 1,\ldots,N$. Given these assumptions, we do not need to know the individual outcomes Y_{ij}, but it suffices to know

$$Z_i = \sum_{j=1}^{n_i} Y_{ij}, \qquad (7.9)$$

the number of successes within a unit, with realized value z_i. Under exchangeability (or equicorrelation), the Bahadur model reduces to

$$f_1(\boldsymbol{y}_i) = \pi_i^{z_i}(1-\pi_i)^{n_i-z_i}$$

and

$$c(\boldsymbol{y}_i) = 1 + \sum_{r=2}^{n_i} \rho_{i(r)} \sum_{s=0}^{r} \binom{z_i}{s} \binom{n_i-z_i}{r-s} (-1)^{s+r} \lambda_i^{r-2s}, \qquad (7.10)$$

with $\lambda_i = \sqrt{\pi_i/(1-\pi_i)}$. The probability mass function of Z_i is given by

$$f(z_i) = \binom{n_i}{z_i} f(\boldsymbol{y}_i).$$

In addition, setting all three- and higher-way correlations equal to zero, the probability mass function of Z_i simplifies further to:

$$f(z_i) \equiv f(z_i|\pi_i, \rho_{i(2)}, n_i) = \binom{n_i}{z_i} \pi_i^{z_i}(1-\pi_i)^{n_i-z_i}$$

$$\times \left[1 + \rho_{i(2)} \left\{ \binom{n_i - z_i}{2} \frac{\pi_i}{1 - \pi_i} - z_i(n_i - z_i) \right. \right.$$
$$\left. \left. + \binom{z_i}{2} \frac{1 - \pi_i}{\pi_i} \right\} \right]. \tag{7.11}$$

This very tractable expression of the Bahadur probability mass function is advantageous over other representations, such as the multivariate probit (Section 7.6) and Dale (Section 7.7) models, for which no closed form solutions, free of integrals, exist. However, a drawback is the fact that the correlation between two responses is highly constrained when the higher order correlations are removed. Even when higher order parameters are included, the parameter space of marginal parameters and correlations is known to be peculiar. Bahadur (1961) discusses restrictions on the correlation parameters. The second-order approximation in (7.11) is only useful if it is a probability mass function. Bahadur indicates that the sum of the probabilities of all possible outcomes is one. However, depending on the values of π_i and $\rho_{i(2)}$, expression (7.11) may fail to be non-negative for some outcomes. The latter results in restrictions on the parameter space, which, in case of the second-order approximation, are described by Bahadur (1961). From these, it can be deduced that the lower bound for $\rho_{i(2)}$ approaches zero as the cluster size increases. However, it is important to note that also the upper bound for this correlation parameter is constrained. Indeed, even though it is one for clusters of size two, the upper bound varies between $1/(n_i - 1)$ and $2/(n_i - 1)$ for larger clusters. Taking a cluster size of, for example, 12, the upper bound is in the range $(0.09; 0.18)$. Kupper and Haseman (1978) present numerical values for the constraints on $\rho_{i(2)}$ for choices of π_i and n_i. Restrictions for a specific version where a third-order association parameter is included as well are studied by Prentice (1988), while a more general situation is studied by Declerck, Aerts, and Molenberghs (1998). See also Aerts *et al* (2002).

The marginal parameters π_i and $\rho_{i(2)}$ can be modeled using a composite link function. Because Y_{ij} is binary, the logistic link function for π_i is a natural choice. In principle, any link function, such as the probit link, the log-log link or the complementary log-log link, could be chosen. A convenient transformation of $\rho_{i(2)}$ is Fisher's z-transform. This leads to the following generalized linear regression relations

$$\begin{pmatrix} \ln\left(\frac{\pi_i}{1-\pi_i}\right) \\ \ln\left(\frac{1+\rho_{i(2)}}{1-\rho_{i(2)}}\right) \end{pmatrix} \equiv \boldsymbol{\eta}_i = X_i \boldsymbol{\beta}, \tag{7.12}$$

where X_i is a design matrix and $\boldsymbol{\beta}$ is a vector of unknown parameters. Note that (7.12) is not encompassed by (6.2).

Denote the log-likelihood contribution of the ith unit by

$$\ell_i = \ln f(z_i|\pi_i, \rho_{i(2)}, n_i).$$

The maximum likelihood estimator $\widehat{\boldsymbol{\beta}}$ for $\boldsymbol{\beta}$ is defined as the solution to the score equations $\boldsymbol{U}(\boldsymbol{\beta}) = \boldsymbol{0}$. The score function $\boldsymbol{U}(\boldsymbol{\beta})$ can be written as

$$\boldsymbol{U}(\boldsymbol{\beta}) = \sum_{i=1}^{N} X'_i (T'_i)^{-1} L_i \qquad (7.13)$$

where

$$T_i = \frac{\partial \boldsymbol{\eta}_i}{\partial \boldsymbol{\Theta}_i} = \begin{pmatrix} \frac{\partial \eta_{i1}}{\partial \pi_i} & \frac{\partial \eta_{i2}}{\partial \pi_i} \\ \frac{\partial \eta_{i1}}{\partial \rho_{(2)}} & \frac{\partial \eta_{i2}}{\partial \rho_{i(2)}} \end{pmatrix} = \begin{pmatrix} \frac{1}{\pi_i(1-\pi_i)} & 0 \\ 0 & \frac{2}{(1-\rho_{i(2)})(1+\rho_{i(2)})} \end{pmatrix},$$

$$L_i = \frac{\partial \ell_i}{\partial \boldsymbol{\Theta}_i} = \begin{pmatrix} \frac{\partial \ell_i}{\partial \pi_i} \\ \frac{\partial \ell_i}{\partial \rho_{i(2)}} \end{pmatrix}$$

and $\boldsymbol{\Theta}_i = (\pi_i, \rho_{i(2)})'$, the set of natural parameters. A Newton-Raphson algorithm can be used to obtain the maximum likelihood estimates $\widehat{\boldsymbol{\beta}}$ and an estimate of the asymptotic covariance matrix of $\widehat{\boldsymbol{\beta}}$ can be obtained from the observed information matrix at maximum.

When including higher order correlations, implementing the score equations and the observed information matrices becomes increasingly cumbersome. Although the functional form (7.13) does not change, the components T_i and L_i become fairly complicated. Fisher's z transform can be applied to all correlation parameters $\rho_{i(r)}$. The design matrix X_i would then extend in a straightforward fashion as well. Unfortunately, fitting a higher order Bahadur model, is not straightforward, due to increasingly complex restrictions on the parameter space.

Observing that interest is often restricted to the marginal mean function and the pairwise association parameter, one can replace a full likelihood approach by estimating equations where only the first two moments are modeled and working assumptions are adopted about third- and fourth-order moments. This is treated as one of the extensions to standard generalized estimating equations in Section 8.5. See also Liang, Zeger, and Qaqish (1992).

7.2.3 Analysis of the NTP Data

Table 7.1 presents parameter estimates and standard errors for the Bahadur model, in the specific context of clustered outcomes as in Section 7.2.2, fitted to several outcomes in three of the NTP datasets, described in Section 2.7. Apart from the external, visceral, and skeletal malformation outcomes, we also consider the so-called collapsed outcome, which is 1 if at least one of the three malformations occur and 0 otherwise.

7.2 The Bahadur Model

TABLE 7.1. *NTP Data. Parameter estimates (standard errors) for the Bahadur model, fitted to various outcomes in three studies. β_0 and β_d are the marginal intercept and dose effect, respectively; β_a is the Fisher z transformed correlation; ρ is the correlation.*

Outcome	Parameter	DEHP	EG	DYME
External	β_0	-4.93(0.39)	-5.25(0.66)	-7.25(0.71)
	β_d	5.15(0.56)	2.63(0.76)	7.94(0.77)
	β_a	0.11(0.03)	0.12(0.03)	0.11(0.04)
	ρ	0.05(0.01)	0.06(0.01)	0.05(0.02)
Visceral	β_0	-4.42(0.33)	-7.38(1.30)	-6.89(0.81)
	β_d	4.38(0.49)	4.25(1.39)	5.49(0.87)
	β_a	0.11(0.02)	0.05(0.08)	0.08(0.04)
	ρ	0.05(0.01)	0.02(0.04)	0.04(0.02)
Skeletal	β_0	-4.67(0.39)	-2.49(0.11)	-4.27(0.61)
	β_d	4.68(0.56)	2.96(0.18)	5.79(0.80)
	β_a	0.13(0.03)	0.27(0.02)	0.22(0.05)
	ρ	0.06(0.01)	0.13(0.01)	0.11(0.02)
Collapsed	β_0	-3.83(0.27)	-2.51(0.09)	-5.31(0.40)
	β_d	5.38(0.47)	3.05(0.17)	8.18(0.69)
	β_a	0.12(0.03)	0.28(0.02)	0.12(0.03)
	ρ	0.06(0.01)	0.14(0.01)	0.06(0.01)

Specifically, a marginal logit model linear in dose and a constant association $\rho_{i(2)} = \rho_{(2)}$ are chosen, implying that X_i in (7.12) takes the form:

$$X_i = \begin{pmatrix} 1 & d_i & 0 \\ 0 & 0 & 1 \end{pmatrix} \quad (7.14)$$

and

$$\boldsymbol{\beta} = \begin{pmatrix} \beta_0 \\ \beta_d \\ \beta_a \end{pmatrix}, \quad (7.15)$$

where β_0 is an intercept, β_d the dose effect, and β_a the Fisher z transformed correlation.

We conclude that the background risk for malformation in all cases is very small, but that it increases with dose. For the external malformation outcome in the DEHP study, for example, the background risk is estimated to be small:

$$\frac{e^{-4.93}}{1 + e^{-4.93}} = 0.0071.$$

When the dose level equals its highest value ($d = 1.0$), the risk becomes

$$\frac{e^{-4.93+5.15}}{1+e^{-4.93+5.15}} = 0.55,$$

implying that more than one out of two foetuses would be malformed.

The dose-response curve that follows from the marginal logistic regression:

$$P(Y_{ij} = 1|d_i) = \frac{e^{-4.93+5.15d_i}}{1+e^{-4.93+5.15d_i}}$$

is supplemented with information on the association. In addition, one obtains a correlation of

$$\widehat{\rho} = \frac{e^{\widehat{\beta}_a} - 1}{e^{\widehat{\beta}_a} + 1} = 0.05.$$

Although small, the within-cluster association is significant, as it is for most but not all outcomes.

7.2.4 Analysis of the Fluvoxamine Trial

The fluvoxamine trial, introduced in Section 2.4, were analyzed in some detail in Chapter 6. In Section 6.6, several two-way contingency tables, either based on a single outcome at two measurement occasions, or side effects and therapeutic effect at the same time, were analyzed. This initial setting was extended to categorical covariates and three-way tables in Sections 6.6.1 and 6.6.2, respectively. Using the Bahadur model, we are able to extend this further to sequences of arbitrary length, and a combination of continuous and categorical covariates. This is true in principle, as the Bahadur model is restrictive due to constraints on the parameter space, as stated before. In Section 7.2.3, we were able to analyze the NTP data, with dose treated as a continuous covariate, in spite of the fact that some litters consist of around 15 littermates, but we could do so only by carefully exploiting the exchangeable nature of the data, with only three regression parameters as a result.

Here, we would like to study three side-effects measures simultaneously, regressed on age and sex of the patient, prior duration of the mental illness, and initial severity of the disease. We are confronted with two stumbling blocks. First, because the Bahadur model is formulated for binary outcomes, we need to collapse the original four-category side effects outcome into a dichotomous variable. This is done by transforming the lower two levels of the side effects variable into 0 and the upper two into 1. Second, due to the parameter restrictions, it was not possible to consider all four covariates simultaneously. Thus, we resrict attention to the sex and prior duration variables. Parameter estimates are given in Table 7.2. The three-way correlation coefficient is set to zero. The effect of the covariates is not significant, but the correlation parameters are. For ease of interpretation,

TABLE 7.2. *Fluvoxamine Study. Longitudinal analysis using Bahadur's model. The side effects at three successive times are regressed on sex and duration. The entries represent the parameter estimates (standard errors).*

	Side effects at time		
Parameter	1	2	3
Intercept	0.81(0.47)	0.15(0.37)	0.57(0.44)
Sex	-0.56(0.26)	0.02(0.20)	0.14(0.24)
Duration	0.008(0.009)	0.01(0.01)	-0.01(0.01)
Association Parameters			
12	13	23	123
Fisher z transformed correlations			
1.42(0.16)	0.84(0.13)	1.37(0.15)	—
Correlations			
0.61(0.05)	0.39(0.05)	0.59(0.05)	—

the Fisher z transformed correlation, as they figure in the model and fitting program, are transformed again to their original scale, supplemented with standard errors obtained by means of the delta method.

Thus, while the Bahadur model can be of some use in a restricted number of situations, including exchangeably clustered outcomes, there are practical limitations when used in multivariate and longitudinal settings. Therefore, in spite of the relatively simple model formulation, there is a need for alternative models, when a full likelihood based analysis of a marginally formulated model is envisaged. In the next section, we will sketch a general framework to achieve this, then consider the probit (Section 7.6) and Dale model (Section 7.7) cases, whereafter we analyze several sets of data. In particular, we return to the fluvoxamine study in Section 7.11.

7.3 A General Framework for Fully Specified Marginal Models

We will now use the contingency table notation laid out in Section 7.1. A marginal model can be built in several ways. In a few cases it is possible to write down the multivariate probability mass function immediately, such as in the Bahadur model of Section 7.2. In most cases, one starts from the univariate margins, on top of which an association structure is assumed, of the second and higher orders, to complete model specification. We will proceed here in this at first sight laborious way.

94   7. Likelihood-based Marginal Models

By means of (7.3), the set of cell probabilities at design level r has been defined. To proceed with modeling, we typically map these onto a set of link functions $\boldsymbol{\eta}_r$, which can then be expressed in terms of parameters of scientific interest. In the Bahadur model for clustered data, this was done by means of (7.12). In general, we map the C_r-vector $\boldsymbol{\mu}_r$ ($C_r = c_1 \cdot c_2 \cdot \ldots \cdot c_{n_r}$) to

$$\boldsymbol{\eta}_r = \boldsymbol{\eta}_r(\boldsymbol{\mu}_r), \qquad (7.16)$$

a C'_r-vector. In many models, $C_r = C'_r$, and $\boldsymbol{\eta}_r$ and $\boldsymbol{\mu}_r$ have the same ordering. A counterexample is provided by the probit model, where the number of link functions is smaller than the number of mean components, as soon as $n_r > 2$, i.e., there are three of more repeated measures [see (7.25)–(7.27)]. As already indicated in Section 6.2.1, an important class of link functions is discussed by McCullagh and Nelder (1989):

$$\boldsymbol{\eta}_r(\boldsymbol{\mu}_r) = C \ln(A\boldsymbol{\mu}_r), \qquad (7.17)$$

a definition in terms of contrasts of log probabilities, where the probabilities involved are linear combinations $A\boldsymbol{\mu}_r$. The same class was presented in (6.2) for the specific case of marginal models for a contingency table.

7.3.1   Univariate Link Functions

We consider particular choices of link functions. To this end, let us abbreviate the univariate marginal probabilities by

$$\mu_{rjk} = \mu_r(c_1, \ldots, c_{j-1}, k, c_{j+1}, \ldots, c_{n_r}),$$

then the logit link becomes

$$\eta_{rjk} = \ln(\mu_{rjk}) - \ln(1 - \mu_{rjk}) = \text{logit}(\mu_{rjk}). \qquad (7.18)$$

Some link functions that are occasionally of interest, such as the probit or complementary log-log link are not supported by (7.17) but they can easily be included in (7.16). The probit link is

$$\eta_{rjk} = \Phi_1^{-1}(\mu_{rjk}),$$

with Φ_1 the univariate standard normal distribution.

7.3.2   Higher-order Link Functions

However, univariate links alone do not fully specify $\boldsymbol{\eta}_r$ and hence leave the joint distribution partly undetermined. Full specification of the association requires addressing the form of pairwise and higher-order probabilities. First, we will consider the pairwise associations. Let us denote the bivariate probabilities, pertaining to the j_1th and j_2th outcomes, by

$$\mu_{r,jh,k\ell} = \mu_r(c_1, \ldots, c_{j-1}, k, c_{j+1}, \ldots, c_{h-1}, \ell, c_{h+1}, \ldots, c_{n_r}).$$

7.3 A General Framework for Fully Specified Marginal Models

TABLE 7.3. *Association structure of selected marginal models.*

Name	Association structure	Equation
Success probability	Logit of joint probability	(7.19)
Bahadur model	Marginal correlation coefficients	(7.5)
Dale model	Global marginal odds ratio	(7.21)–(7.23)
	Local marginal odds ratio	(7.24)
Probit model	Polychoric correlation	(7.25)–(7.27)

Some association parameterizations are summarized in Table 7.3.

The success probability parameterization of Ekholm (1991) consists of choosing a link function for the univariate marginal means (e.g., a logit link) and then applying the same link function to the two- and higher order success probabilities (i.e., the probabilities for observing a single success when looking at one outcome at a time, a pair of successes when looking at pairs of outcomes,...). For categorical data, a logit link for two-way probabilities is given by

$$\eta_{r,jh,k\ell} = \ln(\mu_{r,jh,k\ell}) - \ln(1 - \mu_{r,jh,k\ell}) = \text{logit}(\mu_{i,jh,k\ell}), \qquad (7.19)$$

for $k = 1,\ldots,c_j - 1$ and $\ell = 1,\ldots,c_h - 1$. Ekholm, Smith, and McDonald (1995) and Ekholm, McDonald, and Smith (2000) used these to define dependence ratios, in the specific case of binary data. The marginal correlation coefficient (Bahadur 1961) is defined as

$$\rho_{r,jh,k\ell} = \frac{\mu_{r,jh,k\ell} - \mu_{rjk}\mu_{rh\ell}}{\sqrt{\mu_{rjk}(1 - \mu_{rjk})\mu_{rh\ell}(1 - \mu_{rh\ell})}}. \qquad (7.20)$$

This model has been developed, for binary data, including the higher order correlations, in Section 7.2.

We will put strong emphasis on the marginal global odds ratio, defined by

$$\psi_{r,jh,k\ell} = \frac{(\mu_{r,jh,k\ell})(1 - \mu_{rjk} - \mu_{rh\ell} + \mu_{r,jh,k\ell})}{(\mu_{rh\ell} - \mu_{r,jh,k\ell})(\mu_{rjk} - \mu_{r,jh,k\ell})} \qquad (7.21)$$

and usefully modeled on the log scale as

$$\begin{aligned}\eta_{r,jh,k\ell} &= \ln \psi_{r,jh,k\ell} \\ &= \ln(\mu_{r,jh,k\ell}) - \ln(\mu_{rjk} - \mu_{r,jh,k\ell}) \\ &\quad - \ln(\mu_{rh\ell} - \mu_{r,jh,k\ell}) + \ln(1 - \mu_{rjk} - \mu_{rh\ell} + \mu_{r,jh,k\ell}).\end{aligned}$$

Higher order global odds ratios are easily introduced, for example, using ratios of conditional odds (ratios). Let

$$\mu_{rj|h}(z_h) = P(Z_{rijk_j} = 1 | Z_{rihk_h} = z_h, X_r, \boldsymbol{\beta}) \qquad (7.22)$$

be the conditional probability of observing a success at occasion j, given the value z_h is observed at occasion h, and write the corresponding conditional odds as

$$\psi_{rj|h}(z_h) = \frac{\mu_{rj|h}(z_h)}{1 - \mu_{rj|h}(z_h)}.$$

The pairwise marginal odds ratio, for occasions j and h, is defined as

$$\begin{aligned}\psi_{rjh} &= \frac{\{\text{pr}(Z_{rijk_j} = 1, Z_{rihk_h} = 1)\}\{\text{pr}(Z_{rijk_j} = 0, Z_{rihk_h} = 0)\}}{\{\text{pr}(Z_{rijk_j} = 0, Z_{rihk_h} = 1)\}\{\text{pr}(Z_{rijk_j} = 1, Z_{rihk_h} = 0)\}} \\ &= \frac{\psi_{rj|h}(1)}{\psi_{rj|h}(0)},\end{aligned}$$

in accordance with (7.21). This formulation can be exploited to define the higher order marginal odds ratios in a recursive fashion:

$$\psi_{rj_1\ldots j_m j_{m+1}} = \frac{\psi_{rj_1\ldots j_m | j_{m+1}}(1)}{\psi_{rj_1\ldots j_m | j_{m+1}}(0)}, \qquad (7.23)$$

where $\psi_{rj_1\ldots j_m | j_{m+1}}(z_{m+1})$ is defined by conditioning all probabilities occurring in the expression for $\psi_{rj_1\ldots j_m}$ on $Z_{rij_{m+1}} = z_{j_{m+1}}$. The choice of the variable to condition on is immaterial. Observe that multi-way marginal global odds ratios are defined solely in terms of conditional probabilities. We will return to these in Section 7.7.4, when more detail is given about the multivariate Dale model.

Another type of marginal odds ratios is given by the marginal *local* odds ratios. These were used in Section 6.2.2. This type of odds ratio changes (7.21) to

$$\psi^*_{r,jh,k\ell} = \frac{\mu^*_{r,jh,k\ell}\mu^*_{r,jh,k+1,\ell+1}}{\mu^*_{r,jh,k+1,\ell}\mu^*_{r,jh,k,\ell+1}}, \qquad (7.24)$$

with the cell probabilities as in (7.3). Higher order marginal local odds ratios are constructed in the same way as their global counterparts. The global odds ratio model will be studied further in Section 7.7.

Observe that the multivariate probit model (Ashford and Sowden 1970, Lesaffre and Molenberghs 1991) also fits within the class defined by (7.16). To see this, let $g = h^{-1}$. For three categorical outcome variables, the inverse link is specified by

$$\begin{aligned}\mu_{rjk} &= \Phi_1(\eta_{rjk}), & (7.25) \\ \mu_{r,jh,k\ell} &= \Phi_2(\eta_{rjk}, \eta_{rh\ell}, \eta_{r,jh,k\ell}), & (7.26) \\ \mu_{r,123,k\ell m} &= \Phi_3(\eta_{r1k}, \eta_{r2\ell}, \eta_{r3m}, \eta_{r,12,k\ell}, \eta_{r,13,km}, \eta_{r,23,\ell m}), & (7.27)\end{aligned}$$

where the notation for the three-way probabilities is obvious. The association links $\eta_{r,jh,k\ell}$ represent any transform (e.g., Fisher's z-transform such

7.3 A General Framework for Fully Specified Marginal Models

as in the Bahadur model of Section 7.2) of the correlation coefficient. It is common practice to keep each correlation constant throughout a table, rather than having it depend on the categories: $\eta_{r,jh,k\ell} \equiv \eta_{r,jh}$. Relaxing this requirement may still give a valid set of probabilities, but the correspondence between the categorical variables and a latent multivariate normal variable is lost. Finally, observe that univariate links and bivariate links (representing correlations) fully determine the joint distribution. This implies that the mean vector and the link vector will have a different length, except in the univariate and bivariate cases.

In summary, marginal models are characterized by jointly specifying marginal response functions and marginal association measures. Models can be classified by the association measures, as exemplified in Table 7.3.

Finally, model formulation is completed by constructing appropriate design matrices. Let us give an example to indicate how model assumptions are reflected by choosing particular types of design. We deliberately restrict ourselves to linear predictors, while, in principle, there is no obstacle to include non-linear effects (Chapter 20). The design matrix X_r for the rth design level includes all information which is needed to model both the marginal mean functions and associations. Each row corresponds to an element in the vector of link functions $\boldsymbol{\eta}_r$. Its generality is best illustrated using an example.

Consider the case of three outcomes, recorded on a three-point scale. Let the measurement times be $t_1 \equiv 0$, t_2, and t_3. Assume the recording of four explanatory variables, $x_1, \ldots, x_4$, with only x_3 and x_4 time-varying. We first turn our attention to the marginal distributions. Let x_1 have a constant effect on each outcome, i.e., a single parameter describes the effect of x_1 on the cumulative logits of the three outcome probabilities. On the other hand, the effect of x_2 is allowed to change over time. We also introduce a single parameter to describe the effect of x_3 and three separate parameters to account for the influence of x_4. These assumptions call for the following parameter vector

$$\boldsymbol{\beta}_1 = (\beta_{01}, \beta_{02}, \tau_2, \tau_3, \beta_1, \beta_{21}, \beta_{22}, \beta_{23}, \beta_3, \beta_{41}, \beta_{42}, \beta_{43})',$$

with β_{0k} intercepts, τ_j the effect of measurement time j, β_1 and β_3 the parameters, needed to describe the effect of x_1 and x_3 respectively, and β_{tj} the parameter describing the effect of $x_t^{(j)}$ at time t ($t = 2, 4; j = 1, 2, 3$). Next, assume that the two-way associations depend on the pair of variables they refer to, as well as on the cumulative category within that variable. Finally, assume dependence on the covariate x_{1r}. This introduces extra parameters

$$\boldsymbol{\alpha}_2 = (\gamma, \gamma_{11}, \gamma_{12}, \gamma_{21}, \gamma_{22}, \gamma_{31}, \gamma_{32}, \phi_1, \phi_2, \phi_3)',$$

with γ the intercept, γ_{jk} the dependence on category k of outcome j ($j = 1, 2; k = 1, 2$), and ϕ_j the dependence on x_1. Finally, assume a constant

98   7. Likelihood-based Marginal Models

	β_{01}	β_{02}	τ_2	τ_3	β_1	β_{21}	β_{22}	β_{23}	β_3	β_{41}	β_{42}	β_{43}
$\eta_r(1,3,3)$	1	0	0	0	x_{1r}	x_{2r}	0	0	$x_{3r}^{(1)}$	$x_{4r}^{(1)}$	0	0
$\eta_r(2,3,3)$	0	1	0	0	x_{1r}	x_{2r}	0	0	$x_{3r}^{(1)}$	$x_{4r}^{(1)}$	0	0
$\eta_r(3,1,3)$	1	0	1	0	x_{1r}	0	x_{2r}	0	$x_{3r}^{(2)}$	0	$x_{4r}^{(2)}$	0
$\eta_r(3,2,3)$	0	1	1	0	x_{1r}	0	x_{2r}	0	$x_{3r}^{(2)}$	0	$x_{4r}^{(2)}$	0
$\eta_r(3,3,1)$	1	0	0	1	x_{1r}	0	0	x_{2r}	$x_{3r}^{(3)}$	0	0	$x_{4r}^{(3)}$
$\eta_r(3,3,2)$	0	1	0	1	x_{1r}	0	0	x_{2r}	$x_{3r}^{(3)}$	0	0	$x_{4r}^{(3)}$

FIGURE 7.1. *Design matrix for marginal means and pairwise associations. Marginal means.*

value for the three-way associations, α_3 say. The entire parameter vector is denoted as
$$\boldsymbol{\beta} = (\boldsymbol{\beta}', \boldsymbol{\alpha}_2', \alpha_3)'.$$
The design matrix for design level r, X_r, is block diagonal with blocks X_{r1} (mean functions, shown in Figure 7.1), X_{r2} (pairwise association, shown in Figure 7.2), and X_{r3} (three-way association).

Observe that, apart from the intercepts β_{0k}, the design is identical for each cumulative logit in Figures 7.1 and 7.2. This reflects the proportional odds assumption when marginal logits are used. If this assumption is considered unrealistic, the design can be generalized without any difficulty. Nominal covariates and interactions between covariates are also easily included.

The second block of the design matrix, X_{2r}, corresponds to the pairwise associations and is given by Figure 7.2. Finally, the design for the three-way associations in our example is a 8×1 column vector of ones, corresponding to the 8 link functions $\eta_r(k_1, k_2, k_3)$ ($k_j = 1, 2; j = 1, 2, 3$). Replacing the elements of this vector by zeros has the effect of setting higher order association components equal to one (zero on the log scale).

Generalizations include non-block diagonal designs, and structured association such as exchangeable association, temporal association (as introduced by Fitzmaurice and Lipsitz 1995), and banded association. In many circumstances, the association structure of a given table, representing a two- or multi-way classification of several variables is of direct interest, rather than the dependence of the outcomes on covariates. Association measures are extensively studied in Goodman (1981b). We will discuss these further in Chapter 11. With the current approach, we are also able to explore the association structure of contingency tables. A typical form for the linear predictor, pertaining to a two-way association, is given by

$$\eta_{r,jh,k\ell} = \gamma + \gamma_{jh} + \gamma_{jk} + \gamma_{h\ell} + \delta_{jk}\delta_{h\ell},$$

	γ	γ_{11}	γ_{12}	γ_{21}	γ_{22}	γ_{31}	γ_{32}	ϕ_1	ϕ_2	ϕ_3
$\eta_r(1,1,3)$	1	1	0	1	0	0	0	x_{1r}	0	0
$\eta_r(1,2,3)$	1	1	0	0	1	0	0	x_{1r}	0	0
$\eta_r(2,1,3)$	1	0	1	1	0	0	0	x_{1r}	0	0
$\eta_r(2,2,3)$	1	0	1	0	1	0	0	x_{1r}	0	0
$\eta_r(1,3,1)$	1	1	0	0	0	1	0	0	x_{1r}	0
$\eta_r(1,3,2)$	1	1	0	0	0	0	1	0	x_{1r}	0
$\eta_r(2,3,1)$	1	0	1	0	0	1	0	0	x_{1r}	0
$\eta_r(2,3,2)$	1	0	1	0	0	0	1	0	x_{1r}	0
$\eta_r(3,1,1)$	1	0	0	1	0	1	0	0	0	x_{1r}
$\eta_r(3,1,2)$	1	0	0	1	0	0	1	0	0	x_{1r}
$\eta_r(3,2,1)$	1	0	0	0	1	1	0	0	0	x_{1r}
$\eta_r(3,2,2)$	1	0	0	0	1	0	1	0	0	x_{1r}

FIGURE 7.2. *Design matrix for marginal means and pairwise associations. Pairwise associations.*

including an overall intercept, effects specific to times j and h: γ_{ts}, 'row' and 'column' effects γ_{jk} and $\gamma_{h\ell}$ and multiplicative interactions. Obviously, this model is overparameterizing the association, calling for the usual restrictions.

7.4 Maximum Likelihood Estimation

In the previous section, a general framework for formulating marginal models has been sketched. We will zoom in on specific instances, the multivariate probit and Dale models, in Sections 7.6 and 7.7, respectively. But before doing so, we will discuss a general form for the likelihood equations and discuss algorithms to obtain the maximum likelihood estimator, as well as estimates of precision. When performing maximum likelihood estimation for marginal models, a crucial element is the determination of the joint probabilities. Details on these important but technical aspects are provided in Appendix 7.12.

7.5 An Influenza Study

Consider the following clinical trial. A group of 498 medical students, between 17 and 29 years of age (median 21 years), are randomized to two treatment groups. Those in the HI group receive hepatitis B vaccination (H), followed by influenza vaccination (I), whereas the reverse order is applied in the IH group. For each type of vaccination, vaccines from a company A and a company B are used. In each treatment period, the vaccines are evaluated with respect to the side effects they caused. We are interested in the outcomes *headache* and *respiratory problems*. Because both outcomes are measured in each of the two periods, we obtain a four-dimensional response variable. It is of interest to assess the strength of the association between both headache outcomes, between both respiratory outcomes, as well as to determine whether both complaints are dependent. In addition, a three-point ordinal variable, level of pain, is recorded for six days in row during the first period, supplementing the cross-over study with a longitudinal one. The first three days will be evaluated here. In order to analyze these data, we need tools for longitudinal categorical data, as well as tools for more complex designs, such as cross-over trials with several outcomes in each period. Whereas the association between outcomes is often considered a nuisance characteristic in longitudinal studies, it is usually of direct interest in multivariate settings, such as the bivariate cross-over study considered here.

We analyze the cross-over and longitudinal parts of the influenza study in turn.

7.5.1 The Cross-over Study

Let us now analyze presence/absence of headache (H) and presence/absence of respiratory problems (R), measured in both trial periods. Explicitly, the probability of absence of symptoms will be modeled. We combine marginal logits with marginal log odds ratios. The modeling is in stages. First, period effect is included. Then, a contrast between the two companies, a contrast between the two vaccinations, and an interaction term between companies and treatments is added. Further, the baseline covariates 'age' (in years) and 'sex' (0 =male, 1 =female) are included. There are three types of two-way association: between the two headache outcomes, between the two respiratory problems outcomes, and between a headache and a respiratory outcome. The two-way associations are graphically depicted in Figure 7.3. Three-way and four-way associations are assumed to be constant throughout. The results are presented in Table 7.4.

Respiratory problems are on average very infrequent, as can be seen from the high value of the intercept. For both outcomes, there is a significant period effect: there are less headaches and respiratory problems in the second period. Also, the influenza vaccination causes less headaches, but more respiratory problems. Headaches are more frequently seen in younger people, whereas the opposite holds for respiratory problems. Men suffer more from headaches after vaccination than women. The odds ratio between two respiratory problems is high (7.9), while a somewhat smaller association is

TABLE 7.4. *Influenza Study. Parameter estimates (standard errors) for the cross-over trial.*

Effect	Estimate (s.e.)
Headache	
intercept	0.055 (1.092)
period effect	0.434 (0.140)
company A effect	-0.341 (0.221)
influenza effect	0.132 (0.212)
company A-influenza interaction	-0.053 (0.281)
age	0.052 (0.054)
sex	0.875 (0.217)
Respiratory problems	
intercept	5.217 (1.297)
period effect	0.167 (0.156)
company A effect	-0.229 (0.267)
influenza effect	-0.119 (0.226)
company-influenza interaction	0.257 (0.312)
age	-0.159 (0.063)
sex	0.133 (0.243)
Associations (log odds ratios)	
headache-headache (ψ_{HH})	1.130 (0.251)
respiratory-respiratory (ψ_{RR})	2.061 (0.309)
headache-respiratory (ψ_{HR})	1.090 (0.191)
three-way interaction	0.219 (0.395)
four-way interaction	2.822 (1.462)

seen between the pair of headache measures (3.1) and between the mixed pair (3.0). This is due to the fact that respiratory problems are more severe and probably more strongly related with vaccination than headache, which can have various causes. Extending the two-way association structure to include a company effect was not significant. We found no higher-order association, although the four-way association was close to significance.

7.5.2 The Longitudinal Study

Pain was measured on six consecutive days after vaccination. Changes in response are mainly observed during the first three days. Significant predictors for the evolution of pain level are 'sex,' 'age,' the use of medication ('med'), and the actual vaccination. The effect of all covariates is allowed to change over time. As there are four vaccinations, we decompose them into two factors (company, influenza, and the interaction). At each measurement time, there are two intercepts, corresponding to two cumulative logits [no pain (0) versus pain (1 and 2); no or mild pain (0 and 1) versus moderate

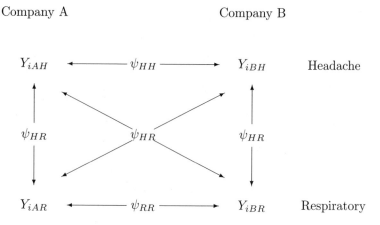

FIGURE 7.3. *Influenza Study. Association structure for the cross-over study.*

pain (2)]. All covariates are allowed to have a different effect at each measurement, presented as 'sex' (overall), 'sex' (linear), and 'sex' (quadratic). The results are presented in Table 7.5. We observe strong quadratic time effects for company A and for the interaction between company A and influenza. Considering the hepatitis vaccine for company B as the baseline, the differences (for each measurement time) on the logit scale between each vaccine and the baseline are: for the influenza vaccine of company A: −5.33, 0.85, and −1.10; for the influenza vaccine of company B: −1.36, 1.95, and 0.43; for the hepatitis vaccine of company A: −4.18, −1.15, and −1.71. The combination of a strong interaction between company and type of vaccine and of the change of the effects over time, yields a complex picture. As the outcomes are modeled via marginal logits, they are interpreted using standard logistic regression methodology. Making comparisons for the three measurement times, we are able to study the evolution of differences over time.

7.6 The Multivariate Probit Model

Section 7.3 presented a general framework to formulate marginal models for categorical data. One of the models mentioned in particular was the multivariate probit model. In this section, we will study this model in more detail. We will refer to the bivariate version as the BPM (bivariate probit

TABLE 7.5. *Influenza Study. Parameter estimates (standard errors) for the longitudinal data.*

	Estimate (s.e.)		
	Marginal parameters		
Effect	Average	Linear	Quadratic
intercept 1	-2.34(1.00)	1.24(0.93)	-0.60(0.36)
intercept 2	0.34(1.00)	0.89(0.93)	-0.80(0.37)
age	0.15(0.05)	-0.01(0.05)	0.05(0.02)
sex	0.43(0.19)	-0.31(0.17)	-0.01(0.07)
medication	-0.47(0.22)	-0.26(0.19)	0.07(0.08)
company A effect	1.23(0.27)	0.37(0.27)	-0.39(0.11)
influenza effect	-0.74(0.21)	0.08(0.19)	-0.11(0.07)
company-influenza interaction	-1.06(0.34)	-0.26(0.32)	0.34(0.12)
Associations (log odds ratios)			
time 1–time 2	1.81(0.21)		
time 1–time 3	0.98(0.26)		
time 2–time 3	3.40(0.41)		
three-way interaction	0.88(0.63)		

model), TPM (trivariate probit model) for the trivariate version, and MPM (multivariate probit model) for the general case.

7.6.1 Probit Models

The bivariate probit methodology will be introduced with the data from the BIRNH study, where smoking and drinking behavior in a general population is studied (Kesteloot, Geboers, and Joossens 1989). Risk factors for these two endpoints are determined but the main interest lies in the association between smoking and drinking. The main question is whether this association changes over demographic variables such as age, sex, and social status. The same data will be analyzed with the bivariate Dale model (BDM).

The BIRNH (Belgian Interuniversity Research on Nutrition and Health) study was conducted in the period 1980–1984 (Kesteloot, Geboers, and Joossens 1989). A stratified random sample from 42 counties of Belgium was taken to study the effect of nutrition on health. We are interested in modeling the relationship between alcohol drinking and smoking habits on the one hand and certain demographic variables on the other hand. Complete data were obtained from 5485 men and 4856 women.

Alcohol is divided into 4 classes according to daily intake: (0, 0–10, 10–30, >30). Smoking is divided into 3 classes: (never smoked, ex-smoker, smoker). Predictors variables are: 'sex' (coded as 1 for males and 2 for females), 'age,' 'weight,' 'height,' body mass index ('BMI'), 'site' within

Belgium (1: Flanders, 2: elsewhere), and social status. Age, weight, and height are categorized using the midpoints of their 10 unit classes, for BMI we chose classes of 5 units. Two variables describe social status: 'social 1' [employment (1) versus unemployment or housework (0)] and 'social 2' [working at home (1) *versus* working outside (0)]. Four questions were of interest:

1. Is there a relationship between drinking and smoking behavior?

2. Is alcohol consumption related to the demographic variables?

3. Is smoking behavior related to the demographic variables?

4. Is the association between smoking and drinking dependent on certain demographic variables, i.e., does the relationship change in certain subgroups?

It will be shown below that the BPM is adequate to answer all those questions.

7.6.2 Tetrachoric and Polychoric Correlation

Assume first that we have divided the study population into drinkers/non-drinkers and smokers/non-smokers. With a homogeneous group, a fourfold table will show whether there is an association between drinking and smoking. For measures of association we can take the cross-product (odds) ratio or the tetrachoric correlation ρ, i.e., the correlation of the underlying, doubly dichotomized bivariate normal, which was introduced almost a century ago (Pearson 1900). For the latter case, we assume that the dichotomous variables smoking (1 =no, 2 =yes) and alcohol drinking (1 =no, 2 =yes) are each discrete categorizations of continuous unobservable random variables. These latent variables follow from a bivariate standard normal (Φ_2) distribution with correlation ρ, and for each variable there is a single threshold that partitions the distribution. The two cutpoints ϕ_1 and ϕ_2 give rise to four quadrants (Figure 7.4). The percentages in the four cells then correspond to the probabilities of the four quadrants under Φ_2, and an estimate of the thresholds is obtained by equating the observed proportions to the theoretical probabilities. The correlation coefficient, called the tetrachoric correlation, is estimated from the thresholds and a series expansion.

If the original classification of drinking and smoking is used, then a 4 × 3-contingency table arises. Similar to the above, we can assume a bivariate normal distribution with correlation ρ. However, there are now three cutpoints in the 'drinking' latent variable and two cutpoints in the 'smoking' variable (see Figure 7.5). The underlying correlation is now called the polychoric correlation. For computational reasons considering a 10% random sample, we obtained a polychoric correlation of 0.25, which is highly

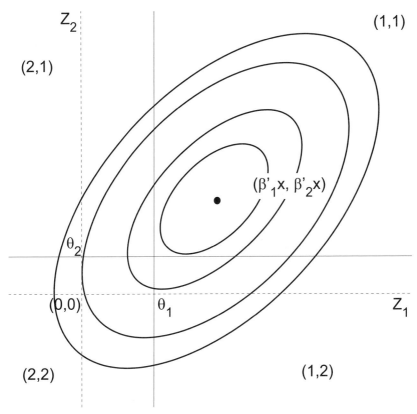

FIGURE 7.4. *Two-dimensional latent space, thresholds θ_1 and θ_2. The bivariate normal density with mean $(\beta'_1 x, \beta'_2 x)'$ and correlation ρ is indicated by the elliptical contours.*

significant ($p < 0.0001$); the p-value is obtained from a Wald test for no correlation.

7.6.3 The Univariate Probit Model

To investigate the relationship between alcohol drinking (yes/no) and the explanatory variables, we would normally use the logistic model. Alternatively, the univariate probit model can be employed. Specifically this model states that the probability of alcohol drinking equals $\Phi(\beta'_1 x)$, where $x = (1, x_1, \ldots, x_{p-1})'$ is the vector of covariates and β_1 the vector of unknown regression parameters. Although not necessary, this model can be justified by the existence of an unobservable latent variable that has a normal distribution with a mean dependent on the covariates. A similar model can be proposed to model smoking behavior. Furthermore, the univariate

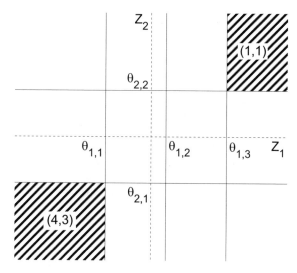

FIGURE 7.5. *Integration areas for a 4×3 BPM. The areas for the response combinations $(1,1)$ and $(4,3)$ are shaded.*

probit model (and the logistic model) can be extended to handle discrete, ordinal response variables.

However, the weakness of this approach lies in the fact that the two response variables are modeled separately, thereby neglecting their association. This will result in less efficient estimates of the parameters even though they are consistent. More importantly, we would obtain severely distorted estimates of the probabilities of combined responses, the so-called joint or union probabilities. This will be illustrated further in Section 7.10.

For the BIRNH study, parameter estimates (standard errors) are presented in Table 7.7. We selected the important risk factors using forward selection based on the score statistic (but the selected models based on the log-likelihood ratio criterion were identical). In Table 7.6, we show the two estimated univariate probit models, next to the bivariate probit model, based on the 10% random sample. The intercepts are the threshold values that determine the classes of the ordinal response variables. The interpretation of these models poses no difficulties, for example, both univariate analyses indicate that women drink and smoke less than men; from the first model we infer that, on average, Flemish people consume less alcohol than elsewhere in the country, and so on.

7.6.4 The Bivariate Probit Model

If there is heterogeneity in the study population, then a single two-by-two or $I \times J$ contingency table, of the type described in Chapter 6, will give a distorted picture of the real association between the two behaviors. The

TABLE 7.6. *BIRNH Study. Univariate and bivariate probit analysis on a 10% random sample of the original set of data.*

	Estimate (s.e.)	
Effect	Univariate	Bivariate
Alcohol		
intercept 1	-1.07 (0.14)	-1.04 (0.14)
intercept 2	-0.69 (0.14)	-0.66 (0.14)
intercept 3	0.07 (0.14)	0.09 (0.14)
sex	0.70 (0.08)	0.69 (0.08)
social 1	-0.29 (0.07)	-0.31 (0.07)
site	0.21 (0.07)	0.21 (0.07)
Smoking		
intercept 1	-3.77 (0.35)	-3.75 (0.35)
intercept 2	-3.18 (0.34)	-3.16 (0.34)
sex	-1.15 (0.09)	-1.15 (0.09)
BMI 2	0.05 (0.01)	0.05 (0.01)
age($\times 10$)	0.12 (0.03)	0.11 (0.03)
social 1	0.23 (0.10)	0.21 (0.10)
social 2	0.25 (0.09)	0.24 (0.09)
Correlation coefficient		
intercept		0.41 (0.13)
sex		-0.30 (0.09)
social 2		0.17 (0.10)
log-likelihood	-2287.06	-2281.01

reason is that part of the association can be "explained" by the confounding effect of the (un)measured variables causing the heterogeneity. The BPM takes account of this effect while calculating the tetrachoric correlation.

In Section 7.3, the multivariate probit model was presented as one member of a general class. Here, we will provide more insight into the genesis of this particular model by first focusing on the bivariate case and then consider the specific approach of an underlying (bivariate) continuous density.

Suppose that there is an underlying but unobservable latent variable $W_s (\equiv W_1)$ that expresses the resistance of an individual to smoking, and further suppose that the individual will smoke if W_s is less than a threshold θ_1. Similarly, we assume that there is a $W_a (\equiv W_2)$ that reflects an individual's attitude toward alcohol consumption and that the individual will be a drinker if W_2 is less than θ_2. We assume that $\boldsymbol{W} = (W_1, W_2)'$ has a bivariate normal density with mean vector $\boldsymbol{\mu} = (\mu_1, \mu_2)'$ and with correlation ρ. Further, assume that each subject has a p-dimensional vector of explanatory variables, $\boldsymbol{x} = (x_0, x_1, \ldots, x_{p-1})'$ with $x_0 \equiv 1$, which has the following effect on the mean vector:

$$\mu_j = \boldsymbol{\beta}'_j \boldsymbol{x}, \quad (j = 1, 2).$$

Thus, by contrast to Section 7.6.2, we now assume that the distribution depends on $\boldsymbol{x}$ and that each individual with covariate vector $\boldsymbol{x}$ is supposed to have a latent bivariate normal attitude distribution with mean vector $(\boldsymbol{\beta}'_1 \boldsymbol{x}, \boldsymbol{\beta}'_2 \boldsymbol{x})'$ and correlation ρ. In other words, the covariates move the mean vector of the two-dimensional Normal density over the plane. This results in the BPM first suggested by Ashford and Sowden (1970).

The cell probabilities for the fourfold table are again given by the probability of a quadrant under a suitable normal distribution. In Figure 7.4, we show the quadrants corresponding to the four cells of the two-by-two contingency table. The probability that a particular combination occurs is then obtained from the volume under the density surface taken in by the corresponding quadrant. For example, the probability of cell $(2, 2)$ in the fourfold table for an individual with covariate vector $\boldsymbol{x}$ is equal to the volume under the normal density $N(\boldsymbol{\beta}'_1 \boldsymbol{x}, \boldsymbol{\beta}'_2 \boldsymbol{x}; \rho)$ for the quadrant $]-\infty, \theta_1[\times]-\infty, \theta_2[$. The quadrant probabilities are also the class of posterior probabilities for each individual once the vector of covariates $\boldsymbol{x}$, is known. Let $\boldsymbol{Y}$ be the two-dimensional vector with first component $Y_1 = 1$ or 2 corresponding to 'non-drinker' or 'drinker,' respectively. The second component Y_2 is defined similarly with respect to smoking. Let $\boldsymbol{y}$ denote the observed values. The class H_y will then contain all cases with the combination of the two response classes corresponding to $\boldsymbol{y}$. We will use

$$\mu_{k_1 k_2}(\boldsymbol{\beta}; \rho | \boldsymbol{x}) = P(Y_1 = k_1, Y_2 = k_2 | \boldsymbol{\beta}, \rho, \boldsymbol{x})$$

to denote the posterior probability of H_y, conditional on $\boldsymbol{x}$. Formally, the BPM assumes

$$\begin{aligned}
\mu_{11}(\boldsymbol{\beta}; \rho | \boldsymbol{x}) &= \Phi_2(\boldsymbol{\beta}'_1 \boldsymbol{x}, \boldsymbol{\beta}'_2 \boldsymbol{x}; \rho), \\
\mu_{12}(\boldsymbol{\beta}; \rho | \boldsymbol{x}) &= \Phi(\boldsymbol{\beta}'_1 \boldsymbol{x}) - p_{11}(\boldsymbol{\beta}; \rho | \boldsymbol{x}), \\
\mu_{21}(\boldsymbol{\beta}; \rho | \boldsymbol{x}) &= \Phi(\boldsymbol{\beta}'_2 \boldsymbol{x}) - p_{11}(\boldsymbol{\beta}; \rho | \boldsymbol{x}), \\
\mu_{22}(\boldsymbol{\beta}; \rho | \boldsymbol{x}) &= 1 - \mu_{12}(\boldsymbol{\beta}; \rho | \boldsymbol{x}) - \mu_{21}(\boldsymbol{\beta}; \rho | \boldsymbol{x}) - \mu_{11}(\boldsymbol{\beta}; \rho | \boldsymbol{x}),
\end{aligned} \quad (7.28)$$

with $\beta_{j0} = \theta_j - \alpha_{j0} (j = 1, 2)$, and $\beta_{js} = -\alpha_{js} (s = 1, \ldots, p; j = 1, 2)$, where $\Phi(a)$ is the standard normal distribution in a and $\Phi_2(a_1, a_2)$ the standard bivariate normal distribution with mean 0 and correlation ρ. Morimune (1979) extended this model by letting ρ depend on $\boldsymbol{x}$, so that $\rho = \rho(\boldsymbol{\alpha}' \boldsymbol{x})$. An immediate generalization of model (7.28) is obtained by allowing more than one cutpoint for each latent variable W_j $(j = 1, 2)$. This corresponds to the analysis of $r_1 \times r_2$ contingency tables. In Figure 7.5, the integration areas are shown for a 4×3 table.

For the binary response model (7.28) we get the marginal probabilities

$$\begin{aligned} \mu_{1+}(\boldsymbol{\beta}_1|\boldsymbol{x}) &= \Phi(\boldsymbol{\beta}_1'\boldsymbol{x}), \\ \mu_{+1}(\boldsymbol{\beta}_2|\boldsymbol{x}) &= \Phi(\boldsymbol{\beta}_2'\boldsymbol{x}), \end{aligned} \qquad (7.29)$$

where the first corresponds to the probability of alcohol drinking for a specific combination of the covariates and the second to the probability of smoking. Observe that these probabilities are identical to those under a univariate probit model. However, with two univariate probit models, the joint probabilities are obtained by simple multiplication of the marginal probabilities, for example the probability of alcohol drinking and smoking is calculated as

$$\Phi(\boldsymbol{\beta}_1'\boldsymbol{x}) \cdot \Phi(\boldsymbol{\beta}_2'\boldsymbol{x}),$$

which corresponds to $\mu_{22}(\boldsymbol{\beta}; \rho|\boldsymbol{x})$ under the BPM only if $\rho = 0$. Thus, by employing two univariate probit models for the analysis of correlated binary response variables, we explicitly assume that $\rho = 0$ in a BPM. Clearly, the same reasoning applies to discrete ordinal responses.

To conclude the model specification, we suppose that there are N independent subsamples, where the rth subsample is characterized by the covariate vector $\boldsymbol{x}_r$. Within the rth subsample, we have N_r independent observations. The corresponding counts are $Z_{r\boldsymbol{y}}$, the number of occurrences of response $\boldsymbol{y}$ in the rth subsample. If $S_j = \{1, 2\}$ denotes the set of levels of the jth characteristic in the binary case, then $S = S_1 \times S_2$ contains all possible combinations of characteristics. Given $\boldsymbol{x}_r$, the counts

$$(Z_{r\boldsymbol{y}}, \boldsymbol{y} \in S)$$

are multinomially distributed with N_r replicates and probability vector

$$(\mu_{r\boldsymbol{y}} = p_{\boldsymbol{y}}(\boldsymbol{\beta}; \rho|\boldsymbol{x}_r), \boldsymbol{y} \in S). \qquad (7.30)$$

To estimate the unknown parameters $\boldsymbol{\beta}$ and ρ, the likelihood of the sample under the model is needed and is given by

$$\ell(\boldsymbol{\beta}, \rho) = \sum_{r=1}^{N} \sum_{\boldsymbol{y} \in S} z_{r\boldsymbol{y}} \ln \mu_{r\boldsymbol{y}}. \qquad (7.31)$$

A maximum likelihood estimate of $(\boldsymbol{\beta}', \rho)$, denoted by $(\widehat{\boldsymbol{\beta}}', \hat{\rho})$, is obtained by maximizing (7.31) with respect to the unknown parameters. The negative inverse of the second derivative of the log-likelihood provides the estimated covariance matrix of the parameters.

For the BIRNH study, a bivariate selection procedure, based on the score statistic, selected the variables: 'sex' ($p < 0.0001$); 'BMI' ($p < 0.0001$); 'age' ($p = 0.0003$); 'social 1' ($p = 0.0033$); 'site' ($p = 0.0071$) and 'social 2' ($p =$

0.0197). Taking these covariates into account, the polychoric correlation coefficient dropped from 0.25 to 0.059 ($p = 0.16$). Thus, it seems that all correlation between drinking and smoking was induced by the confounding effect of the demographic variables.

The score statistic to test the hypothesis of a constant correlation coefficient (that is whether or not Morimune's extension is needed) equals 13.56, which referred to a chi-squared distribution with 4 degrees of freedom, indicating dependence of the correlation on the predictors ($p = 0.035$). Based on the significance of the regression coefficients, both 'sex' ($p = 0.001$) and 'social 2' ($p = 0.048$) seem to have an impact on the polychoric correlation. Thus in the next step, besides the constant, 'sex' and 'social 2' were also included in the model for ρ; the regression coefficients are 0.45 ($p = 0.0004$) for the constant, -0.33 ($p = 0.0004$) for 'sex' and 0.18 ($p = 0.068$) for 'social 2.'

Up to now, the same covariate vector has been employed for both responses. This is not necessary and in a further step we retained only the significant ($p < 0.05$) covariates in modelling the marginal dependencies. As can be seen from Table 7.6, the bivariate probit regression coefficients are very close to those obtained from the univariate probit regressions. This model, applied to the full dataset, gave similar regression coefficients that are not reported here.

For 14 of the 16 combinations of 'sex,' 'social 1,' 'social 2,' and 'site' it was possible to calculate the polychoric correlation locally with only 'age' and 'BMI' as predictors. There is reasonable agreement between global and local estimates, except for the two outlying correlations in the ('sex=female,' 'social 2=1') combination, but these were based on relatively small numbers, 168 and 229 cases, respectively.

Thus, the BPM indicates the same dependence of the responses on the demographic variables as the two univariate probit models, but it has provided extra information about the relationship between alcohol drinking and smoking. We conclude this analysis by observing that the BPM has nicely discerned the predictors affecting the marginal risk of alcohol drinking and smoking from those which affect the relationship between these two habits.

7.6.5 Ordered Categorical Outcomes

As stated before, the probit models can be generalized from binary outcome variables to ordered categorical outcomes. In this case, $\boldsymbol{Y} = (Y_1, Y_2)'$ is a bivariate stochastic vector of discrete ordered variables. Without loss of generality, assume that $Y_j \in S_j \equiv \{1, \ldots, c_j\}$, ($j = 1, 2$).

Again, we assume that $\boldsymbol{Y}$ is a discretized version of an unobservable latent stochastic vector $\boldsymbol{W} = (W_1, W_2)'$ with bivariate normal cumulative distribution function having mean vector $\boldsymbol{\mu} = (\mu_1, \mu_2)'$ standard deviations

7.6 The Multivariate Probit Model

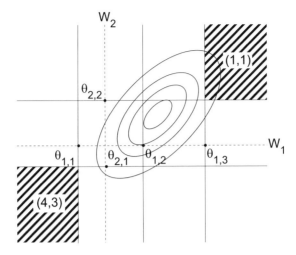

FIGURE 7.6. *Graphical representation of assumed underlying latent space of BPM. The areas for the response combinations (1,1) and (3,4) are shaded. The contours correspond to the surfaces of equal density of the bivariate normal density.*

$\sigma_1 = \sigma_2 = 1$ and correlation coefficient ρ. Then, $c_j - 1$ finite thresholds

$$-\infty \equiv \theta_{j0} < \theta_{j1} < \ldots < \theta_{j,c_j-1} < \theta_{jc_j} \equiv +\infty, \quad (j = 1, 2), \qquad (7.32)$$

result in the vector Y by defining

$$Y_j = k \iff \theta_{j,k-1} \leq W_j < \theta_{jk},$$

with $k \in S_j$. The W-space, the bivariate normal density and its associated subdivision are graphically depicted in Figure 7.6, for $c_1 = 4$ and $c_2 = 3$. The association between Y_1 and Y_2 is expressed as the correlation between the latent variables W_1 and W_2; ρ is called the polychoric correlation (Pearson 1900).

Again, the model description is complete if we specify the link function between x and Y. The probability that $Y = (k_1, k_2)'$, given x, is equal to the probability $p_{k_1 k_2}(x)$ that W lies in the rectangle

$$R_{k_1 k_2}(x) = [\theta_{1,k_1-1}(x), \theta_{1k_1}(x)] \times [\theta_{2,k_2-1}(x), \theta_{2k_2}(x)],$$

where $\theta_{jk}(x) = \theta_{jk} - \boldsymbol{\beta}_j' x$. Specifically, for a BPM where ρ does not depend on the covariates:

$$\mu_{k_1 k_2}(x) = P(Y_1 = k_1, Y_2 = k_2 | x) = \iint_{R_{k_1 k_2}(x)} \phi_2(w, \rho) dw, \qquad (7.33)$$

where $\phi_2(w, \rho)$ denotes the standard bivariate normal density with correlation ρ. If ρ depends on the covariates, it is given by

$$\rho = \rho(\boldsymbol{\alpha}' x). \qquad (7.34)$$

Often, ρ is replaced by Fisher's z transform, as in the second component of (7.12), which takes values in $\mathbb{R}$:

$$\varphi = \ln\left(\frac{1+\rho}{1-\rho}\right).$$

Using such a transformation avoids estimates to jump out of the interval $[-1, +1]$ and is especially useful when covariates are allowed, as in (7.34).

7.6.6 The Multivariate Probit Model

When the latent vector $\boldsymbol{W}$ has an n-dimensional normal distribution, that is when there are n characteristics or repeated measures, and the probability of each diagnostic class conditional on a risk vector $\boldsymbol{x}$ is again an integral over an orthant, the n-dimensional generalization of the quadrant, as in (7.28), we apply a MPM. As for the BPM the n-dimensional response vector can also consist of ordinal discrete responses with integration areas as in Figures 7.5 and 7.6. Anderson and Pemberton (1985) employed a trivariate probit model for the analysis of data on blackbirds. They fitted the model using by fitting the univariate margins independently, supplemented with the correlation parameters assembled from fitting bivariate probit models to all pairs of outcomes. Here, a fully general approach will be presented, but the approximate solution can be a viable option when computations become too cumbersome, e.g., when dimensionality is high.

Thus, a MPM of dimension n actually consists of n marginal probability distributions each corresponding to a particular characteristic and $n(n-1)/2$ polychoric correlations expressing the association between the occurences of the n characteristics. If the correlations equal zero then the marginal probability distributions are sufficient to generate the probabilities of all combinations of characteristics, if not, then the multivariate probability distributions are needed.

In analogy with the bivariate case, we suppose that there is a sample of N independent subsamples available, where the rth subsample is characterized by the covariate vector $\boldsymbol{x}_r$. The observed response vector is denoted by

$$\boldsymbol{y} = (y_1, \ldots, y_n)' \in \prod_{j=1}^{n} S_j.$$

Within the rth subsample, we have N_r independent replications. The number of occurrences of response $\boldsymbol{y}$ in the rth subsample is denoted as $z_{j\boldsymbol{y}}$. Given $\boldsymbol{x}_r$, the counts

$$\left(z_r\boldsymbol{y}, \boldsymbol{y} \in \prod_j S_j\right)$$

are multinomially distributed with N_r replications and probability vector

$$\left(\mu_{ry}(\boldsymbol{\theta}) = \mu_y(\boldsymbol{\theta}|\boldsymbol{x}_r), \boldsymbol{y} \in \prod_j S_j\right),$$

where $\boldsymbol{\theta}$ is the total parameter vector containing both regression and association parameters. Finally, the log-likelihood of the sample under the specified model is given by

$$\ell(\boldsymbol{\theta}) = \sum_{j=1}^N \sum_{\boldsymbol{y} \in \prod_j S_j} z_{ry} \ln p_{ry}(\boldsymbol{\theta}). \tag{7.35}$$

The maximum likelihood estimate of $\boldsymbol{\theta}$, denoted by $\widehat{\boldsymbol{\theta}}$, is obtained by maximizing (7.35) with respect to the unknown parameters.

7.7 The Dale Model

7.7.1 Two Binary Responses

Suppose that for each of N subjects in a study a vector $\boldsymbol{Y}_i = (Y_{i1}, Y_{i2})'$ of two binary responses is observed, together with a vector of covariates $\boldsymbol{x}$. The vector $\boldsymbol{x}$ can be different for each response as in longitudinal studies with time-dependent covariates. Thus, the study subjects are described by $(y_{i1}, y_{i2}, \boldsymbol{x}_{ij}), (i = 1, \ldots, N; j = 1, 2)$. Just as with the bivariate probit model, we want to establish the dependence of each of the two responses on the covariate vector(s), taking the dependence between the responses into account.

Dale (1986) proposed a family of bivariate response models arising from the decomposition of the joint probabilities $\mu_{k_1 k_2}(\boldsymbol{x}) = P(Y_1 = k_1, Y_2 = k_2|\boldsymbol{x}), (k_1, k_2 = 1, 2)$, into 'main effects' and 'interactions.' The marginal probabilities describe the main effect and the log cross-ratio is the interaction term. Formally, this decomposition is given by

$$h_1\left(\mu_{1+}(\boldsymbol{x})\right) = \boldsymbol{\beta}_1'\boldsymbol{x}, \tag{7.36}$$

$$h_2\left(\mu_{+1}(\boldsymbol{x})\right) = \boldsymbol{\beta}_2'\boldsymbol{x}, \tag{7.37}$$

$$h_3\left(\frac{\mu_{11}(\boldsymbol{x})\mu_{22}(\boldsymbol{x})}{\mu_{12}(\boldsymbol{x})\mu_{21}(\boldsymbol{x})}\right) = \boldsymbol{\beta}_3'\boldsymbol{x}, \tag{7.38}$$

where h_1, h_2 and h_3 are link functions in the generalized linear model terminology and $\mu_{1+}(\boldsymbol{x}), \mu_{+1}(\boldsymbol{x})$ are the marginal probabilities for observing $Y_1 = 1$, and $Y_2 = 1$, respectively. The most popular choice for $h_1 \equiv h_2$ is the logit function, whereas for h_3 the natural logarithmic function is commonly used. In that case, one has two marginal logistic regression models and the logarithm of the cross-ratio

$$\ln \psi(\boldsymbol{x}) = \ln\left(\frac{\mu_{11}(\boldsymbol{x})\mu_{22}(\boldsymbol{x})}{\mu_{12}(\boldsymbol{x})\mu_{21}(\boldsymbol{x})}\right) \tag{7.39}$$

is linear in the covariates. Note that (7.39) is in line with (7.21), for the specific situation of two binary outcomes.

The joint probabilities follow from the marginal probabilities in the following way, where we have omitted the dependence of the different terms on $\boldsymbol{x}$ for the ease of notation (Plackett 1965):

$$\mu_{11} = \begin{cases} \dfrac{1 + (\mu_{1+} + \mu_{+1})(\psi - 1) - S(\mu_{1+}, \mu_{+1}, \psi)}{2(\psi - 1)} & \text{if } \psi \neq 1, \\ \mu_{1+}\mu_{+1} & \text{if } \psi = 1, \end{cases} \tag{7.40}$$

and $\mu_{12} = \mu_{1+} - \mu_{11}$, $\mu_{21} = \mu_{+1} - \mu_{11}$, and $\mu_{22} = 1 - \mu_{12} - \mu_{21} - \mu_{11}$, with the function S defined by

$$S(q_1, q_2, \psi) = \sqrt{[1 + (q_1 + q_2)(\psi - 1)]^2 + 4\psi(1 - \psi)q_1 q_2},$$

for $0 \leq q_1, q_2 \leq 1$ and $0 \leq \psi < +\infty$.

Just as in the probit case, above description can also be seen as arising from the discrete realization of a continuous bivariate distribution, the Plackett distribution (Plackett 1965) in this case. Suppose the bivariate random vector $\boldsymbol{W} = (W_1, W_2)'$ has joint distribution function $F(w_1, w_2)$, with marginal distributions $F(w_j)$ $(j = 1, 2)$. Define the (global) cross-ratio function, or global odds ratio function, $\psi(w_1, w_2)$, by

$$\psi(w_1, w_2) = \frac{\mu_{11}\mu_{22}}{\mu_{12}\mu_{21}} = \frac{F(1 - F_1 - F_2 + F)}{(F_1 - F)(F_2 - F)}, \tag{7.41}$$

with $F_j \equiv F_j(w_j)$, $(j = 1, 2)$ and $F \equiv F(w_1, w_2)$. It is clear that $\psi(w_1, w_2)$ satisfies $0 \leq \psi \leq \infty$. The components $\mu_{k_1 k_2}$ in (7.41) are the quadrant probabilities in $\mathbb{R}^2$ with vertex at (w_1, w_2). For a Plackett distribution, the global cross-ratio $\psi(w_1, w_2) \equiv \psi$ is constant. Expression (7.41) can be seen as a defining equation for F, once F_1, F_2, and ψ are known. The Plackett distribution then gives rise to the above bivariate response model if its mean vector $\boldsymbol{\mu} = (\mu_1, \mu_2)'$ depends linearly on the covariate vector and if it is assumed that $\boldsymbol{Z}$ is a discretized version of the continuous vector $\boldsymbol{W}$ in the sense that $Y_j = 1 \iff \theta_j \leq W_j$, for $j = 1, 2$. Here, θ_1, θ_2 are two a priori defined thresholds. In other words, Dale's bivariate response model is obtained if the bivariate response vector $\boldsymbol{Y}$ is a discretized version of $\boldsymbol{W}$ using the threshold vector $\boldsymbol{\theta}$, and if the covariate vector shifts the mean vector of the distribution of $\boldsymbol{W}$ over the plane, thereby possibly changing also the association parameter ψ as a function of $\boldsymbol{x}$.

7.7.2 The Bivariate Dale Model

Dale (1986) generalized above approach to model pairs of ordered categorical variables with c_1 and c_2 levels, respectively, in the presence of explanatory variables $\boldsymbol{x}$. We will refer to this as the (bivariate) *global odds ratio model*, *global cross-ratio model*, or simply *bivariate Dale model* (BDM).

Let $\boldsymbol{Y} = (Y_1, Y_2)'$ be a random vector taking on values (k_1, k_2), where $1 \leq k_j \leq c_j$ $(j = 1, 2)$. The outcomes, corresponding to a given covariate vector $\boldsymbol{x}$, can be arranged as an $c_1 \times c_2$ contingency table $(Z_{k_1 k_2})$ $(k_j = 1, \ldots, c_j; j = 1, 2)$:

z_{11}	$\cdots$	z_{1k_2}	z_{1,k_2+1}	$\cdots$	z_{1c_2}
$\vdots$	$\ddots$	$\vdots$	$\vdots$	$\ddots$	$\vdots$
$z_{k_1 1}$	$\cdots$	$z_{k_1 k_2}$	z_{k_1,k_2+1}	$\cdots$	$z_{k_1 c_2}$
$z_{k_1+1,1}$	$\cdots$	z_{k_1+1,k_2}	z_{k_1+1,k_2+1}	$\cdots$	z_{k_1+1,c_2}
$\vdots$	$\ddots$	$\vdots$	$\vdots$	$\ddots$	$\vdots$
$z_{c_1 1}$	$\cdots$	$z_{c_1 k_2}$	z_{c_1,k_2+1}	$\cdots$	$z_{c_1 c_2}$

(7.42)

Similarly, the probabilities can be represented as a $c_1 \times c_2$ table:

μ_{11}	$\cdots$	μ_{1k_2}	μ_{1,k_2+1}	$\cdots$	μ_{1c_2}
$\vdots$	$\ddots$	$\vdots$	$\vdots$	$\ddots$	$\vdots$
$\mu_{k_1 1}$	$\cdots$	$\mu_{k_1 k_2}$	μ_{k_1,k_2+1}	$\cdots$	$\mu_{k_1 c_2}$
$\mu_{k_1+1,1}$	$\cdots$	μ_{k_1+1,k_2}	μ_{k_1+1,k_2+1}	$\cdots$	μ_{k_1+1,c_2}
$\vdots$	$\ddots$	$\vdots$	$\vdots$	$\ddots$	$\vdots$
$\mu_{c_1 1}$	$\cdots$	$\mu_{c_1 k_2}$	μ_{c_1,k_2+1}	$\cdots$	$\mu_{c_1 c_2}$

(7.43)

This map establishes a lilnk between the regression and table notations (Section 7.1). Note that sparseness of these tables is not an issue, as the essence of the approach is truly of a regression type. When the number of subjects per covariate level $\boldsymbol{x}$ is small, the number of 'tables' increases with sample size, exactly as in a regression setting. However, when the number of covariate levels is small or even bounded (e.g., two sex levels), then the tables fill up, as in ANOVA and genuine contingency tables settings.

Dichotomizing contingency table (7.42) at (k_1, k_2) (double lines) leads to a 2×2 contingency table:

$\{Y_1 \leq k_1, Y_2 \leq k_2\}$	$\{Y_1 \leq k_1, Y_2 > k_2\}$
$\{Y_1 > k_1, Y_2 \leq k_2\}$	$\{Y_1 > k_1, Y_2 > k_2\}$

(7.44)

of which the probabilities are given by

$$P_{11}(k_1, k_2, \boldsymbol{x}) = P(Y_1 \leq k_1, Y_2 \leq k_2 | \boldsymbol{x}),$$

$$P_{12}(k_1, k_2, \boldsymbol{x}) = P(Y_1 \leq k_1, Y_2 > k_2 | \boldsymbol{x}),$$
$$P_{21}(k_1, k_2, \boldsymbol{x}) = P(Y_1 > k_1, Y_2 \leq k_2 | \boldsymbol{x}),$$
$$P_{22}(k_1, k_2, \boldsymbol{x}) = P(Y_1 > k_1, Y_2 > k_2 | \boldsymbol{x}).$$

Marginal probabilities are obtained by summing over subscripts: $P_{1+}(k_1, \boldsymbol{x}) = P(Y_1 \leq k_1 | \boldsymbol{x})$ and $P_{+1}(k_2, \boldsymbol{x}) = P(Y_2 \leq k_2 | \boldsymbol{x})$.

In analogy with (7.36)–(7.38), the link functions are described by

$$h_1[P_{1+}(k_1, \boldsymbol{x})] = \beta_{0,1k_1} + \boldsymbol{\beta}_1' \boldsymbol{x}, \quad (k_1 = 1, \ldots, c_1 - 1), \quad (7.45)$$
$$h_2[P_{+1}(k_2, \boldsymbol{x})] = \beta_{0,2k_2} + \boldsymbol{\beta}_2' \boldsymbol{x}, \quad (k_2 = 1, \ldots, c_2 - 1), \quad (7.46)$$
$$h_3[\psi(k_1, k_2, \boldsymbol{x})] = \boldsymbol{\alpha}' \boldsymbol{x}, \quad (k_j = 1, \ldots, c_j - 1; j = 1, 2), \quad (7.47)$$

where the global cross-ratio $\psi(k_1, k_2, \boldsymbol{x})$ is given by

$$\psi(k_1, k_2, \boldsymbol{x}) = \frac{P_{11}(k_1, k_2, \boldsymbol{x}) P_{22}(k_1, k_2, \boldsymbol{x})}{P_{12}(k_1, k_2, \boldsymbol{x}) P_{21}(k_1, k_2, \boldsymbol{x})}.$$

Note that for every contingency table (7.42) [or, equivalently, table of probabilities (7.43)], a set of $(c_1-1) \times (c_2-1)$ global cross-ratios is obtained:

ψ_{11}	$\cdots$	ψ_{1k_2}	ψ_{1,k_2+1}	$\cdots$	ψ_{1,c_2-1}
$\vdots$	$\ddots$	$\vdots$	$\vdots$	$\ddots$	$\vdots$
$\psi_{k_1 1}$	$\cdots$	$\psi_{k_1 k_2}$	ψ_{k_1,k_2+1}	$\cdots$	ψ_{k_1,c_2-1}
$\psi_{k_1+1,1}$	$\cdots$	ψ_{k_1+1,k_2}	ψ_{k_1+1,k_2+1}	$\cdots$	ψ_{k_1+1,c_2-1}
$\vdots$	$\ddots$	$\vdots$	$\vdots$	$\ddots$	$\vdots$
$\psi_{c_1-1,1}$	$\cdots$	ψ_{c_1-1,k_2}	ψ_{c_1-1,k_2+1}	$\cdots$	ψ_{c_1-1,c_2-1}

More complex choices for the linear predictors on the right hand side of (7.45)–(7.47) are possible. For instance, h_3 can incorporate terms depending on k_1 and k_2, representing row, column, and cell effects. In principle, extensions to non-linear predictors are possible too, although this would make the updating algorithms more cumbersome.

For every table (7.44), we assume that (7.41) holds with ψ replaced by $\psi(k_1, k_2, \boldsymbol{x})$, indicating that ψ is allowed to depend on the cutpoints and on the covariates. Further, $F(.|\boldsymbol{x}) \equiv F_{k_1 k_2}(.|\boldsymbol{x}) = P_{11}(k_1, k_2, \boldsymbol{x})$, and $F(.|\boldsymbol{x})$ can also be expressed in terms of the assumed underlying Plackett distribution: $F(.|\boldsymbol{x}) = P(W_1 \leq \theta_{1k_1}, W_2 \leq \theta_{2k_2}|\boldsymbol{x})$. Observe that for each double dichotomy of the $c_1 \times c_2$ table, a different underlying Plackett distribution is assumed. When it can be assumed that $\psi(k_1, k_2, \boldsymbol{x}) \equiv \psi(\boldsymbol{x})$, for $k_j = 1, \ldots, c_t - 1$ $(j = 1, 2)$, there is a single underlying Plackett distribution, exactly as for the binary response model.

7.7.3 Some Properties of the Bivariate Dale Model

Dale's model has appealing properties. First, there is the flexibility with which the marginal structure is modeled, i.e., the cumulative marginal probabilities can be fitted in the generalized linear models framework. Second, the marginal parameters are orthogonal onto the association parameters in the sense that the corresponding elements in the expected covariance matrix are identically zero (Palmgren 1989). Further, the associations can be modeled in a flexible way including covariate, row, column, and cell specific terms (Dale 1986).

The BDM does not require marginal scores for the responses and is essentially invariant under any monotonic transformation of the marginal response variables. Further, if adjacent marginal categories are combined, the model for the new table has fewer parameters, but they have the same interpretation as they had in the model for the original, expanded table, because the parameters pertain to cutpoints between categories. This is in contrast with models based on local association (Goodman 1981a), as discussed in Chapter 6.

7.7.4 The Multivariate Plackett Distribution

The computational basis of the BDM is the Plackett distribution. Therefore, we first generalize the bivariate Plackett distribution to n dimensions. In this section, we present a general description and some properties. The multivariate Plackett distribution will be the basis for the multivariate Dale model. The genesis of the distribution will automatically lead to an algorithmic way to compute cell probabilities and their derivatives. This is an alternative to the iterative proportional fitting algorithm presented in Section 7.12.3. Other alternatives are given by Lang and Agresti (1994) and Glonek and McCullagh (1995). This rather technical development is deferred to Appendix 7.13.

7.7.5 The Multivariate Dale Model

Given the multivariate Plackett distribution, the multivariate Dale model is a straightforward extension of the BDM. Let $\boldsymbol{W}_{ri} = (W_{ri1}, \ldots, W_{rin})'$ have a multivariate Plackett distribution with univariate marginals F_j, $(r = 1, \ldots, N; i = 1, \ldots, N_r; j = 1, \ldots, n)$ and a particular set of generalized global cross-ratios. Further, let $\boldsymbol{Y}_{ri} = (Y_{ri1}, \ldots, Y_{rin})'$ be a vector of ordered categorical variables with Y_{rij} assuming values $k_j = 1, \ldots, c_j$, $(j = 1, \ldots, n)$. Thus, in analogy with the bivariate case, $\boldsymbol{Y}_{ri}$ is a discrete realization of $\boldsymbol{W}_{ri}$. The covariates at level r are indicated by $\boldsymbol{x}_r$. Both the marginal distributions and the cross-ratios can depend on the covariates.

For each multi-index $\boldsymbol{k} = (k_1, \ldots, k_n)$ with $1 \leq k_j < c_j$, $(j = 1, \ldots, n)$, define a 2^n-*dichotomization table (multiple dichotomy)*:

$$T_{\boldsymbol{k}} = \{\mathcal{O}_{\boldsymbol{s}}(\boldsymbol{k}) | \boldsymbol{s} \in \{-1, 1\}^n\},$$

where

$$\mathcal{O}_{\boldsymbol{s}}(\boldsymbol{k}) = \{\mathbf{Y}_{ri} | Y_{rij} \leq k_j \text{ if } s_j = -1 \text{ and } Y_{rij} > k_j \text{ if } s_j = 1\}.$$

This means that, at every n-dimensional cutpoint, the data table is collapsed into a $2 \times 2 \times \ldots \times 2$ table. Observe the analogy with the bivariate case, as well as with the probit case (Section 7.6). For $n = 2$, $T_{\boldsymbol{k}}$ contains the four corners of the $c_1 \times c_2$ contingency table, split up at $\boldsymbol{k} = (k_1, k_2)$.

Every table is assumed to arise as a discretization of a multivariate Plackett distribution. The n marginal distributions are modeled, together with all pairs of two-way cross-ratios. In addition, three-way up to n-way interactions (generalized cross-ratios) are included to fully specify the joint distribution. Formally, we assume that for each $T_{\boldsymbol{k}}$, (7.69) holds with a cross-ratio possibly depending on $\boldsymbol{k}$ and $\boldsymbol{x}_r$, i.e., $\psi_{1\ldots n}$ is replaced by $\psi(\boldsymbol{k}; \boldsymbol{x}_r)$. Further,

$$\begin{aligned} F \equiv F_{\boldsymbol{k}}(.|\boldsymbol{x}_r) &= P(Y_{ri1} \leq k_1, \ldots, Y_{rin} \leq k_n | \boldsymbol{x}) \\ &= P(W_{ri1} \leq \theta_{1k_1}, \ldots, W_{rin} \leq \theta_{nk_n} | \boldsymbol{x}_r). \end{aligned}$$

The model description is complete by specifying link functions and linear predictors for both the univariate marginals and the association parameters. If we assume a marginal proportional odds model, then the marginal links can be written as:

$$\eta_{rijk}(\boldsymbol{x}_r) = h_j \left[P(Y_{rij} \leq k | \boldsymbol{x}_r) \right] = \beta_{0,jk} + \boldsymbol{\beta}'_j \boldsymbol{x}_r, \qquad (7.48)$$
$$(1 \leq j \leq n, 1 \leq k < c_j).$$

Expression (7.48) can be represented in terms of the latent variables as well:

$$h_j \left[P(W_{rij} \leq \theta_{jk} | \boldsymbol{x}_r) \right] = \beta_{0,jk} + \boldsymbol{\beta}'_j \boldsymbol{x}_r, \quad (1 \leq j \leq n, 1 \leq k < c_j).$$

As in the bivariate case, common choices for the link functions h_j are the logit and the probit link.

The cross-ratios are usually log-linearly modeled. Covariate terms may be included, together with row, column, and cell-specific terms. A possible choice consists of complex models for the bivariate associations and simple ones for the higher order associations. For a fixed pair of variables (j_1, j_2), where $1 \leq j_1 < j_2 \leq n$, one can model the log cross-ratio as

$$\gamma_{j_1 j_2}^{k_1 k_2}(\boldsymbol{x}_r) = \ln \psi_{j_1 j_2}(k_1, k_2, \boldsymbol{x}_r) = \nu + \rho_{k_1} + \kappa_{k_2} + \tau_{k_1 k_2} + \boldsymbol{x}'_r \boldsymbol{\beta}_{j_1 j_2}. \quad (7.49)$$

Here, ν is an intercept parameter, ρ_{k_1} ($k_1 = 1, \ldots, c_1 - 1$) are row-specific parameters, κ_{k_2} ($k_2 = 1, \ldots, c_2 - 1$) are column parameters, and $\tau_{k_1 k_2}$ ($k_1 =$

$1, \ldots, c_1 - 1; k_2 = 1, \ldots, c_2 - 1)$ are cell-specific parameters. Uniqueness constraints need to be imposed on the row, column, and cell parameters. For instance, $\rho_1 = 0$, $\kappa_1 = 0$, $\tau_{k_1 1} = 0, (k_1 = 1, \ldots, c_1 - 1)$, and $\tau_{1 k_2} = 0, (k_2 = 1, \ldots, c_2 - 1)$. The higher order associations usually are assumed to be constant. Parameter estimates are obtained using the maximum likelihood method.

As this model description yields the BDM for $n = 2$, it follows that the attractiveness and the flexibility of the original two-dimensional version is carried over on its n-dimensional version. However, not all properties of the BDM are inherited by the MDM. As mentioned above, Palmgren (1989) shows that the estimated marginal and association parameters are orthogonal. This result does not carry over onto the MDM, although Molenberghs and Lesaffre (1994) have shown it holds approximately for lower order associations, while it fully holds for the n-way association.

Having specified the model, the links and the linear predictors, the model parameters can be estimated by the ML estimation method. The use of the multivariate Plackett distribution makes it easy to compute both the joint probabilities and their derivatives. A Fisher scoring algorithm is a good choice, as it also provides us with the asymptotic expected covariance matrix for the model parameters.

The model formulated above still fits within the general log-contrasts of probabilities framework given by (7.17), as it should be, given the presentation here is merely a more elaborate introduction of the MDM, with an alternative way to compute the cell probabilities.

7.7.6 Maximum Likelihood Estimation

Section 7.4 sketched a general framework for maximum likelihood estimation, using the iterative proportional fitting algorithm. Here, we will specialize to the MDM, using the Plackett probability formulation. Essentially, for every individual or every covariate level, the kernel of a multinomial log-likelihood can be used, considering a highly structured n-way contingency table merely as a collection of multinomial cells.

Despite the fact that the Plackett distribution is only known implicitly, its values can be computed in an efficient way using numerical algorithms. Further, the derivatives of the Plackett cumulative distribution function can be evaluated in an analytical way, using implicit derivation. Based on these results, the score functions and the expected Fisher information matrix can be used to implement a convenient Fisher scoring algorithm. Details are presented in Appendix 7.14.

7.7.7 The BIRNH Study

In this section, we reconsider the BIRNH study, analyzed before in Section 7.6.1. We compare performance of the BPM, the bivariate Dale model

TABLE 7.7. *BIRNH Study. Parameter estimates (standard errors) for the bivariate models [BPM: bivariate probit model; BDM: bivariate Dale model with normal (N) or logistic (L) margins] with constant association parameter (the correlation coefficient for the BPM and the global cross-ratio for the BDM).*

Effect	BPM	BDM-N	BDM-L
	Alcohol		
Intercept 1	-1.07(0.14)	-1.07(0.14)	-1.69(0.23)
Intercept 2	-0.68(0.14)	-0.69(0.14)	-1.07(0.23)
Intercept 3	0.07(0.14)	0.07(0.14)	0.20(0.23)
Sex	0.70(0.08)	0.70(0.07)	1.11(0.12)
Social 1	-0.29(0.07)	-0.29(0.07)	-0.49(0.12)
Site	0.21(0.07)	0.21(0.07)	0.35(0.12)
	Smoking		
Intercept 1	-3.76(0.35)	-3.76(0.35)	-6.24(0.60)
Intercept 2	-3.17(0.34)	-3.18(0.34)	-5.25(0.59)
Sex	1.15(0.09)	1.16(0.09)	1.92(0.15)
BMI	0.04(0.01)	0.04(0.01)	0.07(0.02)
Age(×10)	0.12(0.03)	0.12(0.03)	0.20(0.06)
Social 1	0.22(0.10)	0.22(0.10)	0.36(0.16)
Social 2	0.25(0.08)	0.24(0.09)	0.41(0.15)
Association	0.06(0.04)	0.18(0.12)	0.18(0.11)
Log-likelihood	-2286.12	-2285.87	-2286.58

(BDM) with probit (N) and logistic (L) margins, in modeling the relationship between alcohol drinking and smoking habits on the one hand and certain demographic variables on the other hand.

Tables 7.7–7.9 present the estimates for several models. The BPM column in Table 7.8 coincides with the bivariate column in Table 7.6. The three models in Table 7.7 have a very comparable fit. When comparing the BPM in Table 7.7 with the univariate probit models in Table 7.6 using the likelihood ratio test statistics, we find $G^2 = 0.94$ ($p = 0.1703$). Thus, it would seem there is no need to account for the association. However, this was different when comparing both columns in Table 7.6. It illustrates the point that sometimes careful modeling of the association is necessary, in agreement with several analyses in Chapter 6. Table 7.8 presents the same three models, with the association now depending on the covariates 'sex' and 'social 2,' in line with Table 7.6. Also here, the three models have a comparable fit. Note that in Tables 7.7 and 7.8, the marginal regression parameters for the BPM and the BDM-N are virtually identical, which is to be expected as both models have probit margins. The parameters for the BDM-L are related with the others through the well-known factor $\pi/\sqrt{3}$

7.7 The Dale Model

TABLE 7.8. *BIRNH Study. Parameter estimates (standard errors) for the bivariate models [BPM: bivariate probit model; BDM: bivariate Dale model with normal (N) or logistic (L) margins] with association depending on the covariates (the correlation coefficient for the BPM and the global cross-ratio for the BDM).*

Effect	BPM	BDM-N	BDM-L
\multicolumn{4}{c}{Alcohol}			
Intercept 1	-1.04(0.14)	-1.05(0.14)	-1.65(0.23)
Intercept 2	-0.66(0.14)	-0.67(0.14)	-1.03(0.23)
Intercept 3	0.09(0.14)	0.09(0.14)	0.23(0.23)
Sex	0.69(0.08)	0.70(0.08)	1.09(0.13)
Social 1	-0.31(0.07)	-0.31(0.07)	-0.53(0.12)
Site	0.21(0.07)	0.21(0.07)	0.35(0.12)
Smoking			
Intercept 1	-3.75(0.35)	-3.75(0.35)	-6.21(0.59)
Intercept 2	-3.16(0.34)	-3.16(0.34)	-5.22(0.58)
Sex	1.15(0.09)	1.14(0.09)	1.91(0.15)
BMI	0.05(0.01)	0.05(0.01)	0.08(0.02)
Age($\times 10$)	0.11(0.03)	0.11(0.03)	0.19(0.06)
Social 1	0.21(0.10)	0.21(0.10)	0.34(0.16)
Social 2	0.24(0.09)	0.25(0.09)	0.41(0.15)
Association parameters			
Constant	0.41(0.13)	1.15(0.36)	1.15(0.35)
Sex	-0.30(0.09)	-0.82(0.27)	-0.82(0.27)
Social 2	0.17(0.10)	0.46(0.28)	0.46(0.28)
Log-likelihood	-2281.01	-2280.90	-2281.64

(see also Section 3.4), the standard deviation of the logistic distribution. A similar phenomenon will be observed in Section 7.10. In the three models the association between alcohol and smoking is small but perhaps a bit higher for the Dale models. The association parameters of the BDM-N and BDM-L are similar, as both are framed in terms of odds ratios, in contrast to the correlation-based association in the BPM. The coefficients of the association measures for the variable dependence models are more difficult to compare because of the different reparameterizations used. For the BPM, the Fisher z transform of the correlation ρ depends linearly on the covariates, while for BDM $\log \psi$ depends linearly on x. Nevertheless, from the log-likelihoods it is apparent that again the three models explain the data in virtually the same manner. Table 7.9 further includes row and column effects in the association structure of the BDM models. However, this does not significantly improve the fit of the model.

TABLE 7.9. *BIRNH Study. Parameter estimates (standard errors) for the bivariate Dale model (BDM) with normal (N) and logistic (L) margins, where the association depends both on the covariates and on the cutpoints.*

Effect	BDM-N	BDM-L
Alcohol		
Intercept 1	-1.05(0.14)	-1.66(0.24)
Intercept 2	-0.67(0.14)	-1.03(0.23)
Intercept 3	0.09(0.14)	0.23(0.23)
Sex	0.70(0.08)	1.10(0.13)
Social 1	-0.31(0.07)	-0.52(0.12)
Site	0.21(0.07)	0.35(0.12)
Smoking		
Intercept 1	-3.70(0.35)	-6.13(0.60)
Intercept 2	-3.12(0.34)	-5.14(0.59)
Sex	1.13(0.09)	1.88(0.15)
BMI	0.05(0.01)	0.08(0.02)
Age($\times 10$)	0.11(0.03)	0.18(0.06)
Social 1	0.20(0.10)	0.33(0.16)
Social 2	0.24(0.09)	0.41(0.15)
Association parameters		
Intercept	1.15(0.36)	1.13(0.36)
Sex	-0.72(0.28)	-0.72(0.28)
Social 2	0.45(0.28)	0.45(0.28)
Row 1	-0.19(0.18)	-0.19(0.18)
Row 2	-0.03(0.16)	-0.02(0.16)
Column 1	-0.03(0.11)	-0.03(0.12)
Log-likelihood	-2279.47	-2280.19

7.8 Hybrid Marginal-conditional Specification

The fully specified models in most of this chapter are of a marginal nature. The previous chapter presented marginal models alongside conditionally specified ones, to make a number of points about the advantages of marginal models. Chapter 11 zooms in on conditionally specified models. In this section, we will present a hybrid model family, in the sense that it combines aspects of marginal and conditional models. Because the lower order moments, usually of principal scientific interest, are marginally specified, we have chosen to present it here, rather than in Part III.

Fitzmaurice and Laird (1993) model the marginal mean parameters, together with the canonical interaction parameters in the multivariate exponential family distribution of Cox (1972). Their model is related to the quadratic exponential model of Zhao and Prentice (1990). The distribution of Fitzmaurice and Laird (1993) differs from the previously described distributions because it is specified in terms of a mixture of marginal and conditional parameters.

Molenberghs and Ritter (1996) and Molenberghs and Danielson (1999) proposed a model that combines important advantages of a full marginal model and a mixed marginal-conditional model. The model is parameterized using marginal means, pairwise marginal odds ratios, and higher order conditional odds ratios. These conditional odds ratios are the canonical parameters of the exponential family described by Cox (1972) of which it is known that their interpretation is difficult, especially when the number of measurements per unit is variable. More details on the fully conditional model can be found in Section 11. The mixed parameterization has important advantages. First, it produces lower order parameter estimators that are robust against misspecification of the higher order structure. Second, the likelihood equations are less complex and easier to fit than the ones for the fully marginally specified models of Chapter 7. As such, a hybrid specification is an attractive alternative specification for a full likelihood method. However, one can set higher order association parameters equal to zero, whence they provide an appealing alternative to generalized estimating equations, in particular GEE2, as well (Section 8.7). This last observation was also employed by Heagerty and Zeger (1996), who consider a mixed marginal-conditional parameterization for clustered ordinal data, with the first and the second moments specified through marginal parameters, and who 8propose estimating the model parameters through GEE2, GEE1, or alternating logistic regressions.

7.8.1 A Mixed Marginal-conditional Model

We will use the regression notation. For each individual, subject, or experimental unit i in a study, a series of n categorical measurements Y_{ij}, grouped into a vector $\boldsymbol{Y}_i$ is recorded, together with covariate information $\boldsymbol{x}_i$. The parameters of primary interest are the first- and second-order marginal parameters. The covariate vector can include both time-dependent and time-stationary covariates. Covariate information can be used to model the marginal means, the associations, or both. In this section, we will restrict ourselves to binary outcomes. Section 7.8.2 considers the extension to categorical outcomes. The use of this modeling framework to derive GEE is discussed in Section 8.7 and exemplified in Sections 8.10 and 8.11.

Model building is based on the quadratic version of the joint distribution proposed by Cox (1972) and used by Zhao and Prentice (1990) and Fitzmaurice and Laird (1993). In particular, we write

$$f(\boldsymbol{y}_i|\boldsymbol{\Psi}_i,\boldsymbol{\Omega}_i) = \exp\left\{\boldsymbol{\Psi}_i'\boldsymbol{v}_i + \boldsymbol{\Omega}_i'\boldsymbol{w}_i - A(\boldsymbol{\Psi}_i,\boldsymbol{\Omega}_i)\right\}, \qquad (7.50)$$

with outcomes and pairwise cross-products thereof grouped into

$$v_i = (y_i'; y_{i1}y_{i2}, \ldots, y_{i,n-1}y_{in})',$$

and third and higher order cross-products collected in

$$w_i = (y_{i1}y_{i2}y_{i3}, \ldots, y_{i1}y_{i2}\cdots y_{in})',$$

and Ψ_i and Ω_i the corresponding canonical parameter vectors. Further, let $\mu_i = E(V_i)$ and $\nu_i = E(W_i)$. The distribution is fully parameterized by modeling Ψ_i and Ω_i. However, we choose to model μ_i and Ω_i, enabling us to describe the marginal means and the pairwise marginal odds ratios.

A model for μ_i is specified via a vector of link functions

$$\eta_i = \eta_i(\mu_i), \tag{7.51}$$

An important class of link functions, due to McCullagh and Nelder (1989), is given by (6.2). In particular, the marginal logit link and marginal log odds ratios can be used. The marginal part of the model formulation is complete by specifying the dependence on the covariates. From the covariate vector x_i a design matrix X_i is derived, such that $\eta_i = X_i\beta$, with β a vector of parameters of interest.

Similarly, a model for the conditional higher order parameters needs to be constructed. In agreement with Fitzmaurice and Laird (1993), and because the components of Ω_i can be interpreted as conditonal higher order log odds ratios, we assume an identity link and specify the covariate dependence as $\Omega_i = X_i'\alpha$, with X_i' another design matrix and α a parameter vector. A simple model is found by holding the components of Ω_i constant.

In principle, β and α could be allowed to overlap, making the model slightly more general, but there would typically be little practical relevance to this.

Following derivations in Fitzmaurice and Laird (1993), Fitzmaurice, Laird, and Rotnitzky (1993), and Molenberghs and Ritter (1996), the likelihood equations can be written as:

$$\frac{\partial \ell}{\partial(\beta,\alpha)} = \sum_{i=1}^{N} \begin{pmatrix} \frac{\partial \mu_i}{\partial \beta} & 0 \\ 0 & \frac{\partial \Omega_i}{\partial \alpha} \end{pmatrix}' \begin{pmatrix} M_i^{-1} & 0 \\ -N_i M_i^{-1} & I \end{pmatrix}$$

$$\times \begin{pmatrix} v_i - \mu_i \\ w_i - \nu_i \end{pmatrix}, \tag{7.52}$$

with $M_i = \mathrm{cov}(V_i)$ and $N_i = \mathrm{cov}(V_i, W_i)$.

The form of the derivatives in the first matrix of (7.52) depends on the choice of link functions and linear predictors. Under the assumed linear model for Ω_i, the derivative reduces to X_i'. The computation of $\partial \mu_i / \partial \beta$ is particularly straightforward for link functions of the form (6.2), in agreement with (7.61):

$$\left(\frac{\partial \mu_i}{\partial \beta}\right)' = X'_i(D'_i)^{-1}$$

with

$$D_i = \left(\frac{\partial \eta_i}{\partial \mu_i}\right) = C_i \{\text{diag}(A_i\mu_i)\}^{-1} A_i.$$

As the model is a mixed parameterization of an exponential family model (Barndorff-Nielsen 1978), the parameter vectors β and α are orthogonal in the sense of Cox and Reid (1987). This implies that β and α are asymptotically independent. Indeed, the inverse of the expected information matrix equals:

$$\begin{pmatrix} \Gamma_1^{-1} & 0 \\ 0 & \Gamma_2^{-1} \end{pmatrix}$$

with

$$\Gamma_1 = \sum_{i=1}^N X'_i(D'_i)^{-1} M_i^{-1} D_i^{-1} X_i,$$

$$\Gamma_2 = \sum_{i=1}^N (X'^*_i)'(P_i - N_i M_i^{-1} N'_i) X'^*_i,$$

and $P_i = \text{cov}(W_i)$.

Calculating the joint probabilities can be done in various ways. Fitzmaurice and Laird (1993) proposed the use of the iterative proportional fitting (IPF) algorithm to avoid the computation of Ψ_i. We will proceed similarly. First, the components of μ_i are computed. Let us focus on logit and log odds ratio links. Inverting the logit links, like in (7.18) yields μ_{ij} ($j = 1, \ldots, n$). Given μ_{ij_1}, μ_{ij_2}, and $\psi_{ij_1j_2} = \exp(\eta_{ij_1j_2})$, $\mu_{i_1j_2}$ can be calculated using Plackett's expression (7.40). To obtain higher order probabilities, an initial contingency table is constructed satisfying the third- and higher order conditional odds ratio structure. Then, the set of $n(n-1)/2$ bivariate marginal probabilities is fitted iteratively. This is similar to but different from the IPF algorithm outlined in Section 7.12.3. Although in Section 7.12.3 the algorithm had to be adapted to a marginally specified model for ordinal data, we are faced here with a more conventional application, the higher-order model being specified conditionally and the outcomes of a binary type. The standard algorithm is described in Agresti (2002).

Parameter estimation can be performed using a standard Fisher scoring iteration procedure. The inverse of the Fisher information, with the parameter estimates substituted, provides a variance estimator for $(\hat{\beta}, \hat{\alpha})$. As pointed out in Fitzmaurice, Laird, and Rotnitzky (1993), the consistency of the estimator for β only depends on the correct specification of the marginal part of the model, and not on α. If the α part is misspecified, the model based variance will be inconsistent, so the empirically corrected or 'robust' variance should be used. Apart from inferential advantages (Fitzmaurice, Laird, and Rotnitzky 1993), there are also computational advantages in terms of stability (Cox and Reid 1987). These points are taken up in Section 8.7.

As an alternative to the use of the robust variance estimator, a model checking procedure can be performed to assess whether the model specification is acceptable. If not, the model for the higher order associations can be made more complex in order to improve the fit. When there are only a few categorical covariate levels and the sample size within each level is sufficiently large, a classical model checking procedure such as the Pearson X^2 or the deviance G^2 test can be used (Agresti 1990).

7.8.2 Categorical Outcomes

Like the multivariate probit (Section 7.6) and Dale (Section 7.7) models, the hybrid model can accommodate categorical outcomes just as easily as dichotomous ones.

Let Y_{ij} again be a categorical outcome with c_j (possibly ordered) categories and use the dummy variables formally defined by (7.1) and (7.2). In particular, because we are not making use of the design level indicator r, Z^*_{ijk} indicates outcomes and Z_{ijk} cumulative outcomes. These indicator variables are again grouped into vectors $\boldsymbol{Z}^*_i$ and $\boldsymbol{Z}_i$. The corresponding sets of univariate and pairwise probabilities are

$$\mu^*_{ijk} = P(Y_{ij} = k | \boldsymbol{X}_i, \boldsymbol{\beta}) = P(Z^*_{ijk} = 1 | \boldsymbol{X}_i, \boldsymbol{\beta}),$$

$$\mu^*_{i,jh,k\ell} = P(Y_{ij} = k, Y_{ih} = \ell | \boldsymbol{X}_i, \boldsymbol{\beta}) = P(Z^*_{ijk} = 1, Z^*_{ih\ell} = 1 | \boldsymbol{X}_i, \boldsymbol{\beta}).$$

The cumulative probabilities are

$$\mu_{ijk} = P(Y_{ij} \leq k | \boldsymbol{X}_i, \boldsymbol{\beta}),$$

$$\mu_{i,jh,k\ell} = P(Y_{ij} \leq k, Y_{ih} \leq \ell | \boldsymbol{X}_i, \boldsymbol{\beta})$$

which are grouped in $\boldsymbol{\mu}^*_i$ and $\boldsymbol{\mu}_i$, respectively. The higher order probabilities $\boldsymbol{\nu}^*_i$ and $\boldsymbol{\nu}_i$ are defined similarly. Exponential models, similar to (7.50), are

$$f(\boldsymbol{y}_i | \boldsymbol{\Psi}^*_i, \boldsymbol{\Omega}^*_i) = \exp\left\{ (\boldsymbol{\Psi}^*_i)' \boldsymbol{v}^*_i + (\boldsymbol{\Omega}^*_i)' \boldsymbol{w}^*_i - A^*(\boldsymbol{\Psi}^*_i, \boldsymbol{\Omega}^*_i) \right\}, \qquad (7.53)$$

and

$$f(\boldsymbol{y}_i | \boldsymbol{\Psi}_i, \boldsymbol{\Omega}_i) = \exp\left\{ \boldsymbol{\Psi}_i \boldsymbol{v}_i + \boldsymbol{\Omega}_i \boldsymbol{w}_i - A(\boldsymbol{\Psi}_i, \boldsymbol{\Omega}_i) \right\}, \qquad (7.54)$$

where $\boldsymbol{V}^*_i$ contains the components of $\boldsymbol{Z}^*_i$ and the pairwise cross-products thereof, and $\boldsymbol{W}^*_i$ contains all higher order cross-products. The vectors $\boldsymbol{V}_i$ and $\boldsymbol{W}_i$ are defined similarly. Observe that (7.53) and (7.54) are overparameterized, as sum constraints apply to (7.53) and the variable $Z_{ijc_j} = 1$

in (7.54), which necessitates the use of identifying restrictions. In the case of a single nominal variable, (7.53) is called the multigroup logistic model (Albert and Lesaffre 1986).

With nominal outcomes, the marginal mean functions $\boldsymbol{\mu}_i^*$ will be modeled, together with the higher order conditional association parameters $\boldsymbol{\Omega}_i^*$. A vector of link functions $\boldsymbol{\eta}_i^* = \boldsymbol{\eta}_i^*(\boldsymbol{\mu}_i^*)$ has to be chosen and form (6.2) provides a convenient subclass. Baseline category logits seem very natural, together with local odds ratios. If the outcomes are measured on an ordinal scale it is more convenient to model $\boldsymbol{\mu}_i$, rather than $\boldsymbol{\mu}_i^*$, i.e., link functions $\boldsymbol{\eta}_i = \boldsymbol{\eta}_i(\boldsymbol{\mu}_i)$ are chosen and model (7.54) can be used. Note that this description is equally compatible with (7.53), as $\boldsymbol{\mu}_i^* = \boldsymbol{B}_i \boldsymbol{\mu}_i$ for an appropriate transformation matrix $\boldsymbol{B}_i$, as in (7.4).

The likelihood equations are of the form (7.52). Even more than with binary outcomes, the number of parameters proliferates rapidly with an increasing number of measurements, calling for parsimonious modeling. A simple, but often satisfactory model for the pairwise association is the constant global odds ratio model for ordinal outcomes: the global odds ratio for a pair of variables $(Z_{ijk}, Z_{ih\ell})$ is independent of the 'row' and 'column' indices k and ℓ. Further, one should exploit any additional structure in the outcomes. For exchangeable outcomes, the odds ratios are usually assumed constant for all pairs of variables, whereas for time-ordered measurements, association structures taking into account the time dependence can be investigated. A similar reasoning could be made to simplify the higher order conditional associations. In many instances this effort will be considered of no real benefit, whence one can set $\boldsymbol{\Omega}_i = \boldsymbol{0}$. In order to compute the variance matrix $\boldsymbol{M}_i$, we only need to compute the third- and fourth-order probabilities, which is particularly easy using the iterative proportional fitting algorithm.

7.9 A Cross-over Trial: An Example in Primary Dysmenorrhoea

The data are taken from a cross-over trial that appeared in the paper of Kenward and Jones (1991). Eighty-six subjects were enrolled in a cross-over study that compared placebo (A) with an analgesic at low and high doses (B and C) for the relief of pain in primary dysmenorrhoea. The three treatments were administered in one of six possible orders: ABC, ACB, BAC, BCA, CAB, and CBA. The primary outcome score was the amount of relief coded as none (1), moderate (2), and complete (3). There are 27 possible outcome combinations: $(1, 1, 1), (1, 1, 2), \ldots, (3, 3, 3)$, where (a_1, a_2, a_3) denotes outcome a_j in period j. The data, analyzed before by Kenward and Jones (1991), can be found in Table 7.10. For the analysis of the cross-over data, these authors suggested a subject-specific approach

TABLE 7.10. *Primary Dysmenorrhoea Data.*

Response	ABC	ACB	BAC	BCA	CAB	CBA
(1,1,1)	0	2	0	0	3	1
(1,1,2)	1	0	0	1	0	0
(1,1,3)	1	0	1	0	0	0
(1,2,1)	2	0	0	0	0	0
(1,2,2)	3	0	1	0	0	0
(1,2,3)	4	3	1	0	2	0
(1,3,1)	0	0	1	1	0	0
(1,3,2)	0	2	0	0	0	0
(1,3,3)	2	4	1	0	0	1
(2,1,1)	0	1	1	0	0	3
(2,1,2)	0	0	2	0	1	1
(2,1,3)	0	0	1	0	0	0
(2,2,1)	1	0	0	6	1	1
(2,2,2)	0	2	1	0	0	0
(2,2,3)	1	0	0	0	0	0
(2,3,1)	0	0	0	1	0	2
(2,3,2)	0	0	0	0	0	0
(2,3,3)	0	2	0	0	1	0
(3,1,1)	0	0	0	1	0	2
(3,1,2)	0	0	2	0	2	1
(3,1,3)	0	0	3	0	4	1
(3,2,1)	0	0	0	1	0	0
(3,2,2)	0	0	0	1	0	0
(3,2,3)	0	0	0	0	0	0
(3,3,1)	0	0	0	0	0	1
(3,3,2)	0	0	0	0	0	0
(3,3,3)	0	0	0	0	0	0

based on the Rasch model. Here too, it was of interest to estimate the treatment, period- and carry-over effects.

7.9.1 Analyzing Cross-over Data

Consider a cross-over trial where each patient subsequently receives each of three treatments (A, B, C) in a random order. There are 6 treatment sequences: $ABC, ACB, BAC, BCA, CAB,$ and CBA. Suppose the outcome at time j (corresponding to treatment t) is an ordered categorical variable Y_{jt} with c levels. Then, to each sequence a $c \times c \times c$ table is assigned,

7.9 A Cross-over Trial: An Example in Primary Dysmenorrhoea

containing the joint outcomes for the patients, allocated to that particular sequence. The multivariate Dale model can be used to fit such data. The marginal parameters are used to describe the overall treatment effects, the period- and the carry-over effects. The cross-ratios play a role, similar to the subject specific parameters in the paper of Kenward and Jones (1991).

Given a particular sequence s, let $L^s_{jtk} = \text{logit}\,[P(Y_{jt} \leq k)]$ be the cumulative logit for cutpoint k $(k = 1, \ldots, c-1)$, and time j, which, for sequence s, corresponds to treatment t. In full detail, we have

$$L^{ABC}_{11k}, L^{ABC}_{22k}, L^{ABC}_{33k};$$
$$L^{ACB}_{11k}, L^{ACB}_{23k}, L^{ACB}_{32k};$$
$$L^{BAC}_{12k}, L^{BAC}_{21k}, L^{BAC}_{33k};$$
$$L^{BCA}_{12k}, L^{BCA}_{23k}, L^{BCA}_{31k};$$
$$L^{CAB}_{13k}, L^{CAB}_{21k}, L^{CAB}_{32k};$$
$$L^{CBA}_{13k}, L^{CBA}_{22k}, L^{CBA}_{31k}.$$

The following model for the logits is adopted: $L^s_{jtk} = \mu_k + \tau_t + \rho_j + \lambda_{s(j-1)}$, where μ_k are intercept parameters, τ_t are treatment effects, ρ_j are period effects. $\lambda_{s(j-1)}$ stands for the carry-over effect, corresponding to the treatment at time $j-1$ in sequence s. Given, for instance, sequence CAB, we get

$$L_{13k} = \mu_k + \tau_3 + \rho_1,$$
$$L_{21k} = \mu_k + \tau_1 + \rho_2 + \lambda_3,$$
$$L_{32k} = \mu_k + \tau_2 + \rho_3 + \lambda_1.$$

To avoid overparameterization, the following uniqueness constraints are set:

$$\tau_1 = \rho_1 = \lambda_1 = 0.$$

Let $\gamma^s_{jt,j't'} = \ln \psi^s_{jt,j't'}$ be the log cross-ratio, for the marginal $c \times c$ table, formed by the responses at times j and j' for sequence s (corresponding to treatments t and t' respectively). The simplest model for the cross-ratios is given by

$$\gamma^s_{jt,j't'} = \mu.$$

The most complex model assumes all 18 cross-ratios to be different, which is one by Jones and Kenward (1989) and by Becker and Balagtas (1993). In between these two models there is room for parsimonious modeling. One can think of the following linear models in the log cross-ratios

$$\gamma^s_{jt,j't'} = \mu + \tau_{tt'}, \tag{7.55}$$

$$\gamma^s_{jt,j't'} = \mu + \rho_{jj'}, \tag{7.56}$$

$$\gamma^s_{jt,j't'} = \mu + \tau_{tt'} + \rho_{jj'}, \tag{7.57}$$

where μ is an intercept parameter, $\tau_{tt'}$ are parameters for the joint (t,t')th treatments effects, and $\rho_{jj'}$ describe effects for periods j and j'. In the first model, the log cross-ratio only depends on the treatments, irrespective of their order and the periods they were administered. In the second model, only the periods are of importance. In the third model, the two effects are linearly combined. For instance, for sequence CAB, we get

$$\gamma_{13,21} = \mu + \tau_{13} + \rho_{12},$$
$$\gamma_{13,32} = \mu + \tau_{23} + \rho_{13},$$
$$\gamma_{21,32} = \mu + \tau_{12} + \rho_{23}.$$

Possible uniqueness constraints are $\tau_{12} = \rho_{12} = 0$. The model with association structure (7.56) corresponds to the model introduced in Section 7.7.5. In a model with association structure (7.55) or (7.57), the two-way cross-ratios change with the treatment combination, which is a time-dependent covariate. Finally, the three-way association depends in all six cases on the same periods and treatments, the only difference being the order in which the treatments occur. So the most natural choice is $\gamma_{123}^s = \mu + \mu^s$, ($\mu^{ABC} = 0$), however in most cases it is reasonable to assume $\gamma_{123}^s = \gamma_{123}$ constant over sequences.

No carry-over effects are incorporated in the cross-ratios, as the marginal carry-over parameters have no straightforward generalization. As usual, the different nested models can be tested using the likelihood ratio test statistic, denoted G^2.

7.9.2 Analysis of the Primary Dysmenorrhoea Data

Table 7.11 gives the details concerning the selection of effects for the primary dysmenorrhoea data. As can be seen from this table, the marginal logit modeling yields a highly significant treatment effect. The period and carry-over effects are not significant. The model retained (model I in Table 7.12), consists of two cutpoints μ_k and two treatment parameters τ_t; the estimates are shown in Table 7.12. Up to now no two-way or three-way association is assumed.

Let us turn to the association structure; the three-way association is assumed constant in all cases. First the minimal model is fitted. This model will serve as the basic model against which the other models will be compared. The three different models mentioned in (7.55), (7.56), and (7.57) were fitted to the data. There seems to be evidence that both the treatment terms as well as the period terms are necessary. The maximal model, i.e., with 18 cross-ratios, has a G^2 statistic of 16.27 (13 d.f., $p = 0.2349$) compared to the last model. Model II in Table 7.12 shows the parameter estimates when treatment parameters are included in the two-way cross-ratios. Model III, contains as association parameters: the intercept μ, treatment

TABLE 7.11. *Primary Dysmenorrhoea Data. Selection of effects. The columns describe the model number, the effects included, the log-likelihood of the model, the number of the model to which this model is compared, the likelihood ratio G^2 statistics with the number of degrees of freedom, and the corresponding p-value.*

	Effects	log-lik	Comp.	G^2	d.f.	p-value
		Marginal effects				
1	μ_k	-279.74				
2	μ_k, τ_t	-245.53	1	68.42	2	< 0.0001
3	μ_k, τ_t, ρ_j	-243.78	2	3.50	2	0.1740
4	$\mu_k, \tau_t, \lambda_{s(j-1)}$	-245.40	2	0.26	2	0.8790
		Model 2 + association effects				
5	$\mu_k, \tau_t; \mu, \psi_{123}$	-244.40				
6	$\mu_k, \tau_t; \mu, \tau_{tt'}, \psi_{123}$	-239.54	5	9.66	2	0.0080
7	$\mu_k, \tau_t; \mu, \rho_{jj'}, \psi_{123}$	-239.50	5	9.73	2	0.0077
8	$\mu_k, \tau_t; \mu, \tau_{tt'}, \rho_{jj'}, \psi_{123}$	-236.44	5	15.87	4	0.0032
				6	6.21	2	0.0448
				7	6.14	2	0.0465

effects $\tau_{tt'}$, period parameters $\rho_{jj'}$ and the three-way interaction $\ln \psi_{123}$. This model will be chosen.

Parameter interpretation is as follows. The odds of observing $Y_{jt} \leq k$ ($k = 1, 2$) decreases with factor $\exp(-1.98)$ when the patient is treated with the analgesic at low dose rather than with placebo. A further decrease with factor $\exp(-2.37 + 1.98)$ is observed if the patient is treated with the analgesic at high dose. Further, the association between responses is higher if they are close to each other in time ($\hat{\rho}_{13} = -1.12$). Also, responses from the two analgesic treatments are more associated than responses from one analgesic treatment and placebo ($\hat{\tau}_{23} = 1.32$).

Thus, our analysis confirms the results found by Kenward and Jones (1991). However, the marginal approach here allows the estimation of treatment effects that now are easily interpretable, in contrast with Kenward and Jones (1991) and in contrast with the conditional approach in Jones and Kenward (1989) as well. Confidence intervals for the effects can be found from the estimated standard errors, shown in Table 7.12 for Model III. Finally, the method allows flexible modeling of the association.

7.10 Multivariate Analysis of the POPS Data

The POPS data were introduced in Section 2.6. We will compare the Bahadur model (BAH), introduced in Section 7.2 and applied earlier to

TABLE 7.12. *Primary Dysmenorrhoea Data. Fitted models. Each entry represents the parameter estimates (standard error). The absence of a standard errors corresponds to a preset value.*

Effect	Par.	Model I	Model II	Model III
Marginal effects				
Intercept 1	μ_1	1.07(0.25)	1.07(0.24)	1.08(0.24)
Intercept 2	μ_2	2.71(0.29)	2.70(0.29)	2.72(0.29)
Treatment effect	τ_2	-2.03(0.33)	-2.02(0.35)	-1.98(0.34)
Treatment effect	τ_3	-2.41(0.33)	-2.37(0.36)	-2.37(0.35)
Two-way association effects				
Intercept	μ	0(-)	-0.62(0.47)	-0.46(0.56)
Treatment effect	τ_{13}	0(-)	-0.16(0.65)	-0.10(0.58)
Treatment effect	τ_{23}	0(-)	1.51(0.64)	1.32(0.61)
Period effect	ρ_{13}	0(-)	0(-)	-1.12(0.55)
Period effect	ρ_{23}	0(-)	0(-)	0.51(0.66)
Three-way association				
		1(-)	1.59(0.75)	0.63(0.88)
Log-likelihood				
		-245.53	-239.54	-236.43

the clustered NTP data and the longitudinal fluvoxamine study, with the trivariate probit model (TPM, Section 7.6) and the trivariate Dale model (TDM, Section 7.7), both with probit (normally based, N) and logistic (L) margins. Note that several comparisons are possible: (1) the Bahadur model and the TPM capture the association by means of correlations, whereas the TDM features odds ratios; (2) the Bahadur model and TDM-L have logistic margins, while the TPM and the TDM-N have univariate marginal regressions of a probit type. Finally, the log-likelihood at maximum, or the AIC can be used to compare the models with each other.

From the 8 candidate predictor variables, neonatal seizures, congenital malformations, and highest bilirubin value since birth were retained for analysis. They were selected using a stepwise logistic analysis for each response separately, at significance level 0.05. The first two regressors are dichotomous, the third one is continuous.

Table 7.13 contains the estimated parameters under all four models. In all models, transformed correlation parameters are used to reduce parameter space violations. We present both the transformed parameter (Fisher z transformed correlation and log odds ratio) as well as the parameter expressed on the original scale.

It is seen that the presence of neonatal seizures and/or of congenital malformation significantly decreases the probability of successfully performing

TABLE 7.13. *POPS Study. Parameter estimates (standard errors) for the trivariate Bahadur (BAH), probit (TPM) and Dale models (with probit, TPM-N, or logit, TPM-L, margins). For the associations, correlations [ρ and transformed correlations, using (7.12)] (BAH, TPM) and cross-ratios (ψ) and log cross-ratios for the TDM.*

	BAH	TPM	TDM-N	TDM-L
	First ability score			
Intercept	3.67(0.49)	2.01(0.26)	2.03(0.27)	3.68(0.52)
Neonatal seiz.	-1.94(0.42)	-1.12(0.26)	-1.16(0.26)	-2.06(0.44)
Congenital malf.	-1.21(0.31)	-0.61(0.18)	-0.62(0.18)	-1.17(0.33)
100× Bilirubin	-0.69(0.25)	-0.32(0.14)	-0.32(0.14)	-0.64(0.27)
	Second ability score			
Intercept	4.03(0.51)	2.19(0.27)	2.21(0.27)	4.01(0.54)
Neonatal seiz.	-2.26(0.43)	-1.27(0.26)	-1.29(0.26)	-2.28(0.44)
Congenital malf.	-1.08(0.32)	-0.56(0.19)	-0.59(0.19)	-1.11(0.34)
100× Bilirubin	-0.85(0.26)	-0.42(0.14)	-0.41(0.14)	-0.80(0.27)
	Third ability score			
Intercept	3.32(0.50)	1.84(0.27)	1.91(0.27)	3.49(0.54)
Neonatal seiz.	-1.55(0.44)	-0.88(0.27)	-0.93(0.27)	-1.70(0.46)
Congenital malf.	-0.96(0.32)	-0.47(0.19)	-0.49(0.19)	-0.96(0.35)
100× Bilirubin	-0.44(0.26)	-0.21(0.14)	-0.24(0.14)	-0.49(0.28)
	Association parameters			
	ρ	ρ	ψ	ψ
(1,2): ρ or ψ	0.27(0.05)	0.73(0.05)	17.37(5.19)	17.35(5.19)
(1,2): $z(\rho)$ or $\ln\psi$	0.55(0.11)	1.85(0.23)	2.85(0.30)	2.85(0.30)
(1,3): ρ or ψ	0.39(0.05)	0.81(0.04)	30.64(9.78)	30.61(9.78)
(1,3): $z(\rho)$ or $\ln\psi$	0.83(0.12)	2.27(0.25)	3.42(0.32)	3.42(0.32)
(2,3): ρ or ψ	0.23(0.05)	0.72(0.05)	17.70(5.47)	17.65(5.47)
(2,3): $z(\rho)$ or $\ln\psi$	0.47(0.10)	1.83(0.23)	2.87(0.31)	2.87(0.31)
(1,2,3): ρ or ψ	—	—	0.91(0.69)	0.92(0.69)
(1,2,3): $z(\rho)$ or $\ln\psi$	—	—	-0.09(0.76)	-0.09(0.76)
Log-likelihood	-598.44	-570.69	-567.11	-567.09

any of the three ability tests. A similar effect of bilirubin on the first and second ability score is observed.

The marginal regression parameters agree in pairs: the logit-based Bahadur and TDM-L models on the one hand and the TPM and TDM-N models on the other hand. There is a slight tendency for the Bahadur parameter estimates and standard errors to be a bit smaller. This should not be seen as resulting from a higher efficiency, but rather as downward bias resulting from the model's stringent parameter space restrictions (Declerck, Aerts, and Molenberghs 1998). Upon multiplying the TPM and TDM-N coefficients with the factor $\pi/\sqrt{3}$, the standard deviation of the logistic distribution, all coefficient become very close to each other.

When comparing the association parameters, the (log) odds ratios are clearly very similar between both TDM models. This is less the case when the correlation estimates, obtained from the Bahadur, are compared with their probit model counterparts. A strong downward bias is seen. This is due, again, to the strong parameter space restrictions in the Bahadur case. This effect is magnified by setting the three-way correlation in the Bahadur model equal to zero. Recall that there is no such thing in the TPM, since this model is based on discretizing a multivariate standard normal distribution, which is completely described in terms of its two-way correlations, without the need to separately specifying three-way correlations.

A slight preference for the TDM could be inferred if based either on doubling the negative log-likelihood, or on the AIC. It is not possible to express a preference for either of the TDM models, based on this example. This confirms the well-known univariate result, that logistic and probit regression are hard to distinguish from each other, except when datasets become very large and response probabilities approach zero or one. While the TPM's performance is somewhat worse, the difference is around 5. Bahadur's model, on the other hand, lags behind by about 55 in deviance or AIC. Considering the strength of the association, there is a strong association between each pair of dichotomous responses, but no significant three-way association, as seen from the TDM.

An important feature of the likelihood method is that calculation of individual probabilities can be performed. For example, the method allows to calculate the joint probability of failing at the three tests. This can be quite different from the joint probability obtained by assuming independent responses, as is shown in Figure 7.7, where the probability that the child will fail on all three ability scores is calculated for different bilirubin values, given that both CGM and NSZ are one.

7.11 Longitudinal Analysis of the Fluvoxamine Study

The relationship between the severity of the side effects at the three visits and some baseline characteristics of the patients was established. The response is a trivariate ordered categorical vector with 4 classes, measured at three visits. For the selection of predictors, *age* and *sex* were included by default into the model. The other baseline characteristics were then consid-

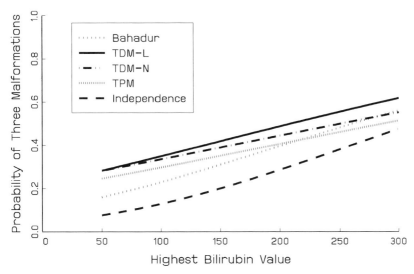

FIGURE 7.7. *POPS Study. probability that a child fails on all three ability scores for a range of bilirubin values, evaluated under five fitted models: the trivariate Bahadur model, the Dale model (TDM) with logistic (L) and normal (N) margins, the trivariate probit model (TPM), and a model assuming independent responses (three logistic regressions).*

ered for selection. Only the *duration* (months) of the disease and the *initial severity* (measured on a 7-point scale) turned out to significantly influence the severity of side effects.

At the second and third visit, a non-negligible portion of the patients dropped out from the study (20%). An ordinary contingency table analysis, as well as a logistic regression of the variable *dropout* on potential covariates showed that the dropout mechanism is heavily depending on the severity of the side-effect reported at the preceding visit. We refer to Part VI for several analysis explicitly addressing the missingness issue.

From the parameter estimates shown in Table 7.14 (Model I), it is seen that the effect of some covariates is almost constant over time. The G^2 test statistic for the hypothesis that both the intercepts and parameters for 'age' and 'sex' are time invariant is 5.37 (10 d.f., $p = 0.8654$). However, 'duration' and 'initial severity' depend on time. ($G^2 = 37.58$, 4 d.f, p< 0.0001). This leads to the more parsimonious Model II. The odds of observing high side-effects increases with 'age' and 'duration' and decreases with 'initial severity.' The influence of 'initial severity' increases over time. There is a strong association between side-effects measured at successive visits. Although significant, the association is less strong between the first and third visit.

TABLE 7.14. *Fluvoxamine Trial. Longitudinal analysis. The side effects at three successive times are regressed on age, duration, initial severity, and sex, using the multivariate Dale model. In Model I, the parameters are assumed to be different over time. In Model II, only duration and initial severity have a time-dependent effect. The entries represent the parameter estimates (standard errors).*

Effect	Side 1	Side 2	Side 3
\multicolumn{4}{c}{Model I}			
\multicolumn{4}{c}{Marginal parameters}			
Intercept 1	-0.41(0.90)	-0.45(0.95)	-0.79(1.06)
Intercept 2	1.78(0.90)	1.64(0.96)	1.64(1.07)
Intercept 3	2.94(0.92)	2.97(0.99)	2.85(1.13)
Age	-0.19(0.09)	-0.22(0.09)	-0.25(0.10)
Duration	-0.14(0.05)	-0.20(0.05)	-0.24(0.06)
In. Severity	0.29(0.14)	0.28(0.15)	0.42(0.17)
Sex	-0.23(0.24)	0.09(0.24)	0.16(0.27)

\multicolumn{4}{c}{Association parameters}			
12	13	23	123
3.20(0.27)	2.49(0.28)	3.71(0.33)	-0.38(0.76)

Effect	Side 1	Side 2	Side 3
\multicolumn{4}{c}{Model II}			
\multicolumn{4}{c}{Marginal parameters}			
Intercept 1		-0.52(0.82)	
Intercept 2		1.67(0.82)	
Intercept 3		2.89(0.84)	
Age		-0.21(0.07)	
Duration	-0.14(0.05)	-0.21(0.05)	-0.24(0.06)
In. Severity	0.27(0.13)	0.33(0.13)	0.42(0.13)
Sex		-0.06(0.22)	

\multicolumn{4}{c}{Association parameters}			
12	13	23	123
3.13(0.26)	2.43(0.27)	3.74(0.33)	-0.29(0.74)

7.12 Appendix: Maximum Likelihood Estimation

We present details on a general expression for the likelihood in marginal models, the corresponding score equations, and how to solve them.

7.12.1 Score Equations and Maximization

Under a multinomial sampling scheme, the kernel of the log-likelihood, in terms of the counts obtained at design level r, $\boldsymbol{Z}_r^*$, and the corresponding cell probabilities $\boldsymbol{\mu}_r^*$ is

$$\ell(\boldsymbol{\beta}; \boldsymbol{Z}^*) = \sum_{r=1}^{N} \boldsymbol{Z}_r^{*'} \ln[\boldsymbol{\mu}_r^*(\boldsymbol{\beta})].$$

When working with the cumulative counts $\boldsymbol{Z}_r$ and the cumulative probabilities $\boldsymbol{\mu}_r$, and knowing that relations (7.4) hold, we can rewrite the log-likelihood as

$$\ell(\boldsymbol{\beta}; \boldsymbol{Z}) = \sum_{r=1}^{N} \ell_r(\boldsymbol{\beta}; \boldsymbol{Z}_r) = \sum_{r=1}^{N} (B_r \boldsymbol{Z}_r)' \ln[B_r \boldsymbol{\mu}_r(\boldsymbol{\beta})]. \tag{7.58}$$

The derivative of the contribution of group r to (7.58) with respect to $\boldsymbol{\mu}_r$ is then given by

$$\begin{aligned}
\frac{\partial \ell}{\partial \boldsymbol{\mu}_r} &= \frac{\partial \ell_r}{\partial \boldsymbol{\mu}_r} \\
&= \left\{ B_r' [\text{diag}(\boldsymbol{\mu}_r^*)]^{-1} B_r \right\} (\boldsymbol{Z}_r - N_r \boldsymbol{\mu}_r) \\
&= \left\{ B_r' \text{cov}(\boldsymbol{Z}_r^*)^{-1} B_r \right\} (\boldsymbol{Z}_r - N_r \boldsymbol{\mu}_r) \\
&= \text{cov}(\boldsymbol{Z}_r)^{-1} (\boldsymbol{Z}_r - N_r \boldsymbol{\mu}_r). \tag{7.59}
\end{aligned}$$

Given (7.59), the score function becomes

$$U(\boldsymbol{\beta}) = \frac{\partial \ell}{\partial \boldsymbol{\beta}} = \sum_{r=1}^{N} \left(\frac{\partial \boldsymbol{\eta}_r}{\partial \boldsymbol{\beta}}\right)' \left[\left(\frac{\partial \boldsymbol{\eta}_r}{\partial \boldsymbol{\mu}_r}\right)'\right]^{-1} V_r^{-1} S_r, \tag{7.60}$$

with $S_r = \boldsymbol{Z}_r - N_r \boldsymbol{\mu}_r$, and $V_r = \text{cov}(\boldsymbol{Z}_r)$. A typical element of V_r is

$$\begin{aligned}
& \text{cov}(z_r(k_1 \ldots k_{n_r}), z_r(\ell_1, \ldots, \ell_{n_r})) \\
&= \mu_r(m_1, \ldots, m_{n_r}) - \mu_r(k_1, \ldots, k_{n_i}) \cdot \mu_r(\ell_1, \ldots, \ell_{n_r}),
\end{aligned}$$

where $m_j = \min(k_j, \ell_j)$.

Computation of the matrix $Q_r = \partial \boldsymbol{\eta}_r / \partial \boldsymbol{\mu}_r$ is extremely simple if the link is of the form (7.17), because then (Grizzle, Starmer, and Koch 1969)

$$Q_r = C \left\{\text{diag}(A\boldsymbol{\mu}_r)\right\}^{-1} A. \tag{7.61}$$

This motivates the choice to compute Q_r and invert it, rather than computing Q_r^{-1} directly, as was done by Molenberghs and Lesaffre (1994) and detailed in Section 7.7.

When we use cumulative probabilities, the component $\mu_r(c_1, \ldots, c_{n_r}) = 1$, whence it can be omitted. This implies that the matrix Q_r is square and can easily be inverted. In case one chooses to use cell probabilities, all components of $\boldsymbol{\mu}_r$ contain information whence the length of $\boldsymbol{\mu}_r^*$ is one more than the length of $\boldsymbol{\eta}_r$, but the probabilities sum to one. This additional equation needs to be added to the list of $\boldsymbol{\eta}_r$, making Q_r square again (McCullagh and Nelder, 1989).

Replacing the univariate marginal link functions in (7.17), $\boldsymbol{\eta}_r^{(1)}$ say, by any other inverse cumulative distribution function F^{-1} with probability density function f, and retaining the specification of the association in terms of a form satisfying (7.17), yields the expression

$$\boldsymbol{\eta} = \boldsymbol{\eta}(\boldsymbol{\mu}) = \begin{pmatrix} F^{-1}(\boldsymbol{\mu}^{(1)}) \\ C_2 \ln(A\boldsymbol{\mu}) \end{pmatrix},$$

with corresponding derivative

$$Q_r = \begin{pmatrix} \text{diag}\{f(\boldsymbol{\eta}^{(1)})\}^{-1} & \mathbf{0} \\ \hline C_2 \{\text{diag}(A\boldsymbol{\mu})\}^{-1} A \end{pmatrix}. \qquad (7.62)$$

The matrix C_2 is similar to the matrix C in (7.17) but now only applies to the association part of the model. Choosing $F = \Phi$ and $f = \phi$, the standard normal distribution and density functions, we obtain a global odds ratio model with univariate probit links.

As discussed in the previous section, the multivariate probit model also fits within the proposed framework. In this case, it might be preferable to compute the matrix Q_r^{-1}, rather than its inverse, unlike with the global odds ratio model, or most other models of the form (7.17). Although in the probit case the matrix Q_r^{-1} is easier to compute than Q_r, the computations are still more complex than calculating (7.62). The components are the derivatives of multivariate standard normal distribution functions. The evaluation of multivariate normal integrals is required. Lesaffre and Molenberghs (1991) chose to use the algorithm proposed by Shervish (1984). In the common case of linear predictors, the derivative of the link vector with respect to $\boldsymbol{\beta}$ is the design matrix X_r. See also Section 7.6.

The maximum likelihood estimator satisfies $\boldsymbol{U}(\widehat{\boldsymbol{\beta}}) = 0$. Two popular fitting algorithms are Fisher scoring and the Newton-Raphson algorithm. In the case of Fisher scoring, one starts with a vector of initial estimates $\boldsymbol{\beta}^{(0)}$ and updates the current value of the parameter vector $\boldsymbol{\beta}^{(t)}$ by

$$\boldsymbol{\beta}^{(t+1)} = \boldsymbol{\beta}^{(t)} + W(\boldsymbol{\beta}^{(t)})^{-1} \boldsymbol{U}(\boldsymbol{\beta}^{(t)}), \qquad (7.63)$$

with

$$W(\boldsymbol{\beta}) = \sum_{i=1}^{N} N_r \left(\frac{\partial \boldsymbol{\eta}_r}{\partial \boldsymbol{\beta}}\right)' \left[\left(\frac{\partial \boldsymbol{\eta}_r}{\partial \boldsymbol{\mu}_r}\right)'\right]^{-1} V_r^{-1} \left[\left(\frac{\partial \boldsymbol{\eta}_r}{\partial \boldsymbol{\mu}_r}\right)\right]^{-1} \left(\frac{\partial \boldsymbol{\eta}_r}{\partial \boldsymbol{\beta}}\right).$$

The expected information matrix assumes the form $W(\boldsymbol{\beta})$, estimated by $W(\widehat{\boldsymbol{\beta}})$. A Newton-Raphson iteration scheme is found by substituting the

7.12 Appendix: Maximum Likelihood Estimation

matrix $W(\boldsymbol{\beta})$ in (7.63) by $H(\boldsymbol{\beta})$, the matrix of second-order derivatives of the log-likelihood. An outline of this procedure for cumulative counts is given next.

7.12.2 Newton-Raphson Algorithm with Cumulative Counts

Replacing the matrix $W(\boldsymbol{\beta})$ in (7.63) by the matrix of second-order derivatives $H(\boldsymbol{\beta})$ of the log-likelihood (7.58) implements a Newton-Raphson algorithm. We present an expression for $H = H(\boldsymbol{\beta})$. It is useful to borrow some notation from McCullagh's (1987) book on tensor methods in statistics. From McCullagh (1987), it follows that the (p, q) element of H is

$$H_{pq} = \sum_{r=1}^{N} \sum_{a,b,c,d} \frac{\partial \eta_{ra}}{\partial \beta_p} \frac{\partial \mu_{rb}}{\partial \eta_{ra}} \frac{\partial^2 \ell}{\partial \mu_{rb} \mu_{rc}} \frac{\partial \mu_{rc}}{\partial \eta_{rd}} \frac{\partial \eta_{rd}}{\partial \beta_q}$$

$$+ \sum_{r=1}^{N} \sum_{a,d,b} \left[\frac{\partial \eta_{ra}}{\partial \beta_p} \frac{\partial \eta_{rd}}{\partial \beta_q} \frac{\partial^2 \mu_{rb}}{\partial \eta_{ra} \partial \eta_{rd}} + \frac{\partial^2 \eta_{ra}}{\partial \beta_p \partial \beta_q} \frac{\partial \mu_{rb}}{\partial \eta_{ra}} \right] \frac{\partial \ell}{\partial \mu_{rb}}.$$

Observing

$$\frac{\partial \ell}{\partial \mu_{rb}} = \sum_k (V_r^{-1})_{bk} S_{rk},$$

$$\frac{\partial^2 \ell}{\partial \mu_{rb} \mu_{rc}} = -N_r * (V_r^{-1})_{bc} - \sum_{e,f,k} (V_r^{-1})_{be} J_{r,c,ef} (V_r^{-1})_{fk} S_{rk},$$

$$J_{r,c,ef} = \delta_{c,\iota(e,f)} - \delta_{ce}\mu_{rf} - \delta_{cf}\mu_{re},$$

where δ is the Kronecker delta function and $\iota(a, d) = c$ if $\min(a_j, d_j) = c_j$ for all components of the index vectors, we can separate the terms involving S_r in the expression for $H(\boldsymbol{\beta})$:

$$H_{pq} = -W_{pq} + \sum_{r=1}^{N} \boldsymbol{\alpha}'_{rpq} S_r,$$

for some vector $\boldsymbol{\alpha}_{rpq}$. Obviously, the second term has expectation zero.

The first and second derivatives of μ_r with respect to ν_r follow from the identities

$$\delta_{bc} = \frac{\partial \mu_{rb}}{\partial \eta_{ra}} \frac{\partial \eta_{ra}}{\partial \mu_{rc}},$$

$$\frac{\partial^2 \mu_{rb}}{\partial \eta_{ra} \partial \eta_{rd}} = -\sum_{c,a,v} \frac{\partial^2 \eta_{rc}}{\partial \mu_{ra} \partial \mu_{rv}} \frac{\partial \mu_{rb}}{\partial \eta_{rc}} \frac{\partial \mu_{ra}}{\partial \eta_{ra}} \frac{\partial \mu_{rv}}{\partial \eta_{rd}}.$$

Note that the first identity merely rephrases that $Q_r Q_r^{-1} = I$.

Opting for linear predictors, we obtain:

$$\frac{\partial \eta_i}{\partial \beta} = X_i \qquad \frac{\partial^2 \eta_{it}}{\partial \beta_p \partial \beta_q} = 0.$$

We are now able to rewrite the Hessian in a concise matrix form

$$H(\beta) = \sum_{r=1}^{N} X'_r \left[F_r + (Q'_r)^{-1} G_r (Q_r)^{-1} \right] X_r$$

with

$$F_r = \left(\sum_b \frac{\partial^2 \mu_{rb}}{\partial \eta_{ra} \partial \eta_{rd}} \frac{\partial \ell}{\partial \mu_{rb}} \right)_{a,d},$$

$$G_r = \frac{\partial^2 \ell}{\partial \mu_r \partial \mu'_r}.$$

Finally, if we again choose a link function of the type (7.17) we can use simple forms

$$Q_r = \frac{\partial \eta_r}{\partial \mu_r} = C \left\{ \text{diag}(A \mu_r) \right\}^{-1} A = C B_r A$$

and

$$\frac{\partial^2 \eta_{ra}}{\partial \mu_r \mu'_r} = -A' B_{ra}^{(2)} A,$$

where the matrix $B_{ra}^{(2)}$ is obtained by multiplying all rows of B_r^2 with the ath row of C.

7.12.3 Determining the Joint Probabilities

To compute the score equations and to implement the updating algorithm, knowledge of the multivariate cumulative probabilities μ_r is required. The choice of a fitting technique will strongly depend on the choice of link functions. For multivariate odds ratio models (multivariate Dale models, see also Section 7.7) several proposals have been made, such as the use of multivariate Plackett probabilities (Plackett 1965, Molenberghs and Lesaffre 1994), the use of Lagrange multipliers (Lang and Agresti 1994), and a Newton iteration mechanism (Glonek and McCullagh 1995). With the Plackett probability approach, we found that for four and higher dimensional problems, the derivatives of high dimensional polynomials can become numerically unstable. Here, the iterative proportional fitting (IPF) algorithm is adapted to produce a quick and reliable tool to compute the cumulative probabilities. A similar use of the IPF algorithm was proposed by Kauermann (1993). Due to the use of score function (7.60), there is no

7.12 Appendix: Maximum Likelihood Estimation

need to compute the *derivatives* of the probabilities directly since Q_r easily follows from (7.61), leaving only the probabilities to be computed.

Given the marginal probabilities and the odds ratio parameters, our IPF algorithm produces a multidimensional table of cell probabilities. The IPF algorithm is known from its use in fitting log-linear models (Bishop, Fienberg, and Holland 1975), where the association is described using *conditional* odds ratios. The algorithm was also applied by Fitzmaurice and Laird (1993) for their mixed marginal-conditional models (Section 7.8). In our fully marginal models, marginal odds ratios are used. We distinguish between two types. Global odds ratios, given in (7.21)–(7.23), are relevant for ordinal responses (Dale 1984), and local odds ratios as in (7.24) are a natural choice for nominal outcomes. Of course, both sets coincide for binary responses.

We will describe our algorithm for global odds ratios first, and then discuss the local odds ratio version in the concluding paragraph of this section. We need to determine the cumulative probabilities $\mu_r(k_1, \ldots, k_{n_r})$ which correspond to cumulative cell count $Z_r(k_1, \ldots, k_{n_r})$. Recall that this notation encompasses not only n_r-way classifications, but also one-way, two-way,... classifications, by setting an appropriate set of indices $k_j = c_j$. Omitting indices for which $k_j = c_j$, we assume without loss of generality that we need to determine a K-way probability $\mu_r(k_1, \ldots, k_K)$, with $k_j < c_j$ for all j.

We will proceed recursively. First, note that the cumulative probabilities $\mu_r(\ell_1, \ldots, \ell_K)$, with $\ell_j \in \{k_j, c_j\}$ for $j = 1, \ldots, K$, completely describe a 2^K contingency table. Second, as soon as at least one $\ell_j = c_j$, we obtain a lower order probability. Our recursion will be based on the assumption that these lower order probabilities have been determined. The starting point of the inductive construction is obtained by setting all but one $\ell_j = c_j$, whence we obtain univariate probabilities μ_{rjk_j} which are of course easy to determine from the marginal links η_{rjk_j}. Drop the index r from notation.

From the cumulative probabilities, we easily determine the cell probabilities $\mu_{k_1 \ldots k_K}^{z_1 \ldots z_K}$, with $z_j = 1, 2$ and adopt the convention that the K-way cumulative cell probabilities are incorporated as:

$$\mu_{k_1 \ldots k_K}^{1 \ldots 1} = \mu(k_1, \ldots, k_K). \tag{7.64}$$

We will explicitly need the cell probabilities of dimension $K - 1$:

$$\mu_{k_1 \ldots k_{j-1} k_{j+1} \ldots k_K}^{z_1 \ldots z_{j-1} z_{j+1} \ldots z_K} = \sum_{z_j=1}^{2} \mu_{k_1 \ldots k_K}^{z_1 \ldots z_K}.$$

The IPF algorithm is started by choosing a table of initial values, e.g.,

$$\mu_{k_1 \ldots k_K}^{z_1 \ldots z_K}(0) = \begin{cases} \psi_r(k_1, \ldots, k_K) & \text{if } (z_1, \ldots, z_K) = (1, \ldots, 1), \\ 1 & \text{otherwise.} \end{cases}$$

with $\psi_r(k_1, \ldots, k_K) = \exp[\eta_r(k_1, \ldots, k_K)]$, the corresponding global odds ratio. This table clearly has the correct association structure, but the marginals are incorrect and the sum of the cell counts is not equal to one. Updating cycle $(m+1)$ requires K substeps, to match each of the $K-1$ dimensional marginal tables:

$$\mu_{k_1\ldots k_K}^{z_1\ldots z_K}\left(m+\frac{j}{K}\right) = \mu_{k_1\ldots k_K}^{z_1\ldots z_K}\left(m+\frac{j-1}{K}\right) \cdot \frac{\mu_{k_1\ldots k_{j-1}k_{j+1}\ldots k_K}^{z_1\ldots z_{j-1}z_{j+1}\ldots z_K}}{\mu_{k_1\ldots k_{j-1}k_{j+1}\ldots k_K}^{z_1\ldots z_{j-1}z_{j+1}\ldots z_K}\left(m+\frac{j-1}{K}\right)},$$

$(j = 1, \ldots, K)$, the argument of μ indicating the iteration subcycle. Upon convergence, (7.64) can be used to identify the required K-way probability.

Convergence of the IPF algorithm is established in Csiszar (1975). However, the parameter space of the marginal odds ratios is constrained, unless in the special case of a constant odds ratio for a bivariate outcome (Liang, Zeger, and Qaqish 1992). A violation of the constraints will be revealed by a cumulative probability vector with negative entries. If this occurs in the course of an updating algorithm, appropriate action (e.g., step halving) has to be taken. We never encountered problems of this kind, suggesting that the constraints are very mild. Practice suggests that these restrictions are much milder than those for the Bahadur model with which a fully satisfactory analysis of the fluvoxamine data (Section 7.2.4) was not possible.

For marginal local odds ratios a slightly adapted and simpler procedure is proposed. Instead of considering subsets of binary variables, we now consider the whole marginal multi-way table directly. With a similar recursive argument, we assume that the full set of marginal tables up to dimension $K-1$ is determined. Then, we construct a K-dimensional initial table

$$\mu_r^*(k_1, \ldots, k_K)(0) = \prod_{c_j > \ell_j \geq k_j} \psi_r^*(\ell_1, \ldots, \ell_K),$$

for all cells $(k_1, \ldots, k_K)$. This table clearly has got the required K-way local association structure. The updating algorithm matches the entries to the K sets of $K-1$ dimensional marginal tables.

7.13 Appendix: The Multivariate Plackett Distribution

Let us start from the bivariate case first. Given the marginal distributions $F_1(w_1)$, $F_2(w_2)$ and the cross-ratio ψ, the Plackett distribution is the solution of the second degree polynomial equation

$$\psi(F - a_1)(F - a_2) - (F - b_1)(F - b_2) = 0, \qquad (7.65)$$

where $a_1 = F_1, a_2 = F_2, b_1 = 0, b_2 = F_1 + F_2 - 1$. The solution of this equation is given by (7.40). To yield a genuine distribution function, the

7.13 Appendix: The Multivariate Plackett Distribution

solution F of (7.65) should satisfy the Fréchet inequalities (Fréchet 1951):

$$\max(b_1, b_2) \leq F \leq \min(a_1, a_2).$$

Now, this approach can be generalized to n dimensions. To define the multivariate Plackett distribution, consider the set of $2^n - 1$ generalized cross-ratios with values in $[0, +\infty]$:

$$\psi_j, \quad (1 \leq j \leq n)$$
$$\psi_{j_1 j_2}, \quad (1 \leq j_1 < j_2 \leq n)$$
$$\vdots$$
$$\psi_{j_1 \ldots j_k}, \quad (1 \leq j_1 < \ldots < j_k \leq n)$$
$$\vdots$$
$$\psi_{1 \ldots n}.$$

The one-dimensional ψ_j's are precisely the odds of the univariate probabilities, i.e.,

$$\psi_j = \frac{\mu_1^j}{\mu_2^j} = \frac{F_j}{1 - F_j}, \tag{7.66}$$

$(1 \leq j \leq n)$. Note that we put the response level in the subscript to μ and the occasions to which they pertain the superscript. Thus, μ_1^j is the probability to observe a '1' at occasion j and μ_2^j is the probability to observe a '2' at this occasion. Similar conventions will be used for the higher orders. The bivariate associations $\psi_{j_1 j_2}$ are defined as in (7.41):

$$\psi_{j_1 j_2} = \frac{\mu_{11}^{j_1 j_2} \mu_{22}^{j_1 j_2}}{\mu_{12}^{j_1 j_2} \mu_{21}^{j_1 j_2}} = \frac{F_{j_1 j_2}(1 - F_{j_1} - F_{j_2} + F_{j_1 j_2})}{(F_{j_1} - F_{j_1 j_2})(F_{j_2} - F_{j_1 j_2})}, \tag{7.67}$$

$(1 \leq j_1 < j_2 \leq n)$. As soon as $\psi_{j_1}, \psi_{j_2}, \psi_{j_1 j_2}$ are known, $F_{j_1 j_2}$ can be calculated. The cross-ratio $\psi_{j_1 j_2}$ can also be viewed as the odds ratio of $\psi_{j_1(1)}, \psi_{j_2(2)}$, computed as in (7.66), within the first and second level of dimension j_2, respectively.

The three-dimensional cross-ratios can be defined in a similar way as the three factor interactions in loglinear models (Agresti 1990) and is analogous to the above extension. They have been considered already in, for example, (7.21), (7.22), and (7.23). Thus, the cross-ratio $\psi_{j_1 j_2 j_3}$ is defined as the ratio of two conditional cross-ratios $\psi_{j_1 j_2 (1)}$ and $\psi_{j_1 j_2 (2)}$. These are the two-dimensional cross-ratios defined within the first and second level of dimension j_3 respectively. The numerator of $\psi_{j_1 j_2 j_3}$ contains $F_{j_1 j_2 j_3}$ with a positive sign and the denominator contains $F_{j_1 j_2 j_3}$ with a negative sign. Again, the knowledge of the cross-ratios enables one to determine $F_{j_1 j_2 j_3}$.

However, care has to be taken when specifying the cross-ratios, since not every combination leads to a valid solution. This is not surprising, and occurred earlier with the Bahadur model (Section 7.2). Also the multivariate probit model of Section 7.6 is subject to such constraints, since the correlation matrix has to be positive definite. In fact, such constraints will show up for every marginal model, because specifying marginal models implies specifying overlapping information, in contrast to conditional models, the genesis of which can be viewed as specifying new model components, conditional upon ones already in the model. Although this may seem a drawback, it is largely compensated by ease of interpretation for the corresponding model parameters, marginal regression functions, etc.

The n-dimensional probabilities can be computed if all lower dimensional probabilities together with the global cross-ratio of dimension n are known. Let $\mu_{k_1\ldots k_m}^{j_1\ldots j_m}$ be the $(k_1,\ldots,k_m)$-orthant probability of the m-dimensional marginal table, formed by dimensions $(j_1,\ldots,j_m)$. We present the defining equation for $F_{m_1\ldots m_k}$:

$$\psi_{j_1\ldots j_m} = \frac{\prod_{(k_1,\ldots,k_m)\in A_m^+} \mu_{k_1\ldots k_m}^{j_1\ldots j_m}}{\prod_{(k_1,\ldots,k_m)\in A_m^-} \mu_{k_1\ldots k_m}^{j_1\ldots j_m}}, \qquad (7.68)$$

where

$$A_m^+ = \{(k_1,\ldots,k_m)\in\{1,2\}^m | 2 \text{ divides } \sum_{\ell=1}^m k_\ell - m\}$$

and

$$A_m^- = \{1,2\}^m \setminus A_m^+,$$

'\' indicating set difference. In particular, for $F_{1\ldots n}$:

$$\psi_{1\ldots n} = \frac{\prod_{(j_1,\ldots,j_n)\in A_n^+} \mu_{j_1\ldots j_n}}{\prod_{(j_1,\ldots,j_n)\in A_n^-} \mu_{j_1\ldots j_n}}. \qquad (7.69)$$

For example, for $n = 3$:

$$\begin{aligned} A_1^+ &= \{1\}, \\ A_2^+ &= \{(1,1),(2,2)\}, \\ A_3^+ &= \{(1,1,1),(1,2,2),(2,1,2),(2,2,1)\}. \end{aligned}$$

Based on these expressions, (7.68) yields (7.66), (7.67), and the three-dimensional odds-ratio

$$\psi_{123} = \frac{\mu_{111}\mu_{122}\mu_{212}\mu_{221}}{\mu_{112}\mu_{121}\mu_{211}\mu_{222}}.$$

The orthant probabilities $\mu_{k_1\ldots k_n}$ are determined by the distribution F. A general expression can be derived, which will be useful for the automated

7.13 Appendix: The Multivariate Plackett Distribution

computation of the orthant probabilities. Some notation is needed. Let $\lambda(\boldsymbol{k}) \equiv \lambda(k_1,\ldots,k_n)$ be the set of places for which k_j is equal to 1, (e.g., $\lambda(1,2,1,1) = \{1,3,4\}$), then

$$\mu_{k_1\ldots k_n} = \sum_{\boldsymbol{s} \supset \lambda(\boldsymbol{k})} \operatorname{sgn}(\boldsymbol{s}) F_{\boldsymbol{s}}, \qquad (7.70)$$

where

$$\operatorname{sgn}(\boldsymbol{s}) = \begin{cases} 1 & \text{if } \#\boldsymbol{s} - \#\beta(\boldsymbol{k}) \text{ is even,} \\ -1 & \text{otherwise,} \end{cases}$$

and $F_{\boldsymbol{s}} = F_{s_1\ldots s_m}$, with $s_1 \leq \ldots \leq s_m$. In the three-dimensional case, the octant probabilities are

$$\begin{aligned}
\mu_{111} &= F_{123}, \\
\mu_{112} &= F_{12} - F_{123}, \\
\mu_{121} &= F_{13} - F_{123}, \\
\mu_{211} &= F_{23} - F_{123}, \\
\mu_{122} &= F_1 - F_{12} - F_{13} + F_{123}, \\
\mu_{212} &= F_2 - F_{12} - F_{23} + F_{123}, \\
\mu_{221} &= F_3 - F_{13} - F_{23} + F_{123}, \\
\mu_{222} &= 1 - F_1 - F_2 - F_3 + F_{12} + F_{13} + F_{23} - F_{123}.
\end{aligned} \qquad (7.71)$$

As an example, consider μ_{212}. In this case, $\lambda(2,1,2) = \{2\}$ and there are 4 possible vectors $\boldsymbol{s}$: (2), (1,2), (2,3) and (1,2,3). Therefore, (7.70) yields the expression for μ_{212} in (7.71).

The set of $2^n - 1$ generalized cross-ratios fully specifies the n-dimensional Plackett distribution. However, from the above reasoning it is not clear whether such a distribution always exists. Further, if existence and uniqueness is guaranteed it is not yet clear how to calculate the distribution since it is only implicitly specified by (7.68). These matters are discussed next.

Let us turn to some computational details. Note that the probabilities in the numerator (denominator) of (7.69) involve $+F_{12\ldots n}$ ($-F_{12\ldots n}$) and that both numerator and denominator contain an even number of factors. Thus, (7.69) may be abbreviated as

$$\psi = \frac{\prod_{i=1}^{2^{n-1}} (F - b_i)}{\prod_{i=1}^{2^{n-1}} (F - a_i)}, \qquad (7.72)$$

where $\psi \equiv \psi_{1\ldots n}$ and $F \equiv F_{1\ldots n}$. The a_i and b_i are functions of the $(n-1)$- and lower-dimensional probabilities (or, equivalently, cross-ratios). A valid solution must satisfy

$$\max_i b_i \leq F \leq \min_i a_i. \qquad (7.73)$$

However, this condition is not satisfied for all choices of a_i and b_i. To see this, take the three-way Plackett distribution. Then, according to (7.73), the one- and two-dimensional marginal distributions have to satisfy the following inequalities:

$$F_{j_1 j_2} + F_{j_1 j_3} \leq F_{j_1} + F_{j_2 j_3}, \quad (j_1 \neq j_2 \neq j_3 \neq j_1)$$
$$F_1 + F_2 + F_3 \leq 1 + F_{12} + F_{13} + F_{23}.$$

Now, as a counterexample, if

$$F_1 = F_2 = F_3 = \frac{1}{2},$$
$$\psi_{12} = 0.05,$$
$$\psi_{13} = 1,$$
$$\psi_{23} = 20,$$

then $F_{13} + F_{23} > F_3 + F_{12}$ and (7.73) cannot be satisfied.

In spite of this, the constraints for this model never were burdensome, neither in the analyses reported in this book, nor for others done by the authors and reported elsewhere. The same holds for the multivariate probit model. This is in contrast to the Bahadur model, where the analysis of the fluvoxamine trial (Section 7.2.4) already posed insurmountable problems.

In case (7.73) is satisfied, existence and uniqueness of a solution is guaranteed by the next lemma. The verification of (7.73) is straightforward, as the functions b_i and a_i are linear functions of the lower order marginal probabilities.

Lemma 7.1 *Let*

$$P(C) = \psi \prod_{i=1}^m (C - a_i) - \prod_{i=1}^m (C - b_i),$$

where m is even, $0 < \psi < +\infty$, and

$$b_1 = \max_{1 \leq i \leq m} b_i < \min_{1 \leq i \leq m} a_i = a_1,$$

then the interval $]b_1, a_1[$ contains exactly one real root of $P(C)$.

Proof. The inequalities

$$P(a_1) = -\prod_{i=1}^m (a_1 - b_i) < 0$$

and

$$P(b_1) = \psi \prod_{i=1}^m (b_1 - a_i) > 0,$$

together with the continuity of $P(C)$, establish the existence. Now,

$$\frac{\partial P}{\partial C} = \psi \sum_{i=1}^{m} \prod_{j \neq i} (C - a_j) - \sum_{i=1}^{m} \prod_{j \neq i} (C - b_j) = \psi \sum_{i} T_i - \sum_{i} S_i.$$

T_i is a product of $(m-1)$ negative factors, whence T_i is negative. S_i is positive, so $P(C)$ is strictly decreasing in $]b_1, a_1[$, establishing the result.

It follows from the proof that the regula falsi method with starting points a_1 and b_1 always leads to the solution. Though in general a_1 and b_1 are close to each other and convergence is quickly reached, it is desirable to look for even faster methods. It is our experience that a Newton iteration with starting point, for example, $\frac{1}{2}(a_1 + b_1)$ converges to the root, generally in 3 or 4 steps (with convergence criterion: $|c_{k+1} - c_k| < 10^{-8}$).

An algebraic solution to the two-dimensional problem is given by Mardia (1970) and Dale (1986). The three-way Plackett distribution can also be solved algebraically using Ferrari's method for solving fourth-degree polynomials. However, the solution cannot be written in a mathematically elegant way. From the four-way Plackett distribution on, one has to rely on numerical techniques. It is a fundamental result of algebra that a polynomial of degree higher than 5 has no algebraic solution. This is not a major disadvantage, since numerical methods for the multivariate Dale model are usually much faster than for the multivariate probit model, which necessitates the calculation of multivariate normal integrals.

7.14 Appendix: Maximum Likelihood Estimation for the Dale Model

We present the basic tools for the computations. We distinguish between the following parts: model description, likelihood function and cell probabilities, and score functions and information matrix.

It is, again, convenient to adopt the contingency table notation, assuming that subjects $i = 1, \ldots, N_r$ are grouped within covariate or design levels $r = 1, \ldots, N$ (Section 7.1). Thus, observations, sharing covariate vector $\boldsymbol{x}_r$, are combined into a single $c_1 \times \ldots \times c_n$ contingency table. The dimension of this table will be abbreviated by $\boldsymbol{c}$. In other words, we adopt the table notation. Denote the entries of this table by $z_{r\boldsymbol{k}}$. Here, $\boldsymbol{k}$ indicates a multi-index: $\boldsymbol{k} = (k_1, \ldots, k_n)$, $(1 \leq k_j \leq c_j, l = 1, \ldots, n)$. In vector notation: $1 \leq \boldsymbol{k} \leq \boldsymbol{c}$. A particular table is indicated by $(z_{r\boldsymbol{k}})_{\boldsymbol{k}}$.

We assume that the tables are sampled from a multinomial distribution, with cell probabilities $(\mu^*_{r\boldsymbol{k}})_{\boldsymbol{k}}$, $(r = 1, \ldots, N)$, given by the MDM. They are derived from the orthant probabilities, defined by (7.70). The model is fully specified by link functions $\eta_{rjk} = \eta_{rj}(\boldsymbol{x}_r)$ given by (7.48), $\gamma_{j_1 j_2}^{k_1 k_2}(\boldsymbol{x}_r)$

given by (7.49), together with the higher-order association parameters. If we denote them by ϕ with an appropriate subscript, then we obtain in vector notation $\ln \psi_h = \phi_h$, with h a vector running through all higher order associations. The parameters γ and ϕ determine the association structure.

Assume that all parameters form a column vector $\boldsymbol{\theta}$. The log-likelihood takes the form:

$$\ell(\boldsymbol{\theta}) = \sum_{r=1}^{N} \sum_{\boldsymbol{k}=1}^{\boldsymbol{c}} z_{r\boldsymbol{k}} \ln \mu_{\boldsymbol{k}}^{*}(\boldsymbol{\theta}, \boldsymbol{x}_r), \tag{7.74}$$

and is fully determined if we indicate in what way the cell probabilities $\mu_{r\boldsymbol{k}}(\boldsymbol{\theta}) = \mu_{\boldsymbol{k}}(\boldsymbol{\theta}, \boldsymbol{x}_r)$ arise from the link functions. Let $\mu_{r\boldsymbol{k}} = \mu_{\boldsymbol{k}}(\boldsymbol{x}_r)$, denote the n-dimensional cumulative Plackett distribution function F, evaluated in the appropriate links:

$$\mu_{r\boldsymbol{k}} = F(\boldsymbol{\eta}_r, \boldsymbol{\gamma}_r, \boldsymbol{\phi}), \tag{7.75}$$

where the arguments are appropriately vectorized forms of the links. Note that $\mu_{r\boldsymbol{k}}$ is the orthant probability of $[-\infty, \eta_{r1k_1}] \times \ldots \times [-\infty, \eta_{rnk_n}]$. To compute the cell probabilities, write the cutpoints for dimension j as:

$$-\infty = \eta_{rj0} < \eta_{rj1} < \ldots < \eta_{rj,c_j-1} < \eta_{rjc_j} = +\infty.$$

If one or more components k_j of $\boldsymbol{k}$ are equal to zero, the corresponding orthant probability $\mu_{r\boldsymbol{k}}$ vanishes. If one or more components of $\boldsymbol{k}$ equal c_j, then $\mu_{r\boldsymbol{k}}$ is an orthant probability of a lower dimensional marginal distribution.

The cell probabilities $\mu_{r\boldsymbol{k}}^{*}$ can be expressed in terms of $\mu_{r\boldsymbol{k}}$:

$$\mu_{r\boldsymbol{k}}^{*} = \sum_{\boldsymbol{h}} (-1)^{S(\boldsymbol{k},\boldsymbol{h})} \mu_{r\boldsymbol{h}}.$$

Summation goes over all indices $\boldsymbol{h}$ satisfying $\boldsymbol{0} \leq \boldsymbol{k} - \boldsymbol{h} \leq \boldsymbol{1}$, and the function S is defined by $S(\boldsymbol{k}, \boldsymbol{h}) = \sum_{j=1}^{n} k_j - h_j$. The computation of $\mu_{\boldsymbol{k}}$ in (7.75) involves the evaluation of the cumulative Plackett distribution. The derivatives are computed by implicit derivation of (7.72).

The derivative of the log-likelihood ℓ with respect to a marginal parameter θ can be written as:

$$\frac{\partial \ell}{\partial \theta} = \sum_{r=1}^{N} \sum_{\boldsymbol{k}=1}^{\boldsymbol{c}} z_{r\boldsymbol{k}} \frac{1}{\mu_{r\boldsymbol{k}}^{*}} \sum_{j=1}^{n} \sum_{m=1}^{c_j-1} \frac{\partial \mu_{r\boldsymbol{m}}^{*}}{\partial \eta_{jm}(\boldsymbol{x}_r)} \frac{\partial \eta_{jm}(\boldsymbol{x}_r)}{\partial \theta}. \tag{7.76}$$

A few conventions will simplify notation. First, assume there is only one covariate vector $\boldsymbol{x}$, thereby dropping the index r. Second, due to model (7.48), a marginal parameter pertains to only one margin, j say. For such a parameter, summation over all $j = 1, \ldots, n$ is replaced by a single j. In principle, we need to distinguish between intercepts $\beta_{0,jm}$, corresponding to

7.14 Appendix: Maximum Likelihood Estimation for the Dale Model

only one cutpoint m, and covariate parameters β, common to all cutpoints $k = 1, \ldots, c_j - 1$ of dimension j. However, we assume that *every* marginal parameter pertains to only one cutpoint, m_j say. The correct formula can be obtained by summing over all cutpoints, if needed. In conclusion, j and $m = m_j$ will be assumed to be fixed. Finally, note that in most formulas, some indices k_j of $\boldsymbol{k}$ will play a particular role and need being mentioned explicitely. The remaining indices will be denoted by $\boldsymbol{k}'$. Accordingly, the upper bound is denoted by $\boldsymbol{c}'$. In subscripts (e.g., $\mu^*_{\boldsymbol{k}}$), only the relevant indices will be mentioned. Applying these conventions to (7.76) yields

$$\frac{\partial \ell}{\partial \theta} = \frac{\partial \eta_{jm}}{\partial \theta} \sum_{\boldsymbol{k}'=1}^{\boldsymbol{c}'} \left(\frac{z_m}{\mu^*_m} - \frac{z_{m+1}}{\mu^*_{m+1}} \right) \sum_{\boldsymbol{h}, h_j = m} (-1)^{S(\boldsymbol{k}'m, \boldsymbol{h})} \frac{\partial \mu_{\boldsymbol{h}}}{\partial \eta_{jm}}.$$

For an intercept or covariate parameter in the two-way association model, we deduce

$$\frac{\partial \ell}{\partial \theta} = \frac{\partial \gamma_{j_1 j_2}}{\partial \theta} \sum_{\boldsymbol{k}} z_{\boldsymbol{k}} \frac{1}{\mu^*_{\boldsymbol{k}}} \psi_{j_1 j_2}^{k_1 k_2} \sum_{\boldsymbol{h}} (-1)^{S(\boldsymbol{k}, \boldsymbol{h})} \frac{\partial \mu_{\boldsymbol{h}}}{\partial \psi_{j_1 j_2}}.$$

Note that a similar form is obtained for higher order associations. For a parameter θ in (7.49) pertaining to a row category m, the score equation is

$$\frac{\partial \ell}{\partial \theta} = \frac{\partial \gamma_{j_1 j_2}}{\partial \theta} \sum_{\boldsymbol{k}'=1}^{\boldsymbol{c}'} \left(\frac{z_m}{\mu^*_m} - \frac{z_{m+1}}{\mu^*_{m+1}} \right) \psi_{j_1 j_2}^{m\, k_2} \sum_{\boldsymbol{h}, h_{j_1} = m} (-1)^{S(\boldsymbol{k}'m, \boldsymbol{h})} \frac{\partial \mu_{\boldsymbol{h}}}{\partial \psi_{j_1 j_2}},$$

while for a cell-specific parameter we find

$$\frac{\partial \ell}{\partial \theta} = \frac{\partial \gamma_{j_1 j_2}}{\partial \theta} \sum_{\boldsymbol{k}'=1}^{\boldsymbol{c}'} \left(\frac{z_{m_1 m_2}}{\mu^*_{m_1 m_2}} - \frac{z_{m_1+1, m_2}}{\mu^*_{m_1+1, m_2}} - \frac{z_{m_1, m_2+1}}{\mu^*_{m_1, m_2+1}} + \frac{z_{m_1+1, m_2+1}}{\mu^*_{m_1+1, m_2+1}} \right)$$
$$\times \psi_{j_1 j_2}^{m_1 m_2} \sum_{\boldsymbol{h}, h_{j_1} = m_1, h_{j_2} = m_2} (-1)^{S(\boldsymbol{k} m_1 m_2, \boldsymbol{h})} \frac{\partial \mu_{\boldsymbol{h}}}{\partial \psi_{j_1 j_2}}.$$

Straightforward but lengthy computations lead to expressions for the elements of the expected information matrix. We do not present them here; they are available as a technical report from the first author. They are used to implement a Fisher scoring algorithm, to maximize (7.74).

8
Generalized Estimating Equations

8.1 Introduction

The main issue with full likelihood approaches for marginal models is the computational complexity they entail. The net benefit can be efficiency gain, but this comes at the cost of an increased risk for model misspecification. Of course, full likelihood methods clearly allow the researcher to calculate joint or union probabilities (such as in the POPS data, Section 7.10) and to make, perhaps subtle, inferences about the association structure. The latter was exemplified in Section 7.7.7. Chapter 7 also made it clear that there is no unambiguous choice for a full distributional specification. For example, while the Bahadur model (Section 7.2) is easy to generate, it suffers from severe restrictions on the parameter space. Other models may become unwieldy in computational terms when the number of repeated measures increases beyond a moderate number.

For all of these reasons, when we are mainly interested in first-order marginal mean parameters and pairwise interactions, a full likelihood procedure can be replaced by quasi-likelihood based methods (McCullagh and Nelder 1989). In quasi-likelihood, the mean response is expressed as a parametric function of covariates, and the variance is assumed to be a function of the mean up to possibly unknown scale parameters. Wedderburn (1974) first noted that likelihood and quasi-likelihood theories coincide for exponential families and that the quasi-likelihood estimating equations provide consistent estimates of the regression parameters β in any generalized linear model, even for choices of link and variance functions that do not correspond to exponential families.

For clustered and repeated data, Liang and Zeger (1986) proposed so-called *generalized estimating equations* (GEE or GEE1) which require only the correct specification of the univariate marginal distributions provided one is willing to adopt 'working' assumptions about the association structure. These models are a direct extension of basic quasi-likelihood theory from cross-sectional to repeated or otherwise correlated measurements. They estimate the parameters associated with the expected value of an individual's vector of binary responses and phrase the working assumptions about the association between pairs of outcomes in terms of marginal correlations. The method combines estimating equations for the regression parameters $\boldsymbol{\beta}$ with moment-based estimation for the correlation parameters entering the working assumptions.

Although Liang and Zeger's (1986) original proposal is undoubtedly the best known one, not in the least due to its implementation in a number of standard software packages, including the SAS procedure GENMOD, a number of alternative proposals have been made as well. Prentice (1988) extended their results to allow joint estimation of probabilities and pairwise correlations. Lipsitz, Laird, and Harrington (1991) modified the estimating equations of Prentice (1988) to allow modeling of the association through marginal odds ratios rather than marginal correlations. When adopting GEE1, one does not use information of the association structure to estimate the main effect parameters. As a result, it can be shown that GEE1 yields consistent main effect estimators, even when the association structure is misspecified. However, severe misspecification may affect the efficiency of the GEE1 estimators. In addition, GEE1 is less adequate when some scientific interest is placed on the association parameters.

Second-order extensions of these estimating equations (GEE2) that include the marginal pairwise association as well, have been studied by Zhao and Prentice (1990), using correlations, and Liang, Zeger, and Qaqish (1992), using odds ratios. They note that GEE2 is nearly fully efficient, as compared to a full likelihood approach, though bias may occur in the estimation of the main effect parameters when the association structure is misspecified. A variation to this theme, using conditional probability ideas, has been proposed by Carey, Zeger, and Diggle (1993). It is referred to as *alternating logistic regressions* and is studied in Section 8.6, alongside second-order GEE. In the same spirit, in Section 8.7, we will show how the hybrid model, combining elements of a marginal and a conditional formulation, introduced in Section 7.8, can be used as the basis for another GEE approach, maintaining computational ease (Fitzmaurice and Laird 1993, Fitzmaurice, Laird, and Rotnitzky 1993).

In Section 8.2, we present the basic GEE theory, while extensions and variations to the theme are the topic of Section 8.3. Some of these are then developed in sections to follow. Prentice's method is reviewed in Section 8.4. Second-order generalized estimating equations are introduced in Section 8.5. GEE based on odds ratios and alternating logistic regressions are discussed in Section 8.6. GEE based on the hybrid marginal-conditional formulation is given in Section 8.7, from which some of the other methods follow as special cases. An alternative approach, based on linearization, is given in Section 8.8. Next, three case studies are analyzed: the NTP data (Section 8.9), the heatshock study, a developmental toxicity study (Section 8.10), and the sports injuries trail (Section 8.11).

8.2 Standard GEE Theory

Let us adopt the regression notation, as outlined in Section 7.1.

In many longitudinal applications, inferences based on mean parameters (e.g., dose effect) are of primary interest. Specifying the full joint distribution would then be unnecessarily cumbersome. When inferences for the parameters in the mean model $E(\boldsymbol{Y}_i)$ are based on classical maximum likelihood theory, full specification of the joint distribution for the vector $\boldsymbol{Y}_i$ of repeated measurements within each unit i is necessary. For discrete data, this implies specification of the first-order moments, as well as of all higher-order moments. For Gaussian data, full-model specification reduces to modeling the first- and second-order moments only, a situation much simpler than in the non-Gaussian case. However, even then can the choice of inappropriate covariance models seriously invalidate inferences for the mean structure.

A technique enabling the researcher to restrict modeling to the first moment only is based on so-called *generalized estimating equations* (GEEs, Liang and Zeger 1986, Zeger and Liang 1986, Diggle *et al* 2002). One way to approach the methodology is by making two observations. First, the score equations for a multivariate marginal normal model $\boldsymbol{Y}_i \sim N(X_i\boldsymbol{\beta}, V_i)$ (Chapter 4; see also Verbeke and Molenberghs 2000, Chapter 5) are given by

$$\sum_{i=1}^N X_i'(A_i^{1/2} R_i A_i^{1/2})^{-1}(\boldsymbol{y}_i - X_i\boldsymbol{\beta}) = \boldsymbol{0}, \tag{8.1}$$

in which the marginal covariance matrix V_i has been decomposed in the form

$$V_i = A_i^{1/2} R_i A_i^{1/2}, \tag{8.2}$$

with A_i the matrix with the marginal variances on the main diagonal and zeros elsewhere, and with R_i equal to the marginal correlation matrix. Decomposition (8.2) is a little unusual in this context, although it is easy to see what it would look like for such structures as, for example, compound symmetry and AR(1). A common decomposition is in terms of a marginalized hierarchical model: $V_i = \Sigma_i + Z_i D Z_i'$ (see Chapter 4). The motivation will become clear before too long.

As a second observation, the score equations to be solved when computing maximum likelihood estimates under a marginal generalized linear model, (Chapter 3) assuming independence of the responses within units (either ignoring the correlation in the repeated measures structure or when truly dealing with uncorrelated measures), takes the form

$$\sum_{i=1}^{N} \frac{\partial \mu_i}{\partial \beta'} (A_i^{1/2} I_{n_i} A_i^{1/2})^{-1} (y_i - \mu_i) = 0, \qquad (8.3)$$

where, again, A_i is again the diagonal matrix with the marginal variances along the main diagonal. The mean μ_i follows from a vector of generalized linear models, specified for each component of the outcome vector. For example, a logistic regression can be specified for each of the components.

Note that expression (8.1) is of the form (8.3) but with the correlations between repeated measures taken into account. A key distinction between both is that A_i (and V_i as a whole) in (8.1) is usually parameterized by a set of parameters, functionally independent of the marginal regression parameters β. On the other hand, A_i in (8.3) is fully specified by the marginal regression parameters β, through the mean-variance link, common to most commonly used generalized linear models, as outlined in Chapter 3. Thus, when measurements are truly uncorrelated, one can restrict model specification to the marginal mean function, as the variance will automatically follow, perhaps up to an overdispersion parameter. These observations are crucial in what follows.

A seemingly straightforward extension of (8.3) that would account for the correlation structure is

$$S(\beta) = \sum_{i=1}^{N} \frac{\partial \mu_i}{\partial \beta'} (A_i^{1/2} R_i A_i^{1/2})^{-1} (y_i - \mu_i) = 0, \qquad (8.4)$$

obtained from replacing the identity matrix I_{n_i} by a correlation matrix R_i. Now, even though (8.4) seems to follow from combining the most general aspects of (8.1) with those of (8.3), matters are not this simple. Although $A_i = A_i(\beta)$ follows directly from the marginal mean model, β commonly contains absolutely no information about R_i, whence R_i is to be parameterized by an additional parameter vector: $R_i = R_i(\alpha)$. Thus, while the first moment completely specified the second (and higher order) moments in the univariate case, this is only partially so in the correlated data setting, the variances are still specified by the marginal means, but the correlations are not. This sets the repeated measures and other correlated data settings fundamentally apart from their univariate counterpart. Simply adding model components (and hence score equations) for the correlation parameters does not solve the problem. To see this, recall that we wanted to restrict model specification to the first moments only, but are faced with the second moments. If we would model the second moments, we would have to address the third and fourth moments as well. Eventually, a full specification of the joint distribution would be obtained, precisely what we wanted to avoid. These observations also underscore the difference between the Gaussian and non-Gaussian settings, as (8.1) is sufficient for the Gaussian case: given the first- and second-order moments, *and assuming multivariate normality*, the joint distribution is fully specified. Thus, in summary, it is too simple to state that the repeated non-Gaussian case is simply a combination of elements from the Gaussian repeated measures case with elements from univariate generalized linear models.

Liang and Zeger (1986) provide a nice way out of this apparent gridlock. While still acknowledging the need for $R_i(\boldsymbol{\alpha})$ in V_i and (8.4), they allowed the modeler to *specify an incorrect structure* or so-called working correlation matrix. Using method of moments concepts, they showed that, when the marginal mean $\boldsymbol{\mu}_i$ has been correctly specified as $h(\boldsymbol{\mu}_i) = X_i\boldsymbol{\beta}$ and when mild regularity conditions hold, the estimator $\widehat{\boldsymbol{\beta}}$ obtained from solving (8.4) is consistent and asymptotically normally distributed with mean $\boldsymbol{\beta}$ and asymptotic variance-covariance matrix covariance matrix

$$\mathrm{Var}(\widehat{\boldsymbol{\beta}}) = I_0^{-1} I_1 I_0^{-1}, \tag{8.5}$$

where

$$I_0 = \sum_{i=1}^{N} \frac{\partial \boldsymbol{\mu}_i'}{\partial \boldsymbol{\beta}} V_i^{-1} \frac{\partial \boldsymbol{\mu}_i}{\partial \boldsymbol{\beta}'}, \tag{8.6}$$

$$I_1 = \sum_{i=1}^{N} \frac{\partial \boldsymbol{\mu}_i'}{\partial \boldsymbol{\beta}} V_i^{-1} \mathrm{Var}(\boldsymbol{Y}_i) V_i^{-1} \frac{\partial \boldsymbol{\mu}_i}{\partial \boldsymbol{\beta}'}. \tag{8.7}$$

Consistent estimates can be obtained by replacing all unknown quantities in (8.5) by consistent estimates. Apart from a working correlation matrix, it is possible to incorporate an overdispersion parameter as well, whence $A_i^{1/2} R_i A_i^{1/2}$ in (8.4) would be replaced by

$$V_i = V_i(\boldsymbol{\beta}, \boldsymbol{\alpha}, \phi) = \phi A_i(\boldsymbol{\beta})^{1/2} R_i(\boldsymbol{\alpha}) A_i(\boldsymbol{\beta})^{1/2}, \tag{8.8}$$

ϕ being the additional overdispersion parameter.

Observe that, when R_i would be correctly specified, $\mathrm{Var}(\boldsymbol{Y}_i) = V_i$ in (8.7) and then $I_1 = I_0$. As a result, (8.5) would reduce to I_0^{-1}, corresponding to full likelihood, i.e., when the first and second moment assumptions would be correct. Thus, (8.5) reduces to full likelihood when the working correlation structure is correctly specified but generally differs from it. There is no price to pay in terms of consistency of asymptotic normality, but there may be efficiency loss when the working correlation structure differs strongly from the true underlying structure.

Thus, whether or not the working correlation structure is correct, point estimates and standard errors based on (8.5) are asymptotically correct. Such standard errors were called 'robust' by Liang and Zeger (1986), while the variance estimator (8.5) is sometimes referred to as the 'sandwich estimator,' for obvious reasons. In the meantime, the terms 'empirically corrected' variance and standard errors found their way to common use, to avoid confusion with methods from robust statistics. In contrast, I_0^{-1} was initially referred to as the 'naive' estimator, but currently the more neutral '(purely) model based' estimator is more common. Note that estimates and standard errors resulting from GEE are often reported in the format 'estimate (empirically corrected standard error; model-based standard error),' in line with the convention used by Liang and Zeger (1986) in their original article. Unless when used for didactical purposes, or when the model-based standard error would be of some scientific interest, this is not necessary. The empirically corrected standard error is the one to be used, the other one generally incorrect. At best, it can be seen as an indication of the 'distance' between the working assumptions for the correlation and the true structure. When both standard errors are far apart, this can be seen as an indication for a poor choice of working assumptions. Once again, a poor working assumption is not wrong, but may hamper efficiency and, when at all possible, it may be of interest to then try alternative working assumptions. The term 'empirical correction' stems from the fact that the data $\boldsymbol{Y}_i$ are used in I_1, not directly following from the likelihood function.

Two further specifications are needed before GEE is operational: $\text{Var}(\boldsymbol{Y}_i)$ on the one hand and $R_i(\boldsymbol{\alpha})$, with in particular estimation of $\boldsymbol{\alpha}$, on the other hand. Full modeling will not be an option, since we would then be forced to do what we want to avoid. First, modeling $\text{Var}(\boldsymbol{Y}_i)$ would imply modeling all components of (8.8) correctly, which we wanted to avoid. Second, fully modeling $R_i(\alpha)$ would, once again, bring in the need to address third and fourth order moments, which we wanted to avoid as well. Let us discuss the pragmatic solutions found to both of these issues in turn.

Turning attention to the empirical covariance of the outcome vector, $\text{Var}(\boldsymbol{Y}_i)$ in (8.5) is typically replaced by

$$(\boldsymbol{y}_i - \boldsymbol{\mu}_i)(\boldsymbol{y}_i - \boldsymbol{\mu}_i)'. \tag{8.9}$$

Although this may seem a natural choice at first sight, also because it is an unbiased estimate at the sole condition that the mean is correctly specified, it is perhaps less so when one realizes it has rank at most one! However, while a poor estimator for $\text{Var}(\boldsymbol{Y}_i)$, it is adequate to estimate I_1 and ultimately (8.5), given the summation over N units in I_1. The deficient rank poses no problems since no inversion takes place within I_1 and, as an extra safety, I_1 does not need to be inverted. It has been reported

TABLE 8.1. *Common choices for the working correlation assumptions in standard generalized estimating equations and moment-based estimators thereof.*

Structure	$\text{Corr}(Y_{ij}, Y_{ik})$	Estimator
Independence	0	—
Exchangeable	α	$\widehat{\alpha} = \frac{1}{N} \sum_{i=1}^{N} \frac{1}{n_i(n_i-1)} \sum_{j \neq k} e_{ij} e_{ik}$
AR(1)	$\alpha^{|j-k|}$	$\widehat{\alpha} = \frac{1}{N} \sum_{i=1}^{N} \frac{1}{n_i-1} \sum_{j \leq n_i-1} e_{ij} e_{i,j+1}$
Unstructured	α_{jk}	$\widehat{\alpha}_{jk} = \frac{1}{N} \sum_{i=1}^{N} e_{ij} e_{ik}$

that replacing (8.9) by $(\boldsymbol{y}_i - \widehat{\boldsymbol{\mu}_i})(\boldsymbol{y}_i - \widehat{\boldsymbol{\mu}_i})'$ may induce some bias into the procedure (Crowder 1995).

Next, regarding the working correlation parameters $\boldsymbol{\alpha}$ and the overdispersion parameter ϕ, Liang and Zeger (1986) proposed moment-based estimates. To this end, first define residuals

$$e_{ij} = \frac{y_{ij} - \mu_{ij}}{\sqrt{v(\mu_{ij})}} \tag{8.10}$$

in line with (7.7), introduced for the Bahadur model. Note that $e_{ij} = e_{ij}(\boldsymbol{\beta})$ through $\mu_{ij} = \mu_{ij}(\boldsymbol{\beta})$ and therefore also through $v(\mu_{ij})$, the variance at time j, and hence the jth diagonal element of A_i. We still assume the variance is decomposed as (8.8). Common choices for the working assumptions are presented in Table 8.1. Similarly, the dispersion parameter can be estimated by

$$\widehat{\phi} = \frac{1}{N} \sum_{i=1}^{N} \frac{1}{n_i} \sum_{j=1}^{n_i} e_{ij}^2. \tag{8.11}$$

Note that the independence structure brings about no additional parameters $\boldsymbol{\alpha}$ and hence, when there is no overdispersion, parameter estimates $\widehat{\boldsymbol{\beta}}$ will not differ from those obtained from logistic regression. Even then, the asymptotic variance covariance matrix, obtained from (8.5), and hence the standard errors, will differ from the ones obtained with logistic regression, the latter stemming from the model-based but incorrect I_1^{-1}. Independence and exchangeable working assumptions can be used in virtually all applications, whether longitudinal, clustered, multivariate, or otherwise correlated. Clearly, AR(1) and unstructured are less relevant for clustered data, longitudinal studies with unequally spaced measurements and/or sequences with differing lengths, etc. However, even though it seems less advisable to use such structures in cases where they are not supported by the study's design, it is strictly speaking not a mistake as, once again, working assumptions *are allowed to be wrong!* Note that the AR(1) parameter is estimated

158   8. Generalized Estimating Equations

using adjacent pairs of measurements only, in contrast to the exchangeable correlation, for which all pairs within a sequence are employed. This is not wrong, but may be somewhat inefficient as, for example, pairs two occasions apart contribute information to α^2 and hence to α. Of course, incorporating such information clutters the moment-based estimators and most implementations still follow Table 8.1, as in Liang and Zeger (1986).

Now, (8.4), conceived to estimate $\boldsymbol{\beta}$, are in need of $\boldsymbol{\alpha}$ and ϕ, while the moment-based estimates for $\boldsymbol{\alpha}$ (Table 8.1) and expression (8.11) for ϕ depend on $\boldsymbol{\beta}$. This circularity is the final stumbling block in the way, but can be circumvented by an iterative procedure. The standard iterative procedure to fit GEE, based on Liang and Zeger (1986), is then as follows:

1. Compute initial estimates for $\boldsymbol{\beta}$, $\boldsymbol{\beta}^{(0)}$ say, using a univariate GLM, i.e., assuming independence or, in other words, using conventional logistic regression.

2. Compute the quantities needed in the estimating equation, i.e., Pearson residuals e_{ij} from (8.10), $\boldsymbol{\alpha}$ from Table 8.1, and ϕ from (8.11).

3. Based on these, $R_i(\boldsymbol{\alpha})$ can be computed, as well as V_i from (8.8).

4. Then, given the current estimate of $\boldsymbol{\beta}$ after t iterations, $\boldsymbol{\beta}^{(t)}$ say, update the estimate for $\boldsymbol{\beta}$:

$$\begin{aligned}\boldsymbol{\beta}^{(t+1)} &= \boldsymbol{\beta}^{(t)} - \left[\sum_{i=1}^{N}\left(\frac{\partial \boldsymbol{\mu}_i}{\partial \boldsymbol{\beta}'}\right)V_i^{-1}\left(\frac{\partial \boldsymbol{\mu}_i}{\partial \boldsymbol{\beta}'}\right)'\right]^{-1}\\&\quad \times \left[\sum_{i=1}^{N}\left(\frac{\partial \boldsymbol{\mu}_i}{\partial \boldsymbol{\beta}'}\right)V_i^{-1}(\boldsymbol{y}_i - \boldsymbol{\mu}_i)\right].\end{aligned} \quad (8.12)$$

The second, third, and fourth steps need to be iterated until convergence.

In conclusion, we have a method at our disposition to obtain valid inferences about a marginal regression model for repeated and otherwise clustered data, without the need to fully specify the joint distribution of the outcomes. This is most useful when the outcomes are of a non-Gaussian nature, as the linear mixed-effects model provides a flexible framework in the latter case (Chapter 4). However, it would still be possible to apply robust inference in the Gaussian case as well (Verbeke and Molenberghs 2000, Section 6.2.4), in case interest is confined to the marginal regression parameters $\boldsymbol{\beta}$, and there is doubt about a correct specification of the covariance structure and/or the random-effects structure. Indeed, the usual estimate for $\boldsymbol{\beta}$ is

$$\widehat{\boldsymbol{\beta}}(\boldsymbol{\alpha}) = \left(\sum_{i=1}^{N}X_i'W_iX_i\right)^{-1}\sum_{i=1}^{N}X_i'W_i\boldsymbol{Y}_i,$$

with α replaced by its ML or REML estimate. Conditional on α, $\widehat{\boldsymbol{\beta}}$ has mean

$$\begin{aligned} E\left[\widehat{\boldsymbol{\beta}}(\boldsymbol{\alpha})\right] &= \left(\sum_{i=1}^{N} X_i' W_i X_i\right)^{-1} \sum_{i=1}^{N} X_i' W_i E(\boldsymbol{Y}_i) \\ &= \left(\sum_{i=1}^{N} X_i' W_i X_i\right)^{-1} \sum_{i=1}^{N} X_i' W_i X_i \boldsymbol{\beta} \\ &= \boldsymbol{\beta}, \end{aligned}$$

provided that $E(\boldsymbol{Y}_i) = X_i \boldsymbol{\beta}$. Hence, for $\widehat{\boldsymbol{\beta}}$ to be unbiased, it is sufficient that the mean of the response is correctly specified. Conditional on α, $\widehat{\boldsymbol{\beta}}$ has covariance

$$\begin{aligned} \operatorname{Var}(\widehat{\boldsymbol{\beta}}) &= \left(\sum_{i=1}^{N} X_i' W_i X_i\right)^{-1} \\ &\quad \times \left(\sum_{i=1}^{N} X_i' W_i \operatorname{Var}(\boldsymbol{Y}_i) W_i X_i\right) \qquad (8.13) \\ &\quad \times \left(\sum_{i=1}^{N} X_i' W_i X_i\right)^{-1} \\ &= \left(\sum_{i=1}^{N} X_i' W_i X_i\right)^{-1}. \qquad (8.14) \end{aligned}$$

Note that (8.14) assumes that the covariance matrix $\operatorname{Var}(\boldsymbol{Y}_i)$ is correctly modeled as $V_i = Z_i D Z_i' + \Sigma_i$, which then again plays the role of the purely model-based estimate. The empirically corrected estimate for $\operatorname{Var}(\widehat{\boldsymbol{\beta}})$, which does not assume the covariance matrix to be correctly specified is obtained from replacing $\operatorname{Var}(\boldsymbol{Y}_i)$ in (8.13) by

$$\left(\boldsymbol{Y}_i - X_i \widehat{\boldsymbol{\beta}}\right)\left(\boldsymbol{Y}_i - X_i \widehat{\boldsymbol{\beta}}\right)', \qquad (8.15)$$

rather than V_i. The sole condition for (8.15) to be unbiased for $\operatorname{Var}(\boldsymbol{Y}_i)$ is that the mean is again correctly specified.

In spite of this potential use for Gaussian outcomes, GEE is most commonly used for non-Gaussian measurement sequences. The need is avoided to specify third- and higher-order moments or, more precisely, third- and higher-order correlations, and two-way correlations are allowed to be misspecified. Should they be correctly specified, and should a set of appropriate third- and higher-order correlations be chosen, together with marginal logit links for binary outcomes, then the Bahadur model (Section 7.2) would follow. Thus, standard GEE can be seen a moment-based version of the Bahadur model. After choosing the marginal response functions, there is always at least one, trivial, Bahadur model that corresponds to the estimating equations, found by setting all correlations to zero, i.e., independence. In general, the working correlations, found upon convergence of GEE, may not necessarily correspond to a valid joint probability mass function, given the severe constraints on the Bahadur model (Section 7.2.2). This need not be a drawback, as the working correlations are merely a device to provide consistent and asymptotically normal point estimates for the marginal regression parameters and, if well chosen, also reasonably efficient. They should not be made a part of formal inference.

The previous statement implies that, strictly speaking, the following two questions should remain unanswered or at least approached cautiously:

- Are particular working correlation values large, moderate, or small?

- Among a set of working correlation matrices under correlation, which one is best?

The first question is a natural one to ask. However, an answer does not come easily, since ordinarily no standard errors are given alongside the working correlations, and neither should they. Indeed, as stated above, they are only devices to support estimation of the regression parameters, with a status almost below the one of nuisance parameter. One can interpret them, informally and with great caution, when the empirically corrected and model-based standard errors are close, for then there usually is good evidence that the working correlation structure has been chosen in line with the true structure (Drum and McCullagh 1993, who present a critical view on the methodology). This may be the case, in particular, when the working correlation structure is fairly general, such as 'unstructured' in the cases of balanced data (with corresponding measurements for different subjects taken at the same time or approximately the same time). Of course, an unstructured covariance matrix is no guarantee for a correct specification since the covariance structure may further depend, for example, on certain covariates.

Turning to the second question, it ought to be clear that there are no formal model comparison tools for the correlation parameters. Because there are no standard errors, Wald-type tests are not possible, and also likelihood-ratio and score tests are not easy to use. Although some model comparison and goodness-of-fit tools have been proposed (Rotnitzky and Jewell 1990), they are for the mean model and not for the association structure, as they should be as, once again, the association is mere nuisance in the GEE philosophy. The worst possible, in fact unscientific, approach that can be taken is to base one's choice for working assumptions on the outcome (significance) for the regression parameters.

Thus, in conclusion, the working correlation structure ought to be left alone or at most used in a very informal way. It is best to specify a single working correlation structure upfront when the need exists to specify a primary analysis. Perhaps some others can be used by way of sensitivity analysis for the regression parameters. It seems best to specify the working correlation structure in agreement with the design of the study (counterexamples being exchangeability for multivariate outcomes or AR(1) for unequally spaced longitudinal measurements), and as general as the data support. The latter is usually a function of the number of subjects in a study, as well as the number of measurements per subject.

When GEE is deemed unsatisfactory in the sense that there is some scientific interest is the association structure, then one should turn to some of the extensions of GEE, reviewed in Section 8.3, in particular to GEE2 (Section 8.5), GEE methods combining a marginal and conditional specification (Section 8.7), or even to alternating logistic regressions (Section 8.6) or pseudo-likelihood (Chapter 9).

Some theoretical considerations regarding problems that may occur with GEE are presented in Crowder (1995), Sutradhar and Das (1999), and Vonesh, Wang, and Majumdar (2001).

8.3 Alternative GEE Methods

In the previous section, standard GEE, as introduced by Liang and Zeger (1986), was discussed. A number of alternatives have been proposed. Prentice (1988) replaced the moment-based estimation for the working correlation parameters by a second set of estimating equations. By making the working assumption that both sets are independent, computational complexity is avoided and, again, the correlation model need not be correctly specified for the marginal regression parameters to be consistent and asymptotically normal. Prentice's method is discussed in Section 8.4. As soon as the two sets of estimating equations are assumed to be correlated, one obtains GEE2, in the sense that the first and second moments are then fully modeled, with working assumptions made about the third and fourth order moments. This method, which is one step up from Prentice's method, is discussed in Section 8.5.

Lipsitz, Laird, and Harrington (1991) adapted Prentice's method to switch from marginal correlation coefficients to marginal odds ratios. These are but two of the association choices from Table 7.3. Thus, while standard GEE and Prentice's method can be seen as derived from the Bahadur model (Section 7.2), the method by Lipsitz, Laird, and Harrington (1991) derives from the multivariate Dale model (Sections 7.3 and 7.7, see also Chapter 6). Of course, GEE2 can be formulated not only with correlations but also based on odds ratios (Liang, Zeger, and Qaqish 1992). GEE with odds ratios (Lipsitz, Laird, and Harrington 1991, Liang, Zeger, and Qaqish 1992), and the link to alternating logistic regression (Carey, Zeger, and Diggle 1993), is discussed in Section 8.6.

Another method, close in spirit to GEE as it also derives from quasi-likelihood ideas, is based on linearizing the link function. It is presented in Section 8.8. A nice feature is that it can be fitted using the SAS procedure GLIMMIX. The method is in fact a special case of a more general approach, that allows the inclusion of random effects into a generalized linear model (Chapter 14).

8.4 Prentice's GEE Method

Prentice (1988) amended the basic GEE or GEE1 of Liang and Zeger (1986), described in Section 8.2. This method allows for estimation of both parameters vectors, $\boldsymbol{\beta}$ and $\boldsymbol{\alpha}$, in the marginal response model and the pairwise correlations, respectively. The key difference with the original GEE is that for both sets of parameters, estimating equations are proposed. Thus, this GEE estimator for $\boldsymbol{\beta}$ and $\boldsymbol{\alpha}$ may be defined as a solution to:

$$\sum_{i=1}^{N} \boldsymbol{D}'_i V_i^{-1}(\boldsymbol{Y}_i - \boldsymbol{\mu}_i) = \boldsymbol{0}, \tag{8.16}$$

$$\sum_{i=1}^{N} \boldsymbol{E}'_i W_i^{-1}(\boldsymbol{Z}_i - \boldsymbol{\delta}_i) = \boldsymbol{0}, \tag{8.17}$$

where $\boldsymbol{Z}_i$ consists of components, doubly indexed by (j_1, j_2) and taking the form:

$$Z_{ij_1 j_2} = \frac{(Y_{ij_1} - \mu_{ij_1})(Y_{ij_2} - \mu_{ij_2})}{\sqrt{\mu_{ij_1}(1 - \mu_{ij_1})\mu_{ij_2}(1 - \mu_{ij_2})}}.$$

The terms carry information about the correlation between measures Y_{ij_1} and Y_{ij_2} on the same subject. In summary,

$$\boldsymbol{Z}_i = (Z_{i12}, Z_{i13}, \ldots, Z_{i,n_i-1,n_i}). \tag{8.18}$$

Further, $\delta_{ij_1 j_2} = E(Z_{ij_1 j_2})$,

$$D_i = \frac{\partial \boldsymbol{\mu}_i}{\partial \boldsymbol{\beta}}, \qquad E_i = \frac{\partial \boldsymbol{\delta}_i}{\partial \boldsymbol{\alpha}},$$

V_i is the variance-covariance matrix of $\boldsymbol{Y}_i$, and W_i is the working variance-covariance matrix of $\boldsymbol{Z}_i$. Strictly speaking, V_i is no working covariance matrix, since the second moments are specified by (8.17). In contrast, W_i does contain working assumptions, usually being that the third- and fourth-order correlations, defined by (7.8), are equal to zero. We will return to these in Section 8.7.

The assumption is made that (8.16) and (8.17) are independent. This would entail a price in terms of efficiency, but has the advantage that, just as in Section 8.2, misspecifying the correlation structure does not hamper consistency and asymptotic normality of the marginal regression parameters. Each set of parameters comes with precision estimates, whence formal inference is possible about the set of parameters for one is prepared to believe the equations have been correctly specified. This could be (8.16), (8.17), or both. The option to make formal inferences about the correlation parameters is a net increase of capabilities over standard GEE1.

The joint asymptotic distribution of $\sqrt{N}(\widehat{\boldsymbol{\beta}} - \boldsymbol{\beta})$ and $\sqrt{N}(\widehat{\boldsymbol{\alpha}} - \boldsymbol{\alpha})$ is Gaussian with mean zero and with variance-covariance matrix consistently estimated by

$$N \cdot \begin{pmatrix} \boldsymbol{A} & \boldsymbol{0} \\ \boldsymbol{B} & \boldsymbol{C} \end{pmatrix} \begin{pmatrix} \Lambda_{11} & \Lambda_{12} \\ \Lambda_{21} & \Lambda_{22} \end{pmatrix} \begin{pmatrix} \boldsymbol{A} & \boldsymbol{B}' \\ \boldsymbol{0} & \boldsymbol{C} \end{pmatrix},$$

where

$$\boldsymbol{A} = \left(\sum_{i=1}^{N} \boldsymbol{D}_i' \boldsymbol{V}_i^{-1} \boldsymbol{D}_i \right)^{-1}, \tag{8.19}$$

$$\boldsymbol{B} = \left(\sum_{i=1}^{N} \boldsymbol{E}_i' \boldsymbol{W}_i^{-1} \boldsymbol{E}_i \right)^{-1} \left(\sum_{i=1}^{N} \boldsymbol{E}_i' \boldsymbol{W}_i^{-1} \frac{\partial \boldsymbol{Z}_i}{\partial \boldsymbol{\beta}} \right) \tag{8.20}$$

$$\times \left(\sum_{i=1}^{N} \boldsymbol{D}_i' \boldsymbol{V}_i^{-1} \boldsymbol{D}_i \right)^{-1}, \tag{8.21}$$

$$\boldsymbol{C} = \left(\sum_{i=1}^{N} \boldsymbol{E}_i' \boldsymbol{W}_i^{-1} \boldsymbol{E}_i \right)^{-1}, \tag{8.22}$$

$$\Lambda_{11} = \sum_{i=1}^{N} \boldsymbol{D}_i' \boldsymbol{V}_i^{-1} \text{Cov}(\boldsymbol{Y}_i) \boldsymbol{V}_i^{-1} \boldsymbol{D}_i, \tag{8.23}$$

$$\Lambda_{12} = \sum_{i=1}^{N} \boldsymbol{D}_i' \boldsymbol{V}_i^{-1} \text{Cov}(\boldsymbol{Y}_i, \boldsymbol{Z}_i) \boldsymbol{W}_i^{-1} \boldsymbol{E}_i, \tag{8.24}$$

$$\Lambda_{21} = \Lambda_{12}, \tag{8.25}$$

$$\Lambda_{22} = \sum_{i=1}^{N} \boldsymbol{E}_i' \boldsymbol{W}_i^{-1} \text{Cov}(\boldsymbol{Z}_i) \boldsymbol{W}_i^{-1} \boldsymbol{E}_i, \tag{8.26}$$

and $\text{Var}(\boldsymbol{Y}_i)$, $\text{Cov}(\boldsymbol{Y}_i, \boldsymbol{Z}_i)$, and $\text{Var}(\boldsymbol{Z}_i)$ are estimated by the quantities

$$(\boldsymbol{Y}_i - \boldsymbol{\mu}_i)(\boldsymbol{Y}_i - \boldsymbol{\mu}_i)', (\boldsymbol{Y}_i - \boldsymbol{\mu}_i)(\boldsymbol{Z}_i - \boldsymbol{\delta}_i)', (\boldsymbol{Z}_i - \boldsymbol{\delta}_i)(\boldsymbol{Z}_i - \boldsymbol{\delta}_i)',$$

respectively, in analogy with GEE1. One may wonder why there is no need to go back and forth between solving the estimating equations and moment-based estimation, as in Section 8.2. In this case, this would mean solving

(8.16) and (8.17), and then switch to moment based estimation for higher moments. However, as stated before, one typically assumes the third and fourth moments are zero. One could call these 'higher-order independence' working assumption, obviating the need for additional parameters.

The above model has a close resemblance with the Bahadur model, as it is based on its first to fourth moments. Williamson, Lipsitz, and Kim (1997) wrote a SAS macro for Prentice's method.

The updating method for Prentice's GEE iterates between solving each of the equations (8.16) and (8.17).

8.5 Second-order Generalized Estimating Equations (GEE2)

Second-order GEE have been proposed by Zhao and Prentice (1990), using correlations, and by Liang, Zeger, and Qaqish (1992), using odds ratios. They are a simple extension of Prentice's (1988) method, described in Section 8.4, by combining the outcome vector Y_i and the pairwise cross-products, Z_i, as in (8.18), into a single outcome vector:

$$W_i = (Y_i', Z_i')'. \qquad (8.27)$$

The vector W_i has $n_i + \binom{n_i}{2}$ components. Further, let

$$\Theta_i = (\mu_i', \delta_i')',$$

the corresponding mean vector, obtained by assembling the means from (8.16) and (8.17). Assuming δ_i depends on a vector of regression parameters β, which now combines the β and α from Section 8.4, the vector β can be estimated by solving the second-order generalized estimating equations:

$$U(\beta) = \sum_{i=1}^{N} U_i(\beta) = \sum_{i=1}^{N} D_i' V_i^{-1} [W_i - E(W_i)] = 0, \qquad (8.28)$$

where

$$D_i = \frac{\partial \Theta_i'}{\partial \beta}.$$

As usual, $V_i = \text{Cov}(W_i)$. Calculation of all matrices involved is straightforward with the exception of the covariance matrix V_i, which contains third- and fourth-order probabilities. Again, as in Section 8.4, the three-way and higher order correlations are set equal to zero. As before, the parameter estimates $\widehat{\beta}$ can then be calculated using, for example, a Fisher scoring algorithm. Provided the first- and second-order models have been correctly specified, $\widehat{\beta}$ is consistent for β and has an asymptotic multivariate normal distribution with mean vector $\boldsymbol{\beta}$ and variance-covariance matrix consistently estimated by:

$$\widehat{V}(\widehat{\boldsymbol{\beta}}) = \left(\sum_{i=1}^N \widehat{D}_i' \widehat{V}_i^{-1} \widehat{D}_i\right)^{-1} \left(\sum_{i=1}^N \boldsymbol{U}_i(\widehat{\boldsymbol{\beta}}) \boldsymbol{U}_i(\widehat{\boldsymbol{\beta}})'\right)$$
$$\times \left(\sum_{i=1}^N \widehat{D}_i' \widehat{V}_i^{-1} \widehat{D}_i\right)^{-1},$$

the usual sandwich estimator.

In principle, there is no reason why one should stop at GEE2. Higher-order GEE is perfectly conceivable. When, moments 1 up to K would be modeled, working assumptions of order $K+1$ up to $2K$ would be needed. Obviously, this will become increasingly cumbersome, not only algebraically, also regarding implementation and computation time. As the order increases, the relative gain will also decrease, as less and less information would be contained in higher moments. When K becomes equal to the length of the response vector $\boldsymbol{Y}_i$, full likelihood is recovered and our specification, carried through to order n_i, would produce the Bahadur model. When higher orders are of interest, this is usually in situations where the joint probabilities need to be calculated and then full likelihood effectively is the only option. Thus, most commonly encountered are GEE1 and GEE2 on the one hand, and then full likelihood on the other hand.

8.6 GEE with Odds Ratios and Alternating Logistic Regression

The GEE versions discussed in Sections 8.2, 8.4, and 8.5 all used correlation as a measure to capture association, either as moment estimated working assumptions, or as part of the estimating equations. Thus, as indicated earlier, all can be seen as deriving from the Bahadur model. The advantage of correlations is that the estimating equations, such as (8.4), include the covariance matrix V_i as in (8.5), and (working) correlation parameters can be used in a particularly straightforward fashion to compose the matrix $R_i(\boldsymbol{\alpha})$. However, many authors have stated that the odds ratio is a particularly straightforward measure to capture association between binary or categorical outcomes (Molenberghs and Lesaffre 1994, 1999, Fitzmaurice, Laird, and Ware 2004, p. 298, see also Chapters 6 and 7). In the context of GEE, the same observation has been made. Lipsitz, Laird, and Harrington (1991) considered GEE1 for binary data with odds ratios, while Liang, Zeger, and Qaqish (1992) did the same for GEE2. The Bahadur-based correlation, expressed as (7.5) and leading to bivariate joint probabilities (7.6), needs to be replaced by the Dale-based odds ratio (7.39), leading to bivariate joint probabilities (7.40). Still focusing on binary outcomes and based on the bivariate probabilities, calculation of V_i in (8.5) is straightforward and follows from observing that

$$V_{i,jj} = \text{Var}(Y_{ij}) = \mu_{ij}(1 - \mu_{ij}),$$
$$V_{i,j_1,j_2} = \text{Cov}(Y_{ij_1}, Y_{ij_2}) = \mu_{ij_1j_2} - \mu_{ij_1}\mu_{ij_2}.$$

Note that the expectation of a component of $\boldsymbol{Z}_i$, $Z_{ij_1j_2}$ say, equals $\mu_{ij_1j_2}$, the probability of a success at occasions j_1 and j_2 at the same time. Assuming a model for the pairwise odds ratios as in (7.39), and working assumptions for the third- and fourth-order log odds ratios (usually by setting them equal to zero), the model specification is complete. Lipsitz, Laird, and Harrington (1991) assumed, for simplicity, W_i in (8.17) to be diagonal, avoiding working assumptions about the third and fourth order; it even avoids calculating the third- and fourth-order probabilities altogether. It is then simple to solve (8.16) and (8.17) with the vector $\boldsymbol{Y}_i$ still equal to the response vector, and with $\boldsymbol{Z}_i$ in (8.18) changed to

$$\boldsymbol{Z}_i = (Y_{i1}Y_{i2}, Y_{i1}Y_{i3}, \ldots, Y_{i,n_i-1}Y_{in_i}). \tag{8.29}$$

The same principles as outlined above can be applied to second-order GEE (8.28). This idea was followed by Liang, Zeger, and Qaqish (1992). While they set the third- and fourth-order log odds ratios equal to zero, obviating the need to invoke additional (moment-based) estimation, they still needed to compute third- and fourth-order probabilities for GEE2, following one of the methods associated with the Dale model, e.g., using the IPF algorithm or the Plackett polynomials (Sections 7.4 and 7.7). This can be computationally less than straightforward, but luckily there is another alternative, termed *alternating logistic regressions* (ALR) and proposed by Carey, Zeger, and Diggle (1993). The method is different from all of the GEE methods considered so far, but has communality with both GEE1 and GEE2 based on odds ratios. In particular, it is almost as efficient as GEE2, and shares the computational ease of conventional GEE1.

Let us first introduce the method, and then provide some further perspective on its advantages. Let μ_{ij} be as before, described by

$$\text{logit}P(Y_{ij} = 1) = \boldsymbol{x}'_{ij}\boldsymbol{\beta}, \tag{8.30}$$

and let $\alpha_{ij_1j_2} = \ln(\psi_{ij_1j_2})$ be the marginal log odds ratio. Then,

$$\text{logit}P(Y_{ij_1} = 1|Y_{ij_2} = y_{ij_2})$$
$$= \ln\left(\frac{\mu_{ij_1} - \mu_{ij_1j_2}}{1 - \mu_{ij_1} - \mu_{ij_2} + \mu_{ij_1j_2}}\right) + \alpha_{ij_1j_2}y_{ij_2}. \tag{8.31}$$

The marginal logistic regression (8.30) is in line with the Bahadur model, the Dale model with logistic margins, and all of the GEEs discussed in

8.6 GEE with Odds Ratios and Alternating Logistic Regression

this chapter. However, rather than further specifying the models by additional marginal description of the pairwise association, a logistic model for an outcome *conditional upon another outcome* is presented, which derives trivially from the expression for the log odds ratio. Logistic regression (8.31) is a little unconventional in the sense that instead of an intercept, there is an offset, i.e., a constant term free of unknown parameters, given the mean model. An example of an offset can be found in Section 3.7. The principle of ALR is to iterate between solving (8.30) and (8.31). Iteration is indeed required because solving (8.30) requires the covariance matrix V_i of $Y_i - \mu_i$, which depends on both β and α, while also (8.31) depends on both. The updating problem can be phrased in terms of simultaneously solving two sets of estimating equations, the first one being exactly equal in form to (8.16), the second one being

$$\sum_{i=1}^{N} \widetilde{E}_i' \widetilde{W}_i^{-1} R_i = 0, \qquad (8.32)$$

where

$$\widetilde{E}_i = \frac{\partial \zeta_i}{\partial \alpha_i'},$$

ζ_i is a vector with elements $\zeta_{ij_1j_2} = P(Y_{ij_1} = 1 | Y_{ij_2} = y_{ij_2})$, $\widetilde{W}_i$ is a diagonal matrix with elements $\zeta_{ij_1j_2}(1 - \zeta_{ij_1j_2})$, and R_i a vector with elements $Y_{ij_1j_2} - \zeta_{ij_1j_2}$.

Note that ALR extends beyond classical GEE, in the sense that precision estimates follow for both the β and the α parameters. However, unlike with GEE2, and even with Prentice's (1988) and Prentice and Zhao (1991) GEE, no working assumptions about the third- and fourth-order odds ratios are required. Thanks to the clever combination of a marginal and a conditional specification, addressing the third and fourth moments is avoided all together, which is strictly different from setting them equal to zero.

In (8.31), arbitrary structures for the log odds ratio parameters $\alpha_{ij_2j_2}$ can be assumed. The odds ratio equivalent of exchangeability would set them all equal to the same constant α. When measurements are taken at fixed time points, an unstructured specification is possible. Further, when measurements are equally spaced, banded structures or other equivalents of autoregressive correlation structures can be entertained.

ALR has been implemented in the SAS procedure GENMOD. More detail is given in Section 10.4.

As was seen here, a combination of marginal and conditional specification can be advantageous. ALR is not the only instance to confirm this. In the next section, a family of hybrid marginal and conditional model specifications is considered.

8.7 GEE2 Based on a Hybrid Marginal-conditional Model

In the previous section, alternating logistic regression combined marginal and conditional aspects of model specification. The hybrid model, combining marginal and conditional aspects, presented in Section 7.8 can be used as a basis for GEE just as easily as the Bahadur and Dale models studied before.

A set of GEE2, proposed also by Heagerty and Zeger (1996), can be derived by specifying only the first and second moments that derive from (7.50):

$$U(\boldsymbol{\beta}) = \sum_{i=1}^{N} \left(\frac{\partial \boldsymbol{\mu}_i}{\partial \boldsymbol{\beta}}\right) \boldsymbol{M}_i^{-1}(\boldsymbol{v}_i - \boldsymbol{\mu}_i) = \boldsymbol{0}, \qquad (8.33)$$

with notation as in Section 7.8.1. Observe that these score equations assume the same form for any fixed value of $\boldsymbol{\Omega}_i$, with $\boldsymbol{\Omega}_i = \boldsymbol{0}$ as a special but important case. However, this leaves $\boldsymbol{M}_i$ partly unspecified. A standard procedure is to replace it by a working covariance matrix, depending on a set of (nuisance) parameters $\boldsymbol{\alpha}$. Heagerty and Zeger (1996) advocated setting the higher order conditional association parameters equal to zero (or, more generally, to a fixed constant). This particular set of GEE2 does not require estimation of extra parameters, a property shared with the GEE2 methods described in Section 8.5 and 8.6. Expression (8.33) can also be seen as the score equations for the likelihood specified by the following member of the quadratic exponential family of Zhao and Prentice (1990):

$$f(y_i|\boldsymbol{\Psi}_i) = \exp\left\{\boldsymbol{\Psi}_i' \boldsymbol{v}_i - A(\boldsymbol{\Psi}_i)\right\}. \qquad (8.34)$$

Another, slightly different set of GEE2, which also does not require estimation of nuisance parameters, is found by setting all three and higher order *marginal* log odds ratios equal to zero, in agreement with GEE2 in Section 8.6 and Liang, Zeger, and Qaqish (1992).

Computing the covariance $\boldsymbol{M}_i$ in (8.33) involves the third and fourth order probabilities. With conditional constraints, they are easily computed using the IPF algorithm, as outlined in Section 7.8.1. To proceed with marginal working assumptions, we first need to define the three- and four-way marginal odds ratios. They can also be introduced using conditional lower order odds ratios. If $\psi_{ij_1j_2|j_3}(y)$ is the conditional odds ratio of outcomes Y_{ij_1} and Y_{ij_2}, given $Y_{ij_3} = y$, then

$$\psi_{ij_1j_2j_3} = \frac{\psi_{ij_1j_2|j_3}(1)}{\psi_{ij_1j_2|j_3}(0)}, \qquad \psi_{ij_1j_2j_3j_4} = \frac{\psi_{ij_1j_2j_3|j_4}(1)}{\psi_{ij_1j_2j_3|j_4}(0)}.$$

To compute the probabilities, again, the IPF algorithm as presented in Section 7.12.3 or the polynomial method of Section 7.7.4 can be used.

When the outcomes are categorical rather than binary, the likelihood presented in Section 7.8.2 can be used and, given the above, GEE2 follows in a straightforward fashion.

8.8 A Method Based on Linearization

All versions of GEE studied sofar can be seen as deriving from the score equations of corresponding likelihood methods, such as the Bahadur model (Section 7.2), the Dale model (Section 7.7), or the hybrid model (Section 7.8). In a sense, GEE results from considering only a subvector of the full vector of scores, corresponding to either the first moments only (the outcomes themselves), or the first and second moments (outcomes and cross-products thereof). On the other hand, they can be seen as an extension of the quasi-likelihood principles, where appropriate modifications are made to the scores to be sufficiently flexible and "work" at the same time. A classical modification is the inclusion of an overdispersion parameter, while in GEE also (nuisance) correlation parameters are introduced.

An alternative approach consists of linearizing the outcome, in the sense of Nelder and Wedderburn (1972), to construct a working variate, to which then weighted least squares is applied. In other words, iteratively reweighted least squares (IRLS) can be used (McCullagh and Nelder 1989). Within each step, the approximation produces all elements typically encountered in a multivariate normal model, and hence corresponding software tools can be used. In case our models would contain random effects as well (Section 14.4), the core of the IRLS could be approached using linear mixed models tools. The SAS procedure GLIMMIX is such a tool and the general case will be taken up in Chapter 14. Here, we restrict attention to the marginal-model situation. Nevertheless, it is important to note that the tools developed here can be approached using the SAS procedure GLIMMIX, as well as with the GLIMMIX macro.

Write the outcome vector in a classical (multivariate) generalized linear models fashion:

$$\boldsymbol{Y}_i = \boldsymbol{\mu}_i + \boldsymbol{\varepsilon}_i \qquad (8.35)$$

where, as usual, $\boldsymbol{\mu}_i = E(\boldsymbol{Y}_i)$ is the systematic component and $\boldsymbol{\varepsilon}_i$ is the random component, typically following from a multinomial distribution. We assume that

$$\text{Var}(\boldsymbol{Y}_i) = \text{Var}(\boldsymbol{\varepsilon}_i) = \Sigma_i. \qquad (8.36)$$

The model is further specified by assuming

$$\boldsymbol{\eta}_i = g(\boldsymbol{\mu}_i),$$
$$\boldsymbol{\eta}_i = X_i \boldsymbol{\beta},$$

where $\boldsymbol{\eta}_i$ is the usual set of linear predictors, $g(.)$ is an inverse vector link function, typically made up of logit components, X_i is a design matrix and $\boldsymbol{\beta}$ are the regression parameters.

Estimation proceeds by iteratively solving

$$\sum_{i=1}^{N} X'_i W_i X_i \boldsymbol{\beta} = \sum_{i=1}^{N} W_i \boldsymbol{Y}^*_i, \qquad (8.37)$$

where a working variate $\boldsymbol{y}^*_i$ has been defined, following from a first-order Taylor series expansion of $\boldsymbol{\eta}_i$ around $\boldsymbol{\mu}_i$:

$$\boldsymbol{Y}^*_i = \widehat{\boldsymbol{\eta}}_i + (\boldsymbol{Y}_i - \widehat{\boldsymbol{\mu}}_i) F_i^{-1},$$

$$F_i = \frac{\partial \boldsymbol{\mu}_i}{\partial \boldsymbol{\eta}_i}. \qquad (8.38)$$

The weights in (8.37) are specified as

$$W_i = F'_i \Sigma_i^{-1} F_i. \qquad (8.39)$$

Note that in the specific case of an identity link, $\boldsymbol{\eta}_i = \boldsymbol{\mu}_i$, $F_i = I_{n_i}$ and $\boldsymbol{Y}_i = \boldsymbol{Y}^*_i$, whence a standard multivariate regression follows.

8.9 Analysis of the NTP Data

The NTP data, introduced in Section 2.7, have been analyzed in Section 7.2.3, by means of the Bahadur model specialized to clustered data (Section 7.2.2). Table 7.1 presented estimates and standard errors for a simple model, with marginal logits linear in dose, and a common correlation parameter, fitted the external, visceral, skeletal, and collapsed outcomes in the DEHP, EG, and DYME studies.

Here, we will consider the same model, but then from the GEE angle. We will apply standard GEE (Section 8.2), Prentice's modification (Section 8.4), and the linearization method (Section 8.8). The first approach was fitted using the SAS procedure GENMOD, the second one with a SAS macro developed by Stuart Lipsitz (Williamson, Lipsitz, and Kim 1997), and the third one using the SAS macro GLIMMIX or, equivalently, with the SAS procedure GLIMMIX. More details on software are deferred to Chapter 10. For all of these analyses, both independence (Table 8.2) and exchangeable (Table 8.3) working assumptions were considered. Other working assumptions, such as AR(1) and unstructured, are less sensible here, given the clustered nature of the data. Several models include, in addition to working assumptions, an overdispersion parameter ϕ.

In addition to these analysis, GEE2 estimates are provided in Table 8.4, based on the same models as in the Bahadur analysis, described by (7.14) and (7.15).

TABLE 8.2. *NTP Data. Parameter estimates (model-based standard errors; empirically corrected standard errors) for GEE1 with independence working assumptions, fitted to various outcomes in the DEHP study. β_0 and β_d are the marginal intercept and dose effect, respectively; ϕ is the overdispersion parameter.*

Outcome	Par.	Standard	Prentice	Linearized
External	β_0	-5.06(0.30;0.38)	-5.06(0.33;0.38)	-5.06(0.28;0.38)
	β_d	5.31(0.44;0.57)	5.31(0.48;0.57)	5.31(0.42;0.57)
	ϕ		0.90	0.74
Visceral	β_0	-4.47(0.28;0.36)	-4.47(0.28;0.36)	-4.47(0.28;0.36)
	β_d	4.40(0.43;0.58)	4.40(0.43;0.58)	4.40(0.43;0.58)
	ϕ		1.00	1.00
Skeletal	β_0	-4.87(0.31;0.47)	-4.87(0.31;0.47)	-4.87(0.32;0.47)
	β_d	4.89(0.46;0.65)	4.90(0.47;0.65)	4.90(0.47;0.65)
	ϕ		0.99	1.02
Collapsed	β_0	-3.98(0.22;0.30)	-3.98(0.22;0.30)	-3.98(0.22;0.30)
	β_d	5.56(0.40;0.61)	5.56(0.40;0.61)	5.56(0.41;0.61)
	ϕ		0.99	1.04

For a given outcome in a given study, results from the Bahadur model, the various GEE1 versions, and GEE2, are very similar. Even though for some parameters the estimated values differ a bit between analyses, they preserve the directionality and, roughly, the magnitude of the effect. This is not surprising, given that all can be seen as deriving from Bahadur's model. However, just as in, for example, Section 7.10, we observe a mild shrinkage. This is, again, due to the parameter constraints on the Bahadur model and, to a lesser extent, on GEE2. For the parameters in the Bahadur model to be allowable, all higher-order probabilities need to be valid, while for GEE2 this is necessary only up to the fourth order, the farthest the working assumptions reach. For GEE1, it is sufficient for the pairwise probabilities to be valid. Thus, it is possible for GEE to provide a valid parameter combination that cannot be reconciled with a Bahadur model, having the same lower order parameters. This does not mean there would be *no* fully specified model corresponding to it. Given the orthogonality properties of the hybrid marginal-conditional model, presented in Section 7.8, there is always a model of this type encompassing the GEE-based parameters.

The constraints on the Bahadur model are very severe indeed. For instance, the allowable range of β_a for the external outcome in the DEHP data is $(-0.0164; 0.1610)$ when β_0 and β_d are fixed at their MLE. This range translates to the very narrow $(-0.0082; 0.0803)$ on the correlation scale, excluding the GEE based values for the correlation ρ.

TABLE 8.3. *NTP Data. Parameter estimates (model-based standard errors; empirically corrected standard errors) for GEE1 with exchangeable working assumptions, fitted various outcomes in the DEHP study. β_0 and β_d are the marginal intercept and dose effect, respectively; ρ is the correlation; ϕ is the overdispersion parameter.*

Outcome	Par.	Standard	Prentice	Linearized
External	β_0	-4.98(0.40;0.37)	-4.99(0.46;0.37)	-5.00(0.36;0.37)
	β_d	5.33(0.57;0.55)	5.32(0.65;0.55)	5.32(0.51;0.55)
	ϕ	0.88		0.65
	ρ	0.11	0.11(0.04)	0.06
Visceral	β_0	-4.50(0.37;0.37)	-4.51(0.40;0.37)	-4.50(0.36;0.37)
	β_d	4.55(0.55;0.59)	4.59(0.58;0.59)	4.55(0.54;0.59)
	ϕ	1.00		0.92
	ρ	0.08	0.11(0.05)	0.08
Skeletal	β_0	-4.83(0.44;0.45)	-4.82(0.47;0.44)	-4.82(0.46;0.45)
	β_d	4.84(0.62;0.63)	4.84(0.67;0.63)	4.84(0.65;0.63)
	ϕ	0.98		0.86
	ρ	0.12	0.14(0.06)	0.13
Collapsed	β_0	-4.05(0.32;0.31)	-4.06(0.35;0.31)	-4.04(0.33;0.31)
	β_d	5.84(0.57;0.61)	5.89(0.62;0.61)	5.82(0.58;0.61)
	ϕ	1.00		0.96
	ρ	0.11	0.15(0.05)	0.11

Comparing model-based and empirically corrected standard errors, there is a clear difference in the case of independence working assumptions, but less so in the exchangeable case. Comparing both analyses is a case in point that the choice of working assumptions, whether right or wrong, is not important for the method's consistency and asymptotic normality. The impact on efficiency is minor. The statement about efficiency continues to hold when comparing all marginal analyses. In case where one is merely interested in assessing the effect of dose, GEE1, being the simplest of all methods, will do fine. When there is additional interest in the association, care is needed with GEE1. Table 8.2 provides no association parameter at all. The correlation in Table 8.3 should be approached cautiously, as the exchangeable correlation is, at best, a nuisance parameter, for which no formal inference is possible. Moreover, because we are allowed to misspecify our association model, there is no *a priori* guarantee that the parameter is trustworthy. However, in this particular case, exchangeability seems reasonable, both on biological grounds and given the design of the study. When more formal inferences about the correlation parameters

TABLE 8.4. *NTP Data. Parameter estimates (empirically corrected standard errors) for GEE2 with exchangeable correlation, fitted to various outcomes in three studies. β_0 and β_d are the marginal intercept and dose effect, respectively; β_a is the Fisher z transformed correlation; ρ is the correlation.*

Outcome	Parameter	DEHP	EG	DYME
External	β_0	-4.98(0.37)	-5.63(0.67)	-7.45(0.73)
	β_d	5.29(0.55)	3.10(0.81)	8.15(0.83)
	β_a	0.15(0.05)	0.15(0.05)	0.13(0.05)
	ρ	0.07(0.02)	0.07(0.02)	0.06(0.02)
Visceral	β_0	-4.49(0.36)	-7.50(1.05)	-6.89(0.75)
	β_d	4.52(0.59)	4.37(1.14)	5.51(0.89)
	β_a	0.15(0.06)	0.02(0.02)	0.11(0.07)
	ρ	0.07(0.03)	0.01(0.01)	0.05(0.03)
Skeletal	β_0	-5.23(0.40)	-4.05(0.33)	
	β_d	5.35(0.60)	4.77(0.43)	
	β_a	0.18(0.02)	0.30(0.03)	
	ρ	0.09(0.01)	0.15(0.01)	
Collapsed	β_0	-5.23(0.40)	-4.07(0.71)	-5.75(0.48)
	β_d	5.35(0.60)	4.89(0.90)	8.82(0.91)
	β_a	0.18(0.02)	0.26(0.14)	0.18(0.12)
	ρ	0.09(0.01)	0.13(0.07)	0.09(0.06)

are required, GEE2 is a viable alternative. This may be less so with the Bahadur model, given the strong parameter space restrictions.

An alternative when the association is of interest is provided by alternating logistic regressions (Section 8.6). Results of fitting ALR to the NTP data are summarized in Table 8.5. The association is in terms of log odds ratios α, as in (8.31). For convenience, we also present the odds ratios ψ. As it is a sensible choice in our case, and for ease of comparison with Tables 8.3 and 8.4, an exchangeable odds ratio structure is chosen, in the sense that all odds ratios are equal. Again, parameter estimates are similar to the ones obtained in Tables 8.2–8.4, and this holds for the standard errors as well. Of course, the association being in terms of (log) odds ratios, comparison with the correlations of the earlier analyses is not straightforward, although the relative magnitudes are roughly preserved. An advantage of the ALR analyses, apart from its implementation in standard software (the SAS procedure GENMOD, see Chapter 10), is that standard errors are provided for the association parameters. In fact, the asymptotic covariance matrix for all estimates together can be obtained.

TABLE 8.5. *NTP Data. Parameter estimates (empirically corrected standard errors) for alternating logistic regression with exchangeable odds ratio, fitted to various outcomes in three studies. β_0 and β_d are the marginal intercept and dose effect, respectively; α is the log odds ratio; ψ is the log odds ratio.*

Outcome	Parameter	DEHP	EG	DYME
External	β_0	-5.16(0.35)	-5.72(0.64)	-7.48(0.75)
	β_d	5.64(0.52)	3.28(0.72)	8.25(0.87)
	α	0.96(0.30)	1.45(0.45)	0.79(0.31)
	ψ	2.61(0.78)	4.26(1.92)	2.20(0.68)
Visceral	β_0	-4.54(0.36)	-7.61(1.06)	-7.24(0.88)
	β_d	4.72(0.57)	4.50(1.13)	6.05(1.04)
	α	1.12(0.30)	0.49(0.42)	1.76(0.59)
	ψ	3.06(0.92)	1.63(0.69)	5.81(3.43)
Skeletal	β_0	-4.87(0.49)	-3.28(0.22)	-4.92(0.34)
	β_d	4.90(0.70)	3.85(0.39)	6.73(0.65)
	α	1.05(0.40)	1.43(0.22)	1.62(0.37)
	ψ	2.86(1.14)	4.18(0.92)	5.05(1.87)
Collapsed	β_0	-4.04(0.31)	-3.19(0.22)	-5.08(0.37)
	β_d	5.93(0.63)	3.86(0.40)	7.98(0.75)
	α	1.17(0.29)	1.40(0.22)	1.26(0.31)
	ψ	3.22(0.93)	4.06(0.89)	3.53(1.09)

8.10 The Heatshock Study

A unique type of developmental toxicity study was originally developed by Brown and Fabro (1981) to assess the impact of heat stress on embryonic development, and adapted by Kimmel *et al* (1993) to investigate effects of both temperature and duration of exposure. In these heatshock experiments, the embryos are explanted from the uterus of the maternal dam during the gestation period and cultured *in vitro*. Each individual embryo is subjected to a short period of heat stress by placing the culture vial into a water bath, involving an increase over body temperature of 3 to 5°C for a duration of 5 to 60 minutes. The embryos are examined 24 hours later for signs of impaired or accelerated development.

This type of developmental toxicity test system has several advantages over the standard Segment II design. First, the exposure is administered directly to the embryo, so controversial issues regarding the unknown (and often non-linear) relationship between the level of exposure to the maternal dam and that received by the developing embryo need not be addressed. While genetic factors are still expected to exert an influence on the vulnerability to injury of embryos from a common dam, direct exposure to

8.10 The Heatshock Study

TABLE 8.6. *Heatshock Study. Hybrid marginal-conditional parameter estimates (model-based standard errors; empirically corrected standard errors) for models fitted to the outcomes MBN, FBN, OLF, and BRB. Covariate effects are allowed to differ across outcomes, and a different association parameter is assumed for each pair. Model 1 presents the estimates under conditional constraints for the higher order association; Model 2 uses marginal constraints. Higher order associations are included in Model 3. Models 1 and 2 are at the same time maximum likelihood and GEE2. Model 3 is full likelihood. Part I: Marginal parameters.*

Parameter	Model 1	Model 2	Model 3
Marginal parameters			
Midbrain (MBN)			
Intercept	-1.81(0.23;0.24)	-1.81(0.23;0.24)	-1.83(0.23;0.24)
'posdur'	-0.12(0.04;0.04)	-0.12(0.04;0.04)	-0.10(0.04;0.04)
'durtemp'	0.04(0.01;0.01)	0.04(0.01;0.01)	0.04(0.01;0.01)
Forebrain (FBN)			
Intercept	-1.73(0.23;0.23)	-1.73(0.23;0.23)	-1.71(0.23;0.22)
'posdur'	-0.09(0.04;0.04)	-0.09(0.04;0.04)	-0.09(0.04;0.04)
'durtemp'	0.04(0.01;0.01)	0.04(0.01;0.01)	0.04(0.01;0.01)
Olfactory system (OLF)			
intercept	-1.43(0.22;0.21)	-1.44(0.22;0.21)	-1.46(0.20;0.21)
'posdur'	-0.21(0.04;0.05)	-0.21(0.04;0.05)	-0.21(0.04;0.05)
'durtemp'	0.07(0.01;0.01)	0.07(0.01;0.01)	0.07(0.01;0.01)
Branchial bars (BRB)			
intercept	-1.19(0.20;0.20)	-1.18(0.20;0.20)	-1.09(0.20;0.20)
'posdur'	-0.13(0.04;0.04)	-0.13(0.04;0.04)	-0.13(0.04;0.04)
'durtemp'	0.04(0.01;0.01)	0.04(0.01;0.01)	0.04(0.01;0.01)

individual embryos reduces the need to account for such litter effects. Thus, the clustering induced by litter effects are not considered in our analysis. A detailed analysis of the clustering aspect can be found in Aerts *et al* (2002). Second, the exposure pattern can be much more easily controlled than in most developmental toxicity studies, as it is possible to achieve target temperature levels in the water bath within one to two minutes. Whereas the typical Segment II study requires waiting eight to twelve days after exposure to assess its impact, information regarding the effects of exposure are quickly obtained in heatshock studies. Finally, this animal test system provides a convenient mechanism for examining the joint effects of both duration of exposure and exposure levels, which until recently have received little attention. The actual study design for the set of experiments is shown in Kimmel *et al* (1994). Of the 327 embryos exposed, 50 did not

TABLE 8.7. *Heatshock Study. Hybrid marginal-conditional parameter estimates (model-based standard errors; empirically corrected standard errors) for models fitted to the outcomes MBN, FBN, OLF, and BRB. Covariate effects are allowed to differ across outcomes, and a different association parameter is assumed for each pair. Model 1 presents the estimates under conditional constraints for the higher order association; Model 2 uses marginal constraints. Higher order associations are included in Model 3. Models 1 and 2 are at the same time maximum likelihood and GEE2. Model 3 is full likelihood. Part II: Association parameters.*

Parameter	Model 1	Model 2	Model 3
Pairwise association			
MBN FBN	3.22(0.38;0.39)	3.22(0.38;0.40)	3.13(0.37;0.38)
MBN OLF	2.69(0.36;0.38)	2.69(0.36;0.37)	2.77(0.36;0.38)
MBN BRB	2.10(0.32;0.33)	2.10(0.32;0.33)	2.17(0.33;0.33)
FBN OLF	3.58(0.41;0.42)	3.59(0.41;0.42)	3.62(0.42;0.44)
FBN BRB	2.54(0.34;0.34)	2.55(0.34;0.34)	2.60(0.34;0.34)
OLF BRB	2.52(0.33;0.34)	2.53(0.33;0.34)	2.61(0.33;0.34)
Higher order association			
MBN FBN OLF			1.30(1.34;1.42)
MBN FBN BRB			0.96(1.19;1.17)
MBN OLF BRB			0.22(1.30;1.38)
FBN OLF BRB			2.12(1.48;1.51)
MBN FBN OLF BRB			3.18(1.77;1.80)
Deviance	946.05	945.15	937.80

survive the heat stress exposure and were excluded from further analysis. The remaining 277 animals have complete data.

Historically, the strategy for comparing responses among exposures of different durations to a variety of environmental agents has relied on a conjecture called Haber's law, which states that adverse response levels should be the same for any equivalent level of dose times duration (Haber 1924). Clearly, the appropriateness of applying Haber's law depends on the pharmacokinetics of the particular agent, the route of administration, the target organ, and the dose/duration patterns under consideration. Although much attention has been focused on documenting exceptions to this rule, it is often used as a simplifying assumption in view of limited testing resources and the multitude of exposure scenarios. However, given the current desire to develop regulatory standards for a range of exposure durations, models flexible enough to describe the response patterns over varying levels of both exposure concentration and duration are greatly needed.

Although a wide variety of statistical methods have been developed for cancer risk assessment, the issue of multiple endpoints does not present

TABLE 8.8. *Heatshock Study. Empirically corrected (e.c.) and model-based (m.b.) Wald test statistics based on Models 1–3. Apart from tests for common covariate effects and common pairwise association, tests for common covariate effects among MBN, FBN, and BRB [indicated by (**)] are presented, as well as a test whether the association splits into two groups: pairs including versus excluding BRB.* indicates $p < 0.05$.*

		Model 1		Model 2		Model 3	
Hypothesis	df	e.c.	m.b.	e.c.	m.b.	e.c.	m.b.
Common 'posdur'	3	*7.95	*9.28	*8.47	*9.85	*9.87	*11.31
Common 'posdur' (**)	2	0.16	0.19	0.17	0.19	0.10	0.07
Common 'durtemp'	3	5.73	7.68	6.13	*8.21	7.39	*9.92
Common 'durtemp' (**)	2	1.36	1.08	1.49	1.14	1.92	1.18
Common pairwise assoc.	5	*12.58	*13.63	*12.55	*13.55	10.16	*11.92
Two groups of pairwise assoc.	4	6.49	6.18	6.52	6.19	4.99	5.65

quite the degree of complexity in this area as it does for developmental toxicity studies. The endpoint of interest in an animal cancer bioassay is typically the occurrence of a particular type of tumor, whereas in developmental toxicity studies there is no clear choice for a single type of adverse outcome. In fact, an entire array of outcomes are needed to define certain birth defect syndromes (Khoury *et al* 1987, Holmes 1988).

The data have been analyzed before by Williams, Molenberghs, and Lipsitz (1996). In line with Molenberghs and Ritter (1996), we will consider a multivariate analysis on four binary morphological parameters: Midbrain (MBN), Forebrain (FBN), Olfactory System (OLF), and Branchial Bars (BRB). They are coded as affected versus normal. If Haber's law is satisfied, the main covariate is 'durtemp,' the product of duration and dose (temperature increase). We found that the main effect 'duration' is also important. However, we expect duration to have no effect at the control dose, therefore it was recoded as 'posdur,' which is equal to 'duration' in the exposed groups and zero in the control group. Including the main effect 'temperature' does not significantly improve the fit.

All of our analyses in this section will be conducted by means of the hybrid between a marginal and conditional model, for which the full likelihood version was given in Section 7.8, with a GEE2 version introduced in Section 8.7. Tables 8.6 and 8.7 show three models fitted to these data. Given the orthogonality between lower-order and higher-order parameters, the estimates can be considered both as stemming from maximum likelihood, as well as from GEE2, depending on whether one views the higher-order association is set equal to zero because this is believed to be the correct structure, or rather merely as a working assumption. In a few models,

178   8. Generalized Estimating Equations

TABLE 8.9. *Heatshock Study. Hybrid marginal-conditional parameter estimates (empirically corrected standard errors) for models fitted to the outcomes MBN, FBN, OLF, and BRB. Covariate effects are allowed to differ across outcomes. Common covariate effects are assumed for MBN, FBN, and BRB. Pairwise associations are grouped in: (1) Group 1, containing all pairs formed from MBN, FBN, and OLF, and (2) Group 2, all pairs containing BRB. Models 4, 5, and 7 are at the same time maximum likelihood and GEE2. Model 6 is full likelihood.*

Parameter	Model 4	Model 5	Model 6	Model 7
Marginal parameters				
Intercepts				
MBN	-1.75(0.20)	-1.75(0.20)	-1.70(0.20)	-1.74(0.20)
FBN	-1.49(0.19)	-1.49(0.19)	-1.47(0.19)	-1.49(0.19)
OLF	-1.40(0.21)	-1.41(0.21)	-1.39(0.21)	-1.45(0.21)
BRB	-1.41(0.19)	-1.41(0.19)	-1.40(0.19)	-1.42(0.19)
Covariates (MBN, FBN, BRB)				
'posdur'	-0.12(0.03)	-0.12(0.03)	-0.12(0.03)	-0.13(0.03)
'durtemp'	0.04(0.01)	0.04(0.01)	0.04(0.01)	0.04(0.01)
Covariates (OLF)				
'posdur'	-0.22(0.05)	-0.22(0.05)	-0.22(0.05)	-0.22(0.04)
'durtemp'	0.07(0.01)	0.07(0.01)	0.07(0.01)	0.07(0.01)
Pairwise association				
Intercepts				
Group 1	3.10(0.29)	3.11(0.29)	3.11(0.29)	3.50(0.40)
Group 2	2.32(0.26)	2.33(0.26)	2.32(0.26)	2.73(0.38)
Covariates				
'posdur'				0.16(0.07)
'durtemp'				-0.05(0.02)
Higher order association				
MBN FBN OLF			0.47(1.35)	
MBN FBN BRB			0.96(1.06)	
MBN OLF BRB			0.19(1.44)	
FBN OLF BRB			1.87(1.50)	
MBN FBN OLF BRB			2.23(1.76)	
Deviance	959.31	959.73	954.24	951.79

higher-order association parameters are included as well (Models 3 and 6), implying they are full likelihood.

Models 1 and 2 do not include higher order associations. Model 1 applies conditional constraints, whereas Model 2 considers its marginal counter-

TABLE 8.10. *Heatshock Study. Estimated odds ratios for Model 7 in Table 8.9. Entries marked with a * correspond to a duration-temperature combination not present in the data.*

	Duration		
Temp.	5	30	60
0.0	33.1	33.1	33.1
3.0	36.1	55.6	93.5
3.5	32.0	26.9	21.8
4.0	28.3	13.0	* 5.1
4.5	25.1	6.3	* 1.2
5.0	22.2	3.0	* 0.3

parts. Model 3 includes the higher-order associations as well. Parameter estimates and standard errors are shown. Clearly, the marginal parameters are virtually the same across models, with the same holding true for the standard errors. Further, it is clear that some of the covariate effects are very similar, and some of the pairwise association parameters are very close to each other.

Table 8.8 presents test statistics based on the model based and robust variance estimators, obtained for Models 1–3. A common 'posdur' effect is clearly not tenable. A common 'durtemp' effect gives p-values that are borderline, as $\chi^2 = 7.68$ corresponds to $p = 0.053$ and $\chi^2 = 7.39$ to 0.061. From the model parameters we observe that the effects of 'posdur' and 'durtemp' are virtually the same for MBN, FBN, and BRB, whereas OLF differs slightly. The test statistics presented in Table 8.8 support these hypotheses. A common pairwise association parameter is not supported, but if the association is divided into two groups (pairs with and without BRB) a simplification which is consistent with the data is achieved.

Reduced models are presented in Table 8.9, where only robust standard errors are shown. Observe that the similarities across Models 4–6 are even greater. Comparing models from Tables 8.6 and 8.7 with their corresponding ones in Table 8.9 using a likelihood ratio statistics yields: 13.26 (Model 4 versus Model 1), 14.58 (Model 5 versus Model 2), and 16.42 (Model 6 versus Model 3), all on 8 degrees of freedom. Only the last one is above the 5 % critical level.

We gathered some evidence for a dependence of pairwise association on the level of exposure. Model 7 in Table 8.9 shows an extension of Model 4, where a common linear effect of 'posdur' and 'durtemp' is included for the pairwise odds ratios. Allowing for a quadratic effect shows no significant improvement. The pairwise association for pairs excluding BRB is described by a log odds ratio of $3.5 + 0.16 *$ 'posdur' $- 0.049 *$ 'durtemp'. The effect of 'temperature' is not significant. The association increases (slightly) with

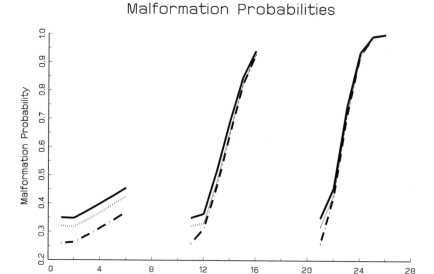

FIGURE 8.1. *Heatshock Study. Malformation probabilities, based on models including three and four outcomes. Ranges of 'durtemp' at three levels of 'duration' are presented. Solid line: MBN, FBN, OLF, BRB; dotted line: FBN, OLF, BRB; dots and dashes: MBN, FBN, OLF.*

'posdur,' but a dramatic decrease is seen with 'durtemp.' A selection of the estimated odds ratios are shown in Table 8.10.

The pairwise associations are important as a tool used to reduce the length of the outcome vector. Indeed, observe that the association between MBN and FBN is very high, and that 'posdur' and 'durtemp' have a similar effect on both. This might imply that considering, e.g., FBN, OLF, and BRB only might yield a similar predicted probability of *any* malformation. In Figure 8.1, we show the malformation probability for a range of 'durtemp' values, at duration levels 5, 30, and 60 minutes. The malformation probabilities are estimated based on three models: Model 1, including all four outcomes, the three-way version with FBN, OLF, and BRB, and the three-way version with MBN, FBN, and OLF. In the latter case, BRB has been omitted. As the association between pairs including BRB is observed to be smaller, it is not surprising that the latter model underestimates the malformation probability as it ignores important independent information. This is best seen at smaller doses, which is important if the models are used for low dose extrapolation.

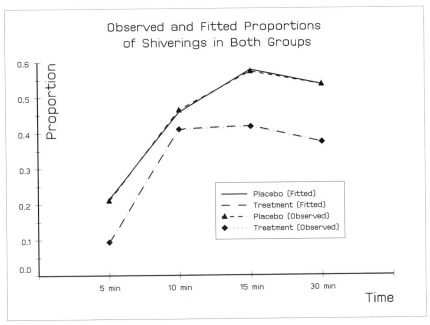

FIGURE 8.2. *Sports Injuries Trial. Observed and fitted proportions of shivering in both arms. Fitted proportions are based on Model 2 in Table 8.11.*

8.11 The Sports Injuries Trial

The sports injuries trial has been introduced in Section 2.8.

We will apply the hybrid marginal and conditional model, introduced in Sections 7.8 and 8.7, in the context of both the longitudinal outcome as well as with repeated measures on the two outcomes, shivering and awakeness. Note that, just as in Section 8.10, two perspectives on the parameter estimates obtained from the hybrid model are possible, maximum likelihood and GEE2. The first one applies when the higher-order association is modeled explicitly or considered to be zero, in line with the working assumptions. The second one applies when the higher-order parameters are set equal to zero by way of working assumption only.

8.11.1 Longitudinal Analysis

The first analysis considers four binary measurements of shivering (at 5, 10, 15, and 20 minutes). Data are presented in Table 2.12. We are interested in a treatment difference and its evolution over time. First, the profiles show a quadratic time trend, as can be seen in Figure 8.2. Next, we need a cubic polynomial to describe the difference between treatment and placebo

TABLE 8.11. *Sports Injuries Trial. Hybrid marginal-conditional model parameter estimates (model based standard errors; empirically corrected standard errors) for models fitted to four binary shivering responses (at 5, 10, 15, and 20 minutes). Model 1 presents unrestricted and Model 2 presents restricted association parameters.*

Parameter	Model 1	Model 2
Marginal parameters		
Intercept	0.15(0.16;0.16)	0.15(0.16;0.16)
Time effect:		
Linear	0.48(0.08;0.08)	0.48(0.08;0.08)
Quadratic	−0.33(0.06;0.06)	−0.33(0.06;0.06)
Treatment effect:		
Main effect	−0.36(0.23;0.23)	−0.36(0.22;0.23)
Linear interaction	−0.52(0.19;0.18)	−0.52(0.19;0.18)
Quadratic interaction	−0.20(0.10;0.10)	−0.20(0.10;0.10)
Cubic interaction	0.28(0.09;0.08)	0.28(0.09;0.08)
Association		
$(1,2)$	3.67(0.73;0.71)	3.71(0.72;0.70)
$(1,3)$	2.54(0.55;0.57)	
$(1,4)$	1.45(0.38;0.39)	
$(2,3)$	2.69(0.31;0.31)	
$(2,4)$	1.48(0.26;0.26)	
$(3,4)$	2.61(0.30;0.30)	
$(1,3)=(2,3)=(3,4)$		2.64(0.21;0.21)
$(1,4)=(2,4)$		1.47(0.25;0.25)
Deviance	1104.09	1104.20

profiles. Not surprisingly, the difference is more marked at later times. Observed an fitted profiles are plotted in Figure 8.2.

Next, we study the association structure. There are six pairwise association parameters, one for each pair of measurement times. There is an extraordinary strong association between the first and second time, the odds ratio equals 39.2. This is explained by the relatively small number of changes in shivering state at the beginning of the trial. Then, association decreases with distance between time points. For the five remaining associations, we consider measurements 1 and 2 to occur virtually together and group the parameters by the difference in time between both measurements: (1,3), (2,3), and (3,4) on the one hand and (1,4) and (2,4) on the other. This reduces the number of association parameters to three, while

TABLE 8.12. *Sports Injuries Trial. Hybrid marginal-conditional model parameter estimates (standard errors) for models fitted to four ordinal shivering responses (at 5, 10, 15, and 20 minutes).*

Parameter	Estimate
Marginal parameters	
First cutpoint:	
Intercept	0.25(0.15)
Linear time	0.47(0.16)
Quadratic time	-0.40(0.06)
Cubic time	0.02(0.07)
Second cutpoint:	
Intercept	-1.42(0.18)
Linear time	0.86(0.22)
Quadratic time	-0.47(0.12)
Cubic time	0.01(0.11)
Treatment effect:	
Main effect	-0.49(0.21)
Linear interaction	-0.46(0.22)
Quadratic interaction	-0.05(0.08)
Cubic interaction	0.22(0.10)
Association	
(1,2)	3.81(0.45)
(1,3)	3.29(0.39)
(1,4)	1.59(0.30)
(2,3)	2.69(0.29)
(2,4)	1.49(0.26)
(3,4)	2.52(0.29)

virtually not changing the quality of the fit. Table 8.11 presents parameter estimates (standard errors) for both unrestricted (Model 1) and restricted (Model 2) associations.

Taking a likelihood perspective, the overall deviance goodness-of-fit statistic is 7.66 on 20 degrees of freedom, providing evidence that there is no need for higher order association. This means that, while a GEE2 perspective is still possible, assuming the higher-order association is left unspecified and replaced by working assumptions, it is fine too to adopt a likelihood point of view, where the first-order and second-order moments have been modeled correctly, and the higher-order associations vanish.

TABLE 8.13. *Sports Injuries Trial. Cross-classification of two pairs of dichotomized shivering and awakeness measurements (at 10 and 20 minutes).*

Shivering	Awakeness			
	(0,0)	(0,1)	(1,0)	(1,1)
	Placebo arm			
(0,0)	14	12	0	20
(0,1)	3	17	0	8
(1,0)	0	12	0	6
(1,1)	3	15	0	28
	Treatment arm			
(0,0)	12	23	0	28
(0,1)	5	9	0	5
(1,0)	2	13	0	9
(1,1)	3	24	0	6

TABLE 8.14. *Sports Injuries Trial. Hybrid marginal-conditional model parameter estimates (model-based standard errors; empirically corrected standard errors) for models fitted to two pairs of shivering/awakeness measurements, at 10 and 20 minutes. When the two sets of standard errors coincide, only one is shown. Part I: Marginal parameters.*

Parameter	Model 1	Model 2	Model 3	Model 4
	Marginal parameters			
Shivering at 10 minutes:				
Intercept	-0.15(0.17;0.17)	-0.15(0.17)	-0.15(0.17)	-0.16(0.17)
Treatment	-0.21(0.24;0.24)	-0.22(0.24)	-0.22(0.24)	-0.21(0.24)
Shivering at 20 Minutes:				
Intercept	0.15(0.17;0.17)	0.15(0.17)	0.15(0.17)	0.14(0.17)
Treatment	-0.67(0.24;0.25)	-0.66(0.24)	-0.66(0.24)	-0.67(0.24)
Awakeness at 10 Minutes:				
Intercept	-0.20(0.17;0.17)	-0.20(0.17)	-0.20(0.17)	-0.20(0.17)
Treatment	-0.45(0.25;0.25)	-0.44(0.25)	-0.44(0.25)	-0.43(0.25)
Awakeness at 20 Minutes:				
Intercept	1.86(0.25;0.26)	1.78(0.24)	1.78(0.24)	1.85(0.24)
Treatment	-0.26(0.33;0.33)	-0.10(0.34)	-0.10(0.34)	-0.23(0.33)

Finally, we reconsidered this analysis, but now on ordinal endpoints. Because category 3 is either empty or very sparse for the four shivering

TABLE 8.15. *Sports Injuries Trial. Hybrid marginal-conditional model parameter estimates (model-based standard errors; empirically corrected standard errors) for models fitted to two pairs of shivering/awakeness measurements, at 10 and 20 minutes. When the two sets of standard errors coincide, only one is shown. Part II: Association parameters.*

Parameter	Model 1	Model 2	Model 3	Model 4
		Pairwise association		
Shivering 1/Shivering 2:				
Intercept	1.48(0.26;0.26)	1.43(0.37)	1.44(0.37)	1.32(0.25)
Treatment		0.08(0.52)	0.08(0.52)	
Shivering 1/Awakeness 1:				
Intercept	0.03(0.25;0.25)	0.62(0.35)	0.62(0.35)	
Treatment		-1.26(0.51)	-1.25(0.51)	
Shivering 1/Awakeness 2:				
Intercept	1.36(0.41;0.42)	1.80(0.65)	1.81(0.64)	1.16(0.36)
Treatment		-0.80(0.85)	-0.81(0.84)	
Shivering 2/Awakeness 1:				
Intercept	-0.28(0.25;0.25)	0.33(0.34)	0.33(0.34)	
Treatment		-1.34(0.53)	-1.34(0.53)	-0.83(0.36)
Shivering 2/Awakeness 2:				
Intercept	0.58(0.36;0.37)	1.15(0.52)	1.15(0.52)	
Treatment		-1.10(0.71)	-1.10(0.71)	
Awakeness 1/Awakeness 2:				
Intercept	$+\infty$	$+\infty$	$+\infty$	$+\infty$
		Higher-order Association		
Shivering 1/Shivering 2/Awakeness 1:				
Intercept			2.58(0.82)	
Treatment			-2.81(1.20)	
Shivering 1/Shivering 2/Awakeness 2:				
Intercept			$-\infty$	
Treatment			0.27(1.18)	
Deviance	1260.03	1249.67	1234.72	1260.82

measures being studied, it is combined with category 2. Consequently, we have two sets of profiles. Potentially, both time and treatment effects can differ depending on the cutpoint. There is evidence for such a difference in the time trend in the form of a Wald test of 10.26 on 3 degrees of freedom ($p = 0.017$). On the other hand, it is plausible to consider a single treatment profile, common to both cutpoints (Wald test of 6.85 on 4 degrees of freedom; $p = 0.14$). Estimates for the corresponding model are presented in Table 8.12.

8.11.2 A Bivariate Longitudinal Analysis

The second analysis considers two pairs of shivering and awakeness outcomes, at 10 and 20 minutes. Data are given in Table 8.13. The main interest lies in the effect of treatment for each outcome, as well as in the association between the outcomes. There is a complication with the association between the two awakeness measures, due to the structural zeros described earlier. Indeed, the corresponding log odds ratio is equal to infinity. If this parameter is estimated along with the others, we obtain a solution on the boundary of the parameter space, invalidating inference. One way out is to set this parameter equal to zero or another arbitrary (finite) value. However, this is unsatisfactory form a theoretical point of view, as we assume independence, knowing that there is an infinitely large association. Alternatively, we can incorporate a log odds ratio of $+\infty$ as a structural feature of the model. Some straightforward technical modifications are required to the fitting program, such as replacing (6.16) by $\mu_{ij_1j_2} = \min(\mu_{ij_1}, \mu_{ij_2})$. The parameter estimates are given in Tables 8.14 and 8.15 (Model 1).

The effect of treatment is clearly seen at the second shivering measurement and only marginally at the first awakeness measurement. Only two of the estimated pairwise associations are strong: between both shivering measurements, and between the first shivering and the second awakeness measurement. Because shivering often occurs as the patient abruptly changes levels of consciousness, this could explain the association.

When computing the goodness-of-fit, one has to take into account that in each $2 \times 2 \times 2 \times 2$ table (one for each treatment group), there are 4 zero cells by design, reducing the data degrees of freedom to 22. Model 1 yields a deviance G^2 statistic of 25.32 on 9 degrees of freedom, which is clearly unacceptable. First, the two-way association can be extended by allowing for differences in association for the two treatment groups. The G^2 statistic reduces to 14.95 on 4 degrees of freedom, which still leaves room for improvement. To extend the model, the higher order associations need to be modeled as well. Recall that, due to the orthogonality of marginal and conditional parameters, this model (Model 2 in Tables 8.14 and 8.15) can be considered satisfactory as it is saturated in the marginal parameters, and the model-based and empirically corrected standard errors coincide (hence only one entry is shown).

As we allowed the pairwise interactions to depend on treatment, a more detailed picture than the one from Model 1 emerges. Apart from a structural $+\infty$ for the association parameter between both awakeness measures, we find a relatively strong odds ratio for the two shiverings (consistent with other analyses), without evidence for a treatment dependence. These two odds ratios describe the longitudinal part of the association, pertaining to two measurements of the same variable at different occasions.

Alternatively, one can seek to estimate the higher order association parameters as well. Here too, we have to take into account the zero cells. It suffices to leave out all higher order interactions containing awakeness measures simultaneously. This leaves two three-way conditional odds ratios to estimate: (shivering 1, shivering 2, awakeness 1) and (shivering 1, shivering 2, awakeness 2). Assuming these are constant yields a G^2 statistic of 9.13 on 2 degrees of freedom. This implies that also the higher order interactions are treatment dependent. Due to a sampling zero, the second one of these log odds ratios is zero. Setting it equal to zero, and estimating the value only in the treatment group, then corresponds to the saturated model (Model 3 in Tables 8.14 and 8.15). It is interesting to note that the first of the three-way interactions (shivering 1, shivering 2, awakeness 1) is significant, at least in the placebo group.

Problems with sampling zeros occur less frequently when the higher order association is described via marginal odds ratios (Molenberghs and Lesaffre 1994). Comparing Models 2 and 3, it might be argued that setting the higher association parameters equal to zero is a sensible choice, especially when scientific interest is limited to the first two moments.

To interpret the two-way association, we observe that some of the associations in Models 2 and 3 do not attain statistical significance. Hence it is useful to consider a more parsimonious model. We simplify Model 2 such that only the following pairwise associations are included: a common log odds ratio for the (shivering 1, shivering 2) and (shivering 1, awakeness 2) pairs and association between shivering 2 and awakeness 1 in the treatment group only. Comparing this model to Model 2 with a likelihood ratio test, of course taking the likelihood perspective on the model, we obtain a G^2 test statistic value of 11.15 on 7 degrees of freedom ($p = 0.13$). Note that the main effect parameters all change less than 0.01 except for awakeness at 20 minutes.

9
Pseudo-Likelihood

9.1 Introduction

Full marginal maximum likelihood, as discussed in Chapters 6 and 7, can become prohibitive in terms of computation when measurement sequences are of moderate to large length. This is one of the reasons why generalized estimating equations (GEE, Chapter 8) have become so popular. One way to view the genesis of GEE is by modifying the score equations to simpler estimating equations, thereby preserving consistency and asymptotic normality, upon using an appropriately corrected variance-covariance matrix. Alternatively, the (log-)likelihood itself can be simplified to a more manageable form. This is, broadly speaking, the idea behind *pseudo-likelihood* (PL). For example, when a joint density is of the Bahadur (Section 7.2), probit (Section 7.6), or Dale (Section 7.7) form, calculating the higher-order probabilities needed to evaluate the score vector and Hessian matrix can be prohibitive while, at the same time, interest can be confined to a small number of lower-order moments. The idea is then to replace the single joint density by, for example, all univariate densities, or all pairwise densities over the set of all possible pairs within a sequence of repeated measures. As a simple illustration, a three-way density

$$L_i = f_i(y_{i1}, y_{i2}, y_{i3}|\boldsymbol{\theta}_i) \tag{9.1}$$

would be replaced by the product

$$L_i^* = f_i(y_{i1}, y_{i2}\boldsymbol{\theta}_i^*) \cdot f_i(y_{i1}, y_{i3}\boldsymbol{\theta}_i^*) \cdot f_i(y_{i2}, y_{i3}|\boldsymbol{\theta}_i^*). \tag{9.2}$$

Such a change is computationally advantageous, asymptotics can be rescued, and modeling (9.2) is equally simple, if not simpler, than modeling (9.1), as the parameter vector $\boldsymbol{\theta}_i^*$ in (9.2) typically is a subvector of $\boldsymbol{\theta}_i$ in (9.1).

Section 9.2 introduces pseudo-likelihood in a formal way, and such that it can be of use, not only here in marginal applications, but also for conditional (Chapter 12) and subject-specific (Chapters 21 and 25) applications. Appropriate test statistics are given in Section 9.3. The specific situation of PL for marginal models is the topic of Section 9.4, and a comparison between marginal PL and GEE is presented in Section 9.5. The methodology is illustrated using the NTP data (Section 9.6).

9.2 Pseudo-Likelihood: Definition and Asymptotic Properties

To formally introduce pseudo-likelihood, we will use the convenient general definition given by Arnold and Strauss (1991). See also Geys, Molenberghs, and Ryan (1999) and Aerts *et al* (2002). Without loss of generality we can assume that the vector $\boldsymbol{Y}_i$ of binary outcomes for subject i ($i = 1, \ldots, N$) has constant dimension n. The extension to variable lengths n_i for $\boldsymbol{Y}_i$ is straightforward.

9.2.1 Definition

Define S as the set of all $2^n - 1$ vectors of length n, consisting solely of zeros and ones, with each vector having at least one non-zero entry. Denote by $\boldsymbol{y}_i^{(s)}$ the subvector of $\boldsymbol{y}_i$ corresponding to the components of s that are non-zero. The associated joint density is $f_s(\boldsymbol{y}_i^{(s)}|\boldsymbol{\theta}_i)$. To define a pseudo-likelihood function, one chooses a set $\delta = \{\delta_s | s \in S\}$ of real numbers, with at least one non-zero component. The log of the pseudo-likelihood is then defined as

$$p\ell = \sum_{i=1}^{N} \sum_{s \in S} \delta_s \ln f_s(\boldsymbol{y}_i^{(s)}|\boldsymbol{\theta}_i). \tag{9.3}$$

Adequate regularity conditions have to be assumed to ensure that (9.3) can be maximized by solving the pseudo-likelihood (score) equations, the latter obtained by differentiation of the logarithm of PL and setting the derivative equal to zero.

The classical log-likelihood function is found by setting $\delta_s = 1$ if s is the vector consisting solely of ones, and 0 otherwise.

9.2.2 Consistency and Asymptotic Normality

Before stating the main asymptotic properties of the PL estimators, we first list the required regularity conditions on the density functions $f_s(\boldsymbol{y}^{(s)}|\boldsymbol{\theta})$.

A0 The densities $f_s(\boldsymbol{y}^{(s)}|\boldsymbol{\theta})$ are distinct for different values of the parameter $\boldsymbol{\theta}$.

A1 The densities $f_s(\boldsymbol{y}^{(s)}|\boldsymbol{\theta})$ have common support, which does not depend on $\boldsymbol{\theta}$.

A2 The parameter space Ω contains an open region ω of which the true parameter value $\boldsymbol{\theta}_0$ is an interior point.

A3 ω is such that for all s, and almost all $\boldsymbol{y}^{(s)}$ in the support of $\boldsymbol{Y}^{(s)}$, the densities admit all third derivatives

$$\frac{\partial^3 f_s(\boldsymbol{y}^{(s)}|\boldsymbol{\theta})}{\partial \theta_{k_1} \partial \theta_{k_2} \partial \theta_{k_3}}.$$

A4 The first and second logarithmic derivatives of f_s satisfy

$$E_{\boldsymbol{\theta}}\left(\frac{\partial \ln f_s(\boldsymbol{y}^{(s)}|\boldsymbol{\theta})}{\partial \theta_k}\right) = 0, \qquad k = 1, \ldots, p,$$

and

$$0 < E_{\boldsymbol{\theta}}\left(\frac{-\partial^2 \ln f_s(\boldsymbol{y}^{(s)}|\boldsymbol{\theta})}{\partial \theta_{k_1} \partial \theta_{k_2}}\right) < \infty, \qquad k_1, k_2 = 1, \ldots, p.$$

A5 The matrix I_0, to be defined in (9.5), is positive definite.

A6 There exist functions $M_{k_1 k_2 k_3}$ such that

$$\sum_{s \in S} \delta_s E_{\boldsymbol{\theta}} \left|\frac{\partial^3 \ln f_s(\boldsymbol{y}^{(s)}|\boldsymbol{\theta})}{\partial \theta_{k_1} \partial \theta_{k_2} \partial \theta_{k_3}}\right| < M_{k_1 k_2 k_3}(\boldsymbol{y})$$

for all $\boldsymbol{y}$ in the support of f and for all $\boldsymbol{\theta} \in \omega$ and $m_{k_1 k_2 k_3} = E_{\boldsymbol{\theta}_0}[M_{k_1 k_2 k_3}(Y)] < \infty$.

Theorem 9.1, proven by Arnold and Strauss (1991), guarantees the existence of at least one solution to the pseudo-likelihood equations, which is consistent and asymptotically normal. Without loss of generality, we can assume $\boldsymbol{\theta}$ is constant. Replacing it by $\boldsymbol{\theta}_i$ and modeling it as a function of covariates is straightforward.

Theorem 9.1 (Consistency and Asymptotic Normality) *Assume that $(\boldsymbol{Y}_1, \ldots, \boldsymbol{Y}_N)$ are i.i.d. with common density that depends on $\boldsymbol{\theta}_0$. Then under regularity conditions (A1)–(A6):*

1. The pseudo-likelihood estimator $\tilde{\boldsymbol{\theta}}_N$, defined as the maximizer of (9.3), converges in probability to $\boldsymbol{\theta}_0$.

2. $\sqrt{N}(\tilde{\boldsymbol{\theta}}_N - \boldsymbol{\theta}_0)$ converges in distribution to

$$N_p[\mathbf{0}, I_0(\boldsymbol{\theta}_0)^{-1} I_1(\boldsymbol{\theta}_0) I_0(\boldsymbol{\theta}_0)^{-1}], \tag{9.4}$$

with $I_0(\boldsymbol{\theta})$ defined by

$$I_{0,k_1 k_2}(\boldsymbol{\theta}) = -\sum_{s \in S} \delta_s E_{\boldsymbol{\theta}} \left(\frac{\partial^2 \ln f_s(\boldsymbol{y}^{(s)}|\boldsymbol{\theta})}{\partial \theta_{k_1} \partial \theta_{k_2}} \right) \tag{9.5}$$

and $I_1(\boldsymbol{\theta})$ by

$$I_{2,k_1 k_2}(\boldsymbol{\theta}) = \sum_{s,t \in S} \delta_s \delta_t E_{\boldsymbol{\theta}} \left(\frac{\partial \ln f_s(\boldsymbol{y}^{(s)}|\boldsymbol{\theta})}{\partial \theta_{k_1}} \frac{\partial \ln f_t(\boldsymbol{y}^{(t)}|\boldsymbol{\theta})}{\partial \theta_{k_2}} \right). \tag{9.6}$$

Similar in spirit to generalized estimating equations (Chapter 8), the asymptotic normality result provides an easy way to consistently estimate the asymptotic covariance matrix. Indeed, the matrix I_0 is found from evaluating the second derivative of the log PL function at the PL estimate. The expectation in I_1 can be replaced by the cross-products of the observed scores. We will refer to I_0^{-1} as the model based variance estimator (which should not be used as it overestimates the precision), to I_1 as the empirical correction, and to $I_0^{-1} I_1 I_0^{-1}$ as the empirically corrected variance estimator. In the context of generalized estimating equations, this is also known as the sandwich estimator.

As discussed by Arnold and Strauss (1991), and exactly the same as with GEE, the Cramèr-Rao inequality implies that $I_0^{-1} I_1 I_0^{-1}$ is greater than the inverse of I (the Fisher information matrix for the maximum likelihood case), in the sense that $I_0^{-1} I_1 I_0^{-1} - I^{-1}$ is positive semi-definite. Strict inequality holds if the PL estimator fails to be a function of a minimal sufficient statistic. Therefore, a PL estimator is always less efficient than the corresponding ML estimator. Note that, for maximum likelihood, the full density f would be used, rather than the pseudo-likelihood contributions.

9.3 Pseudo-Likelihood Inference

The close connection of PL to likelihood is an attractive feature. It enabled Geys, Molenberghs, and Ryan (1999) to construct pseudo-likelihood ratio test statistics that have easy-to-compute expressions and intuitively appealing limiting distributions. In contrast, likelihood ratio test statistics for GEE (Rotnitzky and Jewell 1990) are slightly more complicated.

In practice, one will often want to perform a flexible model selection. Therefore, one needs extensions of the Wald, score, or likelihood ratio test statistics to the pseudo-likelihood framework. Rotnitzky and Jewell (1990) examined the asymptotic distributions of generalized Wald and score tests, as well as likelihood ratio tests, for regression coefficients obtained by generalized estimating equations for a class of marginal generalized linear models for correlated data. Using similar ideas, we derive different test statistics, as well as their asymptotic distributions for the pseudo-likelihood framework. Liang and Self (1996) have considered a test statistic, for one specific type of pseudo-likelihood function, which is similar in form to one of the tests we will present below.

Suppose we are interested in testing the null hypothesis $H_0 : \gamma = \gamma_0$, where γ is an r-dimensional subvector of the vector of regression parameters $\boldsymbol{\theta}$ and write $\boldsymbol{\theta}$ as $(\gamma', \delta')'$. Then, several test statistics can be used.

9.3.1 Wald Statistic

Because of the asymptotic normality of the PL estimator $\tilde{\boldsymbol{\theta}}_N$,

$$W^* = N(\tilde{\gamma}_N - \gamma_0)' \Sigma_{\gamma\gamma}^{-1} (\tilde{\gamma}_N - \gamma_0)$$

has an asymptotic χ_r^2 distribution under the null hypothesis, where $\Sigma_{\gamma\gamma}$ denotes the $r \times r$ submatrix of $\Sigma = I_0^{-1} I_1 I_0^{-1}$. In practice, the matrix Σ can be replaced by a consistent estimator, obtained by substituting the PL estimator $\tilde{\boldsymbol{\theta}}_N$. Although the Wald test is in general simple to apply, it is well-known to be sensitive to changes in parameterization. The Wald test statistic is therefore particularly unattractive for conditionally specified models, as marginal effects are likely to depend in a complex way on the model parameters (Diggle, Heagerty, Liang, and Zeger 2002).

9.3.2 Pseudo-Score Statistics

As an alternative to the Wald statistic, one can propose the *pseudo-score statistic*. A score test has the advantage that it can be obtained by fitting the null model only. Furthermore, it is invariant to reparameterization. Let us define

$$S^*(e.c.) = \frac{1}{N} U_\gamma [\gamma_0, \tilde{\delta}(\gamma_0)]' I_0^{\gamma\gamma} \Sigma_{\gamma\gamma}^{-1} I_0^{\gamma\gamma} U_\gamma [\gamma_0, \tilde{\delta}(\gamma_0)],$$

where 'e.c.' denotes empirically corrected and $\tilde{\delta}(\gamma_0)$ denotes the maximum pseudo-likelihood estimator in the subspace where $\gamma = \gamma_0$, $I_0^{\gamma\gamma}$ is the $r \times r$ submatrix of the inverse of I_0, and $I_0^{\gamma\gamma} \Sigma_{\gamma\gamma}^{-1} I_0^{\gamma\gamma}$ is evaluated under H_0. Geys, Molenberghs, and Ryan (1999) showed that this pseudo-score statistic is asymptotically χ_r^2 distributed under H_0. As discussed by Rotnitzky and Jewell (1990) in the context of generalized estimating equations, such a score statistic may suffer from computational stability problems. A model based test that may be computationally simpler is:

$$S^*(m.b.) = \frac{1}{N} U_\gamma[\gamma_0, \tilde{\delta}(\gamma_0)]' I_0^{\gamma\gamma} U_\gamma[\gamma_0, \tilde{\delta}(\gamma_0)].$$

However, its asymptotic distribution under H_0 is complicated and given by $\sum_{j=1}^{r} \lambda_j \chi^2_{1(j)}$ where the $\chi^2_{1(j)}$ are independently distributed as χ^2_1 variables and $\lambda_1 \geq \ldots \geq \lambda_r$ are the eigenvalues of $(I_0^{\gamma\gamma})^{-1} \Sigma_{\gamma\gamma}$, evaluated under H_0. The score statistic $S^*(m.b.)$ can be adjusted such that it has an approximate χ^2_r distribution, which is much easier to evaluate. Several types of adjustments have been proposed in the literature (Rao and Scott 1987, Roberts, Rao, and Kumar 1987). Similar to Rotnitzky and Jewell (1990), Geys, Molenberghs, and Ryan (1999) proposed an adjusted pseudo-score statistic

$$S^*_a(m.b.) = S^*(m.b.)/\overline{\lambda},$$

where $\overline{\lambda}$ is the arithmetic mean of the eigenvalues λ_j. Note that no distinction can be made between $S^*(e.c.)$ and $S^*_a(m.b.)$ for $r = 1$. Moreover, in the likelihood-based case, all eigenvalues reduce to one and thus all three statistics coincide with the model based likelihood score statistic.

9.3.3 Pseudo-Likelihood Ratio Statistics

Another alternative is provided by the pseudo-likelihood ratio test statistic, which requires comparison of full and reduced model:

$$G^{*2} = 2\left[p\ell(\tilde{\theta}_N) - p\ell(\gamma_0, \tilde{\delta}(\gamma_0))\right].$$

Geys, Molenberghs, and Ryan (1999) showed that the asymptotic distribution of G^{*2} can also be written as a weighted sum $\sum_{j=1}^{r} \lambda_j \chi^2_{1(j)}$, where the $\chi^2_{1(j)}$ are independently distributed as χ^2_1 variables and $\lambda_1 \geq \ldots \geq \lambda_r$ are the eigenvalues of $(I_0^{\gamma\gamma})^{-1} \Sigma_{\gamma\gamma}$. Alternatively, the adjusted pseudo-likelihood ratio test statistic, defined by

$$G^{*2}_a = G^{*2}/\overline{\lambda},$$

is approximately χ^2_r distributed. Their proof shows that G^{*2} can be rewritten as an approximation to a Wald statistic. The covariance structure of the Wald statistic can be calculated under the null hypothesis, but also under the alternative hypothesis. Both versions of the Wald tests are asymptotically equivalent under H_0 (Rao 1973, p. 418). Therefore, it can be argued that the adjustments in G^{*2}_a can also be evaluated under the null as well as under the alternative hypothesis. These adjusted statistics will then be denoted by $G^{*2}_a(H_0)$ and $G^{*2}_a(H_1)$, respectively. In analogy with the Wald test statistic, we expect $G^{*2}_a(H_1)$ to have high power. A similar reasoning suggests that the score test $S_a^*(m.b.)$ might closely correspond to $G_a^{*2}(H_0)$, as both depend strongly on the fitted null model. Analogous results were obtained by Rotnitzky and Jewell (1990). Aerts *et al* (2002) reported on extensive simulations to compare the behavior of the various test statistics.

The asymptotic distribution of the pseudo-likelihood based test statistics are weighted sums of independent χ_1^2 variables where the weights are unknown eigenvalues. In Aerts and Claeskens (1999) it is shown theoretically that the parametric bootstrap leads to a consistent estimator for the null distribution of the pseudo-likelihood ratio test statistic. The bootstrap approach does not need any additional estimation of unknown eigenvalues and automatically corrects for the incomplete specification of the joint distribution in the pseudo-likelihood. Similar results hold for the robust Wald and robust score test. The simulation study of Aerts and Claeskens (1999) indicates that the χ^2 tests often suffer from inflated type I error probabilities, which are nicely corrected by the bootstrap. This is especially the case for the Wald statistic, whereas the asymptotic χ^2 distribution of the robust score statistic test is performing quite well. The parametric bootstrap is expected to break down if the likelihood of the data is grossly misspecified. Aerts *et al* (2002, Chapter 11) present a more robust semiparametric bootstrap, based on resampling the score and differentiated score values.

9.4 Marginal Pseudo-Likelihood

A marginally specified odds ratio model (Molenberghs and Lesaffre 1994, 1999, Glonek and McCullagh 1995, Lang and Agresti 1994, see also Section 7.7) becomes prohibitive in computational terms when the number of replications within a unit gets moderate to large. In such a situation, both GEE and PL are viable alternatives. The connection between GEE based on odds ratios (Section 8.6) and the corresponding PL is strong and will be developed in Section 9.5. Marginal PL methodology has been proposed, among others, by le Cessie and van Houwelingen (1994) and Geys, Molenberghs, and Lipsitz (1998).

9.4.1 Definition of Marginal Pseudo-Likelihood

Again, assume there are $i = 1, \ldots, N$ units with $j = 1, \ldots, n_i$ measurements per unit. We will start with a general form and then focus on clustered binary data, where the outcomes Y_{ij} are replaced by a summary statistic $Z_i = \sum_{j=1}^{n_i} Y_{ij}$, the total number of successes within the ith cluster.

9.4.1.1 First Form

le Cessie and van Houwelingen (1994) replace the true contribution of a vector of correlated binary data to the full likelihood, written as $f(y_{i1}, \ldots, y_{in_i})$, by the product of all pairwise contributions $f(y_{ij_1}, y_{ij_2})$ $(1 \leq j_1 < j_2 \leq n_i)$, to obtain a *pseudo-likelihood function*. Grouping the outcomes for subject i into a vector $\boldsymbol{Y}_i$, the contribution of the ith cluster to the log pseudo-likelihood is

$$p\ell_i = \sum_{1 \leq j_1 < j_2 \leq n_i} \ln f(y_{ij_1}, y_{ij_2}), \tag{9.7}$$

if it contains more than one observation. Otherwise $p\ell_i = f(y_{i1})$. In what follows, we restrict our attention to clusters of size larger than 1. Units of size 1 contribute to the marginal parameters only. This specific version of pseudo-likelihood is often referred to as pairwise likelihood.

Using a bivariate Plackett distribution (Plackett 1965, Section 7.7.1), the joint probabilities $f(y_{ij_1}, y_{ij_2})$, denoted by $\mu_{ij_1 j_2}$, can be specified using (7.40), with the pairwise odds ratio as in (7.39). The contributions of the form $f(y_{ij_1}, y_{ij_2})$ can then be combined into a pseudo-likelihood function $p\ell$ (9.7), which can be maximized as if it where a genuine bivariate log-likelihood. The asymptotic variance-covariance matrix of the parameter estimates then follows from (9.4).

9.4.1.2 Under Exchangeability

For binary data and taking the exchangeability assumption into account, the log pseudo-likelihood contribution $p\ell_i$ can be formulated as:

$$p\ell_i = \binom{z_i}{2} \ln \mu^*_{i11} + \binom{n_i - z_i}{2} \ln \mu^*_{i00} + z_i(n_i - z_i) \ln \mu^*_{i10}. \tag{9.8}$$

In this formulation, μ^*_{i11} and μ^*_{i00} denote the bivariate probabilities of observing two *successes* or two *failures*, respectively, and μ^*_{i10} is the probability for the first component being 1 and the second being 0. Under exchangeability, this is identical to the probability μ^*_{i01} for the first being 0 and the second being 1. If we consider the following reparameterization:

$$\mu_{i11} = \mu^*_{i11},$$
$$\mu_{i10} = \mu^*_{i11} + \mu^*_{i10} = \mu_{01},$$
$$\mu_{i00} = \mu^*_{i11} + \mu^*_{i10} + \mu^*_{i01} + \mu^*_{i00} = 1,$$

then this one-to-one reparameterization maps the three, common within-cluster, two-way marginal probabilities $(\mu^*_{i11}, \mu^*_{i10}, \mu^*_{i00})$ to two one-way marginal probabilities (which under exchangeability are both equal to μ_{i10}) and one two-way probability $\mu_{i11} = \mu^*_{i11}$. Hence, equation (9.8) can be reformulated as:

$$p\ell_i = \binom{z_i}{2} \ln \mu_{i11} + \binom{n_i - z_i}{2} \ln(1 - 2\mu_{i10} + \mu_{i11})$$

$$+z_i(n_i - z_i)\ln(\mu_{i10} - \mu_{i11}), \tag{9.9}$$

and the pairwise odds ratio ψ_{ijk} reduces to:

$$\psi_i = \frac{\mu_{i11}(1 - 2\mu_{i10} + \mu_{i11})}{(\mu_{i10} - \mu_{i11})^2}.$$

To enable model specification, we assume a composite link function $\boldsymbol{\eta}_i = (\eta_{i1}, \eta_{i2})'$ with a mean and an association component:

$$\eta_{i1} = \ln(\mu_{i10}) - \ln(1 - \mu_{i10}),$$
$$\eta_{i2} = \ln(\psi_i) = \ln(\mu_{i11}) + \ln(1 - 2\mu_{i10} + \mu_{i11}) - 2\ln(\mu_{i10} - \mu_{i11}).$$

From these links, the univariate and pairwise probabilities are easily derived (Plackett 1965), leading to a specific version of (7.40):

$$\mu_{i10} = \frac{\exp(\eta_{i1})}{1 + \exp(\eta_{i1})}$$

and

$$\mu_{i11} = \begin{cases} \frac{1 + 2\mu_{i10}(\psi_i - 1) - S_i}{2(\psi_i - 1)}, & \text{if } \psi_i \neq 1 \\ \mu_{i10}^2 & \text{if } \psi_i = 1, \end{cases}$$

with

$$S_i = \sqrt{[1 + 2\mu_{i10}(\psi_i - 1)]^2 + 4\psi_i(1 - \psi_i)\mu_{i10}^2}.$$

Finally, we can assume a linear model $\boldsymbol{\eta}_i = X_i\boldsymbol{\theta}$, with X_i a known design matrix and $\boldsymbol{\theta}$ a vector of unknown regression parameters. The maximum pseudo-likelihood estimator $\widehat{\boldsymbol{\theta}}$ of $\boldsymbol{\theta}$ is then defined as the solution to the pseudo-score equations $\boldsymbol{U}(\boldsymbol{\theta}) = \boldsymbol{0}$. Using the chain rule, $\boldsymbol{U}(\boldsymbol{\theta})$ can be written as:

$$\boldsymbol{U}(\boldsymbol{\theta}) = \sum_{i=1}^{N} X_i'(T_i^{-1})' \frac{\partial p\ell_i}{\partial \boldsymbol{\mu}_i} \tag{9.10}$$

with $\boldsymbol{\mu}_i = (\mu_{i10}, \mu_{i11})'$ and $T_i = \partial \boldsymbol{\eta}_i / \partial \boldsymbol{\mu}_i$. Newton-Raphson starts with a vector of initial estimates $\boldsymbol{\theta}^{(0)}$ and updates the current value of the parameter vector $\boldsymbol{\theta}^{(s)}$ by

$$\boldsymbol{\theta}^{(s+1)} = \boldsymbol{\theta}^{(s)} + W(\boldsymbol{\theta}^{(s)})^{-1}\boldsymbol{U}(\boldsymbol{\theta}^{(s)}).$$

Here, $W(\boldsymbol{\theta})$ is the matrix of the second derivatives of the log pseudo-likelihood with respect to the regression parameters $\boldsymbol{\theta}$:

$$W(\boldsymbol{\theta}) = \sum_{i=1}^{N} X_i' \left[F_i + (T_i^{-1})' \frac{\partial^2 p\ell_i}{\partial \boldsymbol{\mu}_i \partial \boldsymbol{\mu}_i'} (T_i^{-1}) \right] X_i,$$

and F_i is defined by (McCullagh 1987, p. 5; Molenberghs and Lesaffre 1999, see also Section 7.12.2):

$$(F_i)_{pq} = \sum_s \sum_{a,b,c} \frac{\partial^2 \eta_{ia}}{\partial \mu_{ib} \partial \mu_{ic}} \frac{\partial \mu_{is}}{\partial \eta_{ia}} \frac{\partial \mu_{ib}}{\partial \eta_{ip}} \frac{\partial \mu_{ic}}{\partial \eta_{iq}} \frac{\partial p\ell_i}{\partial \mu_{is}}.$$

The Fisher scoring algorithm is obtained by replacing the matrix $W(\boldsymbol{\theta})$ by its expected value:

$$E[W(\boldsymbol{\theta})] = \sum_{i=1}^N X_i'(T_i^{-1})' A_i (T_i^{-1}) X_i,$$

with A_i the expected value of the matrix of second derivatives of the log pseudo-likelihood $p\ell_i$ with respect to $\boldsymbol{\mu}_i$.

The sandwich estimator (9.4) can now be written as:

$$W(\widehat{\boldsymbol{\theta}})^{-1} \left[\sum_{i=1}^N \boldsymbol{U}_i(\widehat{\boldsymbol{\theta}}) \boldsymbol{U}_i(\widehat{\boldsymbol{\theta}})' \right] W(\widehat{\boldsymbol{\theta}})^{-1}.$$

9.4.1.3 Second Form

A non-equivalent specification of the pseudo-likelihood contribution (9.7) is:

$$p\ell_i^* = p\ell_i/(n_i - 1).$$

The factor $1/(n_i - 1)$ corrects for the feature that each response Y_{ij} occurs $n_i - 1$ times in the ith contribution to the PL, and it ensures that the PL reduces to full likelihood under independence, as then (9.9) simplifies to:

$$p\ell_i = (n_i - 1) \left[z_i \ln(\mu_{i10}) + (n_i - z_i) \ln(1 - \mu_{i10}) \right].$$

We can replace $p\ell_i$ by $p\ell_i^*$. However, if $(n_i - 1)$ is considered random it is not obvious that the expected value of $U_i(\boldsymbol{\theta})/(n_i - 1)$ equals zero. To ensure that the solution to the new pseudo-score equation is consistent, we have to assume that n_i is independent of the outcomes given the covariates for the ith unit. When all n_i are equal, the PL estimator $\boldsymbol{\theta}$ and its variance-covariance matrix remain the same, no matter whether we use $p\ell_i$ or $p\ell_i^*$ in the definition of the log pseudo-likelihood.

9.4.2 A Generalized Linear Model Representation

To obtain the pseudo-likelihood function described in Section 9.4.1, we replaced the true contribution $f(y_{i1}, \ldots, y_{in_i})$ of the ith unit to the full likelihood by the product of all pairwise contributions $f(y_{ij_1}, y_{ij_2})$ with

$1 \leq j_1 < j_2 \leq n_i$. This implies that a particular response y_{ij} occurs $n_i - 1$ times in $p\ell_i$. Therefore, it is useful to construct for each response y_{ij}, $n_i - 1$ replicated $y_{ij_1}^{(j_2)}$ with $j_2 \neq j_1$. The dummy response $y_{ij_1}^{(j_2)}$ is to be interpreted as the particular replicate of y_{ij} that is paired with the replicate $y_{ij_2}^{(j_1)}$ of y_{ij_2} in the pseudo-likelihood function. Using this at first sight odd but convenient device, we are able to rewrite the gradient of the log pseudo-likelihood $p\ell$ in an appealing generalized linear model type representation. With notation introduced in the previous section, the gradient can now be written as

$$U(\boldsymbol{\theta}) = \sum_{i=1}^{N} X_i'(T_i^{-1})' V_i^{-1}(\boldsymbol{Z}_i - \boldsymbol{\mu}_i),$$

or, using the second representation $p\ell_i^*$, as

$$U(\boldsymbol{\theta}) = \sum_{i=1}^{N} \frac{1}{n_i - 1} X_i'(T_i^{-1})' V_i^{-1}(\boldsymbol{Z}_i - \boldsymbol{\mu}_i),$$

where we now define

$$\boldsymbol{Z}_i = \begin{pmatrix} \sum_{j_1=1}^{n_i} \sum_{j_2 \neq j_1} Y_{ij_1}^{(j_2)} \\ \frac{1}{2} \sum_{j_1=1}^{n_i} \sum_{j_2 \neq j_1} Y_{ij_1}^{(j_2)} Y_{ij_2}^{(j_1)} \end{pmatrix}, \quad \boldsymbol{\mu}_i = \begin{pmatrix} n_i(n_i - 1)\mu_{i10} \\ \binom{n_i}{2}\mu_{i11} \end{pmatrix},$$

and V_i is the covariance matrix of $\boldsymbol{Z}_i$. Geys, Molenberghs, and Lipsitz (1998) have shown that the elements of V_i take appealing expressions and are easy to implement. One only needs to evaluate first- and second-order probabilities. Under independence, the variances reduce to well-known quantities. To obtain a suitable PL estimator for $\boldsymbol{\theta}$, we can use the Fisher-scoring algorithm where the matrix A_i in the previous section is now replaced by the inverse of V_i. The asymptotic covariance matrix of $\widehat{\boldsymbol{\theta}}$ is estimated in a similar fashion as before.

9.5 Comparison with Generalized Estimating Equations

In the previous sections, we described one alternative estimating procedure for full maximum likelihood estimation in the framework of a marginally specified odds ratio model, which is easier and much less time consuming. Several questions arise such as to how the different methods compare in terms of efficiency and in terms of computing time and what the mathematical differences and similarities are. At first glance, there is a fundamental difference. A pseudo-likelihood function is constructed by modifying a joint density. Parameters are estimated by setting the first derivatives of this function equal to zero. On the contrary, generalized estimating equations follow from specification of the first few moments and by adopting assumptions about the higher order moments. We will explore similarities and differences in some detail.

In Section 9.4.2, we have rewritten the PL score equations as contrasts of observed and fitted frequencies, establishing some agreement between PL and GEE2. Both procedures lead to similar estimating equations. The most important difference is in the evaluation of the matrix $V_i = \text{Cov}(Z_i)$. This only involves first- and second-order probabilities for the pseudo-likelihood procedure. In this respect, PL resembles GEE1. In contrast, GEE2 also requires evaluation of third- and fourth-order probabilities. This makes the GEE2 score equations harder to evaluate and also more time consuming.

Both pseudo-likelihood and generalized estimating equations yield consistent and asymptotically normally distributed estimators, provided an empirically corrected variance estimator is used and provided the model is correctly specified. This variance estimator is similar for both procedures, the main difference being the evaluation of V_i.

If we define the log of the pseudo-likelihood contribution for clusters with size larger than one as $p\ell_i^* = p\ell_i/(n_i - 1)$, the first component of the PL vector contribution $\boldsymbol{S}_i = \boldsymbol{Z}_i - \boldsymbol{\mu}_i$ equals that of GEE2. On the contrary, the association component differs by a factor of $1/(n_i - 1)$. Yet, if we would define the log pseudo-likelihood as $p\ell = \sum_{i=1}^N p\ell_i$, then the second components would be equal, while the first components would differ by a factor of $n_i - 1$. Therefore, in studies where the main interest lies in the marginal mean parameters, one would prefer $p\ell^*$ over $p\ell$. However, if primary interest focuses on the estimation of the association parameters, we advocate the use of $p\ell$ instead. GEE1 in that case should be avoided, as its goal is limited to estimation of the mean model parameters, whereas GEE2 is computationally more complex.

Aerts et al (2002) compared PL, GEE1, and GEE2 in terms of asymptotic and small sample relative efficiency. It was found that the behavior of PL is generally highly acceptable. In particular, the behavior of PL was very similar to GEE2, while in terms of computational complexity it is closer to GEE1 than to GEE2. Liang, Zeger, and Qaqish (1992) suggested GEE1, GEE2, and PL may be less efficient when the number of repeated measures per unit are unequal.

9.6 Analysis of NTP Data

We apply the PL and first- and second-order GEE estimating procedures to data from the DEHP and DYME studies, described in Section 2.7 and analyzed, using the Bahadur model, in Section 7.2.3 and, using a number of GEE methods (GEE1, GEE2, and ALR), in Section 8.9. The model

TABLE 9.1. *NTP Data. Parameter estimates (empirically corrected standard errors) for pseudo-likelihood (PL), GEE1, and GEE2 with exchangeable odds ratio, fitted to the collapsed outcome in the DEHP and DYME studies. β_0 and β_d are the marginal intercept and dose effect, respectively; α is the log odds ratio; ψ is the odds ratio.*

Study	β_0	β_d	α	ψ
	Newton-Raphson PL Estimates			
DEHP	-3.98(0.30)	5.57(0.61)	1.10(0.27)	3.00(0.81)
DYME	-5.73(0.46)	8.71(0.94)	1.42(0.31)	4.14(1.28)
	Fisher scoring PL Estimates			
DEHP	-3.98(0.30)	5.57(0.61)	1.11(0.27)	3.03(0.82)
DYME	-5.73(0.47)	8.71(0.95)	1.42(0.35)	4.14(1.45)
	GEE2 Estimates			
DEHP	-3.69(0.25)	5.06(0.51)	0.97(0.23)	2.64(0.61)
DYME	-5.86(0.42)	8.96(0.87)	1.36(0.34)	3.90(1.32)
	GEE1 Estimates			
DEHP	-4.02(0.31)	5.79(0.62)	0.41(0.34)	1.51(0.51)
DYME	-5.89(0.42)	8.99(0.87)	1.46(0.75)	4.31(3.23)

used in the earlier analyses is retained, using intercept (β_0) and dose (β_d) parameters. The log odds ratio ψ_i is modeled as $\ln \psi_i = \alpha$, in agreement with, for example, Table 8.5. Table 9.1 shows that the parameter estimates, obtained by either the pseudo-likelihood or the generalized estimating equations approach, are comparable. Note that the GEE1 and GEE2 parameter estimates differ somewhat from the ones obtained in Tables 8.2–8.5, as here the odds ratio is used to measure association, whereas we used the correlation coefficient in Tables 8.2–8.4. Table 8.5 used the odds ratio as well, but there ALR was used as estimation method. Because main interest is focused on the dose effect, we used $p\ell^*$ rather than $p\ell$. Dose effects and association parameters are, again, significant throughout, except for the GEE1 association estimates. For this procedure, β_a is not significant for the DEHP study and marginally significant for the DYME study. The GEE1 standard errors for β_a are much larger than for their PL and GEE2 counterparts. The GEE2 standard errors are the smallest among the different estimating approaches, which is in agreement with findings in previous sections. Furthermore, it is observed that the standard errors of the Newton-Raphson PL algorithm are generally slightly smaller than those obtained using Fisher scoring, which is in line with other empirical findings. On the other hand, the Newton-Raphson procedure is computationally slightly more complex in this case. The time gain of Fisher scoring, however, is negligible. PL based on the classical representation of Section 9.4.1 only needs 11% of the computation time needed for GEE2. For the GLM, based representation of Section 9.4.2, this becomes 7%. The corresponding figure for GEE1 is 2.5%.

10
Fitting Marginal Models with SAS

10.1 Introduction

In this chapter, we present software tools to estimate parameters and make inferences for marginal models, as introduced in Chapters 6–9. Although a large number of methods have been introduced, we will focus on selected approaches. The emphasis will be on methods that can be fitted using the SAS system. A number of software tools for GEE is presented. Basic GEE1, with moment-based estimation for the correlations, is discussed in Section 10.3. Alternating logistic regression, of course based on odds ratios, is presented in Section 10.4. The linearization-based method of Section 8.8 is discussed in Section 10.5. In Section 10.6, we present selected programs and output for the NTP studies analyzed before in Section 8.9.

Some alternative approaches are briefly discussed in Section 10.7.

10.2 The Toenail Data

We will use the toenail data, introduced in Section 2.3, as a running example. We are interested in the analysis of the severity of infection. SAS Version 9.1 will be the basis for our analysis. The outcome of interest is the binary indicator reflecting severity of the infection. Frequencies at each visit for both treatments is presented in Figure 10.1. We will consider the model:

$$Y_{ij} \sim \text{Bernoulli}(\pi_{ij}), \tag{10.1}$$

204   10. Fitting Marginal Models with SAS

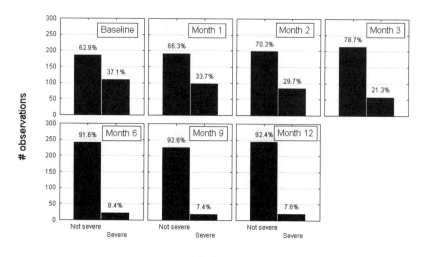

FIGURE 10.1. *Toenail Data. Frequencies of patients with severe and non-severe toenail infections, at 7 occasions.*

$$\log\left(\frac{\pi_{ij}}{1-\pi_{ij}}\right) = \beta_0 + \beta_1 T_i + \beta_2 t_{ij} + \beta_3 T_i t_{ij}, \qquad (10.2)$$

where T_i is the treatment indicator for subject i (1 for the experimental arm, 0 for the standard arm), t_{ij} is the time point at which the jth measurement is taken for the ith subject. Note that, strictly speaking, the randomization would allow to set β_1 equal to 0, but it will be kept in the model for generality. If necessary, more complex mean models can be considered as well, including polynomial time effects, additional covariate effects, etc.

10.3   GEE1 with Correlations

Within SAS, GEE1 as in Section 8.2, with moment-based estimation for the working correlation parameters, can be fitted by means of the GENMOD procedure. We will fit Model (10.1)–(10.2) using three sets of working assumptions: (1) independence, (2) exchangeable, and (3) unstructured. Note that, while in principle also AR(1) could be considered, this set of working assumptions is less in line with the design, as the measurement occasions are not equally spaced.

10.3.1 The SAS Program

The SAS procedure GENMOD has been conceived to fit generalized linear models, including logistic regression, probit regression, Poisson regression, classical linear regression, etc. The REPEATED statement can be invoked when a GEE analysis is required. All other statements refer to the standard generalized linear model application of the procedure.

A typical program to fit Model (10.1)–(10.2) is:

```
proc genmod data=test descending;
class idnum timeclss;
model onyresp = treatn time treatn*time
            / dist=binomial;
repeated subject=idnum / withinsubject=timeclss
                      type=ind covb corrw modelse;
run;
```

The option 'descending' in PROC GENMOD is to require modeling of $P(Y_{ij} = 1)$ rather than $P(Y_{ij} = 0)$, to align ourselves with the more standard practice in logistic regression. The distribution is specified as binomial, using the 'dist=' option in the MODEL statement. No link function is specified, implying that we are happy with the default link for the binomial distribution, i.e., the logit link.

The variable 'timeclss' is an exact copy of 'time.' The difference is that we will consider 'time' to be a continuous variable, allowing to consider a linear time effect and time by treatment interaction, while properly using 'timeclss' as an ordinal variable, specifying the within-subject ordering of measurements.

Without the REPEATED statement, we would have specified standard logistic regression. The REPEATED statement, together with the 'type=' option, specifies standard GEE1, with working correlations that are estimated using moment-based methods (Section 8.2). In Section 10.4, it will be shown how the same procedure, but with different option in the REPEATED statement, can be used for alternating logistic regression (ALR) as well.

The independent blocks, e.g., the subjects in a longitudinal study, are indicated by means of the 'subject=' option. The order of measurements within a subject are either assumed to be presented chronologically, by default, or specified by means of the 'withinsubject=' option. The working assumptions are specified by the 'type=' option. This option has defining status for this particular GEE1 method, as the other possible choice, the 'logor=' option, will be used for alternating logistic regressions (Section 10.4). By default, only the empirically corrected standard errors accompany the parameter estimates, but in case one is interested in exploring the model-based ones as well, the 'modelse' option should be used. The 'covb' option provides the entire variance-covariance matrix of the model parameters.

Also here, a model-based and empirically corrected version is given. Note that the 'covb' option restricts attention to the regression parameters $\boldsymbol{\beta}$, which is $(\beta_0, \beta_1, \beta_2, \beta_3)'$ in (10.2). In the ALR case (Section 10.4) the log odds ratio parameters are included as well.

10.3.2 The SAS Output

We will discuss some of the output produced by the program presented in Section 10.3.1 and present a selection of it.

First, a number of tables are presented, containing information about the distribution, link function, response, and model specification. The procedure then specifies:

```
PROC GENMOD is modeling the probability that onyresp='1'.
```

in line with the 'descending' option. Next, a map is presented between generic names for parameters and actual effects:

```
Parameter Information
```

Parameter	Effect
Prm1	Intercept
Prm2	treatn
Prm3	time
Prm4	treatn*time

One has to be very careful with the two panels that are presented next. The first of these panels is:

```
           Criteria For Assessing Goodness Of Fit
```

Criterion	DF	Value	Value/DF
Deviance	1904	1811.8260	0.9516
Scaled Deviance	1904	1811.8260	0.9516
Pearson Chi-Square	1904	1995.2107	1.0479
Scaled Pearson X2	1904	1995.2107	1.0479
Log Likelihood		-905.9130	

It is tempting to interpret the goodness-of-fit table. However, this information is correct only in the context of cross-sectional data. Now, we are applying the method to analyze repeated measures, hence this information has to be ignored. It cannot even be used for approximate purposes. Next, the initial estimates, obtained with ordinary logistic regression as in Section 3.6, are presented:

```
           Analysis Of Initial Parameter Estimates
```

Parameter	DF	Estimate	Standard Error	Wald 95% Confidence Limits		Chi-Square
Intercept	1	-0.5571	0.1090	-0.7708	-0.3433	26.10
treatn	1	0.0240	0.1565	-0.2827	0.3307	0.02
time	1	-0.1769	0.0246	-0.2251	-0.1288	51.91
treatn*time	1	-0.0783	0.0394	-0.1556	-0.0010	3.95
Scale	0	1.0000	0.0000	1.0000	1.0000	

These estimates are obtained from fitting the model, ignoring the correlation structure. In other words, a standard GLM, which in this case is a logistic regression, is fitted. Note that these parameters correspond to independence working assumptions, which is what we are considering here. We will return to this in what follows. Of course, the standard errors are based on assuming the measurements are uncorrelated. Here, and when other working assumptions are used, these estimates are used as initial estimates for GEE, as in the first step of the GEE algorithm outlined on page 158. Hence, upon obtaining the initial table, GEE can be started. This initial analysis is identical to the one in Section 3.6, presented as an example of ordinary logistic regression.

Some of the model information, shown at the beginning of the output, reads:

Model Information

Distribution	Binomial
Link Function	Logit
Dependent Variable	onyresp
Number of Events	408
Number of Trials	1908

which is typical information for logistic regression. From the perspective of the initial analysis, there would be a sample size of 1908, with 408 successes on the outcome variable 'onyresp.' Now, this information is refined from a GEE, i.e., correlated data, setting:

GEE Model Information

Correlation Structure	Independent
Within-Subject Effect	timeclss (7 levels)
Subject Effect	idnum (294 levels)
Number of Clusters	294
Correlation Matrix Dimension	7
Maximum Cluster Size	7
Minimum Cluster Size	1

It is now acknowledged that the overall sample size is $N = 294$ rather than $N = 1908$ and that, in addition, the number of measurements per patient varies between $n_i = 1$ and $n_i = 7$. Indeed, though 7 measurements are planned for everyone enrolled into the trial, some do not complete the study. Then, two sets of parameter estimates, standard errors, confidence limits, Z-statistic values, and corresponding p-values are presented:

```
            Analysis Of GEE Parameter Estimates
             Empirical Standard Error Estimates

                        Standard    95% Confidence
Parameter    Estimate    Error         Limits              Z  Pr > |Z|

Intercept    -0.5571    0.1713   -0.8929  -0.2212       -3.25   0.0011
treatn        0.0240    0.2506   -0.4672   0.5152        0.10   0.9236
time         -0.1769    0.0302   -0.2361  -0.1178       -5.86   <.0001
treatn*time  -0.0783    0.0546   -0.1854   0.0287       -1.43   0.1515


            Analysis Of GEE Parameter Estimates
            Model-Based Standard Error Estimates

                        Standard    95% Confidence
Parameter    Estimate    Error         Limits              Z  Pr > |Z|

Intercept    -0.5571    0.1090   -0.7708  -0.3433       -5.11   <.0001
treatn        0.0240    0.1565   -0.2827   0.3307        0.15   0.8780
time         -0.1769    0.0246   -0.2251  -0.1288       -7.20   <.0001
treatn*time  -0.0783    0.0394   -0.1556  -0.0010       -1.99   0.0470
```

Both sets of parameter estimates are identical. This is in line with the GEE algorithm presented on page 158, only the asymptotic covariance matrices differ. The empirically corrected standard errors are quite a bit larger than the model-based ones. This implies that ignoring the correlation in these data could lead to invalid conclusions. Based on our analyses, the model-based standard errors would declare the treatment by time interaction significant ($p = 0.0470$), but the empirically corrected ones contradict this ($p = 0.1515$). Further, the model-based results coincide with the initial analysis, which is entirely due to the use of independence working assumptions. This will not be the case in what follows.

Apart from the standard errors, the full asymptotic variance-covariance matrices can be obtained. Again, there are two versions, a model-based and an empirically corrected on.

```
              Covariance Matrix (Model-Based)

          Prm1            Prm2            Prm3            Prm4
```

```
Prm1       0.01189      -0.01189     -0.001809     0.001809
Prm2      -0.01189       0.02449      0.001809    -0.004097
Prm3      -0.001809      0.001809     0.0006031   -0.000603
Prm4       0.001809     -0.004097    -0.000603     0.001555
```

```
                    Covariance Matrix (Empirical)

                 Prm1           Prm2           Prm3           Prm4

Prm1        0.02936       -0.02936       -0.002328       0.002328
Prm2       -0.02936        0.06281        0.002328      -0.006720
Prm3       -0.002328       0.002328       0.0009102     -0.000910
Prm4        0.002328      -0.006720      -0.000910       0.002982
```

Next, the estimated working correlation matrix is printed. In this case this is the identity matrix, not shown here.

Next, we will consider exchangeable and unstructured working assumptions, which is done by replacing 'type=ind' in the program in Section 10.3.1 by 'type=exch' and 'type=un,' respectively. In these cases, the initial estimates are, of course, the same as before.

The results for the exchangeable working correlation structure are as follows:

```
              Analysis Of GEE Parameter Estimates
                Empirical Standard Error Estimates

                       Standard    95% Confidence
Parameter    Estimate    Error         Limits            Z   Pr > |Z|

Intercept    -0.5840    0.1734    -0.9238   -0.2441    -3.37    0.0008
treatn        0.0120    0.2613    -0.5001    0.5241     0.05    0.9633
time         -0.1770    0.0311    -0.2380   -0.1161    -5.69   <.0001
treatn*time  -0.0886    0.0571    -0.2006    0.0233    -1.55    0.1208


              Analysis Of GEE Parameter Estimates
               Model-Based Standard Error Estimates

                       Standard    95% Confidence
Parameter    Estimate    Error         Limits            Z   Pr > |Z|

Intercept    -0.5840    0.1344    -0.8475   -0.3204    -4.34   <.0001
treatn        0.0120    0.1866    -0.3537    0.3777     0.06    0.9486
time         -0.1770    0.0209    -0.2180   -0.1361    -8.47   <.0001
treatn*time  -0.0886    0.0362    -0.1596   -0.0177    -2.45    0.0143
```

The parameter estimates are still equal across both tables, but different from the initial ones, given that there is a parameterized working correlation structure and hence iteration is required between steps 2, 3, and

4 on page 158. The treatment by time interaction still is non-significant ($p = 0.1208$). The asymptotic variance-covariance matrices of the parameter estimates have changed to

Covariance Matrix (Model-Based)

	Prm1	Prm2	Prm3	Prm4
Prm1	0.01808	-0.01808	-0.000192	0.0001916
Prm2	-0.01808	0.03482	0.0001916	-0.000115
Prm3	-0.000192	0.0001916	0.0004365	-0.000436
Prm4	0.0001916	-0.000115	-0.000436	0.001309

Covariance Matrix (Empirical)

	Prm1	Prm2	Prm3	Prm4
Prm1	0.03006	-0.03006	-0.002476	0.002476
Prm2	-0.03006	0.06826	0.002476	-0.007883
Prm3	-0.002476	0.002476	0.0009676	-0.000968
Prm4	0.002476	-0.007883	-0.000968	0.003264

Just as in the independence case, these matrices are relatively far apart. This indicates that, although the methods are consistent and asymptotically normal, efficiency may be questioned and, especially in a case like this where the sample size $N = 254$ is considerable and the number of measurements per subject $n_i = 7$ is relatively small, it would be sensible to consider unstructured working correlations instead of exchangeable ones. The exchangeable working correlation is estimated as

Exchangeable Working
         Correlation

Correlation   0.420259237

and the request to print the working correlation matrix merely produces a 7×7 matrix with ones on the diagonal and 0.4203 in the off-diagonal elements.

Turning attention to unstructured working assumptions, the parameter estimates now become:

Analysis Of GEE Parameter Estimates
Empirical Standard Error Estimates

Parameter	Estimate	Standard Error	95% Confidence Limits		Z	Pr > |Z|
Intercept	-0.7204	0.1733	-1.0600	-0.3807	-4.16	<.0001

```
treatn          0.0721   0.2461  -0.4102   0.5544   0.29   0.7695
time           -0.1413   0.0291  -0.1982  -0.0843  -4.86   <.0001
treatn*time    -0.1135   0.0515  -0.2145  -0.0126  -2.20   0.0275
```

Analysis Of GEE Parameter Estimates
Model-Based Standard Error Estimates

```
                         Standard    95% Confidence
Parameter     Estimate    Error         Limits            Z  Pr > |Z|

Intercept     -0.7204    0.1655    -1.0448   -0.3959    -4.35   <.0001
treatn         0.0721    0.2352    -0.3889    0.5331     0.31   0.7592
time          -0.1413    0.0277    -0.1956   -0.0870    -5.10   <.0001
treatn*time   -0.1135    0.0470    -0.2057   -0.0214    -2.41   0.0158
```

We now find a significant difference in evolution between both treatment groups ($p = 0.0275$), in contrast to what was obtained earlier. This confirms the fact that GEE may suffer from efficiency problems when the working correlation structure is not correct. The model-based and empirically corrected standard errors are now much closer to each other and, in addition, the empirically corrected standard errors are somewhat smaller than their counterparts under the independence and exchangeable assumptions. Once again, it is sensible to seek working assumptions that are sufficiently in line with the correct structure, for reasons of efficiency. The asymptotic covariance matrices confirm that our choice is reasonable:

Covariance Matrix (Model-Based)

	Prm1	Prm2	Prm3	Prm4
Prm1	0.02740	-0.02740	-0.002170	0.002170
Prm2	-0.02740	0.05532	0.002170	-0.004603
Prm3	-0.002170	0.002170	0.0007671	-0.000767
Prm4	0.002170	-0.004603	-0.000767	0.002211

Covariance Matrix (Empirical)

	Prm1	Prm2	Prm3	Prm4
Prm1	0.03003	-0.03003	-0.002486	0.002486
Prm2	-0.03003	0.06055	0.002486	-0.006017
Prm3	-0.002486	0.002486	0.0008447	-0.000845
Prm4	0.002486	-0.006017	-0.000845	0.002652

Table 10.1 presents an overview of the various GEE model fits to the toenail data.

The working correlation structure entertains 21 correlations, made up by the $\binom{7}{2}$ that can be formed from the 7 outcomes:

Working Correlation Matrix

	Col1	Col2	Col3	Col4	Col5	Col6	Col7
Row1	1.0000	0.8772	0.7003	0.4901	0.2368	0.1802	0.1475
Row2	0.8772	1.0000	0.8131	0.5864	0.2782	0.2081	0.2148
Row3	0.7003	0.8131	1.0000	0.7507	0.2927	0.2158	0.2166
Row4	0.4901	0.5864	0.7507	1.0000	0.3680	0.2876	0.2683
Row5	0.2368	0.2782	0.2927	0.3680	1.0000	0.5274	0.4561
Row6	0.1802	0.2081	0.2158	0.2876	0.5274	1.0000	0.8242
Row7	0.1475	0.2148	0.2166	0.2683	0.4561	0.8242	1.0000

As stated in Section 8.2, no formal inference can be made about the correlation structure, neither here nor in the exchangeable structure. At best, one can make informal statements, such as that the exchangeable correlation is moderate, and the unstructured matrix seems to exhibit, more or less, a decrease of the correlation when pairs are further apart, i.e., a banded or AR(1) structure. To make formal inferences about the correlation, at least Prentice's GEE (Section 8.4), or GEE2 (Section 8.5) is needed.

When the association can be modeled in terms of odds ratios, alternating logistic regressions come into view (Section 8.6). These can be fitted with the SAS procedure GENMOD as well and are the topic of the next section.

10.4 Alternating Logistic Regressions

Alternating logistic regressions, presented in Section 8.6, are a convenient tool to fit a marginal model based on odds ratios in such a way that inferences can be made, not only about the marginal parameters, but about the pairwise associations as well. The method has conveniently been implemented in the SAS procedure GENMOD. Fitting Model (10.1)–(10.2) to the toenail data, can be done by removing the 'type=' statement in the REPEATED statement of the program presented in Section 10.3.1, and replacing it by the 'logor=' option. A number of choices are available, including exchangeability ('logor=exch') or unstructured ('logor=fullclust,' which stands for 'full clustering'). Some other structures exist, including the ability to create one's own design, as will be presented in Section 17.5.

The GEE portion of the output is slightly modified to accommodate this technique, different from but similar to standard GEE (Section 10.3). In particular, the GEE model information, which should perhaps have been labeled 'ALR model information,' now is:

10.4 Alternating Logistic Regressions

TABLE 10.1. *Toenail Data. Parameter estimates (model-based standard errors; empirically corrected standard errors) for GEE1 under independence (IND), exchangeable (EXCH), and unstructured (UN) working assumptions; for ALR under EXCH; for the linearization-based approach for IND, EXCH, and UN.*

Effect	Par.	IND	EXCH	UN
		GEE1		
Int.	β_0	-0.557(0.109;0.171)	-0.584(0.134;0.173)	-0.720(0.166;0.173)
T_i	β_1	0.024(0.157;0.251)	0.012(0.187;0.261)	0.072(0.235;0.246)
t_{ij}	β_2	-0.177(0.025;0.030)	-0.177(0.021;0.031)	-0.141(0.028;0.029)
$T_i \cdot t_{ij}$	β_3	-0.078(0.039;0.055)	-0.089(0.036;0.057)	-0.114(0.047;0.052)
		ALR		
Int.	β_0		-0.524(0.157;0.169)	
T_i	β_1		0.017(0.222;0.243)	
t_{ij}	β_2		-0.178(0.023;0.030)	
$T_i \cdot t_{ij}$	β_3		-0.084(0.039;0.052)	
Ass.	α		3.222(;0.291)	
		Linearization-based method		
Int.	β_0	-0.557(0.112;0.171)	-0.585(0.142;0.174)	-0.630(0.171;0.172)
T_i	β_1	0.024(0.160;0.251)	0.011(0.196;0.262)	0.036(0.242;0.242)
t_{ij}	β_2	-0.177(0.025;0.030)	-0.177(0.022;0.031)	-0.204(0.038;0.034)
$T_i \cdot t_{ij}$	β_3	-0.078(0.040:0.055)	-0.089(0.038;0.057)	-0.106(0.058;0.058)

```
                 GEE Model Information

Log Odds Ratio Structure                  Exchangeable
Within-Subject Effect              timeclss (7 levels)
Subject Effect                       idnum (294 levels)
Number of Clusters                                 294
Correlation Matrix Dimension                         7
Maximum Cluster Size                                 7
Minimum Cluster Size                                 1
```

The initial parameter estimates are exactly as in GEE1, and the parameter estimates and standard errors, produced upon convergence, are

```
              Analysis Of GEE Parameter Estimates
               Empirical Standard Error Estimates

                       Standard    95% Confidence
Parameter   Estimate     Error         Limits           Z Pr > |Z|

Intercept    -0.5244    0.1686    -0.8548   -0.1940   -3.11   0.0019
```

```
treatn          0.0168   0.2432  -0.4599   0.4935    0.07   0.9448
time           -0.1781   0.0296  -0.2361  -0.1200   -6.01  <.0001
treatn*time    -0.0837   0.0520  -0.1856   0.0182   -1.61   0.1076
Alpha1          3.2218   0.2908   2.6519   3.7917   11.08  <.0001
```

Analysis Of GEE Parameter Estimates
Model-Based Standard Error Estimates

```
                         Standard    95% Confidence
Parameter    Estimate      Error         Limits          Z   Pr > |Z|

Intercept    -0.5244      0.1567   -0.8315  -0.2173   -3.35   0.0008
treatn        0.0168      0.2220   -0.4182   0.4519    0.08   0.9395
time         -0.1781      0.0233   -0.2238  -0.1323   -7.63  <.0001
treatn*time  -0.0837      0.0392   -0.1606  -0.0068   -2.13   0.0329
```

A key difference with GEE1 is that the association parameters, in this exchangeable case a single log odds ratio α, is added to the empirical panel, but not to the purely model-based one. We obtain a non-significant p-value for the treatment by time interaction ($p = 0.1076$), close to but a bit smaller than its counterpart from the exchangeable analysis in GEE1. This underscores the somewhat higher efficiency of a GEE2 method, to which family ALR can be considered to belong. Similarly, the empirically corrected asymptotic variance-covariance matrix encompasses the α parameter:

Covariance Matrix (Model-Based)

	Prm1	Prm2	Prm3	Prm4
Prm1	0.0245554	-0.024555	-0.000945	0.0009447
Prm2	-0.024555	0.0492659	0.0009447	-0.00229
Prm3	-0.000945	0.0009447	0.0005442	-0.000544
Prm4	0.0009447	-0.00229	-0.000544	0.0015399

Covariance Matrix (Empirical)

	Prm1	Prm2	Prm3	Prm4	Alpha1
Prm1	0.0284159	-0.028416	-0.002133	0.0021329	0.0017753
Prm2	-0.028416	0.0591554	0.0021329	-0.005708	0.0033175
Prm3	-0.002133	0.0021329	0.0008764	-0.000876	0.0003229
Prm4	0.0021329	-0.005708	-0.000876	0.0027053	-0.002278
Alpha1	0.0017753	0.0033175	0.0003229	-0.002278	0.0845464

We are now in a position to assert that the association is strongly significant ($p < 0.0001$), provided it has been correctly specified, a statement we could not make in the corresponding exchangeable GEE1 analysis, where the working correlation was estimated to be $\widehat{\rho} = 0.42$. Of course, it is still possible for the working correlation structure to be misspecified. For example, as was hinted from the unstructured GEE1 analysis, the correlations could be stronger when measurement occasions are closer to each other. Unfortunately, the set of 21 log odds ratio parameters makes the ALR method difficult to converge. The results of the exchangeable model can be found in the second panel of Table 10.1.

10.5 A Method Based on Linearization

The linearization-based method, presented in Section 8.8, can be fitted using the SAS macro GLIMMIX. As of SAS Version 9.1, there is an experimental GLIMMIX procedure as well. Both will be explained here.

10.5.1 The SAS Program for the GLIMMIX Macro

Fitting Model (10.1)–(10.2) with, for example, exchangeable working assumptions, can be effectuated using the following program:

```
%glimmix(data=test, procopt=%str(method=ml empirical),
   stmts=%str(
      class idnum timeclss;
      model onyresp = treatn time treatn*time / solution;
      repeated timeclss / subject=idnum type=cs rcorr;
   ),
   error=binomial,
   link=logit);
```

The macro is based on fitting the iterative procedure, outlined in Section 8.8. The 'generalized linear models' shell linearizes the outcome and computes the weights, as in (8.38) and (8.39). Specific statements that govern this procedure are the 'error=' and 'link=' statement. We need to choose the binomial error structure. The logit link is the default for this option, but we have still chosen to explicitly specify it, for clarity. The inner core of the procedure is based on the MIXED procedure, used to solve iteratively reweighted least squares equations (8.37). Virtually all statements, available in the MIXED procedure, can be used. They are passed on, in string form, to the macro via the 'stmts=' option. Note that 'type=cs,' referring to compound symmetry, has to be used here rather than 'type=exch' or 'logor=exch,' in Sections 10.3 and 10.4, respectively. For unstructured working assumptions, we have to use 'type=un,' for AR(1) this would be 'type=ar(1),' and for independence assumptions, 'type=simple' needs to be used. One set of assumptions, corresponding to the PROC MIXED statement, are passed on via a separate statement, i.e., the 'procopt=' string.

Note that we have inserted the 'empirical' option, to ensure the empirically corrected standard errors are produced. Leaving this one out produces the model-based standard errors. We have a choice between the updating methods that are available in the MIXED procedure. In the GLIMMIX procedure, a set of updating methods is available that have been devised for the evaluation of the integral that occurs in the likelihood of random-effects models for non-Gaussian data (see Chapter 14).

In case one is interested in receiving the MIXED output at every step in the iteration process, this can be obtained by adding the option 'printall' in the 'options=' option. Arguably, the latter is primarily useful for debugging purposes.

10.5.2 The SAS Output from the GLIMMIX Macro

The typical GLIMMIX output consists of tables copied from the MIXED output, as well as some additional information. Typical output includes book keeping information such as model information, dimensions, number of observations. Because we included the 'rcorr' option in the REPEATED statement, the fitted correlation matrix of the measurements is given, which is to be interpreted as the working correlation matrix. In our case, this is a 7×7 correlation matrix with off-diagonal elements equal to 0.4283, the exchangeable working correlation. The panel 'Covariance Parameter Estimates' has to be interpreted with caution. In our case, it reads:

```
Covariance Parameter Estimates

Cov Parm     Subject     Estimate

CS           idnum       0.4711
Residual                 0.6289
```

The working correlation is obtained from the usual compound-symmetry equation:

$$\frac{0.4711}{0.4711 + 0.6289} = 0.4283.$$

In the 'GLIMMIX Model Statistics' panel, the residual value is copied as the extra-dispersion parameter:

```
GLIMMIX Model Statistics

Description                     Value

Deviance                        1812.6701
Scaled Deviance                 2882.1849
Pearson Chi-Square              2091.2017
Scaled Pearson Chi-Square       3325.0561
```

```
Extra-Dispersion Scale            0.6289
```

It is best not to use this panel, as it is not appropriately adapted to the combination of generalized linear model and the repeated measures nature of the data. In case we would have used independence working assumptions, there would be a single covariance parameter only:

```
Covariance Parameter Estimates

Cov Parm     Subject     Estimate

timeclss     idnum       1.0457
```

which is then considered the overdispersion parameter. Arguably, there is little basis to do so, and it is unlikely to see almost no overdispersion with independence and strong underdispersion with exchangeability. It might make more sense to consider the total variance in the exchangeable case, i.e., $0.4711 + 0.6289$, the overdispersion parameter. Similarly, the fit statistics panel, copied from the MIXED procedure, is best not used.

The most relevant panel is the 'Solution for Fixed Effects' table:

```
             Solution for Fixed Effects

                           Standard
Effect         Estimate    Error       DF    t Value    Pr > |t|

Intercept      -0.5849     0.1735      292   -3.37      0.0008
treatn          0.01142    0.2617      292    0.04      0.9652
time           -0.1771     0.03114    1612   -5.69      <.0001
treatn*time    -0.08885    0.05721    1612   -1.55      0.1206
```

with its associated F-tests. Because all effects are based on a single degrees of freedom, the F-tests reproduce the p-values of the above table and hence we do not show it. These estimates, together with the ones for other working assumptions, and with both model-based and empirically corrected standard errors, are given in the third panel of Table 10.1. Clearly, the estimates under independence are equal to the ones of GEE1, as in both cases they are the ones that would be obtained from standard logistic regression. The ones under exchangeability are very similar, but the estimates for unstructured working assumptions are a little different, although the conclusions would not change.

In terms of inference for the treatment by time interaction effect, none of the linearization-based analyses produce significant p-values. The values for exchangeability ($p = 0.1206$) and independence ($p = 0.1517$) are extremely close to their GEE1 counterparts, but for unstructured working assumptions ($p = 0.0668$) the difference is not only a bit larger than the value for GEE1 ($p = 0.0275$), it also lands at the other side of the 0.05 border.

10.5.3 The Program for the SAS Procedure GLIMMIX

Equivalently to the above, the SAS procedure GLIMMIX can be used. The procedure can fit models of a marginal type, of a subject-specific type, as well as models with subject-specific effects and residual association in addition to that. A general treatment of the procedure will be given in Section 15.2. The program, equivalent to the GLIMMIX macro program in Section 10.5.1 equals:

```
proc glimmix data=test method=RSPL empirical;
class idnum;
model onyresp (event='1') = treatn time treatn*time
                          / dist=binary solution;
random _residual_ / subject=idnum type=cs;
run;
```

Even though the program is rather different, at first sight, from the one in Section 10.5.1, the correspondence is almost immediate.

The 'method=RSPL' is explained in more detail in Section 15.2. Suffice it to say here that it corresponds to PQL, combined with REML. The MODEL statement is self-explanatory given the earlier GLIMMIX macro program. The REPEATED statement of the macro corresponds to the 'RANDOM _residual_' statement here. SAS refers to this as the 'R-side' of the random statement. It is useful to think about it as the variance-covariance matrix of the outcome vector Y_i, of which the variances follow from the mean-variance link, but the correlation structure needs to be specified, as in GEE. In case random effects are present, then this structure refers to the residual correlation, in addition to the correlation induced by the random effects. Changing the 'type=' option in the RANDOM statement to 'simple,' 'cs,' and 'un,' respectively, combined with either omission or inclusion of the 'empirical' option in the GLIMMIX statement, produces exactly the same results as with the GLIMMIX macro, i.e., as reported in the third panel of Table 10.1.

10.5.4 Output from the GLIMMIX Procedure

The output from the procedure, although structured differently from the macro output, is largely equivalent. The fact that the empirically corrected standard errors are produced is properly acknowledged:

```
The GLIMMIX Procedure

                 Model Information

Fixed Effects SE Adjustment      Sandwich - Classical
```

The fact that we are using a marginal model, i.e., a model without random effects, is acknowledged through reference to the so-called 'R-side' covariance parameters:

```
                    Dimensions

R-side Cov. Parameters               2
```

The procedure took 9 iterations to converge, and then produces covariance parameters that are equivalent to the ones found above, up to numerical accuracy:

```
            Covariance Parameter Estimates

                                        Standard
Cov Parm    Subject     Estimate         Error

CS          idnum        0.4749         0.04800
Residual                 0.6300         0.02219
```

The procedure then goes on to produce the fixed-effects parameters, again equivalent, up to numerical accuracy, to their GLIMMIX macro counterparts:

```
               Solutions for Fixed Effects

                        Standard
Effect       Estimate    Error      DF    t Value    Pr > |t|

Intercept    -0.5851    0.1735      292    -3.37     0.0008
treatn        0.01130   0.2618      292     0.04     0.9656
time         -0.1771    0.03115    1612    -5.69     <.0001
treatn*time  -0.08889   0.05723    1612    -1.55     0.1206
```

together with associated F-tests. As long as the procedure is experimental, which it is at this point, it is cautious to consider the macro as an option as well. Also, having the macro as a backup may increase one's changes to reach convergence.

10.6 Programs for the NTP Data

By way of summary, a few sample programs for the NTP data, as analyzed in Section 8.9, are presented. We focus on the visceral outcome in the DEHP study, under exchangeable working assumptions. Standard GEE1 can be fitted using:

```
proc genmod data=m.dehp33 descending;
```

```
class litter;
model visceral = dose / dist=binary;
repeated subject=litter / type=exch covb corrw modelse;
run;
```

Alternating logistic regression require the following program:

```
proc genmod data=m.dehp33 descending;
class litter;
model visceral = dose / dist=binary;
repeated subject=litter / logor=exch covb corrw modelse;
run;
```

For the linearization-based method, we can use, for example, the following GLIMMIX macro code:

```
%include 'glimmix.sas';
```

```
%glimmix(
   data=m.dehp33,
   procopt=method=reml empirical,
   stmts=%str(
      class litter;
      model visceral=dose / solution;
      repeated / subject=litter type=cs r;),
   error=binomial,
   link=logit,
   options=mixprintlast
   );
```

Alternatively, the SAS procedure GLIMMIX can be used:

```
proc glimmix data=m.dehp33 method=RSPL empirical;
class litter;
model visceral (event='1') = dose
                            / dist=binary solution;
random _residual_ / subject=litter type=cs;
run;
```

For these data, we also fitted Prentice's GEE, introduced in Section 8.4, and reported in Tables 8.2 and 8.3. To this end, the gee1corr.mac macro, written by Stuart Lipsitz (Williamson, Lipsitz, and Kim 1997), was used. It produces the following output:

```
Correlation Structure: Exchangeable

PARAMETER ESTIMATES with naive variance

VARIABLE   ESTIMATE     SE_EST          Z         P
```

```
INTERCEP -4.507824 0.3958657 -11.38726           0
DOSE      4.5890696 0.5845582  7.8504921  4.108E-15


PARAMETER ESTIMATES with robust variance

VARIABLE   ESTIMATE   SE_EST         Z         P
INTERCEP  -4.507824 0.3685713 -12.23053         0
DOSE       4.5890696 0.5932811  7.735068  1.033E-14


    CORR      SECORR        Z          P
0.1100235  0.0455011  2.4180411  0.0156043
```

The output is in agreement with what is found in Table 8.3.

10.7 Alternative Software Tools

Many commonly used and commercially available software packages these days have GEE modules. These include SPlus, R, SPSS, Stata, and SUDAAN. It is, of course, very important to understand the syntax requirements and conventions when applying GEE fitting code, just as with any other software application. Arguably, it is equally important to understand which of the many GEE versions has been implemented. It should have been clear from Chapter 8 that there is no such thing as 'the' GEE approach. One can choose between correlations and odds ratios to model the association, but in the literature other measures have been used as well, such as the κ coefficient (Agresti 2002), etc. One can use GEE1 or GEE2, or one of the many alternatives, such as the linearization-based method, or a method based on a hybrid marginal-conditional specification, rather than on the Bahadur model (correlations) or the Dale model (odds ratios), etc.

Given the variety of GEE-based methods, it is not surprising that a colorful collection of user-defined macros and programs exist to supplement the implementations in standard software. Trying to describe this ever changing collection is aiming at a moving target. It is recommended that the interested user conduct a careful search of the available methodology, either through dedicated statistical libraries, or via the Internet in general.

Obviously, this chapter has focused on the non-likelihood-based marginal models. Although many of the likelihood-based marginal approaches have existed longer than their non-likelihood counterparts, there is little or no standard software available, in spite of a wide variety of user-defined tools. We have chosen not to discuss this dynamic conglomerate of *ad hoc* tools and rather refer to statistical and general search tools.

Part III

Conditional Models

11
Conditional Models

11.1 Introduction

Chapter 5 presented the three main modeling families: marginal models, conditional models, and subject-specific models. In particular, it was indicated that there are strong differences between the model families, unless outcomes are of a Gaussian type. Part II was devoted to marginal modeling. It is clear that a wide variety of marginal models is available, whether a likelihood-based view is taken (Chapters 6 and 7) on the one hand, or the focus is on alternative methods on the other hand, such as generalized estimating equations (Chapter 8) and pseudo-likelihood methods (Chapter 9).

Section 5.3.2 introduced the concept of conditional models as one where outcomes are modeled, conditional upon the value of other outcomes on the same unit. The other outcomes could encompass the entire set of measurements, like in a classical log-linear model (Agresti 2002), or a subset. In a longitudinal study, such a subset can usefully be chosen as all measurements prior to the measurement being modeled, or perhaps a subset of the most recent measurements. We then refer to such models as transition models.

As alluded to in Section 5.3.2, conditional models have been heavily criticized, a point that we will expand in Section 11.3. To be able to do so, we first will need a good concept of conditional models. Section 11.2 introduces a general family of conditional models, which is studied in the specific situation of clustered outcomes in Section 11.2.2. Returning to Section 11.3, a comparison between marginal and conditional models is made, based on the models introduced here, on general insights, and on the developments in Chapter 6. The models introduced in Sections 11.2.2 and 11.2.3 are then fitted to the NTP data, introduced in Section 2.7 and analyzed, using marginal models, in Sections 7.2.3, 8.9, and 9.6, and are now analyzed by means of a conditional model in Section 11.4. Using pseudo-likelihood methods, we will return to these data in Section 12.4. Although there are strong similarities between all of the marginal models, it will be shown that there are strong differences between the conditional and marginal models.

Finally, Section 11.5 briefly discusses the special, important, and somewhat different case of transition models.

11.2 Conditional Models

In a conditional model, the parameters describe a feature (probability, odds, logit,...) of (a set of) outcomes, given values for the other outcomes (Cox 1972). The best known example is undoubtedly the log-linear model. Rosner (1984) described a conditional logistic model.

Conditional models have already been studied in Chapter 6. Section 6.2.2 introduced Goodman's association model, a model with a strong conditional flavor. In a number of case studies, such as the British Occupational Study (Section 6.3), the Caithness data (Section 6.4), and the fluvoxamine trial (Section 6.5), it was shown that the marginal Dale model (Section 6.2.3) outperformed Goodman's model. Moreover, the Dale model held more perspective for the inclusion of covariates from a general nature and more easily allowed for measurement sequences longer than two, as was shown in Section 6.6. Both models could be linked to different underlying latent densities: the normal density for Goodman's model and the Plackett (1965) density for the Dale model (Section 6.7).

Further, Section 7.8, in the heart of Chapter 7 on marginal models, introduced a full model specification of a hybrid form, in the sense that marginal and conditional aspects are combined. The starting point was the exponential family formulation (7.50). The model is hybrid because for the lower-order moments, the mean or dual parameters are modeled, while for the higher-order moments, the natural or canonical parameters are modeled. The former are marginal in nature, the latter conditional. Moreover, the two sets are orthogonal onto each other. When the set of mean parameters would be empty, a purely conditional model results and when the set of canonical parameters is empty, a fully marginal model obtains. The orthogonality of the two sets of parameters makes the hybrid practically useful, together with the fact that the conditional parameters are not subject to parameter-space constraints.

Molenberghs and Ryan (1999) and Aerts *et al* (2002) discuss, in the specific context of exchangeable binary data, some advantages of conditional models and show how, with appropriate care, the disadvantages can be overcome for their setting. They constructed the joint distribution for clustered multivariate binary outcomes, based on the multivariate exponential family model. A slightly different approach, also based on the exponential family, is presented in Fitzmaurice, Laird, and Tosteson (1996). An advantage of such a likelihood-based approach is that, under correct model specification, efficiency can be gained over other procedures such as generalized estimating equations (GEE). Molenberghs and Ryan (1999) use the method primarily in view of quantitative risk assessment. Some of the quantities used, such as the probability that an entire cluster is free of malformations, are framed in terms of joint probabilities, making such techniques as generalized estimating equations less suitable. When computations become cumbersome, pseudo-likelihood for this particular model can be used, as outlined in Chapter 12.

Attention will be restricted to binary data. We assume the regression notation, outlined in Section 7.1, but need a slight extension, in the sense that there are N units, the ith of which contains n_i measurements *on each of M outcomes*. Thus, M describes the multivariate nature of the problem, while n_i refers to the repeated, longitudinal, or clustered nature of the study. Write $Y_{ikj} = 1$ when the jth individual in unit i exhibits the kth response and 0 otherwise. Let $\boldsymbol{Y}_i$ represent the vector of outcomes for the ith unit, and $\boldsymbol{x}_i$ an associated vector of unit level covariates. We can now consider a general conditional exponential family model, for repeated multivariate data. However, it is instructive to start with two special cases. In Section 11.2.1, we assume $n_i = 1$, in other words, there is no repeated aspect to the study. In Section 11.2.2, $M = 1$, i.e., a single repeated outcome is considered, removing the multivariate aspect of the problem. Section 11.2.3 presents the general case.

11.2.1 A Pure Multivariate Setting

Let us first suppose data are not repeated ($n_i = 1; k = 1, \ldots, M$). Because $j \equiv 1$ in this setting, we drop this index temporarily from our notation. The observable outcome is thus $\boldsymbol{Y}_i = (Y_{i1}, \ldots, Y_{iM})'$. Consider the following probability mass function proposed by Cox (1972):

$$f_i(\boldsymbol{y}_i; \boldsymbol{\Theta}_i) = \exp\left\{\sum_{k=1}^{M} \theta_{ik} y_{ik} + \sum_{k<k'} \omega_{ikk'} y_{ik} y_{ik'} + \ldots \right.$$
$$\left. + \omega_{i1\ldots M} y_{i1} \ldots y_{iM} - A(\boldsymbol{\Theta}_i)\right\}. \quad (11.1)$$

The θ parameters can be thought of as 'main effects,' whereas the ω parameters are association parameters or interactions. There is a strong connection with (7.50) even though here we consider a multivariate problem and (7.50) is for repeated data. Equating M here with n in (7.50) establishes equivalence. Of course, we should note that the parameters here are partitioned differently than in Section 7.8.1, the relationship being:

$$\Psi_i = (\theta_{i1}, \ldots, \theta_{in}; \omega_{i12}, \ldots, \omega_{i,M-1,M})', \qquad (11.2)$$
$$\Omega_i = (\omega_{i123}, \ldots, \omega_{i1\ldots M})'. \qquad (11.3)$$

The reason is that here, we tend to focus on the split between marginal (regression type) parameters versus association, whereas in expression 7.50 the seizure was between second and higher-order association parameters.

Note that the model has a marginal appearance, rather than a conditional one. However, in line with Section 7.8, the parameters have a conditional interpretation. For example, the main effects describe logits of a particular outcome, conditional on the level of all others. Similar interpretations hold for the association parameters and therefore it is sensible to classify the model as a conditional one.

Models that do not include all interactions are derived, for example, by omitting all ω terms from a certain order onwards. A useful special case is found by setting all three and higher order parameters equal to zero, which is a member of the quadratic exponential family discussed by Zhao and Prentice (1990). Thélot (1985) studied the case where $M = 2$. If $M = 1$, the model reduces to ordinary logistic regression.

We will briefly outline standard procedures for likelihood based parameter estimation in this setting. Modeling in terms of a parsimonious parameter vector of interest can be achieved, as usual, using a linear model of the form $\Theta_i = X_i \beta$, where Θ_i is a vector of natural parameters, X_i is a $q \times p$ design matrix and β a $p \times 1$ vector of unknown regression coefficients. Let the mean parameter be μ_i. Then the duality property of exponential families (e.g., Brown 1986, p. 36) states that μ_i is related to the natural parameter Θ_i by $\mu_i = \partial A(\Theta_i)/\partial \Theta_i$. Here, $A(\Theta_i)$ is the normalizing constant. Next, the log-likelihood can be written as

$$\ell = \sum_{i=1}^{N} \ln f(y_i; \Theta_i) = \sum_{i=1}^{N} \left[\beta' X_i' w_i - A(X_i \beta) \right],$$

and the score function is

$$U(\beta) = \sum_{i=1}^{N} X_i'(w_i - \mu_i).$$

Here, w_i is the vector made up of all outcomes y_{ik}, and their pairwise and higher-order cross products. The maximum likelihood estimator for β is defined as the solution to $U(\beta) = 0$. It is usually found by applying a Newton-Raphson procedure which, of course, coincides with a Fisher scoring algorithm for exponential family models with canonical link functions.

11.2.2 A Single Repeated Outcome

Let us now consider a single repeated outcome. Because here the index k always equals 1, we drop it temporarily from notation. We re-introduce however the subscript j to indicate an observation within a cluster.

A model for a single repeated outcome can now be written as:

$$f_i(\boldsymbol{y}_i; \boldsymbol{\Theta}_i) = \exp\left\{\sum_{j=1}^{n_i} \theta_{ij} y_{ij} + \sum_{j<j'} \delta^*_{ijj'} y_{ij} y_{ij'} + \cdots \right.$$
$$\left. + \omega_{i1\ldots n_i} y_{i1} \cdots y_{in_i} - A(\boldsymbol{\Theta}^*_i)\right\}. \qquad (11.4)$$

Recall, in agreement with the comment made in Section 11.2.1, that the model is classified as conditional, in spite of its marginal appearance, because the parameters have a conditional interpretation.

This model is equivalent to (7.50), through (11.2)–(11.3), where the δ^* play the role of the ω's. Similar in spirit to Zhao and Prentice (1990), Thélot (1985), and Molenberghs and Ryan (1999) we can simplify (11.4) to a quadratic version:

$$f_i(\boldsymbol{y}_i; \boldsymbol{\Theta}_i^*, n_i) = \exp\left\{\sum_{j=1}^{n_i} \theta^*_i y_{ij} + \sum_{j<j'} \delta^*_i y_{ij} y_{ij'} - A(\boldsymbol{\Theta}^*_i)\right\}, \qquad (11.5)$$

with δ^*_i now describing the association between pairs of measurements within the ith unit only.

It is useful to code the outcomes as 1 and -1, rather than 1 and 0, whenever the number of measurements per unit is variable. The 0/1 coding does not preserve the model when the coding is reversed to 1/0, unless all n_i are equal (Cox and Wermuth 1994a). Arguably, this and related drawbacks are stumbling blocks on the way to general use of conditional models of this type.

Focusing on an exchangeable situation, define once more the number of measurements from unit i with positive response to be z_i, (11.5) then becomes

$$f_i(\boldsymbol{y}_i; \boldsymbol{\Theta}_i^*, n_i)$$
$$= \exp\left\{\theta^*_i z_i - \theta^*_i (n_i - z_i)\right.$$
$$\left. + \delta^*_i\left[\binom{z_i}{2} + \binom{n_i - z_i}{2} - z_i(n_i - z_i)\right] - A(\boldsymbol{\Theta}^*_i)\right\}$$
$$= \exp\left\{\theta^*_i(2z_i - n_i) + \delta^*_i\left[\binom{n_i}{2} - 2z_i n_i + 2z_i^2\right] - A(\boldsymbol{\Theta}^*_i)\right\}. \qquad (11.6)$$

Upon absorbing constant terms into the normalizing constant and using the reparametrization $\theta_i = 2\theta_i^*$ and $\delta_i = 2\delta_i^*$, this becomes

$$f_i(\boldsymbol{y}_i; \boldsymbol{\Theta}_i, n_i) = \exp\left\{\theta_i z_i^{(1)} + \delta_i z_i^{(2)} - A(\boldsymbol{\Theta}_i)\right\}, \qquad (11.7)$$

with $z_i^{(1)} = z_i$ and $z_i^{(2)} = -z_i(n_i - z_i)$.

Note that this model contains the same building blocks as the Bahadur model for clustered data (Section 7.2.2; see also Section 9.4.1).

For model (11.7), independence corresponds to $\delta_i = 0$. A positive δ_i corresponds to classical clustering or overdispersion, whereas a negative parameter value occurs in the underdispersed case. It is worthwhile to note that even for underdispersion, no restrictions exist on the parameter space. Molenberghs and Ryan (1999) show that model (11.7) has several noteworthy properties. First, the model is clearly invariant to interchanging the codes of successes and failures, whence both estimation and testing will be invariant for this change as well. Second, the conditional probability of observing a positive response in a unit of size n_i, given that the remaining littermates yield $z_i - 1$ successes, is given by:

$$P(Y_{ij} = 1 | z_i - 1, n_i) = \frac{\exp[\theta_i - \delta_i(n_i - 2z_i + 1)]}{1 + \exp[\theta_i - \delta_i(n_i - 2z_i + 1)]}, \qquad (11.8)$$

which decreases to zero when n_i increases and z_i is bounded, and approaches unity for increasing n_i and bounded $n_i - z_i$, whenever there is a positive association between outcomes. From (11.8) it is clear that the conditional logit of an additional success, given $z_i - 1$ successes, equals $\theta_i - \delta_i(n_i - 2z_i + 1)$. Thus, upon noting that the second term vanishes if $z_i - 1 = (n_i - 1)/2$, θ_i is seen to be the conditional logit for an additional success when about half of the measurements are a success already. Similarly, the log odds ratio for the responses between two measurements is equal to $2\delta_i$, confirming the association parameter interpretation of the δ-parameter. Finally, the marginal success probability in a unit of size n_i is clearly a (non-linear) function of n_i:

$$E\left(\frac{Z_i}{n_i}\right) = \frac{\sum_{z=0}^{n_i} z \binom{n_i}{z} \exp\{\theta_i z - \delta_i z(n_i - z)\}}{\sum_{z=0}^{n_i} n_i \binom{n_i}{z} \exp\{\theta_i z - \delta_i z(n_i - z)\}}. \qquad (11.9)$$

Because this model is conditional in nature, this marginal quantity does not simplify in general. Nevertheless, (11.9) can easily be calculated and plotted to explore the relationship between cluster size and response probability.

11.2.3 Repeated Multivariate Outcomes

Suppose again that $Y_{ikj} = 1$ when at the jth occasion in unit i response k is observed and -1 otherwise. It is convenient to group the outcomes for the

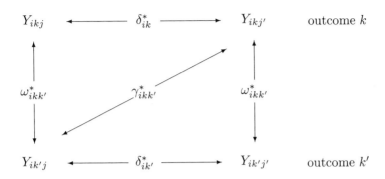

FIGURE 11.1. *Association structure for outcomes k and k' on measurement occasions j and j' in unit i.*

ith unit into an Mn_i vector $\boldsymbol{Y}_i = (Y_{i11}, \ldots, Y_{i1n_i}, \ldots, Y_{iMn_i})$. Molenberghs and Ryan (1999) proposed the following model for the joint distribution of clustered multivariate binary data:

$$f_i(\boldsymbol{y}_i; \boldsymbol{\Theta}_i^*) = \exp\left\{ \sum_{k=1}^{M} \sum_{j=1}^{n_i} \theta_{ik}^* y_{ikj} + \sum_{k=1}^{M} \sum_{j<j'} \delta_{ik}^* y_{ikj} y_{ikj'} \right.$$
$$+ \sum_{k<k'} \sum_{j=1}^{n_i} \omega_{ikk'}^* y_{ikj} y_{ik'j}$$
$$\left. + \sum_{k<k'} \sum_{j\neq j'} \gamma_{ikk'}^* y_{ikj} y_{ik'j'} - A(\boldsymbol{\Theta}_i^*) \right\}, \quad (11.10)$$

where $A(\boldsymbol{\Theta}_i^*)$ is the normalizing constant, resulting from summing (11.10) over all 2^{Mn_i} possible outcome vectors. The building blocks of this model are clearly the main effects (θ^*) and three types of association parameters, reflecting three different types of association. For example, δ_{ik}^* refers to the association between two different measurement occasions within the same unit on the same outcome k, $\omega_{ikk'}^*$ refers to the association between outcomes k and k' for a single measurement occasion within unit i and $\gamma_{ikk'}^*$ gives the association between outcomes k and k' for two different measurement occasions within the same unit. The three different types of associations captured in the model are depicted in Figure 11.1.

The absence of observation-specific subscripts reflects the implicit exchangeability assumption between any two measurement occasions within the same unit. This is sensible whenever the same mean is assumed across occasions, for a given outcome, and the association does not depend on the particular pair of measurement occasions. When measurement occasions refer to littermates within a litter, for example, such an assumption is sensible and can lead to further model simplification. Further, all third and higher-order associations have been omitted. In principle, they can be included as well, although even writing them down in the current multivariate clustered setting would be a challenging endeavor.

The exchangeability assumption will now be used to simplify the model. Defining z_{ik} as the number of measurement occasions in unit i, positive on outcome k and $z_{ikk'}$ as the number of occasions within unit i, positive on both outcomes k and k', Molenberghs and Ryan (1999) derived (after reparameterization):

$$f_i(\boldsymbol{y}_i; \boldsymbol{\Theta}_i)$$

$$= \exp\left\{\sum_{k=1}^{M} \theta_{ik} z_{ik}^{(1)} + \sum_{k=1}^{M} \delta_{ik} z_{ik}^{(2)}\right.$$

$$\left. + \sum_{k<k'} \omega_{ikk'} z_{ikk'}^{(3)} + \sum_{k<k'} \gamma_{ikk'} z_{ikk'}^{(4)} - A(\boldsymbol{\Theta}_i)\right\}, \quad (11.11)$$

where

$$\begin{aligned} z_{ik}^{(1)} &= z_{ik}, \\ z_{ik}^{(2)} &= -z_{ik}(n_i - z_{ik}), \\ z_{ikk'}^{(3)} &= 2z_{ikk'} - z_{ik} - z_{ik'}, \\ z_{ikk'}^{(4)} &= -z_{ik}(n_i - z_{ik'}) - z_{ik'}(n_i - z_{ik}) - z_{ikk'}^{(3)}. \end{aligned} \quad (11.12)$$

Advantages of this model are the flexibility with which both main effects and associations can be modeled, and the absence of constraints on the parameter space, which eases interpretability. Success probabilities at both the measurement occasion level, as well as on the unit level as whole, have simple expressions (Aerts *et al* 2002, Chapter 10). This aspect is important when using the model in a dose-response setting.

The fact that the probability model depends explicitly [see (11.12)] and implicitly on the cluster size is an advantage in some cases, and a disadvantage in others. For example, it can be advantageous when the number of measurements made is informative in its own right for the effect of a certain covariate, such as dose or exposure. Also note that Model (11.11) is conditional in nature, as it describes a feature of (a set of) outcomes conditional on the other outcomes. It implies conditional odds and conditional odds ratios that are log-linear in the natural parameters. Molenberghs and Ryan (1999) construct the conditional logit associated with the presence and absence of outcome k for an occasion j in unit i, given all other outcomes in the same cluster, and they show that this function depends on cluster size and on the observed pattern of the remaining outcomes. Let $\kappa_{ikj} = 1$ if at the jth measurement occasion a success is seen on the kth outcome variable and 0 otherwise. Then

$$\ln \frac{\text{pr}(Y_{ikj} = 1 | y_{ik'j'}, k' \neq k \text{ or } j' \neq j)}{\text{pr}(Y_{ikj} = -1 | y_{ik'j'}, k' \neq k \text{ or } j' \neq j)}$$
$$= \theta_{ik} + \delta_{ik}(2z_{ik} - n_i - 1)$$
$$+ \sum_{k' \neq k} \omega_{ikk'}(2\kappa_{ik'j} - 1)$$
$$+ \sum_{k' \neq k} \gamma_{ikk'}(2z_{ik'} - n_i - 2\kappa_{ik'j} + 1). \quad (11.13)$$

Marginal quantities are fairly complicated functions of the parameters and are best represented graphically.

11.3 Marginal *versus* Conditional Models

Having introduced marginal and conditional models, we are now in a position to discuss points of meaningfulness of one relative to the other. It will be clear from the briefest comparison, that fitting a marginal model is typically more involved than fitting the conditional model of the previous section. Most marginal models have constrained parameter spaces. This is often cited as an interpretational disadvantage. However, the same is true for the multivariate normal model, as the covariance matrix has to be positive definite. Except for the bivariate case, the various correlations constrain each other to ensure positive definiteness. Exactly the same constraint applies to the multivariate probit model, and similar but less tractable constraints apply to the Dale model. In contrast, the parameters of (11.1), (11.4), and (11.10) can take on any value in the Euclidean space whilst still producing valid probabilities. Also, marginal models differ one from the other in terms of the severity of the restrictions. Although in the Bahadur model the association parameter is restricted, even when $n_i = n = 2$, this is not the case in the Dale model where the odds ratio can range over the entire parameter space $[0, +\infty]$. Restrictions in the higher dimensional case exist but are rather weak.

One of the main interpretational advantages of marginal models is their so-called upward compatibility or reproducibility (Liang, Zeger, and Qaqish 1992). This means that when a marginal model (e.g., the Dale, probit, or Bahadur model) is used to model a response vector, the appropriate submodel applies to any subvector of the response vector. Such a sub-vector still follows a model of the same structure, with as parameter vector the corresponding sub-vector. In particular, the univariate margins of the marginal models discussed above are typically of the logistic type, the probit model the obvious exception.

In this sense, model (11.4) is often not meaningful when the number of measurement occasions n_i are unequal. Indeed, when $n_i = 1$ then $\theta_{i1} = \text{logit}[P(Y_{ij} = 1)]$, whereas, when $n_i = 2$, $\theta_{i1} = \text{logit}[P(Y_{ij} = 1|Y_{ij} = 0)]$. Thus, the same parameter would change its interpretation depending on the cluster size. When $n_i = n$ for all i, and the design is balanced (i.e., measurement occasions are common to all clusters), then the model is mathematically principled. The question then is whether the investigator is interested in a response to a conditional question rather than to, for example, a marginal one. A marginal question might be whether the probability of side effects in the fluvoxamine trial increases or decreases with time; a conditional question might consider the probability of side effects at the second occasion, given there were none at the first occasion.

Ideally, marginal models should be chosen whenever there are marginal research questions, e.g., pertaining to one or a few occasions, or the evolution between them (e.g., the time evolution of the response in the toenail data). They are also useful when not only the strength of association between occasions, but also a quantification of this association is of interest. Of course, when the number of measurement occasions within a subject grows, such models become intractable from a likelihood perspective. One can then resort to alternative approaches, such as generalized estimating equations (Chapter 8) or pseudo-likelihood (Chapters 9 and 12).

Chapter 6 provided a thorough comparison of the marginal Dale model and the more conditionally natured Goodman association model. It is clear from this chapter that a marginal approach, in particular when the global odds ratio is featured as a measure of association, often leads to well fitting, parsimonious, and convenient to interpret models.

11.4 Analysis of the NTP Data

To illustrate conditional models in practice, we apply the univariate and multivariate clustered models of Sections 11.2.2 and 11.2.3, respectively, to the NTP data. Reports on marginal analyses can be found in Sections 7.2.3, 8.9, and 9.6. The data were introduced in Section 2.7. We fitted Model (11.7) to 4 outcomes in each of the 3 datasets, in line with earlier analyses. Maximum likelihood estimates (model-based standard errors; empirically corrected standard errors) are presented in Table 11.1. The natural parameters were modeled as:

$$\theta_i = \beta_0 + \beta_d d_i,$$

TABLE 11.1. *NTP Data. Maximum likelihood estimates (model based standard errors; empirically corrected standard errors) of the conditional model for univariate clustered data, fitted to various outcomes in three studies. β_0 and β_d are the marginal intercept and dose effect, respectively; β_a is the conditional log odds ratio association parameter.*

Outcome	Par.	DEHP	EG	DYME
External	β_0	-2.81(0.58;0.52)	-3.01(0.79;1.01)	-5.78(1.13;1.23)
	β_d	3.07(0.65;0.62)	2.25(0.68;0.85)	6.25(1.25;1.41)
	β_a	0.18(0.04;0.04)	0.25(0.05;0.06)	0.09(0.06;0.06)
Visceral	β_0	-2.39(0.50;0.52)	-5.09(1.55;1.51)	-3.32(0.98;0.89)
	β_d	2.45(0.55;0.60)	3.76(1.34;1.20)	2.88(0.93;0.83)
	β_a	0.18(0.04;0.04)	0.23(0.09;0.09)	0.29(0.05;0.05)
Skeletal	β_0	-2.79(0.58;0.77)	-0.84(0.17;0.18)	-1.62(0.35;0.48)
	β_d	2.91(0.63;0.82)	0.98(0.20;0.20)	2.45(0.51;0.82)
	β_a	0.17(0.04;0.05)	0.20(0.02;0.02)	0.25(0.03;0.03)
Collapsed	β_0	-2.04(0.35;0.42)	-0.81(0.16;0.16)	-2.90(0.43;0.51)
	β_d	2.98(0.51;0.66)	0.97(0.20;0.20)	5.08(0.74;0.96)
	β_a	0.16(0.03;0.03)	0.20(0.02;0.02)	0.19(0.03;0.03)

where d_i is the dose level applied to the ith cluster, and where the association model equals

$$\delta_i = \beta_a,$$

i.e., a constant association model is assumed.

Fitting the trivariate clustered model of Section 11.2.3 is not feasible with maximum likelihood. This issue will be taken up in Section 12.4, using pseudo-likelihood. There, we will also present the PL counterpart to Table 11.1, and discuss similarities and differences.

Clearly, parameter estimates for β_0 and β_d, as well as their corresponding standard errors, are uniformly smaller than their counterparts obtained from the marginal model. This is not surprising. Although all marginal models, whether likelihood based or rooted in GEE, model the marginal logit of success, given dose, this model considers the conditional logit of a success in littermate j, not only given dose, but also given values for the other littermates. It is clear from (11.8) that, with the $-1/+1$ coding, θ_i corresponds to the logit, given there are $z_i = (n_i + 1)/2$ successes. For all other logits, a correction in terms of $\delta_i = \beta_a$ enters the equation. In a sense, specifying the values for other littermates "ties the hands" of the success probability we focus on, hence a dilution of the parameters. Arguably, the parameters are much more difficult to interpret than their marginal counterparts, and models like this one may be more useful for hypothesis testing

11.5 Transition Models

A very specific class of conditional models are so-called transition models. In a transition model, a measurement Y_{ij} in a longitudinal sequence is described as a function of previous outcomes, or history $\boldsymbol{h}_{ij} = (Y_{i1}, \ldots, Y_{i,j-1})$ (Diggle et al 2002, p. 190). One can write a regression model for the outcome Y_{ij} in terms of $\boldsymbol{h}_{ij}$, or alternatively the error term ε_{ij} can be written in terms of previous error terms. In the case of linear models for Gaussian outcomes, one formulation can be translated easily into another one and specific choices give rise to well-known marginal covariance structures such as, for example, AR(1). Specific classes of transition models are also called Markov models (Feller 1968). The order of a transition model is the number of previous measurements that is still considered to influence the current one. A model is called stationary if the functional form of the dependence is the same regardless of the actual time at which it occurs. An example of a stationary first-order autoregressive model for continuous data is:

$$Y_{i1} = \boldsymbol{x}'_{i1}\boldsymbol{\beta} + \varepsilon_{i1}, \qquad (11.14)$$
$$Y_{ij} = \boldsymbol{x}'_{ij}\boldsymbol{\beta} + \alpha Y_{i,j-1} + \varepsilon_{ij}. \qquad (11.15)$$

Assuming $\varepsilon_{i1} \sim N(0, \sigma^2)$ and $\varepsilon_{ij} \sim N(0, \sigma^2(1-\alpha^2))$ yields, after some simple algebra: $\text{var}(Y_{ij}) = \sigma^2$ and $\text{cov}(Y_{ij}, Y_{ij'}) = \alpha^{|j'-j|}\sigma^2$. In other words, this model produces a marginal multivariate normal model with AR(1) variance-covariance matrix. It makes most sense for equally spaced outcomes, of course. Upon including random effects into (11.14)–(11.15), and varying the assumptions about the autoregressive structure, it is clear that the general linear mixed-effects model formulation with serial correlation encompasses wide classes of transition models.

Serial processes can be built into random-effects models for categorical data as well, as will be discussed in Chapter 22. There is a relatively large literature on the direct formulation of Markov models for binary, categorical, and Poisson data as well (Diggle et al 2002, pp. 190–207).

For outcomes of a general type, generalized linear model ideas (Chapter 3) can be followed to formulate transition models. Decomposing an outcome as $Y_{ij} = \mu^c_{ij} + \varepsilon^c_{ij}$ ('c' referring to conditional), the first and second moment of a GLM can now be written in terms of the history $\boldsymbol{h}_{ij}$:

$$\mu^c_{ij} = E(Y_{ij}|\boldsymbol{h}_{ij}), \qquad (11.16)$$
$$\phi v^c(\mu^c_{ij}) = \text{var}(Y_{ij}|\boldsymbol{h}_{ij}), \qquad (11.17)$$

where, as in Section 3.2, $v^c(\mu^c_{ij})$ is a function allowing to the variance in terms of the mean, and ϕ is an overdispersion parameter. The only difference is that, by including h_{ij}, an outcome is described in terms of its predecessors. Exactly as in Section 3.3, a function of the mean components is equated to a linear function of the predictors:

$$\eta_{ij}(\mu_{ij}^c) = x'_{ij}\boldsymbol{\beta} + \kappa(h_{ij}, \boldsymbol{\beta}, \boldsymbol{\alpha}), \qquad (11.18)$$

where κ is a function, often linear, of the history. This model is quite simple and the contributions for Y_{ij}, given the history h_{ij}, lead to independent GLM contributions. This is due to the law of total probability:

$$f(y_{i1}, \ldots, y_{in_i}) = f(y_{i1}) \cdot f(y_{i2}|y_{i1}) \cdot f(y_{i3}|y_{i1}, y_{i2}) \cdot f(y_{in_i}|y_{i1}, \ldots, y_{i,n_i-1}),$$

which can be re-written as:

$$f(y_{i1}, \ldots, y_{in_i}) = f(y_{i1}) \cdot \prod_{j=2}^{n_i} f(y_{ij}|h_{ij}), \qquad (11.19)$$

$$= f(y_{i1}, \ldots, y_{iq}) \cdot \prod_{j=q+1}^{n_i} f(y_{ij}|h_{ij}), \qquad (11.20)$$

the latter decomposition being relevant when the history h_{ij} contains the q immediately preceding measurements. It is now clear that the the product in (11.20) yields $n_i - q$ independent univariate GLM contributions. Clearly, a separate model may need to be considered for the first q measurements, as these are left undescribed by the conditional GLM. Note that this was different in the normal case where the formulation of (11.14) and (11.15) produces the marginal distribution in an elegant way, by virtue of full distributional assumptions and their multivariate normal nature.

A logistic-regression type example would be:

$$\text{logit}[P(Y_{ij} = 1|x_{ij}, Y_{i,j-1} = y_{i,j-1}, \boldsymbol{\beta}, \alpha)] = x'_{ij}\boldsymbol{\beta} + \alpha y_{i,j-1}. \qquad (11.21)$$

This model is of the stationaly first-order autoregressive type. Evaluating (11.21) to $y_{i,j-1} = 0$ and $y_{i,j-1} = 1$, respectively, produces the so-called transition probabilities between occasions $j-1$ and j. In this model, when there would be no covariates, these would be constant across the population. When there are time-independent covariates only, the transition probabilities change in a relatively straightforward way with level of covariate. For example, a different transition structure may apply to the standard and experimental arms in a two-armed clinical study.

To ensure a fully separate model is fitted between both groups defined by $y_{i,j-1}$ in (11.21), the model can be extended to:

$$\text{logit}[P(Y_{ij} = 1|x_{ij}, Y_{i,j-1} = y_{i,j-1}, \boldsymbol{\beta}, \boldsymbol{\alpha}] = x'_{ij}\boldsymbol{\beta} + y_{i,j-1}x'_{ij}\boldsymbol{\alpha}. \qquad (11.22)$$

Model (11.21) is a special case of (11.22), found by setting the components of $\boldsymbol{\beta}$ and $\boldsymbol{\alpha}$ equal to each other, except for the intercept.

When κ in (11.18) does not depend on the parameters $\boldsymbol{\beta}$, standard GLM software, such as the SAS procedures LOGISTIC and GENMOD, can be used without any problem. When κ depends on both $\boldsymbol{\beta}$ and $\boldsymbol{\alpha}$, it might be necessary in some, but not all, cases to write the regression function in a user-defined fashion, for which then the SAS procedure NLMIXED can be used.

Whereas the Gaussian transition model (11.14)–(11.15) produces a simple marginal model, this is not true in the general case. In the logistic case, such as in (11.21), and from specification (11.16)–(11.17), it follows that recursive formulas for the marginal means and variances are:

$$\mu_{ij} = \mu_{ij}^c(0)[1 - \mu_{i,j-1}] + \mu_{ij}^c(1)\mu_{i,j-1}, \qquad (11.23)$$

$$v_{ij} = [\mu_{ij}^c(1) - \mu_{ij}^c(0)]^2 v_{i,j-1}$$
$$+ v_{ij}^c(0)[1 - \mu_{i,j-1}] + v_{ij}^c(1)\mu_{i,j-1}. \qquad (11.24)$$

Here, $\mu_{ij}^c(y)$ is shorthand for the conditional mean when $Y_{i,j-1} = y$, with the same convention for the variances. Expressions (11.23) and (11.24) will generally not be constant across measurement occasions, not even for constant levels of the covariates, except in very special and in limiting cases (Feller 1968). As a result, explicit calculation of the marginal variance function can be a challenge and one would have to resort to numerical methods.

11.5.1 Analysis of the Toenail Data

We will illustrate the ideas developed here using the toenail data, analyzed before in Chapter 10. We will adapt Model (10.1)–(10.2) to the transition model context:

$$Y_{ij} \sim \text{Bernoulli}(\mu_{ij}), \qquad (11.25)$$

$$\text{logit}\left(\frac{\mu_{ij}}{1 - \mu_{ij}}\right) = \beta_0 + \beta_1 T_i + \beta_2 t_{ij} + \beta_3 T_i t_{ij} + \alpha_1 y_{i,j-1}. \qquad (11.26)$$

This model is found in the first column of Table 11.2 (Model I). It is clear that there is a very strong dependence on the previous measurement and, before looking into the model further, one may wonder whether there is a dependence on the measurement two occasions prior to the current one as well. This model is given by updating (11.26) as follows:

$$\text{logit}\left(\frac{\mu_{ij}}{1 - \mu_{ij}}\right) = \beta_0 + \beta_1 T_i + \beta_2 t_{ij} + \beta_3 T_i t_{ij} + \alpha_1 y_{i,j-1} + \alpha_2 y_{i,j-2}. \qquad (11.27)$$

The fit of this model is given in the third column of Table 11.3. Obviously, there is no need for an extension in this direction. However, following the

11.5 Transition Models   239

TABLE 11.2. *Toenail Data. Parameter estimates (standard errors) for a first- and second-order stationary autoregressive model. For the first-order case, a model with a common (I) and two separate (II) autoregressive parameters is considered.*

Effect	Par.	First order I	First order II	Second order
Intercept	β_0	-3.14(0.27)	-3.77(0.34)	-3.28(0.34)
T_i	β_1	0.00(0.31)	-0.08(0.32)	0.13(0.39)
t_{ij}	β_2	-0.09(0.04)	0.03(0.05)	-0.05(0.04)
$T_i \cdot t_{ij}$	β_3	-0.08(0.06)	-0.06(0.06)	-0.09(0.07)
Dep. on $Y_{i,j-1}$	α_1	4.48(0.22)	3.59(0.29)	4.01(0.39)
Dep. on $Y_{i,j-1}$	α_{1a}		1.56(0.35)	
Dep. on $Y_{i,j-2}$	α_2			0.25(0.38)

ideas in (11.22), one can consider two separate models, depending on the level of the previous outcome. This model is found by rewriting (11.26) as

$$\text{logit}\left(\frac{\mu_{ij}}{1-\mu_{ij}}\right)$$
$$= (\beta_{00} + \beta_{10}T_i + \beta_{20}t_{ij} + \beta_{30}T_i t_{ij})I_{Y_{i,j-1}=0}$$
$$+ (\beta_{01} + \beta_{11}T_i + \beta_{21}t_{ij} + \beta_{31}T_i t_{ij})I_{Y_{i,j-1}=1}. \qquad (11.28)$$

The dependence on the previous outcome is not included as an explicit parameter into (11.28), but rather as the difference between the two parameters corresponding to the same effect. For example, the main treatment effect is β_{10} in the group with previous measurement equal to zero and to β_{11} in the group with previous measurement equal to one. The fit of this model is given in Table 11.3.

There is quite a bit of difference between the submodels for the two levels of the previous outcome even though, apart from the dependence on the previous outcome itself, there is very little evidence for significance of the various effects, except for the time effect when the previous level of the response is equal to one. Turning to the dependence on the previous outcome, reparameterizing the model indicates that only the main effect of the dependence is significant (results not shown).

A final issue to consider is the spacing of the outcomes. Recall that measurements are taken one month apart in the first quarter (0, 1, 2, and 3 months) and quarterly thereafter (6, 9, and 12 months). Hence, it is cautious to allow for a different transition effect in the first quarter versus the others. Model II in Table 11.2 covers this case. The parameter α_1 describes the transition effect for the later measurements, whereas α_{1a} is the 'excess' during the first quarter, implying that the autoregressive effect

TABLE 11.3. *Toenail Data. Parameter estimates (standard errors) for a first-order stationary autoregressive model with all parameters dependent on the level of the previous outcome.*

Effect	$Y_{i,j-1}=0$		$Y_{i,j-1}=1$	
	Par.	Estimate (s.e.)	Par.	Estimate (s.e.)
Intercept	β_{00}	-3.92(0.56)	β_{01}	1.56(1.26)
T_i	β_{10}	0.45(0.70)	β_{11}	-0.01(0.37)
t_{ij}	β_{20}	-0.06(0.09)	β_{21}	-0.20(0.06)
$T_i \cdot t_{ij}$	β_{30}	0.07(0.10)	β_{31}	0.04(0.07)

at months 1, 2, and 3 is given by $\alpha_1 + \alpha_{1a}$. Clearly, both parameters are significant, showing there are autoregressive effects in both periods of the study and moreover that they are different from each other. Hence, Model II in Table 11.2 would be our preferred choice.

When comparing the estimates in Tables 11.2 and 11.3 on the one hand, with those reported in Table 10.1 on the other hand, it is clear that no direct comparison is possible. Unlike in the Gaussian case, marginal and conditional model parameters cannot be compared directly. The same phenomenon was observed in Section 11.4 for the NTP data. For similar reasons, marginal and random-effects model parameters are typically different in magnitude, as is studied in Chapter 16.

11.5.2 Fitting Transition Models in SAS

Fitting transition models as in Section 11.5.1 is easy, because subsequent measurements, given their past history, are independent of each other, and hence standard GLM software can be used, such as the SAS procedures GENMOD and LOGISTIC. One only needs to ensure that the previous measurement(s) can be used as a covariate. Preparing this covariate in a longitudinally organized dataset (one record per measurement rather than per subject) is straightforward, using the DROPOUT macro described in Section 32.5. Because we used the two most recent measurements, the macro needs to be called twice. The macro returns its input dataset, supplemented with the variables 'prev' and 'dropout.' The second one is immaterial. To call the macro a second time, it is wise to rename 'prev' to, for example, 'prev1,' since otherwise two columns with the same name would result, implying confusing and error prone data manipulation. We then call the result of the second run 'prev2.' Code to perform these actions is

```
%dropout(data=test,id=idnum,time=time,
  response=onyresp,out=test2);
```

11.5 Transition Models

```
data test2a;
set test2;
prev1=prev;
drop prev;
run;

%dropout(data=test2a,id=idnum,time=time,
 response=prev1,out=test3);

data test3a;
set test3;
prev2=prev;
drop prev;
run;
```

The result for the first subject is

Obs	idnum	time	treatn	onyresp	prev1	prev2
1	1	0	1	1	.	.
2	1	1	1	1	1	.
3	1	2	1	1	1	1
4	1	3	1	0	1	1
5	1	6	1	0	0	1
6	1	9	1	0	0	0
7	1	12	1	0	0	0

Then, code to fit (11.25)–(11.26) is

```
proc genmod data=test3a descending;
model onyresp = treatn time treatn*time prev1
                / dist=binomial;
run;
```

which is ordinary logistic regression code. When both predecessors are used, one merely adds 'prev2' to the MODEL statement. The MODEL statement needed to produce Table 11.3 is

```
model onyresp = prev1 treatn*prev1 time*prev1
                treatn*time*prev1
                / noint dist=binomial;
```

where now the variables 'treatn' and 'prev1' are treated as class variables.

To fit Model II from Table 11.2, an additional variable 'prev1a' needs to be created:

```
data test3b;
set test3a;
prev1a=prev1;
```

11. Conditional Models

```
if time>3 then prev1a=0;
run;
```

which is then added to the logistic regression, next to 'prev1.'

12
Pseudo-Likehood

12.1 Introduction

The conditional model introduced in Section 11.2, with clustered data versions in Sections 11.2.2 and 11.2.3, rests on the exponential family framework. This implies the models are elegant from a mathematical point of view, even though there may be serious interpretational concerns (Section 11.3). Nevertheless, maximum likelihood estimation can be unattractive, due to excessive computational requirements. For example, with multivariate exponential family models, the normalizing constant can have a cumbersome expression, rendering it hard to evaluate (Arnold and Strauss 1991). Several suggestions have been made to overcome this problem, such as Monte Carlo integration (Tanner 1991). For example, Geyer and Thompson (1992) use Markov Chain Monte Carlo simulations to construct a Monte Carlo approximation to the analytically intractable likelihood. Arnold and Strauss (1991) and Arnold, Castillo, and Sarabia (1992) propose the use of a so-called *pseudo-likelihood* (PL). A general framework for pseudo-likelihood estimation and inference has been introduced in Chapter 9. Applications in a marginal modeling context were the topic of Sections 9.4–9.6.

In the context of a general exponential-family model like the one discussed in the previous chapter, a conditional form of pseudo-likelihood is sensible and attractive in computational terms. Geys, Molenberghs, and Ryan (1997, 1999) implemented a pseudo-likelihood method for the model described in Section 11.2, replacing the joint distribution of the responses by an appropriate product of conditional densities that do not necessarily multiply to the joint distribution. A bivariate distribution $f(y_1, y_2)$, for example, can be replaced by the product $f(y_1|y_2) \cdot f(y_2|y_1)$ of both conditionals. The key advantage of this approach is that the general form of the normalizing constant cancels, thus greatly simplifying computations, especially when there is a large number of repeated measures per unit, such as in a clustered, multivariate setting. For three outcomes, each measured 20 times, the normalizing constant is made up of 2^{60} terms. The PL approach replaces the joint distribution by 60 univariate distributions of a logistic regression type, of which the normal constant is trivial to evaluate. Although the method achieves important computational economies by changing the method of estimation, it does not affect model interpretation. Model parameters can be chosen in the same way as with full likelihood and retain their meaning. This method converges quickly with only minor efficiency losses, especially for a range of realistic parameter settings.

In Section 12.2, pseudo-likelihood is developed for a single repeated (clustered) outcome, building upon the model in Section 11.2.2, and Section 12.3 presents a similar approach for the multivariate repeated setting of Section 11.2.3. The NTP data are analyzed in Section 12.4, building upon the analyses conducted in Section 11.4.

12.2 Pseudo-Likelihood for a Single Repeated Binary Outcome

A convenient pseudo-likelihood function for exponential family models such as (11.5) with a single clustered outcome is found by replacing the joint density $f_i(\boldsymbol{y}_i; \boldsymbol{\Theta}_i)$ by the product of univariate "full" conditional densities $f(y_{ij}|\{y_{ij'}\}, j' \neq j; \boldsymbol{\Theta}_i)$ for $j = 1, \ldots, n_i$, obtained by conditioning each observed response on all others. This idea can be put into the framework (9.3) by choosing $\delta_{1_{n_i}} = n_i$ and $\delta_{s_j} = -1$ for $j = 1, \ldots, n_i$ where $\mathbf{1}_{n_i}$ is a vector of ones and s_j consists of ones everywhere, except for the jth entry. For all other vectors s, δ_s equals zero. We refer to this particular choice as the *full conditional pseudo-likelihood function*. This pseudo-likelihood has the effect of replacing a joint mass function with a complicated normalizing constant by n_i univariate functions.

If we can assume that outcomes within a unit are exchangeable, there are only two types of contributions: (1) the conditional probability of an additional success, given there are $z_i - 1$ successes and $n_i - z_i$ failures (this contribution occurs with multiplicity z_i):

$$p_{is} = \frac{\exp\{\theta_i - \delta_i(n_i - 2z_i + 1)\}}{1 + \exp\{\theta_i - \delta_i(n_i - 2z_i + 1)\}},$$

and (2) the conditional probability of an additional failure, given there are z_i successes and $n_i - z_i - 1$ failures (with multiplicity $n_i - z_i$):

$$p_{if} = \frac{\exp\{-\theta_i + \delta_i(n_i - 2z_i - 1)\}}{1 + \exp\{-\theta_i + \delta_i(n_i - 2z_i - 1)\}}.$$

The log PL contribution for unit i can then be expressed as

$$p\ell_i = z_i \ln p_{is} + (n_i - z_i) \ln p_{if}.$$

The contribution of unit i to the pseudo-likelihood score vector takes the form

$$\begin{pmatrix} z_i(1-p_{is}) - (n_i-z_i)(1-p_{if}) \\ -z_i(n_i - 2z_i + 1)(1-p_{is}) + (n_i - z_i)(n_i - 2z_i - 1)(1-p_{if}) \end{pmatrix}.$$

Note that, if $\delta_i \equiv 0$, then $p_{is} \equiv 1 - p_{if}$ and the first component of the score vector is a sum of terms $z_i - n_i p_{is}$, i.e., standard logistic regression follows. In the general case, we have to account for the association, but this non-standard system of equations can be solved using logistic regression software as follows. Represent the contribution for cluster i by two separate records, with repetition counts z_i for the success case and $n_i - z_i$ for the failure case, respectively. All interaction covariates need to be multiplied by $-(n_i - 2z_i + 1)$ in the success case and $-(n_i - 2z_i - 1)$ in the failure case.

12.3 Pseudo-Likelihood for a Multivariate Repeated Binary Outcome

For repeated multivariate binary data, several formulations can be adopted. One convenient PL function is found by replacing the joint density (11.11) by the product of Mn_i univariate conditional densities describing outcome k for the jth occasion within a unit, given all other outcomes in the unit:

$$PL(1) = \prod_{i=1}^{N} \prod_{k=1}^{M} \prod_{j=1}^{n_i} f(y_{ikj}|y_{ik'j'}, k' \neq k \text{ or } j' \neq j; \Theta_i). \quad (12.1)$$

This fits into framework (9.3) by choosing $\delta_{\mathbf{1}_{Mn_i}} = Mn_i$ and $\delta_{s_{kj}} = -1$ for $j = 1, \ldots, n_i$ and $k = 1, \ldots, M$ where $\mathbf{1}_{Mn_i}$ is a vector of ones and s_{kj} is a $Mn_i \times 1$ vector, obtained by applying the vec operator to an $M \times n_i$ matrix, consisting of ones everywhere, except for entry (k, j), which is 0. If the members of each unit are assumed to be exchangeable on every outcome separately, there are only $M2^M$ different contributions. Subsequently, one can model components of Θ as a function of covariates, and take derivatives of the log PL function with respect to the regression parameters β to derive the score functions.

Equation (12.1) is one convenient definition of the PL function but certainly not the only one. For example, one might want to preserve the multivariate nature of the data on each measurement occasion by considering the product of n_i conditional densities of the M outcomes for occasion j, given the outcomes for the other subjects:

$$PL(2) = \prod_{i=1}^{N}\prod_{j=1}^{n_i} f(y_{ikj}, k=1,\ldots,M|y_{ikj'}, j \neq j', k=1,\ldots,M). \quad (12.2)$$

This satisfies (9.3) by taking $\delta_{\mathbf{1}_{Mn_i}} = n_i$ and $\delta_{\mathbf{s}_j} = -1$ for $j = 1,\ldots,n_i$. Here, $\mathbf{1}_{Mn_i}$ denotes the Mn_i dimensional vector of ones, and $\mathbf{s}_j$ is the $(Mn_i \times 1)$ vector, obtained by applying the vec operator to an $(n_i \times M)$ matrix, consisting of ones everywhere, except for the jth row, which consists of zeros.

Computational convenience may be the primary reason for choosing one PL definition over another. Let us discuss the relative merits of definitions (12.1) and (12.2). The former procedure is straightforward and natural when interest is focused on the estimation of main effect parameters. Furthermore, it is slightly easier to evaluate. If, however, interest lies in the estimation of multivariate associations then approach (12.2) would be more natural. Geys, Molenberghs, and Ryan (1999) have shown that both procedures are roughly equally efficient.

Further, it should be noted that, in general, it is not guaranteed that a $p\ell$ function corresponds to an existing and uniquely defined probability mass function. However, because PL(1) and PL(2) are derived from (11.11), existence is guaranteed. In addition, both definitions (12.1) and (12.2) satisfy the conditions of the theorem presented in Gelman and Speed (1993), and hence uniqueness is guaranteed as well.

12.4 Analysis of the NTP Data

Section 11.4 presented maximum-likelihood based inference for the univariate clustered data model presented in Section 11.2.2. Here, we will present the corresponding estimates based on pseudo-likelihood. In addition, a trivariate analysis, based on the model of Section 11.2.3 will be presented. Fitting this model with maximum likelihood is prohibitive. In Section 12.4.1, parameter estimation is discussed. Inference and model selection is illustrated in Section 12.4.2.

TABLE 12.1. *NTP Data. Pseudo-likelihood estimates (empirically corrected standard errors) of the conditional model for univariate clustered data, fitted to various outcomes in three studies. β_0 and β_d are the marginal intercept and dose effect, respectively; β_a is the conditional log odds ratio association parameter.*

Outcome	Parameter	DEHP	EG	DYME
External	β_0	-2.85(0.53)	-2.61(0.88)	-5.04(0.94)
	β_d	3.24(0.60)	2.14(0.71)	5.52(1.01)
	β_a	0.18(0.04)	0.30(0.06)	0.13(0.05)
Visceral	β_0	-2.30(0.50)	-5.10(1.55)	-3.34(0.99)
	β_d	2.55(0.53)	3.79(1.18)	2.91(0.91)
	β_a	0.20(0.04)	0.23(0.10)	0.29(0.06)
Skeletal	β_0	-2.41(0.73)	-1.18(0.14)	-2.20(0.27)
	β_d	2.52(0.81)	1.43(0.19)	3.22(0.49)
	β_a	0.21(0.05)	0.21(0.01)	0.25(0.02)
Collapsed	β_0	-1.80(0.35)	-1.11(0.14)	-3.08(0.47)
	β_d	2.95(0.56)	1.41(0.19)	5.20(0.97)
	β_a	0.20(0.03)	0.21(0.01)	0.19(0.02)

12.4.1 Parameter Estimation

Table 12.1 considers exactly the same model, Model (11.7), as in Section 11.4 (see Table 11.1). The methods can be compared based on the parameter estimates, their standard errors (model-based likelihood, empirically corrected likelihood, and pseudo-likelihood), or a combination of both (e.g., the Z statistic, defined as the ratio of estimate and standard error). Obviously, the development of methods to assess the fit of the proposed methods is necessary. However, classical tools cannot be used within the pseudo-likelihood framework without modification. We will return to this in Section 12.4.2, using methods developed in Section 9.3.

Maximum likelihood and pseudo-likelihood dose parameter estimates agree fairly closely, except for the skeletal and collapsed outcomes in the EG study. No method systematically leads to larger parameter estimates (each one yields the largest value in about half of the cases). Pairwise comparisons of the test statistics (estimates divided by standard errors; details not shown) reveal again that no procedure systematically yields larger values. Indeed, in all three comparisons, the magnitude of one statistic is larger than the other in approximately 50% of the cases. These results are in line with findings reported in Aerts *et al* (2002), showing that in realistic settings both the asymptotic relative efficiency and the small sample relative efficiency of the PL method, compared to maximum likelihood, is extremely high.

TABLE 12.2. *NTP Data. Pseudo-likelihood estimates (empirically corrected standard errors) of the conditional model for trivariate clustered data (different main dose effects).*

Parameter	DEHP	EG	DYME
θ parameters			
β_{01}	-2.13(0.64)	-1.64(1.04)	-5.67(1.16)
β_{02}	-2.38(0.63)	-5.04(1.75)	-2.34(1.26)
β_{03}	-2.76(0.72)	-0.39(0.51)	-2.97(0.90)
β_{d1}	2.70(0.66)	1.12(0.86)	6.48(1.26)
β_{d2}	2.63(0.66)	3.63(1.04)	1.66(1.36)
β_{d3}	2.70(0.76)	1.42(0.19)	4.29(0.99)
Association parameters			
δ_1	0.14(0.07)	0.18(0.13)	0.15(0.04)
δ_2	0.18(0.04)	0.12(0.17)	0.30(0.06)
δ_3	0.29(0.06)	0.20(0.01)	0.25(0.02)
ω_{12}	0.06(0.25)	-0.05(0.57)	-0.45(0.20)
ω_{13}	0.60(0.20)	0.11(0.31)	0.25(0.31)
ω_{23}	0.36(0.29)	0.86(0.34)	0.35(0.31)
γ_{12}	0.11(0.06)	0.14(0.13)	0.07(0.04)
γ_{13}	-0.06(0.05)	0.08(0.04)	-0.11(0.05)
γ_{23}	-0.14(0.06)	-0.09(0.04)	0.01(0.05)

When considering all three outcomes jointly (external, visceral, and skeletal, respectively indexed by 1, 2, and 3 in the tables), ML becomes prohibitively difficult to fit. Some analyses are very sensitive to initial values and take hours to converge. Therefore, we abandoned ML and concentrated solely on the PL method, which took a little time to converge.

For all three NTP studies, we considered (1) a model with a different dose effect per outcome and (2) a common dose effect model, both of which are tested for the null hypothesis of no dose effect. In both cases, all association parameters are held constant. Results of these analyses are tabulated in Tables 12.2 and 12.3 and indicate, based on Wald tests, that all dose effect parameters are significant (except for the external outcome in the EG study and visceral malformations in the DYME study). In addition, Tables 12.2 and 12.3 show that by fitting a relatively simple model with different dose effects for each outcome and constant association parameters, the three different main dose effect parameters in the DEHP study all seem to be relevant and of similar magnitude. This suggests that the use of a common main dose parameter is desirable, hereby increasing the

TABLE 12.3. *NTP Data. Pseudo-likelihood estimates (empirically corrected standard errors) of the conditional model for trivariate clustered data (common main dose effects).*

Parameter	DEHP	EG	DYME
θ parameters			
β_{01}	-2.10(0.51)	-1.97(0.56)	-3.89(0.83)
β_{02}	-2.42(0.50)	-2.96(0.87)	-4.77(0.87)
β_{03}	-2.74(0.49)	-0.27(0.55)	-3.21(0.81)
β_d	2.67(0.48)	1.50(0.20)	4.31(0.85)
Association parameters			
δ_1	0.14(0.07)	0.18(0.13)	0.22(0.03)
δ_2	0.18(0.04)	0.17(0.17)	0.25(0.06)
δ_3	0.29(0.05)	0.20(0.01)	0.25(0.02)
ω_{12}	0.06(0.24)	-0.05(0.57)	-0.46(0.19)
ω_{13}	0.60(0.20)	0.11(0.30)	0.29(0.30)
ω_{23}	0.36(0.28)	0.97(0.37)	0.28(0.31)
γ_{12}	0.11(0.06)	0.13(0.13)	0.05(0.04)
γ_{13}	-0.06(0.05)	0.06(0.04)	-0.09(0.04)
γ_{23}	-0.14(0.06)	-0.07(0.03)	-0.03(0.05)

efficiency (Lefkopoulou and Ryan 1993). The estimated clustering parameters δ_k ($k = 1, 2, 3$) are all significant, except for external and visceral malformation outcomes in the EG study. In contrast, the other association parameters often do not reach the 5% significance level.

12.4.2 Inference and Model Selection

In this section, we focus on the EG study. The goal is to construct an appropriate dose-response model. This will be achieved by fitting Model (11.11) and modeling the natural parameters Θ in this model as fractional polynomial functions of dose (Royston and Altman 1994), as fractional polynomials provide more flexibly shaped curves than conventional polynomials. More details on this approach can be found in Aerts *et al* (2002, Chapter 8) and Verbeke and Molenberghs (2000, Section 10.3 and 24.5). See also page 373 in this text. Attempts to use conventional low-order polynomials of the form $\beta_0 + \sum_{\ell=1}^{m} \beta_\ell d^\ell$ to express the model parameters Θ as a function of dose (d) are not successful for the EG data. Royston and Altman (1994) argue that conventional low-order polynomials offer only a limited family of shapes and that high-order polynomials may fit poorly at the extreme values of the covariates. Moreover, polynomials do not have finite

TABLE 12.4. *NTP Data. EG Study. Model selection. (All effects are constant except the ones mentioned.)*

Model	Description	# Pars.
1	$\neq \sqrt{d}$ trends on $\theta_1, \theta_2, \theta_3$; d trend on θ_3; $\neq \sqrt{d}$ trends on $\delta_1, \delta_2, \delta_3$	19
2	$\neq \sqrt{d}$ trends on $\theta_1, \theta_2, \theta_3$; d trend on θ_3	16
3	$\neq \sqrt{d}$ trends on $\theta_1, \theta_2, \theta_3$	15
4	$= \sqrt{d}$ trend on $\theta_1, \theta_2, \theta_3$; d trend on θ_3	14
5	$\neq \sqrt{d}$ trends on $\theta_1, \theta_2, \theta_3$; d trend on θ_3;No ω, γ pars.	10

Comparison	df	$\overline{\lambda}(H_0)$	$\overline{\lambda}(H_1)$	$S^*(e.c.)$	$S_a^*(m.b.)$	$G_a^{*2}(H_0)$	$G_a^{*2}(H_1)$
1–2	3	1.27	0.89	3.77	2.84	2.84	4.06
2–3	1	0.45	0.78	15.19	15.19	18.55	10.68
2–4	2	0.79	0.70	5.76	8.03	8.05	9.09
2–5	6	1.48	1.44	7.71	9.18	9.68	10.01

asymptotes and cannot fit the data where limiting behavior is expected. This is a severe limitation when low dose extrapolation is envisaged. As an alternative, Royston and Altman (1994) propose an extended family of curves, which they call fractional polynomials.

Again, estimation is by pseudo-likelihood rather than maximum likelihood, due to the latter's excessive computational requirements. The following strategy is adopted. First, we select a suitable set of dose transformations for each of the three developmental outcomes (skeletal, visceral, and external) separately, using the method described by Royston and Altman (1994). The resulting set of transformations is then used to construct more elaborate (multivariate) models that can be scrutinized further by means of the formal tests proposed in Section 9.3 (Geys, Molenberghs, and Ryan 1999).

Our most complex model (Model 1) allows different $\sqrt{d}$ trends on the external, visceral, and skeletal main effect parameters, an additional d trend on the skeletal main effect parameter:

$$\theta_1 = \beta_{01} + \beta_{\sqrt{d}1}\sqrt{d},$$
$$\theta_2 = \beta_{02} + \beta_{\sqrt{d}2}\sqrt{d},$$
$$\theta_3 = \beta_{03} + \beta_{\sqrt{d}3}\sqrt{d} + \beta_{d3}d,$$

and different $\sqrt{d}$ trends to the clustering parameters (δ). All other association parameters (ω and γ) are held constant.

From Table 12.4, it is clear that the clustering parameters do not depend on $\sqrt{d}$ (confirming our preliminary, univariate findings). Hence, Model 2 is now selected. The d trend on the skeletal main effect parameter cannot be

12.4 Analysis of the NTP Data

TABLE 12.5. *NTP Data. EG Study. Pseudo-likelihood estimates (standard errors) for the final model.*

Effect	Outcome	Parameter	Est. (s.e.) Model 2	Est. (s.e.) Model 5
θ Main	Ext.	β_{01}	-2.27 (1.16)	-3.58 (1.10)
		$\beta_{\sqrt{d}1}$	1.71 (0.99)	3.07 (0.97)
	Visc.	β_{02}	-6.98 (2.36)	-7.17 (2.26)
		$\beta_{\sqrt{d}2}$	5.54 (1.71)	5.83 (1.96)
	Skel.	β_{03}	-2.81 (0.95)	-3.61 (0.84)
		$\beta_{\sqrt{d}3}$	7.73 (2.32)	7.59 (2.22)
		β_{d3}	-4.01 (1.50)	-3.89 (1.43)
δ Clustering	Ext.	δ_1	0.18 (0.13)	0.29 (0.06)
	Visc.	δ_2	0.12 (0.17)	0.22 (0.09)
	Skel.	δ_3	0.18 (0.01)	0.19 (0.01)
ω Assoc.	Ext.-Visc.	ω_{12}	-0.06 (0.57)	
	Ext.-Skel.	ω_{13}	0.11 (0.29)	
	Skel.-Visc.	ω_{23}	0.81 (0.34)	
γ Assoc.	Ext.-Visc.	γ_{12}	0.14 (0.13)	
	Ext.-Skel.	γ_{13}	0.08 (0.04)	
	Skel.-Visc.	γ_{23}	-0.08 (0.04)	

removed (comparing Models 2 and 3), nor can the different $\sqrt{d}$ trends on the external, visceral, and skeletal main effects be replaced by a common trend (comparing Models 2 and 4). Therefore, we select Model 2 for the time being. Table 12.5 shows parameter estimates for this model.

A key tool to gain insight in this model and to assess its fit in an informal way is the qualitative study of the dose-response relationship. In the area of developmental toxicity, there is generally little understanding about the complex processes that relate maternal exposure to adverse fetal impacts. For developmental toxicity studies where offspring are clustered within litters, there are several ways to define an adverse effect. A foetus-based approach considers the malformation probability of an individual offspring while a litter-based approach is based on the probability that at least one adverse effect has occurred within a litter. Here, we restrict attention to the litter-based approach. To this end, moment-based methods such as GEE cannot be used, while the Molenberghs and Ryan (1999) model allows flexible modeling for both the main effects and the association structure. Given the number of viable foetuses n_i, the probability of observing at least one abnormal foetus in a cluster is $1 - \exp[-A_{n_i}(\Theta_i)]$. Integrating

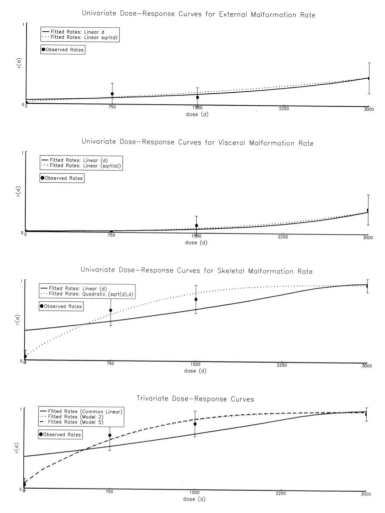

FIGURE 12.1. *NTP Data. EG Study. Dose-response curves. (a) Univariate dose-response curve for external malformations based on a model with $\sqrt{d}$ trend on main effect parameter θ and constant clustering parameter δ. (b) Univariate dose-response curve for visceral malformations based on a model with $\sqrt{d}$ trend on main effect parameter θ and constant clustering parameter δ. (c) Univariate dose-response curve for skeletal malformations based on the quadratic $(\sqrt{d}, d)$ trend on main effect parameter θ and constant clustering parameter δ. (d) Trivariate dose-response curves based on Models 2 and 5.*

over all possible values of n_i, we obtain the following *risk function*:

$$r(d) = \sum_{n_i=0}^{\infty} P(n_i)\{1 - \exp[-A_{n_i}(\boldsymbol{\Theta}_i)]\}, \qquad (12.3)$$

where $P(n_i)$ is the probability of observing n_i viable foetuses in a pregnant dam. (We use the empirical distribution of $P(n_i)$.) One of the major challenges of a teratology study lies in characterizing the relationship between dose and event probability (12.3) by means of a dose-response curve. Here, Model 2 is used to construct dose-response curves representing the probability of observing an adverse event as a function of dose (d). The risk function $r(d)$ is calculated using PL parameter estimates.

Figures 12.1 (a) and (b) show the observed frequencies of malformed litters at the selected dose levels for external and visceral malformations and the (univariate) dose-response curves for models with constant association and $\sqrt{d}$ trends on the main effects. The observed malformation rates are supplemented with pointwise 95% confidence intervals. The dose-response curve for skeletal malformation [Figure 12.1(c)] is based on the quadratic $(\sqrt{d}, d)$-model for the main effect parameter and constant clustering. Figure 12.1 (d) shows the trivariate dose-response curve based on all three outcomes simultaneously (Model 2). Both the univariate and the trivariate fits are excellent. All curves gradually increase when dams are exposed to larger quantities of the toxic substance, before finally reaching an asymptotic. Note that there is a fundamental difference in the dose-response curve for external and visceral outcomes on the one hand, and skeletal malformation on the other, the latter showing a much more pronounced dose-response relationship. This is in line with the different functional form for these responses. Further, the joint dose-response curve is clearly driven by skeletal malformation.

These observations suggest to explore additional model simplification. Candidates for removal are the dose trends on the external and visceral outcomes, as well as one or more association parameters. Table 12.4 shows that the ω and γ association parameters are redundant (compare Model 2–Model 5). However, the clustering parameters could not be removed from the model without a substantial decrease in fit. Furthermore, the dose trends on the external and visceral main effects are also important. Because the goal of selecting a good-fitting model is to perform risk assessment, merely concentrating on formal model selection criteria is insufficient. Arguably, the excellent fit of the dose-response curves that have been achieved should not be compromised. However, Figure 12.1 shows that the simplified Model 5 produces essentially the same dose-response curve as Model 3. Therefore, Model 5 will be treated as our final model. The parameter estimates are tabulated in Table 12.5. It is important to remember that the model parameters have a conditional interpretation. For example it can be derived from (11.13) that, in Model 5, the main effect parameter θ_{ij} can be interpreted as the conditional logit, associated with an additional malformation of type j in the ith cluster, given the cluster contains already $z_{ij} = (n_i + 1)/2$ foetuses with malformations of that type. Similarly, δ_{ij} can be interpreted as the conditional log odds ratio for a pair of foetuses, exhibiting malformation j, given all other outcomes. Thus, if interest is in marginal quantities, such as the dose-response curve, they have to be obtained as non-linear functions of the parameters. Computationally, this is a very feasible task. In contrast, conditional questions can be answered in terms of linear functions of the parameters.

Part IV

Subject-specific Models

13
From Subject-specific to Random-effects Models

13.1 Introduction

The aim of any longitudinal analysis is to study how subjects change over time and what characteristics influence such changes. When interest is in marginal population-averaged evolutions, marginal models as discussed in Part II are the obvious choice. However, one may also be interested in describing the evolution of each subject separately or in predicting subject-specific evolutions. This has already been illustrated in Chapter 4, in the context of linear mixed models for continuous data, and will now be extended to models with subject-specific parameters, for discrete longitudinal data. Section 13.2 introduces the general model with subject-specific parameters, and Section 13.3 discusses three general procedures to handle subject-specific parameters. Finally, in Section 13.4, some frequently used random-effects models are presented.

13.2 General Model Formulation

A general framework for subject-specific models can be expressed as follows. As before, let $\boldsymbol{Y}_i$ denote the n_i-dimensional vector of repeated measurements for cluster (subject) i, $i = 1, \ldots, N$; in other words, the regression notation, introduced in Section 7.1. It will be assumed that $\boldsymbol{Y}_i$ (possibly appropriately transformed) satisfies

$$\boldsymbol{Y}_i | \boldsymbol{b_i} \;\sim\; F_i(\boldsymbol{\theta}, \boldsymbol{b_i}), \qquad (13.1)$$

i.e., conditional on b_i, Y_i follows a pre-specified distribution F_i, possibly depending on covariates, and parameterized through a vector θ of unknown parameters, common to all subjects, and a vector b_i which is cluster-specific. Let the corresponding density be denoted by $f_i(y_i|b_i, \theta)$.

The distribution F_i can be any n_i-dimensional distribution, such as any of the models discussed in Chapter 7. In practice however, it is often assumed that, conditionally on b_i, the components Y_{ij} in Y_i are independent such that it suffices to specify the univariate distributions of all responses Y_{ij}. The distribution function F_i in (13.1) then becomes a product over the n_i independent elements in Y_i. In the case of a linear model for continuous data, this would correspond to specifying $\Sigma_i = \sigma^2 I_{n_i}$ in (4.3). Unless explicitly stated otherwise, this so-called assumption of conditional independence will be made in the sequel of this book.

13.3 Three Ways to Handle Subject-specific Parameters

13.3.1 Treated as Fixed Unknown Parameters

Once the model in (13.1) has been specified, an obvious approach toward estimation is based on maximizing the likelihood $\prod_i f_i(y_i|b_i, \theta)$ with respect to θ and all b_i. However, Neyman and Scott (1948) showed that the so-obtained ML estimates may be inconsistent due to the fact that the number of unknown parameters increases with the sample size, i.e., with the number N of clusters. This is a well-known result in the context of logistic regression for matched binary data, where, in the case of an increasing number of strata, the ML estimator $\widehat{\psi}$ for the odds ratio converges to ψ^2 rather than to ψ. We refer to Breslow and Day (1989, Section 7.1) for an extensive discussion in this context.

This shows that the subject-specific parameters b_i should not be treated as fixed, unknown parameters, and that procedures are required to eliminate the b_i from the estimation process. Two such procedures will now be discussed in turn.

13.3.2 Conditional Inference

A first alternative to classical ML estimation, also applied in the above discussed example of a logistic model for matched data, is conditional inference. One then considers the subject-specific parameters b_i as nuisance, and estimation of θ is done by maximizing the likelihood of the data y_i, conditional on sufficient statistics for the b_i.

The main advantage of conditional inference is that no additional assumptions are needed with respect to the nuisance parameters b_i. This is in contrast to the random-effects approach discussed in Section 13.3.3. A disadvantage is clearly that sufficient statistics for the b_i need to be found, and that the likelihood of the data conditional on these statistics needs to be calculated and maximized. Also, all information on the b_i is lost. As discussed in Section 4.5, these subject-specific parameters indicate how evolutions differ among subjects, and can be used to highlight special profiles or to look for (groups of) individuals evolving differently in time. The main disadvantage however is the fact that information may also be lost for the estimation of certain elements in θ. An easy example is found in the context of the linear model for continuous outcomes. Elimination of the subject-specific intercepts b_{i0} and slopes b_{i1} in model (4.2) would also eliminate the population-averaged intercept β_0 and slope β_1. Verbeke, Spiessens, and Lesaffre (2001) use the conditional approach to eliminate subject-specific intercepts, while the subject-specific slopes are dealt with using the random-effects approach to be discussed in Section 13.3.3. An example of the conditional approach in the context of the logistic model can be found in Diggle *et al* (2002, Section 9.3).

13.3.3 Random-effects Approach

If interest is also in drawing inferences with respect to the b_i, including making subject-specific predictions, a random-effects approach can be followed. The key idea is that, simultaneously with randomly drawing subjects from a general population of subjects, parameters b_i are drawn from a population of subject-specific parameters. Hence, the b_i can be considered random vectors, drawn independently from a distribution function $Q(b_i)$, called the mixing distribution. Elimination of the parameters b_i is then obtained from integrating them out, over their assumed distribution. More specifically, estimation and inference for θ is obtained from ML estimation, based on the marginal density for Y_i given by

$$f_i(y_i|\theta, Q) = \int f_i(y_i|b_i, \theta) dQ(b_i). \qquad (13.2)$$

Note that this random-effects approach can be interpreted as a flexible way of deriving multivariate marginal likelihoods. In this respect, it can be viewed as a competitor to, e.g., the probit model, the Bahadur model, and the Dale model, discussed in Chapter 7.

It follows from the classical maximum likelihood theory that, if Q is assumed to belong to some parametric family of distributions (i.e., a set of distributions indexed by a finite number of parameters), all parameter estimators are consistent and asymptotically normally distributed. However, it is also possible not to make any assumptions about the mixing distribution, and to estimate Q by the distribution that yields the highest likelihood of all distributions. This is referred to as the nonparametric maximum likelihood estimator (NPMLE) of the mixing distribution. Kiefer and Wolfowitz

(1956) have shown that the corresponding estimator $\widehat{\boldsymbol{\theta}}$ is strongly consistent and also that $\widehat{Q}$ converges with probability one to Q at every point of continuity of the latter. Later, Laird (1978) gave sufficient conditions such that the NPMLE would be a step function, and Lindsay (1983a–c) showed that, under general regularity conditions, the NPMLE exists, is discrete, and an upper bound for the number of points of support can be given. In some contexts, such as the Rasch model, conditions can be derived under which the nonparametric estimate for the population parameters coincide with the estimate obtained from a conditional approach (if estimable). More details on the relation between a NPML approach and the conditional inference approach can be found in Lindsay (1983b) and Lindsay, Clogg, and Grego (1991).

A disadvantage of the NPMLE is that it is computationally intensive, especially for multivariate random effects, but also that it results in a discrete estimate of a possibly continuous mixing distribution. One therefore often assumes a parametric model for the random-effects distribution $Q(\boldsymbol{b}_i)$. In many cases, the $\boldsymbol{b}_i$ are assumed to be sampled from a (multivariate) normal distribution, but alternatives are possible. We refer to Section 13.4.2 for an example. With a normal mixing distribution, it is usually assumed that the mean is incorporated in the population parameter $\boldsymbol{\theta}$ such that it can be assumed that the $\boldsymbol{b}_i$ have mean zero. This is in analogy with the linear mixed model discussed in Section 4.3.

13.4 Random-effects Models: Special Cases

13.4.1 The Linear Mixed Model

It is important to realize that the linear mixed model introduced and discussed in Section 4.3 is a special case of our general random-effects model. Indeed, let F_i in (13.1) be the n_i-dimensional normal model with mean $X_i\boldsymbol{\beta} + Z_i\boldsymbol{b}_i$ and covariance Σ_i. We then obtain a random-effects model with $\boldsymbol{\theta}$ equal to $\boldsymbol{\beta}$ together with all parameters in Σ_i, and with normally distributed random effects $\boldsymbol{b}_i \sim N(\boldsymbol{0}, D)$.

13.4.2 The Beta-binomial Model

Let $\boldsymbol{Y}_i$ be a n_i-dimensional vector of Bernoulli-distributed outcomes, with success probability b_i. Assuming the elements in $\boldsymbol{Y}_i$ to be independent, conditionally on b_i, we have that the conditional density of $\boldsymbol{Y}_i$, given b_i is proportional to the density of $Z_i = \sum_j Y_{ij}$ which, conditionally on b_i is binomial with n_i trials and success probability b_i. The beta-binomial model (Skellam 1948, Kleinman 1973) assumes the parameters b_i to be sampled from a beta distribution with parameters α and β (which can depend on covariates, but this dependence is temporarily dropped from notation), i.e., the density of b_i equals

$$f(b_i|\alpha,\beta) = \frac{b_i^{\alpha-1}(1-b_i)^{\beta-1}}{B(\alpha,\beta)},$$

where $B(.,.)$ denotes the beta function. The marginal density of Z_i is then given by

$$\begin{aligned}f_i(z_i|\alpha,\beta) &= \int \binom{n_i}{z_i} b_i^{z_i}(1-b_i)^{n_i-z_i} f(b_i|\alpha,\beta) db_i \\ &= \binom{n_i}{z_i}\frac{B(z_i+\alpha, n_i-z_i+\beta)}{B(\alpha,\beta)},\end{aligned} \qquad (13.3)$$

the so-called beta-binomial density. The average value equals

$$\mu_i = \mathrm{E}(Z_i) = n_i\frac{\alpha}{\alpha+\beta}, \qquad (13.4)$$

and it can be shown that the correlation between any two outcomes Y_{ij} and Y_{ik}, $j \neq k$, from the same cluster i equals

$$\rho = \mathrm{Corr}(Y_{ij}, Y_{ik}) = \frac{1}{\alpha+\beta+1}. \qquad (13.5)$$

In terms of $\pi = \mu_i/n_i$ and ρ, we have

$$\alpha = \pi(\rho^{-1}-1), \qquad \beta = (1-\pi)(\rho^{-1}-1)$$

such that

$$\mathrm{Var}(Z_i) = n_i\pi(1-\pi)[1+(n_i-1)\rho],$$

and density (13.3) can be re-parameterized as

$$f_i(z_i|\pi,\rho) = \binom{n_i}{z_i}\frac{B[z_i+\pi(\rho^{-1}-1), n_i-z_i+(1-\pi)(\rho^{-1}-1)]}{B[\pi(\rho^{-1}-1), (1-\pi)(\rho^{-1}-1)]},$$

in terms of the average proportion π of successes and the within-cluster correlation ρ.

In case subpopulations need to be compared, or in case the effect of cluster-specific covariates needs to be investigated, π and/or ρ will have to be rewritten as π_i and ρ_i, which can then be modeled through, e.g., a logit and a Fisher's z transformation, respectively. An example will be given in Section 16.5. Kupper and Haseman (1978) compare the Bahadur model (Section 7.2) with the beta-binomial model. They conclude that the models perform similarly in three clustered data experiments, whereas they both outperform the (naive) binomial model. The similar performance will also be observed in the example in Section 16.5. Declerck et al (1998) however, report better performance of the beta-binomial model in comparison to the Bahadur model.

13.4.3 The Probit-normal Model

As in the beta-binomial model, let $\boldsymbol{Y}_i$ be a n_i-dimensional vector of Bernoulli-distributed outcomes. Let π_{ij} be the success probability for outcome Y_{ij}, which is assumed to be of the form $\pi_{ij} = \Phi(\boldsymbol{x}'_{ij}\boldsymbol{\beta} + \boldsymbol{z}'_{ij}\boldsymbol{b}_i)$, in which Φ is the distibution function of the standard normal $N(0,1)$ distribution, and where $\boldsymbol{x}_{ij}$ and $\boldsymbol{z}_{ij}$ are vectors of known covariate values. Further, it is assumed that the elements in $\boldsymbol{Y}_i$ are independent, conditionally on $\boldsymbol{b}_i$. The model is finalized by assuming the subject-specific parameters $\boldsymbol{b}_i$ to be sampled from a multivariate normal distribution with mean $\boldsymbol{0}$ and covariance D, the density of which is denoted by $f(\boldsymbol{b}_i|D)$.

This model has a latent variable interpretation since it can be viewed as being generated from the dichotomization at zero of underlying continous outcomes $\tilde{Y}_{ij} = \boldsymbol{x}'_{ij}\boldsymbol{\beta} + \boldsymbol{z}'_{ij}\boldsymbol{b}_i + \tilde{\varepsilon}_{ij}$, where all $\tilde{\varepsilon}_{ij}$ are independent $N(0,1)$ variables. Indeed,

$$\pi_{ij} = P(Y_{ij} = 1|\boldsymbol{b}_i) = P(-\tilde{\varepsilon}_{ij} < \boldsymbol{x}'_{ij}\boldsymbol{\beta} + \boldsymbol{z}'_{ij}\boldsymbol{b}_i)$$
$$= P(\tilde{Y}_{ij} > 0).$$

The conditional density $f_i(\boldsymbol{y}_i|\boldsymbol{b}_i)$ is equal to $P(\tilde{\boldsymbol{Y}}_i \in \mathcal{C}_i|\boldsymbol{b}_i)$ where $\mathcal{C}_i$ equals the appropriate quadrant in the n_i-dimensional Euclidean space with vertex at the origin, and where $\tilde{\boldsymbol{Y}}_i = X_i\boldsymbol{\beta} + Z_i\boldsymbol{b}_i + \tilde{\boldsymbol{\varepsilon}}_i$, where X_i and Z_i are the design matrices with rows $\boldsymbol{x}'_{ij}$ and $\boldsymbol{z}'_{ij}$ respectively, and where $\tilde{\boldsymbol{\varepsilon}}_i \sim N(\boldsymbol{0}, I_{n_i})$. The unconditional (marginal) density $f_i(\boldsymbol{y}_i)$ is given by

$$f_i(\boldsymbol{y}_i|\boldsymbol{\beta}, D) = \int P(\tilde{\boldsymbol{Y}}_i \in \mathcal{C}_i|\boldsymbol{\beta}, \boldsymbol{b}_i) f(\boldsymbol{b}_i|D) d\boldsymbol{b}_i$$
$$= \int d\boldsymbol{b}_i \int_{\mathcal{C}_i} f_i(\tilde{\boldsymbol{y}}_i|\boldsymbol{\beta}, \boldsymbol{b}_i) f(\boldsymbol{b}_i|D) d\tilde{\boldsymbol{y}}_i$$
$$= \int_{\mathcal{C}_i} f_i(\tilde{\boldsymbol{y}}_i|\boldsymbol{\beta}, D) d\tilde{\boldsymbol{y}}_i, \tag{13.6}$$

where $f_i(\tilde{\boldsymbol{y}}_i|\boldsymbol{\beta}, D)$ is the marginal density corresponding to the linear mixed model $\tilde{\boldsymbol{Y}}_i = X_i\boldsymbol{\beta} + Z_i\boldsymbol{b}_i + \tilde{\boldsymbol{\varepsilon}}_i$, i.e., the density of the $N(X_i\boldsymbol{\beta}, Z_iDZ'_i + I_{n_i})$ distribution.

Note that, in practice, calculation of ML estimates based on (13.6) requires evaluation of (high dimensional) multivariate integrals of normal densities over regions $\mathcal{C}_i$. Further, the assumption of uncorrelated errors $\tilde{\varepsilon}_{ij}$ can be relaxed, which is the topic of Chapter 22.

13.4.4 The Generalized Linear Mixed Model

The generalized linear mixed model is the most frequently used random-effects model for discrete outcomes. Conditionally on random effects $\boldsymbol{b}_i$, it assumes that the elements Y_{ij} of $\boldsymbol{Y}_i$ are independent, following a generalized linear model as introduced in Section 3.3, but with the linear predictor extended with subject-specific regression parameters b_i. More specifically, it is assumed that all Y_{ij} have densities of the form

$$f_i(y_{ij}) \equiv f_i(y_{ij}|\theta_{ij}, \phi) = \exp\left\{\phi^{-1}[y_{ij}\theta_{ij} - \psi(\theta_{ij})] + c(y_{ij}, \phi)\right\},$$

where the mean μ_{ij} is modeled through a linear predictor containing fixed regression parameters β as well as subject-specific parameters b_i, i.e., $\eta(\mu_{ij}) = x'_{ij}\beta + z'_{ij}b_i$ for a known link function $\eta(\cdot)$, and for x_{ij} and z_{ij} two vectors containing known covariate values. With the natural link function, this becomes $\theta_{ij} = x'_{ij}\beta + z'_{ij}b_i$. The model is completed by assuming that, conditionally on the subject-specific effects b_i, the responses Y_{ij} are independent and by assuming that the b_i are $N(\mathbf{0}, D)$ distributed.

The examples discussed in Section 3.4 for univariate settings immediately extend, leading to, for example, the linear mixed model for continuous data, the logistic-normal model for binary data, and the Poisson-normal model for counts. Note that, in the case of binary data, with probit link function, the probit-normal model discussed in Section 13.4.3 is obtained as special case.

13.4.5 The Hierarchical Generalized Linear Model

As will be discussed in Chapter 14, the normality assumption for the random effects in generalized linear mixed models leads, in general, to intractable likelihood functions, except in the case of the linear mixed model for continuous data. This is because the normal random-effects distribution is conjugate to the normal distribution for the outcome, conditional on the random effects. Lee and Nelder (1996, 2001, 2003) have extended this idea, and propose using conjugate random-effects distributions in contexts other than the classical normal linear model.

14
The Generalized Linear Mixed Model (GLMM)

14.1 Introduction

The generalized linear mixed model is the most frequently used random-effects model in the context of discrete repeated measurements. Not only is it a rather straightforward extension of the generalized linear model for univariate data to the context of clustered measuerements, there is also a wide range of software tools available for fitting these models. In this chapter, we will therefore discuss estimation and inference for this class of random-effects models in particular. In Section 14.2, the model is introduced, and some general issues on estimation are presented. Afterwards, the Sections 14.3, 14.4, and 14.5 discuss three different approach toward maximum likelihood estimation in generalized linear mixed models. Inference will be handled in Section 14.6. Finally, the Sections 14.7 and 14.8 present two examples.

14.2 Model Formulation and Approaches to Estimation

14.2.1 Model Formulation

As before, Y_{ij}, is the jth outcome measured for cluster (subject) i, $i = 1, \ldots, N$, $j = 1, \ldots, n_i$ and $\boldsymbol{Y}_i$ is the n_i-dimensional vector of all measurements available for cluster i. As introduced in Section 13.4.4, it is assumed that, conditionally on q-dimensional random effects $\bm{b}_i$, assumed to be drawn independently from the $N(\bm{0}, D)$, the outcomes Y_{ij} are independent with densities of the form

$$f_i(y_{ij}|\bm{b}_i, \bm{\beta}, \phi) = \exp\left\{\phi^{-1}[y_{ij}\theta_{ij} - \psi(\theta_{ij})] + c(y_{ij}, \phi)\right\},$$

with $\eta(\mu_{ij}) = \eta[E(Y_{ij}|\bm{b}_i)] = \bm{x}'_{ij}\bm{\beta} + \bm{z}'_{ij}\bm{b}_i$ for a known link function $\eta(\cdot)$, with $\bm{x}_{ij}$ and $\bm{z}_{ij}$ p-dimensional and q-dimensional vectors of known covariate values, with $\bm{\beta}$ a p-dimensional vector of unknown fixed regression coefficients, and with ϕ a scale parameter. Finally, let $f(\bm{b}_i|D)$ be the density of the $N(\bm{0}, D)$ distribution for the random effects $\bm{b}_i$.

14.2.2 Bayesian Approach to Model Fitting

The hierarchical model formulation where the outcome Y is modeled conditionally on random effects, which are then modeled in an additional step, makes Bayesian methodology very appealing for fitting generalized linear mixed models. Prior distributions then need to be specified for $\bm{\beta}$, ϕ, and D, usually assuming prior independence. The corresponding densities are denoted by $f(\bm{\beta})$, $f(\phi)$, and $f(D)$, respectively. For $\bm{\beta}$, one commonly chooses either normal distributions or flat, noninformative priors. Standard noninformative priors for D and ϕ are Jeffreys priors (Gelman et al 1995). Fahrmeir and Tutz (2001) report that such choices can lead to improper posteriors (see also Hobert and Casella 1996). Besag et al (1995) proposed the use of proper but highly dispersed inverted Wishart priors for the random-effects covariance matrix D, i.e., $D \sim IW(\xi, \Psi)$, where the hyperparameters ξ and Ψ have to be selected very carefully.

Once priors have been specified, the posterior distribution can be expressed as

$$f(\bm{\beta}, D, \phi, \bm{b}_1, \ldots, \bm{b}_N | Y_1, \ldots, Y_N)$$
$$\propto \prod_{i=1}^{N}\prod_{j=1}^{n_i} f_i(y_{ij}|\bm{\beta}, \phi, \bm{b}_i) \prod_{i=1}^{N} f(\bm{b}_i|D)f(D)f(\bm{\beta})f(\phi).$$

Full conditionals for the fixed effects $\bm{\beta}$, the random effects $\bm{b}_i$, and the variance components in D and ϕ often take simple forms and standard algorithms can be used for drawing samples from the posterior distribution (Ripley 1987). Zeger and Karim (1991) used Gibbs sampling with rejection sampling for the fixed and random effects. Gamerman (1997) proposed a more efficient algorithm, exploiting the computational advantage of one-step Fisher scoring.

14.2.3 Maximum Likelihood Estimation

As explained in Section 13.3.3, random-effects models can be fitted by maximization of the marginal likelihood, obtained by integrating out the

14.2 Model Formulation and Approaches to Estimation

random effects. The likelihood contribution (13.2) of subject i then becomes

$$f_i(\boldsymbol{y}_i|\boldsymbol{\beta},D,\phi) = \int \prod_{j=1}^{n_i} f_{ij}(y_{ij}|\boldsymbol{b}_i,\boldsymbol{\beta},\phi)\, f(\boldsymbol{b}_i|D)\, d\boldsymbol{b}_i, \quad (14.1)$$

from which the likelihood for $\boldsymbol{\beta}$, D, and ϕ is derived as

$$\begin{aligned} L(\boldsymbol{\beta},D,\phi) &= \prod_{i=1}^{N} f_i(\boldsymbol{y}_i|\boldsymbol{\beta},D,\phi) \\ &= \prod_{i=1}^{N} \int \prod_{j=1}^{n_i} f_{ij}(y_{ij}|\boldsymbol{b}_i,\boldsymbol{\beta},\phi)\, f(\boldsymbol{b}_i|D)\, d\boldsymbol{b}_i. \end{aligned} \quad (14.2)$$

The key problem in maximizing (14.2) is the presence of N integrals over the q-dimensional random effects $\boldsymbol{b}_i$. In some special cases, these integrals can be worked out analytically. For example, it has been shown in Section 4.3 on linear mixed models for continuous outcomes that (14.1) is the density of a n_i-dimensional multivariate normal distribution with mean $X_i\boldsymbol{\beta}$ and covariance V_i of the form $V_i = Z_i D Z_i' + \Sigma_i$. Another example where the integrals can be solved analytically is the probit-normal model discussed in Section 13.4.3, where (14.1) was shown to be given by (13.6). In the latter case, however, calculation of the marginal likelihood still involves integration of n_i-dimensional normal densities over the quadrants $\mathcal{C}_i$.

In general, no analytic expressions are available for the integrals in (14.2) and numerical approximations are needed. There is a large statistical literature on various methods to do so. Here, we will focuss on the most-frequently used ones, also implemented in commercially available software packages. In general, the numerical approximations can be subdivided in those that are based on the approximation of the integrand, those based on an approximation of the data, and those that are based on the approximation of the integral itself. These families of approaches will be discussed in the Sections 14.3, 14.4, and 14.5, respectively. Emphasis will be on summarizing the key ideas on which the various estimation methods are based, rather than on technical details. Also, small differences can be found between implementations (software packages), if for example Hessian matrices are replaced by their expectations (Fisher scoring rather than Newton-Raphson). An extensive overview of the currently available approximations can be found in Tuerlinckx *et al* (2004), Pinheiro and Bates (2000), and Skrondal and Rabe-Hesketh (2004). Finally, in order to simplify notation, it will be assumed that natural link functions are used, but straightforward extensions can be applied.

14.2.4 Empirical Bayes Estimation

Although in practice one is usually primarily interested in estimating the parameters in the marginal distribution for Y_i, i.e., in estimating β, D, and ϕ, it is often useful to calculate estimates for the random effects b_i as well. They reflect between-subject variability, which makes them helpful for detecting special profiles (i.e., outlying individuals) or groups of individuals evolving differently in time. Also, estimates for the random effects are needed whenever interest is in prediction of subject-specific evolutions. As for the linear mixed model (Section 4.5), estimation of the random effects will be based on their posterior distribution with density given by

$$f_i(b_i|y_i, \beta, D, \phi) = \frac{f_i(y_i|b_i, \beta, \phi)\, f(b_i|D)}{\int f_i(y_i|b_i, \beta, \phi)\, f(b_i|D)\, db_i}. \qquad (14.3)$$

Unlike in the linear case, this posterior density is, in general, not a normal one. Therefore, the posterior mode, rather than posterior mean, is used as point estimator for b_i. More specifically, the estimator $\widehat{b}_i$ is the value for b_i that maximizes $f_i(b_i|y_i, \beta, D, \phi)$, in which the unknown parameters have been replaced by their estimates obtained from maximum likelihood estimation. The obtained estimates are again called empirical Bayes (EB) estimates.

14.3 Estimation: Approximation of the Integrand

When integrands are approximated, the goal is to obtain a tractable integral such that closed-form expressions can be obtained, making the numerical maximization of the approximated likelihood feasible. Several methods have been proposed, but basically all come down to Laplace-type approximations of the function to be integrated. The Laplace method (Tierny and Kadane 1986) has been designed to approximate integrals of the form

$$I = \int e^{Q(b)}\, db \qquad (14.4)$$

where $Q(b)$ is a known, unimodal, and bounded function of a q-dimensional variable b. Let $\widehat{b}$ be the value of b for which Q is maximized. We then have that the second-order Taylor expansion of $Q(b)$ is of the form

$$Q(b) \approx Q(\widehat{b}) + \frac{1}{2}(b - \widehat{b})' Q''(\widehat{b})(b - \widehat{b}), \qquad (14.5)$$

for $Q''(\widehat{b})$ equal to the Hessian of Q, i.e., the matrix of second-order derivative of Q, evaluated at $\widehat{b}$. Replacing $Q(b)$ in (14.4) by its approximation in (14.5), we obtain

$$I \approx (2\pi)^{q/2} \left| -Q''(\widehat{b}) \right|^{-1/2} e^{Q(\widehat{b})}.$$

Clearly, each integral in (14.2) is proportional to an integral of the form (14.4), for functions $Q(\boldsymbol{b})$ given by

$$Q(\boldsymbol{b}) = \phi^{-1} \sum_{j=1}^{n_i} [y_{ij}(\boldsymbol{x}'_{ij}\boldsymbol{\beta} + \boldsymbol{z}'_{ij}\boldsymbol{b}) - \psi(\boldsymbol{x}'_{ij}\boldsymbol{\beta} + \boldsymbol{z}'_{ij}\boldsymbol{b})] - \frac{1}{2}\boldsymbol{b}'D^{-1}\boldsymbol{b}$$

such that Laplace's method can be applied here. Note that the mode $\widehat{\boldsymbol{b}}$ of Q depends on the unknown parameters $\boldsymbol{\beta}$, ϕ, and D, such that in each iteration of the numerical maximization of the likelihood, $\widehat{\boldsymbol{b}}$ will be recalculated conditionally on the current values for the estimates for these parameters.

The Laplace approximation will be exact when $Q(\boldsymbol{b})$ is a quadratic function of $\boldsymbol{b}$, i.e., if the integrands in (14.2) are exactly equal to normal kernels. Interpreting these integrands as unnormalized posterior distributions of the random effects $\boldsymbol{b}_i$, it is known from the Bayesian literature (Gelman et al 1995) that this will be the case only in very special examples such as linear models, or provided that the number n_i of repeated measurements for all subjects are sufficiently large.

Raudenbush, Yang, and Yosef (2000) have extended the above Laplace method by including higher-order terms in the Taylor expansion (14.5) for Q, up to the order 6. In a simulation study, they show that this considerably improves the approximation, and they find results comparable to those obtained from methods based on the approximation of the integrals, to be discussed in Section 14.5.

14.4 Estimation: Approximation of the Data

A second class of approaches is based on a decomposition of the data into the mean and an appropriate error term, with a Taylor series expansion of the mean that is a non-linear function of the linear predictor. All methods in this class differ in the order of the Taylor approximation and/or the point around which the approximation is expanded.

More specifically, one considers the decomposition

$$Y_{ij} = \mu_{ij} + \varepsilon_{ij} = h(\boldsymbol{x}'_{ij}\boldsymbol{\beta} + \boldsymbol{z}'_{ij}\boldsymbol{b}_i) + \varepsilon_{ij} \qquad (14.6)$$

in which $h(\cdot)$ equals the inverse link function, and where the error terms have the appropriate distribution with variance equal to $\text{Var}(Y_{ij}|\boldsymbol{b}_i) = \phi v(\mu_{ij})$ for $v(\cdot)$ the usual variance function in the exponential family (Section 3.2). Note that, with the natural link function, $v(\mu_{ij}) = h'(\boldsymbol{x}'_{ij}\boldsymbol{\beta} + \boldsymbol{z}'_{ij}\boldsymbol{b}_i)$. As an illustration of this decomposition, consider binary outcomes with the logistic natural link function. One then has

$$\mu_{ij} = P(Y_{ij} = 1) = \pi_{ij} = \frac{\exp(\boldsymbol{x}'_{ij}\boldsymbol{\beta} + \boldsymbol{z}'_{ij}\boldsymbol{b}_i)}{1 + \exp(\boldsymbol{x}'_{ij}\boldsymbol{\beta} + \boldsymbol{z}'_{ij}\boldsymbol{b}_i)},$$

270   14. The Generalized Linear Mixed Model (GLMM)

and ε_{ij} equals $1-\pi_{ij}$ with probability π_{ij} and equals $-\pi_{ij}$ with probability $1-\pi_{ij}$.

14.4.1 Penalized Quasi-Likelihood (PQL)

Several approximations of the mean μ_{ij} in (14.6) can be considered. We first discuss a linear Taylor expansion of (14.6) around current estimates $\widehat{\boldsymbol{\beta}}$ and $\widehat{\boldsymbol{b}}_i$ of the fixed effects and random effects, respectively. This yields

$$\begin{aligned}
Y_{ij} &\approx h(\boldsymbol{x}'_{ij}\widehat{\boldsymbol{\beta}} + \boldsymbol{z}'_{ij}\widehat{\boldsymbol{b}}_i) \\
&\quad + h'(\boldsymbol{x}'_{ij}\widehat{\boldsymbol{\beta}} + \boldsymbol{z}'_{ij}\widehat{\boldsymbol{b}}_i)\boldsymbol{x}'_{ij}(\boldsymbol{\beta} - \widehat{\boldsymbol{\beta}}) \\
&\quad + h'(\boldsymbol{x}'_{ij}\widehat{\boldsymbol{\beta}} + \boldsymbol{z}'_{ij}\widehat{\boldsymbol{b}}_i)\boldsymbol{z}'_{ij}(\boldsymbol{b}_i - \widehat{\boldsymbol{b}}_i) + \varepsilon_{ij} \\
&= \widehat{\mu}_{ij} + v(\widehat{\mu}_{ij})\boldsymbol{x}'_{ij}(\boldsymbol{\beta} - \widehat{\boldsymbol{\beta}}) + v(\widehat{\mu}_{ij})\boldsymbol{z}'_{ij}(\boldsymbol{b}_i - \widehat{\boldsymbol{b}}_i) + \varepsilon_{ij}
\end{aligned}$$

where $\widehat{\mu}_{ij}$ equals the current predictor $h(\boldsymbol{x}'_{ij}\widehat{\boldsymbol{\beta}} + \boldsymbol{z}'_{ij}\widehat{\boldsymbol{b}}_i)$ for the conditional mean $E(Y_{ij}|\boldsymbol{b}_i)$. In vector notation, this becomes

$$\boldsymbol{Y}_i \approx \widehat{\boldsymbol{\mu}}_i + \widehat{V}_i X_i(\boldsymbol{\beta} - \widehat{\boldsymbol{\beta}}) + \widehat{V}_i Z_i(\boldsymbol{b}_i - \widehat{\boldsymbol{b}}_i) + \boldsymbol{\varepsilon}_i,$$

for appropriate design matrices X_i and Z_i, and with $\widehat{V}_i$ equal to the diagonal matrix with diagonal entries equal to $v(\widehat{\mu}_{ij})$. Re-ordering the above expression yields

$$\boldsymbol{Y}_i^* \equiv \widehat{V}_i^{-1}(\boldsymbol{Y}_i - \widehat{\boldsymbol{\mu}}_i) + X_i\widehat{\boldsymbol{\beta}} + Z_i\widehat{\boldsymbol{b}}_i \approx X_i\boldsymbol{\beta} + Z_i\boldsymbol{b}_i + \boldsymbol{\varepsilon}_i^*, \quad (14.7)$$

for $\boldsymbol{\varepsilon}_i^*$ equal to $\widehat{V}_i^{-1}\boldsymbol{\varepsilon}_i$, which still has mean zero. Note that (14.7) is of the form (4.3), and hence can be viewed as a linear mixed model for the pseudo data $\boldsymbol{Y}_i^*$, with fixed effects $\boldsymbol{\beta}$, random effects $\boldsymbol{b}_i$, and error terms $\boldsymbol{\varepsilon}_i^*$.

This immediately yields an algorithm for fitting the original generalized linear mixed model. Given starting values for the parameters $\boldsymbol{\beta}$, D, and ϕ in the marginal likelihood, empirical Bayes estimates are calculated for $\boldsymbol{b}_i$, and pseudo data $\boldsymbol{Y}_i^*$ are computed. Then, the approximate linear mixed model (14.7) is fitted, yielding updated estimates for $\boldsymbol{\beta}$, D and ϕ. These are then used to update the pseudo data and this whole scheme is iterated untill convergence is reached.

The resulting estimates are called *penalized quasi-likelihood* estimates (PQL) because they can be obtained from optimizing a quasi-likelihood function which only involves first- and second-order conditional moments, augmented with a penalty term on the random effects. We refer to Breslow and Clayton (1993) and Wolfinger and O'Connell (1993) for more details.

14.4.2 Marginal Quasi-Likelihood (MQL)

An alternative approximation is very similar to the PQL method, but is based on a linear Taylor expansion of the mean μ_{ij} in (14.6) around the current estimates $\widehat{\boldsymbol{\beta}}$ for the fixed effects and around $\boldsymbol{b}_i = \boldsymbol{0}$ for the random effects. This yields very similar expressions as derived in Section 14.4.1, only is the current predictor $\widehat{\mu}_{ij}$ now of the form $h(\boldsymbol{x}'_{ij}\widehat{\boldsymbol{\beta}})$ rather than $h(\boldsymbol{x}'_{ij}\widehat{\boldsymbol{\beta}} + \boldsymbol{z}'_{ij}\widehat{\boldsymbol{b}}_i)$, as was the case before. The pseudo-data are now of the form $\boldsymbol{Y}_i^* \equiv \widehat{V}_i^{-1}(\boldsymbol{Y}_i - \widehat{\boldsymbol{\mu}}_i) + X_i\widehat{\boldsymbol{\beta}}$ and satisfy the approximate linear mixed model

$$\boldsymbol{Y}_i^* \approx X_i\boldsymbol{\beta} + Z_i\boldsymbol{b}_i + \boldsymbol{\varepsilon}_i^*. \tag{14.8}$$

Again, model fitting is done by iterating between the calculation of the pseudo-data and the fitting of the approximate linear mixed model for these pseudo-data.

The resulting estimates are called *marginal quasi-likelihood* estimates (MQL). As with the PQL estimates, they can be obtained by optimizing a quasi-likelihood function which only involves first- and second-order moments, but now evaluated in the marginal linear predictor $\boldsymbol{x}'_{ij}\widehat{\boldsymbol{\beta}}$ rather than the conditional linear predictor $\boldsymbol{x}'_{ij}\widehat{\boldsymbol{\beta}} + \boldsymbol{z}'_{ij}\widehat{\boldsymbol{b}}_i$. We refer to Breslow and Clayton (1993) and Goldstein (1991) for more details.

14.4.3 Discussion and Extensions

The essential difference between PQL and MQL is that the latter do not incorporate the random effects $\boldsymbol{b}_i$ in the linear predictor, but both methods are based on the same key idea and will, in general, have very similar properties. Obviously the accuracy of both approximations depends on the accuracy of the linear mixed model for the pseudo data $\boldsymbol{Y}_i^*$. In each step of the iterative process, $\prod_j f_{ij}(y_{ij}|\boldsymbol{b}_i, \boldsymbol{\beta}, \phi)$ in (14.2) is replaced by the multivariate normal density of $\boldsymbol{Y}_i^*$. Note that

$$\prod_j f_{ij}(y_{ij}|\boldsymbol{b}_i, \boldsymbol{\beta}, \phi)$$

$$= \exp\left\{\sum_j \phi^{-1}[y_{ij}\theta_{ij} - \psi(\theta_{ij})] + \sum_j c(y_{ij}, \phi)\right\}$$

$$= \exp\left\{\phi^{-1}\left[\boldsymbol{\beta}'\sum_j \boldsymbol{x}_{ij}y_{ij} + \boldsymbol{b}_i'\sum_j \boldsymbol{z}_{ij}y_{ij} - \psi(\theta_{ij})\right] + \sum_j c(y_{ij}, \phi)\right\}.$$

The sufficient statistics for $\boldsymbol{\beta}$ and $\boldsymbol{b}_i$ are $\sum_j \boldsymbol{x}_{ij}y_{ij}$ and $\sum_j \boldsymbol{z}_{ij}y_{ij}$, respectively. Hence, the approximation will be accurate whenever these sufficient statistics are approximately normally distributed, i.e., whenever the responses y_{ij} are 'sufficiently continuous' and/or if the number n_i of measurements per subject is sufficiently large. This explains why, as for the Laplace method, PQL and MQL perform poorly in cases with binary repeated observations, with a relatively small number of repeated observations available for all persons (Wolfinger 1998). Rodríguez and Goldman

(1995) demonstrate that PQL and MQL may be seriously biased when applied to binary response data. Their simulations reveal that both fixed effects and variance components may suffer from substantial, if not severe, attenuation bias in certain situations.

Although similar in underlying key ideas, there are also some important differences between MQL and PQL. Obviously, MQL completely ignores the random-effects variability in the linearization of the mean. Therefore, it will only provide a reasonable approximation when the variance of the random effects is (very) small. Even with increasing numbers of measurements per cluster, the bias in MQL remains. This is not the case for PQL which can be shown to be consistent when both the number of subjects as well as the number of measurements per subject approach infinity, even for binary outcomes. The differences between MQL and PQL will be further illustrated in our examples in the Sections 16.4 and 16.5. See also Breslow and Lin (1995) and Vonesh et al (2002) for more details.

One way to improve the accuracy of the approximations is the inclusion of a second-order term in the Taylor expansions. This leads to the PQL2 and MQL2 methods, discussed in, e.g., Goldstein and Rasbash (1996) and Rodríguez and Goldman (1995). It was shown that MQL2 performs only slightly better than MQL, but that PQL2 leads to a substantial improvement when compared to PQL. Also, MQL uses a linear expansion around the current fixed effects and zeros for all random effects. This explains why this method is considerably worse than PQL in situations with much between-subject heterogeneity, i.e., with large random-effects variances (Browne and Draper 2003). This will be illustrated in Section 16.4 in the context of the toenail data. Finally, besides using higher orders in the Taylor expansions, some authors have advised the introduction of bias-correction terms (Breslow and Lin 1995, Lin and Breslow 1996) or the use of iterative bootstrap (Kuk 1995).

Because the linearizations in the PQL and the MQL methods lead to linear mixed models, the implementation of these procedures is often based on feeding updated pseudo data into software for the fitting of linear mixed models. However, it should be emphasized that outputs resulting from such fittings, which are sometimes reported intermediately, should be interpreted with great care. For example, reported (log-)likelihood values correspond to the assumed normal model for the pseudo data and should not be confused with (log-)likelihood for the generalized linear mixed model for the actual data at hand.

Also, as discussed in Chapter 4, fitting of linear mixed models can be based on maximum likelihood (ML) as well as restricted maximum likelihood (REML) estimation. Hence, within the PQL and MQL frameworks, both methods can be used for the fitting of the linear model to the pseudo data, yielding (slightly) different results.

Finally, the quasi-likelihood methods discussed here are very similar to the method of linearization discussed in Section 8.8 for fitting generalized estimating equations (GEE). The difference is that here, the correlation between repeated measurements is modeled through the inclusion of random effects, conditionally on which repeated measures are assumed independent, while, in the GEE approach, this association is modeled through a marginal working correlation matrix. Some software packages, including SAS, even allow to combine both ideas by allowing a working correlation matrix for the residual components in (14.6). Examples can be found in Chapters 22 and 24.

14.5 Estimation: Approximation of the Integral

Especially in cases where the above approximation methods fail, approximations to the integral, i.e., numerical integration, proof to be very useful. Of course, a wide toolkit of numerical integration tools, available from the optimization literature, can be used. Several of those have been implemented in various software tools for generalized linear mixed models. A general class of quadrature rules selects a set of abscissas and constructs a weighted sum of function evaluations over those. In the particular context of random-effects models, so-called *adaptive* quadrature rules can be used (Pinheiro and Bates 1995, 2000), were the numerical integration is centered around the EB estimates of the random effects, and the number of quadrature points is then selected in terms of the desired accuracy.

To illustrate the main ideas, we consider Gaussian and adaptive Gaussian quadrature, designed for the approximation of integrals of the form

$$\int f(z)\phi(z)dz, \qquad (14.9)$$

for an known function $f(z)$ and for $\phi(z)$ the density of the (multivariate) standard normal distribution. We will therefore first standardize the random effects such that they get the identity covariance matrix. Let $\boldsymbol{\delta}_i$ be equal to $\boldsymbol{\delta}_i = D^{-1/2}\boldsymbol{b}_i$. We then have that $\boldsymbol{\delta}_i$ is normally distributed with mean $\mathbf{0}$ and covariance I, and the linear predictor becomes $\theta_{ij} = \boldsymbol{x}'_{ij}\boldsymbol{\beta} + \boldsymbol{z}'_{ij}D^{1/2}\boldsymbol{\delta}_i$. Hence, the variance components in D have been moved to the linear predictor. The likelihood contribution for subject i equals

$$\begin{aligned} f_i(\boldsymbol{y}_i|\boldsymbol{\beta}, D, \phi) &= \int \prod_{j=1}^{n_i} f_{ij}(y_{ij}|\boldsymbol{b}_i, \boldsymbol{\beta}, \phi) \, f(\boldsymbol{b}_i|D) \, d\boldsymbol{b}_i \\ &= \int \prod_{j=1}^{n_i} f_{ij}(y_{ij}|\boldsymbol{\delta}_i, \boldsymbol{\beta}, D, \phi) \, f(\boldsymbol{\delta}_i) \, d\boldsymbol{\delta}_i. \quad (14.10) \end{aligned}$$

Obviously, (14.10) is of the form (14.9) as required to apply (adaptive) Gaussian quadrature.

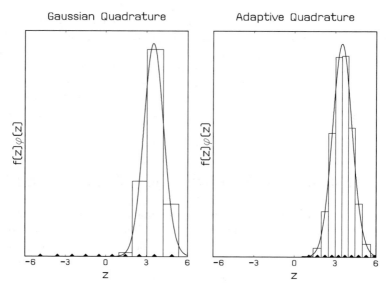

FIGURE 14.1. *Graphical illustration of Gaussian (left window) and adaptive Gaussian (right window) quadrature of order $Q = 10$. The black triangles indicate the position of the quadrature points, and the rectangles indicate the contribution of each point to the integral.*

14.5.1 Gaussian Quadrature

In Gaussian quadrature, $\int f(z)\phi(z)dz$ is approximated by the weighted sum

$$\int f(z)\phi(z)dz \approx \sum_{q=1}^{Q} w_q f(z_q).$$

Q is the order of the approximation. The higher Q, the more accurate the approximation will be. Further, the so-called nodes (or quadrature points) z_q are solutions to the Qth order Hermite polynomial, while the w_q are appropriately chosen weights. The nodes z_q and weights w_q are reported in tables. Alternatively, an algorithm is available for calculating all z_q and w_q for any value Q (Press et al 1992).

In case of univariate integration, the approximation consists of subdividing the integration region into intervals, and approximating the surface under the integrand by the sum of surfaces of the so-obtained approximating rectangles. An example is given in the left hand window of Figure 14.1, for the case of $Q = 10$ quadrature points. A similar interpretation is possible for the approximation of multivariate integrals.

Note that the figure immediately highlights one of the main disadvantages of (non-adaptive) Gaussian quadrature, i.e., the fact that the quadrature points z_q are chosen based on $\phi(z)$, independent of the function $f(z)$ in the integrand. Depending on the support of $f(z)$, the z_q will or will not lie in the region of interest. Indeed, the quadrature points are selected to perform well in case $f(z)\phi(z)$ approximately behaves like $\phi(z)$, i.e., like a standard normal density function. This will be the case, for example, if $f(z)$ is a polynomial of a sufficiently low order. In our applications however, the function $f(z)$ will take the form of a density from the exponential family, hence an exponential function. It may then be helpful to rescale and shift the quadrature points such that more quadrature points lie in the region of interest. This is shown in the right hand window of Figure 14.1, and is called adaptive Gaussian quadrature.

14.5.2 Adaptive Gaussian Quadrature

With adaptive Gaussian quadrature, the quadrature points are centered and scaled as if $f(z)\phi(z)$ were a normal distribution. The mean of this normal distribution would be the mode $\hat{z}$ of $\ln[f(z)\phi(z)]$, and the variance would equal

$$\left[-\frac{\partial^2}{\partial z^2} \ln[f(z)\phi(z)] \bigg|_{z=\hat{z}} \right]^{-1}.$$

Hence, the new (adaptive) quadrature points are given by

$$z_q^+ = \hat{z} + \left[-\frac{\partial^2}{\partial z^2} \ln[f(z)\phi(z)] \bigg|_{z=\hat{z}} \right]^{-1/2} z_q$$

with corresponding weights

$$w_q^+ = \left[-\frac{\partial^2}{\partial z^2} \ln[f(z)\phi(z)] \bigg|_{z=\hat{z}} \right]^{-1/2} \frac{\phi(z_q^+)}{\phi(z_q)} w_q.$$

As before, the integral is now approximated by

$$\int f(z)\phi(z)dz \approx \sum_{q=1}^{Q} w_q^+ f(z_q^+).$$

Note that, when Gaussian or adaptive Gaussian quadrature is used in the fitting of generalized linear mixed models, an approximation is applied to the likelihood contribution of each of the N subjects (units) in the dataset. In general, the higher the order Q, the better the approximation will be of the N integrals in the likelihood. Typically, adaptive Gaussian quadrature needs (much) less quadrature points than classical Gaussian quadrature. On the other hand, adaptive Gaussian quadrature requires calculation of $\hat{z}$ for each unit in the dataset, hence the numerical maximization of N functions of the form (14.9). This implies that adaptive Gaussian quadrature is much more time consuming. Moreover, as these functions (14.9) depend on the unknown parameters $\boldsymbol{\beta}$, D, and ϕ, the quadrature points, as well as the weights used in adaptive Gaussian quadrature depend on those parameters, and hence need to be updated in every step of the iterative estimation procedure. The differences between Gaussian and adaptive Gaussian quadrature, and the effects of different numbers of quadrature points will be further discussed and illustrated in Section 14.8.

A special case occurs when adaptive Gaussian quadrature is applied of the order 1, $Q = 1$. Denote $\ln[f(z)\phi(z)]$ by $Q(z)$. Because, for $Q = 1$, $z_1 = 0$ and $w_1 = 1$, we get $z_1^+ = \widehat{z}$, which is the maximum of $Q(z)$. Further, the adaptive weight equals

$$w_1^+ = |Q''(\widehat{z})|^{-1/2} \frac{\phi(\widehat{z})}{\phi(0)} = (2\pi)^{q/2} |Q''(\widehat{z})|^{-1/2} \frac{e^{Q(\widehat{z})}}{f(\widehat{z})}.$$

Hence, the approximation becomes

$$\int f(z)\phi(z)dz = \int e^{Q(z)}dz$$
$$\approx w_1^+ f(z_1^+) = (2\pi)^{q/2}|Q''(\widehat{z})|^{-1/2}e^{Q(\widehat{z})},$$

showing that adaptive Gaussian quadrature with one node is equivalent to approximating the integrand using the Laplace approximation (Section 14.3).

14.6 Inference in Generalized Linear Mixed Models

Because fitting of generalized linear mixed models is based on maximum likelihood principles, inferences for the parameters are readily obtained from classical maximum likelihood theory. Indeed, assuming the fitted model is appropriate, the obtained estimators are asymptotically normally distributed with the correct values as means, and with the inverse Fisher information matrix as covariance matrix. Hence, Wald-type tests, comparing standardized estimates to the standard normal distribution can easily be performed. Composite hypotheses can be tested using the more general formulation of the Wald statistic which is a standardized quadratic form, which is then compared to the chi-squared distribution. Alternatively, likelihood ratio and score tests can be used as well.

As discussed in Section 14.4, the parameters in generalized linear mixed models are often estimated by fitting linear mixed models to pseudo-data. Therefore, precision estimates for the fixed effects and for the random effects are often calculated using linear mixed model methodology as discussed in Sections 4.4 and 4.5, yielding for example Z-, t- and F-tests for the fixed effects. We refer to Verbeke and Molenberghs (2000, Chapter 6) for more details on inference in linear mixed models. Note that, although this yields valid precision estimates, correctness of the inferences also depends on the assumed sampling distribution. In linear mixed models, the normal t- or F- distributions immediately follow from the normality of the response vectors $\boldsymbol{Y}_i$. For the fixed effects, aymptotic normality follows from applying the central limit theorem on $\widehat{\boldsymbol{\beta}}$ in (4.8). For the empirical Bayes estimates, underlying normality may be more questionable, especially since their posterior distribution may be skewed (Section 14.2.4). Further, as discussed before, one should be careful in using outputs from the linear mixed model that was fitted to the pseudo data. For example, likelihood ratio tests should be based on the likelihood (14.2) of the observed data, and not on the likelihood corresponding to the linear mixed model for the pseudo data.

Finally, when interest is also in inference for some of the variance components in D, classical asymptotic Wald, likelihood ratio, and score tests can be used, as long as the hypotheses to be tested are not on the boundary of the parameter space. For example, suppose one wishes to test whether the variance τ^2 of a single random effect in a generalized linear mixed model equals zero, one has to test the null-hypothesis $H_0 : \tau^2 = 0$ versus the alternative $H_A : \tau^2 > 0$. Obviously, the null-hypothesis is on the boundary of the parameter space $\tau^2 \geq 0$. None of the classical Wald, likelihood ratio, or score tests are still valid. This can most easily be seen from considering the classical Wald test that would be based on the standard normal approximation to the standardized maximum likelihood estimate $\widehat{\tau}^2$. Obviously, this Z-statistic cannot be normally distributed with mean zero because the estimation of τ^2 is restricted to positive values only. Hence, under H_0, this Z-statistic follows the positive normal distribution in 50% of the cases, and will equal zero in the other 50% of the cases. This leads to the well-known mixture of chi-squared distributions as null distribution. Similar properties can be derived for the one-sided likelihood ratio test and the one-sided score test. This has been well-documented in the context of the linear mixed model (Stram and Lee 1994, 1995, Verbeke and Molenberghs 2000 Chapter 6, and Verbeke and Molenberghs 2003). However, the general theory on tests of hypotheses on the boundary of the parameter space (Self and Liang 1987, Silvapulle and Silvapulle 1995, and Hall and Præstgaard 2001) is much more general, and can be applied equally well to the present context of generalized linear mixed models.

14.7 Analyzing the NTP Data

We have applied the various estimation methods to the outcome 'external malformation' in the DEHP study, introduced in Section 2.7.2. As before, let Y_{ij} be the binary outcome (absent/present) for littermate j in litter i. It is assumed that

$$Y_{ij}|b_i \sim \text{Bernoulli}(\pi_{ij}),$$

TABLE 14.1. *NTP Data. External malformations in DEHP Study. Parameter estimates and associated standard errors for the parameters in Model (14.11), obtained using various estimation methods: Laplace approximation, adaptive Gaussian quadrature (QUAD) with 50 quadrature points, penalized quasi-likelihood (PQL) under REML as well as ML estimation, and marginal quasi-likelihood (MQL) under REML as well as ML estimation.*

Effect	Parameter	Laplace	QUAD
Intercept	β_0	-6.02 (0.59)	-5.97 (0.57)
Dose effect	β_d	6.50 (0.86)	6.45 (0.84)
Intercept var.	τ^2	1.42 (0.70)	1.27 (0.62)
Effect	Parameter	PQL (REML)	PQL (ML)
Intercept	β_0	-5.32 (0.40)	-5.30 (0.40)
Dose effect	β_d	5.73 (0.65)	5.71 (0.64)
Intercept var.	τ^2	0.95 (0.40)	0.89 (0.38)
Effect	Parameter	MQL (REML)	MQL (ML)
Intercept	β_0	-5.18 (0.40)	-5.17 (0.39)
Dose effect	β_d	5.70 (0.66)	5.67 (0.65)
Intercept var.	τ^2	1.20 (0.53)	1.10 (0.50)

$$\text{logit}(\pi_{ij}) = \beta_0 + b_i + \beta_d d_i, \tag{14.11}$$

in which d_i equals the dose applied to litter i, and b_i is a litter-specific intercept assumed to be sampled from a normal distribution with mean 0 and variance τ^2. Table 14.1 summarizes the results obtained from the Laplace method, PQL and MQL based on ML as well as REML fitting of the linear mixed models for the pseudo data, as well as obtained with adaptive Gaussian quadrature with 50 quadrature points.

All results are different with substantial differences for some of the parameters. For example, the estimates for the random intercepts variance τ^2 range from 0.89 to 1.42. For both PQL as well as MQL, we observe smaller estimates for τ^2 obtained under ML than under REML. This is a direct implication of the difference between ML and REML in the linear mixed models for the pseudo data: The REML estimates correctly account for the fact that the regression parameters β_0 and β_d are unknown and need to be estimated as well. See Section 4.4 for more details.

14.8 Analyzing the Toenail Data

In Section 14.5, adaptive and non-adaptive Gaussian quadrature were discussed as approximation methods to the integral in the likelihood function. As an illustration of the difference between both methods, and of the impact

TABLE 14.2. *Toenail Data. Summary of parameter estimates and associated standard errors obtained from fitting Model (14.12), for varying numbers Q of quadrature points, and for adaptive as well as non-adaptive Gaussian quadrature. The obtained maximized approximate log-likelihood is denoted by ℓ.*

	Gaussian quadrature				
	$Q = 3$	$Q = 5$	$Q = 10$	$Q = 20$	$Q = 50$
β_0	-1.52 (0.31)	-2.49 (0.39)	-0.99 (0.32)	-1.54 (0.69)	-1.65 (0.43)
β_1	-0.39 (0.38)	0.19 (0.36)	0.47 (0.36)	-0.43 (0.80)	-0.09 (0.57)
β_2	-0.32 (0.03)	-0.38 (0.04)	-0.38 (0.05)	-0.40 (0.05)	-0.40 (0.05)
β_3	-0.09 (0.05)	-0.12 (0.07)	-0.15 (0.07)	-0.14 (0.07)	-0.16 (0.07)
τ	2.26 (0.12)	3.09 (0.21)	4.53 (0.39)	3.86 (0.33)	4.04 (0.39)
-2ℓ	1344.1	1259.6	1254.4	1249.6	1247.7
	Adaptive Gaussian quadrature				
	$Q = 3$	$Q = 5$	$Q = 10$	$Q = 20$	$Q = 50$
β_0	-2.05 (0.59)	-1.47 (0.40)	-1.65 (0.45)	-1.63 (0.43)	-1.63 (0.44)
β_1	-0.16 (0.64)	-0.09 (0.54)	-0.12 (0.59)	-0.11 (0.59)	-0.11 (0.59)
β_2	-0.42 (0.05)	-0.40 (0.04)	-0.41 (0.05)	-0.40 (0.05)	-0.40 (0.05)
β_3	-0.17 (0.07)	-0.16 (0.07)	-0.16 (0.07)	-0.16 (0.07)	-0.16 (0.07)
τ	4.51 (0.62)	3.70 (0.34)	4.07 (0.43)	4.01 (0.38)	4.02 (0.38)
-2ℓ	1259.1	1257.1	1248.2	1247.8	1247.8

of the number of quadrature points, we fitted a single model, for varying numbers of quadrature points, and for adaptive as well as non-adaptive Gaussian quadrature. As before, let Y_{ij} be the binary outcome indicating severity of the toenail infection. A logistic model will be assumed, with linear time trends, for both treatment groups separately. The association between repeated measurements will be modeled through inclusion of random intercepts. More specifically, the model is given by

$$Y_{ij}|b_i \sim \text{Bernoulli}(\pi_{ij}),$$
$$\text{logit}(\pi_{ij}) = \beta_0 + b_i + \beta_1 T_i + \beta_2 t_{ij} + \beta_3 T_i t_{ij}, \quad (14.12)$$

in which T_i is the treatment indicator for subject i, t_{ij} is the time-point at which the jth measurement is taken for the ith subject, and b_i is the random intercept assumed to be normally distributed with mean zero and variance τ^2.

The results of the various analyses are shown in Table 14.2. First, it should be emphasized that each reported log-likelihood value equals the maximum of the approximation to the model log-likelihood, which implies that log-likelihoods corresponding to different estimation methods and/or different numbers of quadrature points are not necessarily comparable. Indeed, differences in log-likelihood values reflect differences in the quality of the numerical approximations, and thus higher log-likelihood values not necessarily correspond to better approximations. Further, we find that different values for Q can lead to considerable differences in estimates as well as standard errors. For example, using non-adaptive quadrature, with $Q = 3$, and looking at β_3, we found no difference in time effect between both treatment groups ($t = -0.09/0.05, p = 0.0833$). Using adaptive quadrature, with $Q = 50$, this interaction between the time effect and the treatment was found to be statistically significant ($t = -0.16/0.07$, $p = 0.0255$). Finally, assuming that $Q = 50$ is sufficient, the 'final' results are well approximated with smaller Q under adaptive quadrature, but not under non-adaptive quadrature.

15
Fitting Generalized Linear Mixed Models with SAS

15.1 Introduction

Nowadays, many software packages allow for fitting of generalized linear mixed models, using one or several of the estimation procedures discussed in Chapter 14. Amongst the commercially available packages, SAS is the most flexible package, with most of the discussed methods included. In this chapter, we will show how the various methods can be implemented in the SAS package. The examples will be worked out using SAS version 9.1. It is by no means the intention to give a full detailed overview of all available options. Instead, emphasis will be on general guidelines with respect to the choice of the appropriate SAS procedures as well as with respect to how models are specified in the various available procedures. We refer to the online SAS manuals for a full description of the available procedures and their possible options.

As a guiding example, we reconsider the toenail data, with the same random-effects model as used in Section 14.8. More specifically, it will be assumed that, conditionally on subject-specific, random, intercepts b_i, Y_{ij} is Bernoulli distributed with mean π_{ij}, modeled as

$$\text{logit}(\pi_{ij}) \quad = \quad \beta_0 + b_i + \beta_1 T_i + \beta_2 t_{ij} + \beta_3 T_i t_{ij}, \qquad (15.1)$$

in which T_i is the treatment indicator for subject i (1 for group B, 0 for group A), t_{ij} is the time point at which the jth measurement is taken for the ith subject, and b_i is the random intercept assumed to be normally distributed with mean zero and variance τ^2. Note that the marginal version of this model was used in Chapter 10 to illustrate how marginal models can be fitted within the SAS environment.

As in Chapter 10, it will be assumed that the data have been stored in the SAS data file 'test,' which contains the variables 'onyresp,' 'treatn,' 'time,' and 'idnum.' The variable 'response' is the binary outcome variable defined as 1 for a severe toenail infection, and equal to 0 otherwise. Further, 'treat' is a binary treatment indicator to be 1 for group B and 0 for group A. The variable 'time' contains the time-point at which the outcome has been measured, and 'idnum' is the variable containing the subject's identification label. Finally, it will be assumed that the data are organized such that each record corresponds to the information available for one specific subject, at one specific point in time, and it will be assumed that the data have been ordered according to the variable 'idnum.' For example, our toenail data set is set up in the following way:

Obs	time	treatn	idnum	onyresp
1	0	1	1	1
2	1	1	1	1
3	2	1	1	1
4	3	1	1	0
5	6	1	1	0
6	9	1	1	0
7	12	1	1	0
....	..	.	...	.
1903	0	1	383	1
1904	1	1	383	1
1905	2	1	383	1
1906	3	1	383	1
1907	6	1	383	0
1908	9	1	383	0

Note that subject #383 left the study prematurely after 9 months of follow-up, but before month 12.

15.2 The GLIMMIX Procedure for Quasi-Likelihood

The marginal and penalized quasi-likelihood methods have been implemented in the SAS procedure GLIMMIX, which is still experimental under SAS version 9.1. As an example, we will fit Model (15.1) using the PQL method. The procedure has many more statements and options than those

15.2 The GLIMMIX Procedure for Quasi-Likelihood

TABLE 15.1. *SAS Procedure GLIMMIX. Available options for specification of the estimation method.*

GLIMMIX option	Quasi-likelihood type PQL/MQL	Inference pseudo-data ML/REML
'method=RSPL'	PQL	REML
'method=MSPL'	PQL	ML
'method=RMPL'	MQL	REML
'method=MMPL'	MQL	ML

presented here, but we restrict to the basic statements needed to fit a generalized linear mixed model.

15.2.1 The SAS Program

The following SAS code can be used to fit Model (15.1) using PQL based on REML estimation for the linear mixed models for the pseudo data:

```
proc glimmix data=test method=RSPL ;
class idnum;
model onyresp (event='1') = treatn time treatn*time
                         / dist=binary solution;
random intercept / subject=idnum;
run;
```

Users of the SAS procedure MIXED for linear mixed models will recognize that the code here is very similar to that used in PROC MIXED. As explained in Section 14.4, this is because the estimation methods implemented in the GLIMMIX procedure iteratively fit linear mixed models to newly updated pseudo data.

A very important option is 'method=' in the GLIMMIX statement. Here, the type of quasi-likelihood is specified. In our example, the model is fitted using PQL, based on REML for the linear mixed models. This corresponds to the option 'method=RSPL.' An overview of the other available options is given in Table 15.1.

The CLASS statement specifies which variables should be considered as factors. Such classification variables can be either character or numeric. Internally, each of these factors will correspond to a set of dummy variables in the manner described in the SAS manual on linear models (1991, Section 5.5).

The MODEL statement names the response variable and all covariates corresponding to the fixed effects. By default, an intercept is added. In case no intercept is needed, the option 'noint' can be inserted. The option '(event='1')' has been added here in order to specify that the probability to be modeled is $P(Y_{ij} = 1)$ (the probability of a severe infection), rather than $P(Y_{ij} = 0)$. The 'solution' option is used to request printing of the estimates of all the fixed effects in the model, together with standard errors, t-statistics, corresponding p-values and confidence intervals. The 'dist=' is used to specify the conditional distribution of the data, given the random effects. Various distributions are available, including the normal, Bernoulli, binomial, and Poisson distribution. In our example, the Bernoulli distribution is specified as 'dist=binary.' The link function is then by default the natural link. In our example, this is the logit link. Others, such as probit, log-log, log, or identity, can be requested by adding an appropriate 'link=' option.

The RANDOM statement defines the vectors z_{ij} corresponding to the random effects in the model. Note that, when random intercepts are required (as in our example), this should be specified explicitly, which is in contrast to the MODEL statement where an intercept is included by default. The 'subject=' option is used to identify the subjects in our dataset. Here, 'subject=idnum' means that all records with the same value for 'idnum' are assumed to be from the same subject, whereas records with different values for 'idnum' are assumed to contain independent data. The variable 'idnum' is permitted to be continuous as well as categorical (specified in the CLASS statement). However, when 'idnum' is continuous, PROC GLIMMIX considers a record to be from a new subject whenever the value of 'idnum' is different from the previous record.

Suppose that random slopes for the time trend were to be included as well. This could be obtained by replacing the RANDOM statement in the above program by

```
random intercept time / subject=idnum type=un;
```

in which the option 'type=un' now specifies that the random-effects covariance matrix D is a general unstructured 2×2 matrix. Special structures are available, such as models that assume equal variance for the intercepts and slopes, or models that assume independent intercepts and slopes.

15.2.2 The SAS Output

We now discuss some of the output produced by the original program presented in Section 15.2.1.

First, a table is given with some information about the fitted model and the estimation procedure. The 'Residual PL' estimation technique refers to PQL with REML (restricted or residual maximum likelihood) for the fitting of the linear models for the pseudo data:

Model Information

Data Set   WORK.TEST

```
Response Variable            onyresp
Response Distribution        Binary
Link Function                Logit
Variance Function            Default
Variance Matrix Blocked By   idnum
Estimation Technique         Residual PL
Degrees of Freedom Method    Containment

Number of Observations Read      1908
Number of Observations Used      1908
```

The table labeled 'Response Profile' summarizes the number of severe and non-severe infections in the dataset, and reports that the probability that will be modeled is $P(Y_{ij} = 1)$, the probability of a severe infection.

```
            Response Profile

Ordered                        Total
 Value      onyresp           Frequency

   1          0                 1500
   2          1                  408
```

The GLIMMIX procedure is modeling the probability that onyresp='1'.

The 'Iteration History' table gives a summary of the different steps in the iterative optimization procedure. Depending on the numerical optimization algorithm chosen, this table will contain different entries. The most important ones are:

```
               Iteration History

             Objective                        Max
Iteration    Function         Change       Gradient

    0       8517.0833042     0.97407150    0.000272
    1       9474.2004261     1.19238147    0.000682
    2      10389.283759      2.00000000    1.148E-6

   ..       ...........     ..........    ........

   11      11147.900904     0.00001765    7.376E-8
   12      11147.902006     0.00000000    3.708E-6

Convergence criterion (PCONV=1.11022E-8) satisfied.
```

At each intermediate step, minus the log-likelihood evaluated in the current parameter values is reported, together with how much this value differs from the value in the previous step. Further, the column labeled 'Max Gradient' reports the largest absolute value of the components in the gradient. At the optimum, this value equals zero.

```
                    Fit Statistics

-2 Res Log Pseudo-Likelihood            11147.90
Pseudo-AIC   (smaller is better)        11149.90
Pseudo-AICC  (smaller is better)        11149.90
Pseudo-BIC   (smaller is better)        11153.59
Pseudo-CAIC  (smaller is better)        11154.59
Pseudo-HQIC  (smaller is better)        11151.38
Pearson Chi-Square                       1455.03
Pearson Chi-Square / DF                     0.76
```

The table termed 'Fit Statistics' gives minus twice the residual log-pseudo-likelihood value evaluated in the final solution, together with a number of information criteria, including the Akaike information criterion (AIC) and the Schwarz (BIC) information criterion. When REML estimation is used for the fitting of the linear mixed models for the pseudo-data, an objective function is maximized, which is called residual log-likelihood function, while, strictly speaking, the function is not a log-likelihood, and should not be used as a log-likelihood. We refer to Verbeke and Molenberghs (2000, Chapters 5 and 6) for a more detailed discussion with examples. Further, information criteria are statistics that are sometimes used to compare non-nested models that cannot be compared based on a formal testing procedure. The main idea behind information criteria is to compared models based on their maximimized (residual) log-likelihood value (or equivalently minimized minus twice the log-likelihood value), but to penalize for the use of too many parameters. They should by no means be interpreted as formal statistical tests of significance. In specific examples, different information criteria can even lead to different model selections. An example of this is given in Section 6.4 of Verbeke and Molenberghs (2000) in the context of linear mixed models. More details about the use of information criteria can be found in Akaike (1974), Schwarz (1978), and Burnham and Anderson (1998). Finally, the 'Pearson Chi-Square' value and derived ratio over the degrees of freedom are based on the marginal distribution of the pseudo-data as well. It should be emphasized that, as all statistics in the above output table are based on the underlying model for the pseudo data, rather than on the model for the actually observed outcomes, they should be interpreted with extreme caution.

```
              Covariance Parameter Estimates
```

			Standard
Cov Parm	Subject	Estimate	Error
Intercept	idnum	4.7116	0.6031

In the table called 'Covariance Parameter Estimates,' estimates and associated standard errors are given voor de variance components in the model, i.e., for the elements in the random-effects covariance matrix D. In our example, this is the random-intercepts variance τ^2.

Finally, two tables are reported containing estimates and inferences for the fixed effects in the model. As discussed in Section 14.6, the reported inferences immediately result from the linear mixed model fitted to the pseudo-data in the last step of the iterative estimation procedure.

Solutions for Fixed Effects

Effect	Estimate	Standard Error	DF	t Value	Pr > |t|
Intercept	-0.7239	0.2370	292	-3.05	0.0025
treatn	0.000918	0.3363	1612	0.00	0.9978
time	-0.2883	0.03349	1612	-8.61	<.0001
treatn*time	-0.1106	0.05366	1612	-2.06	0.0395

Type III Tests of Fixed Effects

Effect	Num DF	Den DF	F Value	Pr > F
treatn	1	1612	0.00	0.9978
time	1	1612	74.10	<.0001
treatn*time	1	1612	4.25	0.0395

15.3 The GLIMMIX Macro for Quasi-Likelihood

The GLIMMIX procedure can be viewed as a formal procedure, although still experimental in SAS version 9.1, which has grown out of the SAS macro GLIMMIX, applied earlier in Section 10.5 for fitting generalized estimating equations (GEE) based on linearization (Section 8.8). In GEE, the association between repeated measures is modeled through a marginal working correlation matrix. In our context, this correlation is modeled via the inclusion of random effects, conditionally on which repeated measures are assumed independent. This similarity implies that the same macro can be used for fitting generalized linear mixed models as well. Without going into much detail, we present here the SAS code needed to repeat the analysis from Section 15.2 with the GLIMMIX macro. Afterwards, some selected output is shown.

15.3.1 The SAS Program

Before the GLIMMIX macro can be called, one has to specify where the code can be obtained from:

```
%inc 'path\glmm800.sas' / nosource;
run;
```

The following SAS code can now be used to repeat the analysis from Section 15.2 with the GLIMMIX macro:

```
%glimmix(
   data=test,
   stmts=%str(
      class idnum;
      model onyresp = treatn time treatn*time  / solution;
      random intercept / subject=idnum;
      parms (4) (1) / hold=2;
      ),
   error=binomial
)
run;
```

The statements that appear in the STMTS statement are directly fed into the PROC MIXED calls needed for fitting the linear mixed models to the pseudo-data. Note that the GLIMMIX macro by default includes a residual overdispersion parameter. If the corresponding generalized linear mixed model does not contain such a parameter, it should explicitly be kept equal to one by the user. This is done using the 'hold=' option in the PARMS statement.

Because the MIXED procedure uses REML estimation by default, the above program requests PQL estimation, based on REML fitting for the pseudo-data. If ML fitting is required, this can be specified by adding the line

```
procopt=%str(method=ml),
```

into the above '%glimmix' call. In case MQL is required, rather than the default PQL, this can be specified by adding the line

```
options=MQL,
```

15.3.2 Selected SAS Output

Without discussing the output from the GLIMMIX macro in much detail, we here present some output tables, which are to be compared with the output from the GLIMMIX procedure, discussed in Section 15.2.2.

Covariance Parameter Estimates

Cov Parm	Subject	Estimate
Intercept	idnum	4.7116
Residual		1.0000

Fit Statistics

-2 Res Log Likelihood	11147.9
AIC (smaller is better)	11149.9
AICC (smaller is better)	11149.9
BIC (smaller is better)	11153.6

Solution for Fixed Effects

Effect	Estimate	Standard Error	DF	t Value	Pr > |t|
Intercept	-0.7239	0.2370	292	-3.05	0.0025
treatn	0.000918	0.3363	1612	0.00	0.9978
time	-0.2883	0.03349	1612	-8.61	<.0001
treatn*time	-0.1106	0.05366	1612	-2.06	0.0395

Type 3 Tests of Fixed Effects

Effect	Num DF	Den DF	F Value	Pr > F
treatn	1	1612	0.00	0.9978
time	1	1612	74.10	<.0001
treatn*time	1	1612	4.25	0.0395

Note that, indeed, the residual overdispersion parameter was kept equal to one, and the results are the same as obtained earlier from the GLIMMIX procedure.

15.4 The NLMIXED Procedure for Numerical Quadrature

Gaussian and adaptive Gaussian quadrature, as approximations to the integral in the marginal likelihood (Section 14.5) have been implemented in the SAS procedure NLMIXED. As an example, we will reproduce the results reported in Table 14.2 for (non-adaptive) Gaussian quadrature with 3 quadrature points. The procedure has many more statements and options than those presented here, but we restrict to the basic statements needed to fit a generalized linear mixed model.

15.4.1 The SAS Program

The following SAS code can be used to fit Model (15.1) using Gaussian quadrature with 3 quadrature points:

```
proc nlmixed data=test noad qpoints=3;
parms beta0=-1.6 beta1=0 beta2=-0.4 beta3=-0.5 tau=3.9;
teta = beta0 + b + beta1*treatn + beta2*time
     + beta3*time*treatn;
expteta = exp(teta);
p = expteta/(1+expteta);
model onyresp ~ binary(p);
random b ~ normal(0,tau**2) subject=idnum;
run;
```

Before presenting the results of this analysis, we briefly discuss the statements and options used in the above program. It is clear from the above code that the NLMIXED procedure requires completely different model-specifications than most other SAS procedures. The main advantage is that the user is given a very high degree of flexibility in the way the model is specified and parameterized. One of the consequences of this flexibility is that the user not only needs to specify the model but also has to specify names for all the parameters in the model. In this respect, it is important to know that SAS considers all symbols in the model specification that are not referring to variables in the input dataset as unknown parameters, to be estimated from the data.

The option 'noad' in the NLMIXED statement is needed to request non-adaptive quadrature as, by default, adaptive quadrature is used. The option 'qpoints=' specifies the number of quadrature points. If this option is omitted, the number of quadrature points is selected adaptively by evaluating the log-likelihood function at the starting values of the parameters until two successive evaluations show sufficiently small relative change. Remember that model fitting based on the Laplace approximation for the integrals

15.4 The NLMIXED Procedure for Numerical Quadrature

in the marginal likelihood (Section 14.3) can be specified by choosing adaptive Gaussian quadrature with one quadrature point.

The PARMS statement is used to specify starting values for all parameters in the model. Parameters not listed in the PARMS statement are given an initial value of 1. Here we are confronted with one of the major drawbacks of the current version of the NLMIXED procedure, i.e., the fact that the procedure does not automatically generate starting values, except for the default value of 1 for all the parameters that do not occur in the PARMS statement. In complex models however, convergence of the numerical optimization algorithms may highly depend on the specified starting values.

The MODEL statement is used to specify the conditional distribution of the data, given the random effects. Various distributions are available, including the normal, Bernoulli, binomial, and Poisson distributions. In our example, the Bernoulli distribution is specified as 'binary(p)' in which p is the success probability that has been specified in the program lines prior to the MODEL statement. The user has full flexibility over the way the model is specified as well as the number of intermediate steps that are used to define the success probability. For example, the above program corresponds to the parameterization as given in (15.1). A different parameterization of the same model would be

$$\text{logit}(\pi_{ij}) = \begin{cases} \beta_0 + b_i + \beta_1 t_{ij}, & \text{Treatment A} \\ \beta_2 + b_i + \beta_3 t_{ij}, & \text{Treatment B} \end{cases}$$

This can be specified using the statements

```
teta = beta0*(1-treatn) + beta2*treatn + b
     + beta1*(1-treatn)*time + beta3*treatn*time;
expteta = exp(teta);
p = expteta/(1+expteta);
```

or, equivalently,

```
if treatn=0 then teta=beta0 + b + beta1*time;
if treatn=1 then teta=beta2 + b + beta3*time;
expteta = exp(teta);
p = expteta/(1+expteta);
```

In case models are needed that do not fit within any of the classical distributions, user-defined likelihoods can be specified through the option 'model onyresp $\sim$ general($\ell\ell$)' in which $\ell\ell$ is the user-defined log-likelihood.

The RANDOM statement defines the random effects in the model. In our example, if the RANDOM statement had been omitted, the parameter b would have been considered a fixed intercept, and this would have led to an over-parameterized model. Now, b is specified to be normally distributed with mean 0 and standard deviation τ. Again, the user has full flexibility here. For example, if one wishes to estimate the random-intercepts variance rather than the standard deviation, this can be achieved by specifying

```
random b ~ normal(0,tau2) subject=idnum;
```

Also, a mean model can be specified for the random effect b. For example, our original model can also be specified as

```
proc nlmixed data=test noad qpoints=3;
parms beta0=-1.6 beta1=0 beta2=-0.4 beta3=-0.5 tau=3.9;
teta =  b + beta1*treatn + beta2*time + beta3*time*treatn;
expteta = exp(teta);
p = expteta/(1+expteta);
model onyresp ~ binary(p);
random b ~ normal(beta0,tau**2) subject=idnum;
run;
```

in which the overall intercept β_0 is now incorporated as average of the random effects. Inclusion of random slopes in Model (15.1) can be done with the following code:

```
proc nlmixed data=test qpoints=10 noad;
parms beta0=-1.6 beta1=0 beta2=-0.4 beta3=-0.5
      d11=16 d12=0 d22=0.1;
teta = beta0 + b1 + beta1*treatn + beta2*time
             + b2*time + beta3*time*treatn;
expteta = exp(teta);
p = expteta/(1+expteta);
model onyresp ~ binary(p);
random b1 b2 ~ normal([0, 0], [d11,d12,d22]) subject=idnum;
run;
```

with obvious parameterization for the means of all components in the random-effects vector, and with the random-effects covariance specified through its lower triangle. If for example, one wishes to incorporate independence of random intercepts and slopes, this is done by replacing the RANDOM statement in the above program by

```
random b1 b2 ~ normal([0, 0], [d11,0,d22]) subject=idnum;
```

When one wishes to directly estimate the correlation between random intercepts and slopes, rather than their covariance, the following PARMS and RANDOM statements can be used:

```
parms beta0=-1.6 beta1=0 beta2=-0.4 beta3=-0.5
      d11=16 rho=0 d22=0.1;
random b1 b2 ~ normal([0, 0],
                      [d11,rho*sqrt(d11)*sqrt(d22),d22])
               subject=idnum;
```

The 'subject=' option determines when new realizations of the random effects occur. The procedure assumes the occurrence of a new realization whenever the value of the variable specified in the 'subject=' option changes from the previous observation. This is why the input dataset needs to be sorted according to this variable (Section 15.1). Further, the RANDOM statement allows inclusion of an output option of the form 'out=dataset' which requests an output dataset containing empirical Bayes estimates for the random effects, together with their approximate standard errors.

The current version of the NLMIXED procedure allows one RANDOM statement only, which poses some restrictions to flexibly specifying random-effects models with random effects at different levels. In the examples considered so far, we had two levels in the design: A first level representing the subjects, and a second level representing the measurements within the subjects. An example where more than two levels would be required would be the analysis of longitudinal profiles from children randomly sampled from randomly sampled schools. In order to correctly account for the different sources of sampling variability, random effects might be needed for schools as well as for children within the schools. Such multi-level models can, to some extent, be fitted within the NLMIXED procedure, but non-standard coding is required.

15.4.2 The SAS Output

We now discuss some of the output produced by the original program presented in Section 15.4.1. The parameter estimates and associated standard errors have already been reported in Table 14.2.

First, two tables are given, containing information about the specified model, the observations in the dataset, and the numerical optimization algorithms used in the model fitting process:

```
                    Specifications

Data Set                                    WORK.TEST
Dependent Variable                          onyresp
Distribution for Dependent Variable         Binary
Random Effects                              b
Distribution for Random Effects             Normal
Subject Variable                            idnum
Optimization Technique                      Dual Quasi-Newton
Integration Method                          Gaussian Quadrature

                    Dimensions

Observations Used                   1908
Observations Not Used                  0
Total Observations                  1908
```

Subjects	294
Max Obs Per Subject	7
Parameters	5
Quadrature Points	3

The table labeled 'Parameters' lists the parameters in the model, their starting values, and minus the log-likelihood evaluated in these initial parameter values:

Parameters

beta0	beta1	beta2	beta3	tau	NegLogLike
-1.6	0	-0.4	-0.5	3.9	760.941002

The 'Iteration History' table gives a summary of the different steps in the iterative optimization procedure. Depending on the chosen numerical optimization algorithm, this table will contain different entries. The most important ones are:

Iteration History

Iter	NegLogLike	Diff	MaxGrad
1	747.757703	13.1833	129.7817
2	728.271809	19.48589	133.3329
3	686.505096	41.76671	116.594
..	....	....	....
10	672.074434	0.000686	0.012941
11	672.074433	8.32E-7	0.000319

NOTE: GCONV convergence criterion satisfied.

At each intermediate step, minus the log-likelihood evaluated in the current parameter values is reported, together with how much this value differs from the value in the previous step. Further, the column labeled 'MaxGrad' reports the largest absolute value of the components in the gradient. At the optimum, this value equals zero.

Fit Statistics

-2 Log Likelihood	1344.1
AIC (smaller is better)	1354.1
AICC (smaller is better)	1354.2
BIC (smaller is better)	1372.6

The table termed 'Fit Statistics' gives minus twice the log-likelihood value evaluated in the final solution, together with the information criteria of Akaike (AIC) and Schwarz (BIC), as well as a finite-sample corrected version of AIC (AICC). They have the same interpretation as discussed earlier in Section 15.2.2. However, the information criteria are now defined in terms of the maximized likelihood (obtained from numerical integration) for the assumed model for the actually observed data, rather than on the likelihood for the underlying pseudo-data, as was the case in Section 15.2.2.

The final part of the output is the table labeled 'Parameter Estimates,' which contains estimates and associated inferences for all the parameters in the marginal likelihood:

Parameter Estimates

Parameter	Estimate	Standard Error	DF	t Value	Pr > |t|	Alpha
beta0	-1.5221	0.3063	293	-4.97	<.0001	0.05
beta1	-0.3932	0.3812	293	-1.03	0.3031	0.05
beta2	-0.3198	0.03481	293	-9.19	<.0001	0.05
beta3	-0.09098	0.05236	293	-1.74	0.0833	0.05
tau	2.2555	0.1217	293	18.54	<.0001	0.05

Parameter	Lower	Upper	Gradient
beta0	-2.1250	-0.9192	-0.00007
beta1	-1.1433	0.3570	-0.00002
beta2	-0.3883	-0.2513	0.000058
beta3	-0.1940	0.01207	0.000319
tau	2.0161	2.4950	-0.00003

As discussed in Section 14.6, the reported standard errors are obtained from the inverse Fisher information matrix. The ratio of the estimate over its standard error produces a t-value that is compared to a t-distribution in order to obtain a formal test of significance. One hereby uses an *ad hoc* number of degrees freedom equal to the number of subjects in the dataset, minus the number of random effects. In our example, this results in t-tests based on $294 - 1 = 293$ degrees of freedom. In case one wishes classical Wald-type tests (Z-tests), these can be obtained by pre-specifying a large number of degrees of freedom. This is done through the 'df=' option in the NLMIXED statement. Based on the chosen t-approximation to the standardized parameter estimate, lower and upper confidence limits are reported based on the $(1 - \text{Alpha})100\%$ confidence level. The default 'Alpha'-value can be changed using the 'alpha=' option in the NLMIXED statement. Finally, the column labeled 'Gradient' contains the first-order derivative of the objective function with respect to each of the parameters in the marginal likelihood. Note that the maximal gradient value of 0.000319 reported previously in the 'Iteration History' table is the gradient value for the parameter β_3, i.e., for the interaction between the time trend and the treatment indicator. Finally, it should be emphasized that, in general, the reported p-values for variance components should be interpreted with great care, due to possible occurrence of boundary problems, as explained in Section 14.6.

15.5 Alternative Software Tools

In this chapter, we have extensively illustrated the use of the SAS package for fitting generalized linear mixed models. Many other statistical software packages offer tools for fitting these models, including HLM (Raudenbush *et al* 2001), EGRET (Cytel Software Corpration 2000), *gllamm* in Stata (Rabe-Hesketh, Pickles, and Skrondal 2001), and MIXOR and MIXREG (Hedeker and Gibbons 1994, 1996).

As discussed in Chapter 14, there is a variety of methods available for fitting generalized linear mixed models. They differ in the type of approximation or in the order of the approximation. When using software, it is therefore very important to be aware of what precisely has been implemented. A full description of software tools can be found in Tuerlinckx *et al* (2004) and in Skrondal and Rabe-Hesketh (2004).

16
Marginal *versus* Random-effects Models

16.1 Introduction

The most frequently used models for discrete repeated measurements are of the marginal or random-effects type, and most of them can be viewed as direct extensions of general linear models introduced in Chapter 3 for independent observations to the context of correlated data. Despite the severe similarities between marginal and random-effects model specifications, both families often produce very different results, confusing many statisticians less familiar with these types of models. The aim of the current chapter is therefore to investigate why such strong differences occur in so many applications. In Section 16.2, marginal and random-effects results are compared for the toenail data. Section 16.3 provides some theoretical arguments about the observed differences between both modeling approaches. Finally, the Sections 16.4 and 16.5 will apply these ideas to the toenail and the NTP data, respectively.

16.2 Example: The Toenail Data

Table 16.1 summarizes the parameter estimates and standard errors for a marginal model and a random-effects model, fitted to the toenail data. Both models include linear time-effects, with treatment-specific intercepts and slopes. The marginal model parameter estimates are obtained using generalized estimating equations (GEE1), where a marginal logit function

TABLE 16.1. *Toenail Data. Parameter estimates (standard errors) for a generalized linear mixed model (GLMM) and a marginal model (GEE), as well as the ratio between both sets of parameters.*

	GLMM	GEE	
Parameter	Estimate (s.e.)	Estimate (s.e.)	Ratio
Intercept group A	−1.63 (0.44)	−0.72 (0.17)	2.26
Intercept group B	−1.75 (0.45)	−0.65 (0.17)	2.69
Slope group A	−0.40 (0.05)	−0.14 (0.03)	2.87
Slope group B	−0.57 (0.06)	−0.25 (0.04)	2.22
SD random intercept (τ)	4.02 (0.38)		

is combined with unstructured working assumptions about the association structure. The random-effects model is of the logistic-normal type, with no other random effects than intercepts with variance τ^2, fitted using adaptive Gaussian quadrature with 50 quadrature points. The models are reparameterized versions for the models used earlier in the Chapters 10 and 15, for the same data. Obviously, both analyses produce very different results in the sense that the estimates from the generalized linear mixed model analysis are much bigger in magnitude.

16.3 Parameter Interpretation

The severe differences in results obtained from marginal and random-effects models follow from the fact that the parameters in both models have completely different interpretations. To see the nature of the difference between both model families, consider a binary outcome variable and assume a random-intercepts logistic model with linear predictor logit$[P(Y_{ij} = 1|b_i)] = \beta_0 + b_i + \beta_1 t$, where t is the time covariate. This model was used in Section 16.2 for each treatment group separately. The conditional means $E(Y_{ij}|b_i)$, as functions of t, are given by

$$E(Y_{ij}|b_i) = \frac{\exp(\beta_0 + b_i + \beta_1 t)}{1 + \exp(\beta_0 + b_i + \beta_1 t)}. \qquad (16.1)$$

The model assumes that the conditional means all satisfy a logistic model, with the same slope β_1 but with different intercepts $\beta_0 + b_i$ for all subjects. The marginal average evolution $E(Y_{ij})$ is obtained from averaging (16.1) over the random effects, i.e.,

$$\begin{aligned} E(Y_{ij}) &= E[E(Y_{ij}|b_i)] \\ &= E\left[\frac{\exp(\beta_0 + b_i + \beta_1 t)}{1 + \exp(\beta_0 + b_i + \beta_1 t)}\right] \end{aligned} \qquad (16.2)$$

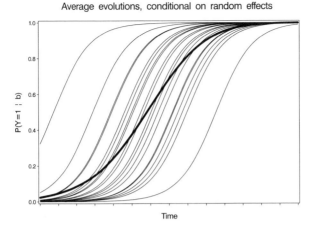

FIGURE 16.1. *Graphical representation of a random-intercepts logistic curve, across a range of levels of the random intercept, together with the corresponding marginal curve.*

$$\neq \frac{\exp(\beta_0 + \beta_1 t)}{1 + \exp(\beta_0 + \beta_1 t)}.$$

A graphical representation of both (16.1) and (16.2) is given in Figure 16.1. Obviously, the marginal time trend is much less steep than each of the individual time trends. Intuitively, it is to be expected that this effect strongly depends on the amount of between-subject variability: In case the random-intercepts variability is large, parameters from fitting marginal models and random-effects models will be very different, while equal parameter values hold if the variance of the random-effects equals zero.

Figure 16.1 clearly shows that the regression parameters in marginal and random-effects models have a completely different inerpretation. Therefore, it may be helpful to denote them differently, such as $\boldsymbol{\beta}^{\mathrm{RE}}$ for the parameter vector in the random-effects model, and $\boldsymbol{\beta}^{\mathrm{M}}$ for the parameter vector in the marginal model. The vector $\boldsymbol{\beta}^{\mathrm{RE}}$ models the evolution of each individual subject separately, whereas $\boldsymbol{\beta}^{\mathrm{M}}$ expresses how, on average, the success probability evolves in the population.

This phenomenon holds more generally for any generalized linear mixed model, and there is no straightforward relation between the parameter vector $\boldsymbol{\beta}^{\mathrm{RE}}$ in the random-effects model and the parameter vector $\boldsymbol{\beta}^{\mathrm{M}}$ in the marginal model, except in a few special cases. For example, consider the linear mixed model introduced in Section 4.3, where the random-effects model $\boldsymbol{Y}_i|\boldsymbol{b}_i \sim N(X_i\boldsymbol{\beta} + Z_i\boldsymbol{b}_i, \Sigma_i)$ implies that, marginally, $\boldsymbol{Y}_i$ has mean $E(Y_{ij}) = E[E(Y_{ij}|b_i)] = X_i\boldsymbol{\beta}$, showing that, in this case $\boldsymbol{\beta}^{\mathrm{RE}} = \boldsymbol{\beta}^{\mathrm{M}}$. Another example is the above discussed logistic model with random intercepts,

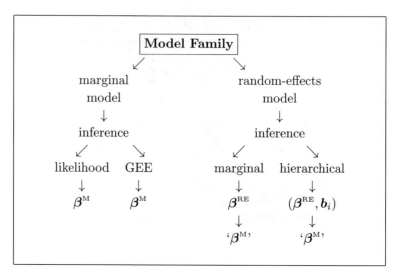

FIGURE 16.2. *Representation of model families and corresponding inferences. A superscript 'M' stands for marginal, 'RE' for random effects. A parameter between quotes indicates that marginal functions but no direct marginal parameters are obtained.*

for which it can be derived that

$$\left|\frac{\beta^{RE}}{\beta^{M}}\right| \approx \sqrt{c^2\tau^2 + 1} > 1 \qquad (16.3)$$

where τ^2 is the variance of the random intercepts and with $c = 16\sqrt{3}/(15\pi)$ (Diggle *et al* 2002, Section 7.4). Note that (16.3) implies our heuristically obtained result that β^{RE} is not smaller than β^{M}, with equality when the random-intercepts variance τ^2 is zero.

The fact that parameters from marginal and random-effects models need to be interpreted completely differently shows that the choice between these model families has important consequences and should be reflected upon very carefully. A schematic display of the possible choices is given in Figure 16.2. Whenever a marginal model is fitted, one directly obtains estimates and inferences for the components in β^{M}, the regression vector that models the average trend in the population. Within this class of approaches, fitting and inference can be based on full maximum likelihood principles, or on methods that only require correct specification of a number of moments (GEE and related methods). In case a random-effects model is fitted, one should realize that, even when estimation and inference is based on likelihood principles for the marginal likelihood (14.2) where the random effects have been integrated out, the parameters keep their original random-effects interpretation, such that estimates as well as inferences are obtained for the components in β^{RE} rather than β^{M}. Note that, under the random-effects model family, one can also obtain inferences for the random effects, under the assumption that the hierarchical model formulation was correct, i.e., under the assumption that the correlation between repeated measurements was indeed implied by an underlying random-effects structure. Alternatively, one may consider the generalized linear mixed model as just one approach to construct a marginal likelihood, without having any interests in possible presence of underlying latent variables b_i.

Note that, because the random-effects approach results in a marginal likelihood, hereby completely specifying the distribution of Y_i, it is possible to derive the marginal average trends in the data. As is indicated in (16.2), this requires averaging the conditional means in (16.1), over the random effects b_i. Again, numerical integration methods can be used, but it is often much easier to use numerical averaging by sampling a large number M of random-effects vectors b_i from their fitted distribution $N(\mathbf{0}, \widehat{D})$, and to estimate $E(Y_{ij})$ at a specific point t in time by

$$\widehat{E}(Y_{ij}) = \frac{1}{M} \sum_i^M \frac{\exp(\widehat{\beta}_0^{\text{RE}} + b_i + \widehat{\beta}_1^{\text{RE}} t)}{1 + \exp(\widehat{\beta}_0^{\text{RE}} + b_i + \widehat{\beta}_1^{\text{RE}} t)}.$$

This can be calculated for a fine grid of time-points t, such that a graphical representation for the average trend can be obtained. An example, including SAS code for averaging over the fitted random-effects distribution can be found in Section 19.4. It should be emphasized that, in general, the average trend $E(Y_{ij})$ is not of the same parametric form as the conditional means $E(Y_{ij}|b_i)$. Hence, the averaging over the random effects will not yield formal estimates for the elements in $\boldsymbol{\beta}^M$. They can only provide a plot of the population-averaged trends. This explains why, in Figure 16.2, the marginal trends obtained from the random-effects approach are indicated as '$\boldsymbol{\beta}^M$.'

16.4 Toenail Data: Marginal *versus* Mixed Models

We reconsider the toenail data, with the results from a GEE analysis and a random-effects analysis summarized in Table 16.1. The generalized linear mixed model is logistic with random intercepts only, hence, the approximate relation (16.3) holds and yields as approximate ratio

$$\sqrt{[16\sqrt{3}/(15\pi)]^2 (4.02)^2 + 1} = 2.56$$

302   16. Marginal *versus* Random-effects Models

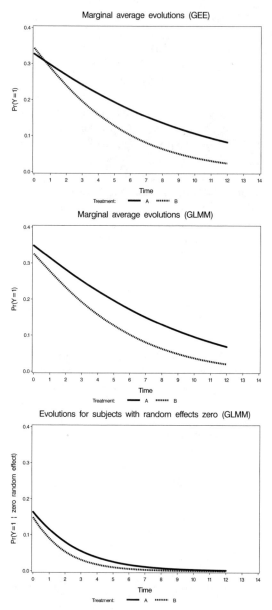

FIGURE 16.3. *Toenail Data. Treatment-arm specific evolutions. (a) Marginal evolutions as obtained from a marginal (GEE) model, (b) marginal evolutions as obtained from integrating out a GLMM, and (c) evolutions for an "average" subject from a GLMM, i.e., a subject with $b_i = 0$.*

16.4 Toenail Data: Marginal versus Mixed Models

which is in line with the observed ratio reported in Table 16.1. The fitted average evolutions, directly obtained from the GEE analysis, are given by

$$P(Y_{ij} = 1) = \begin{cases} \dfrac{\exp(-0.72 - 0.14t)}{1 + \exp(-0.72 - 0.14t)}, & \text{Treatment A} \\[2ex] \dfrac{\exp(-0.65 - 0.25t)}{1 + \exp(-0.65 - 0.25t)}, & \text{Treatment B}, \end{cases}$$

and are shown in the top graph in Figure 16.3. The middle panel of Figure 16.3 shows the marginal trends implied by the mixed model, i.e.,

$$P(Y_{ij} = 1) = \begin{cases} E\left[\dfrac{\exp(-1.63 + b_i - 0.40t)}{1 + \exp(-1.63 + b_i - 0.40t)}\right], & \text{Treatment A} \\[2ex] E\left[\dfrac{\exp(-1.75 + b_i - 0.57t)}{1 + \exp(-1.75 + b_i - 0.57t)}\right], & \text{Treatment B}, \end{cases}$$

where the expectation is taken over the fitted random-effects distribution $N(0, 4.02^2)$. Note that very similar trends are obtained, except maybe early in the study (first 2 months). This may be due to sampling variability, or due to the fact that not all subjects have been followed until the end of the experiment. Indeed, as discussed in Section 2.3, 72 (24%) out of the 298 participants left the study prematurely, due to a variety of, often unknown, reasons. As will be discussed in Part VI, GEE and random-effects analyses make different assumptions about the relation between missingness and the longitudinal response of interest. This may result in (slightly) different fitted average trends. Finally, the bottom plot in Figure 16.3 shows the expected trends for 'average' patients, i.e., for patients with random intercept $b_i = 0$. This again illustrates that, unlike for linear mixed models, the population-averaged trends cannot be obtained by setting random effects in a generalized linear mixed model, equal to zero.

As a summary and conclusion, we now compare the results from various models and estimation techniques applied to the toenail data. Table 16.2 summarizes the results from the marginal model and the random-effects model, considered earlier in Section 16.2: Both models include linear time-effects, with treatment-specific intercepts and slopes. The marginal model parameter estimates are obtained using generalized estimating equations (GEE1), where a marginal logit function is combined with unstructured working assumptions about the association structure. The random-effects model is of the logistic-normal type, with no other random effects than intercepts with variance τ^2. The mixed model has been fitted using MQL and PQL (both with REML for fitting the linear mixed models to the pseudo-data), as well as with adaptive Gaussian quadrature with 50 quadrature points. A selection of the results was shown before in Table 16.1. We now clearly observe that the estimates obtained from PQL and MQL are situated somewhat in between the estimates obtained from QUAD and GEE,

TABLE 16.2. *Toenail Data. Parameter estimates (standard errors) for a generalized linear mixed model and a marginal model (GEE). The mixed model has been fitted using MQL and PQL (both with REML for fitting the linear mixed models to the pseudo-data), as well as with adaptive Gaussian quadrature with 50 quadrature points (QUAD).*

Parameter	QUAD	PQL
Intercept group A	−1.63 (0.44)	−0.72 (0.24)
Intercept group B	−1.75 (0.45)	−0.72 (0.24)
Slope group A	−0.40 (0.05)	−0.29 (0.03)
Slope group B	−0.57 (0.06)	−0.40 (0.04)
Var. random intercepts (τ^2)	15.99 (3.02)	4.71 (0.60)

Parameter	MQL	GEE
Intercept group A	−0.56 (0.17)	−0.72 (0.17)
Intercept group B	−0.53 (0.17)	−0.65 (0.17)
Slope group A	−0.17 (0.02)	−0.14 (0.03)
Slope group B	−0.26 (0.03)	−0.25 (0.04)
Var. random intercepts (τ^2)	2.49 (0.29)	

where MQL is closest to GEE. As has been discussed in Section 14.4, MQL is based on a Taylor series expansion of the mean μ_{ij} around current estimates of the fixed effects and around random effects equal to zero. Therefore it produces estimates relatively close to those from marginal models, which do not contain any random effects at all (i.e., which have all $b_i \equiv 0$). PQL, on the other hand, explicitly accounts for the random effects in its Taylor series expansion and therefore yields estimates closer to those obtained under Gaussian quadrature.

16.5 Analysis of the NTP Data

As discussed in Chapter 13, the generalized linear mixed model (GLMM) is not the only model in the class of random-effects models. An alternative model is the beta-binomial model, introduced in Section 13.4.2. We will now fit a beta-binomial model and compare it to the results obtained from previous analyses. It will be assumed that the success probability π_i and the within-cluster correlation ρ_i satisfy

$$\ln\left(\frac{\pi_i}{1-\pi_i}\right) = \beta_0 + \beta_d d_i \qquad (16.4)$$

$$\ln\left(\frac{1+\rho_i}{1-\rho_i}\right) = \beta_a, \qquad (16.5)$$

16.5 Analysis of the NTP Data

TABLE 16.3. *NTP Data. Parameter estimates (standard errors) for the beta-binomial model, fitted to various outcomes in three studies. β_0 and β_d are the marginal intercept and dose effect, respectively; β_a is the Fisher z transformed correlation; ρ is the correlation.*

Outcome	Parameter	DEHP	EG	DYME
External	β_0	-4.91(0.42)	-5.32(0.71)	-7.27(0.74)
	β_d	5.20(0.59)	2.78(0.81)	8.01(0.82)
	β_a	0.21(0.09)	0.28(0.14)	0.21(0.12)
	ρ	0.10(0.04)	0.14(0.07)	0.10(0.06)
Visceral	β_0	-4.38(0.36)	-7.45(1.17)	-6.21(0.83)
	β_d	4.42(0.54)	4.33(1.26)	4.94(0.90)
	β_a	0.22(0.09)	0.04(0.09)	0.45(0.21)
	ρ	0.11(0.04)	0.02(0.04)	0.22(0.10)
Skeletal	β_0	-4.88(0.44)	-2.89(0.27)	-5.15(0.47)
	β_d	4.92(0.63)	3.42(0.40)	6.99(0.71)
	β_a	0.27(0.11)	0.54(0.09)	0.61(0.14)
	ρ	0.13(0.05)	0.26(0.04)	0.30(0.06)
Collapsed	β_0	-3.83(0.31)	-2.51(0.09)	-5.42(0.45)
	β_d	5.59(0.56)	3.05(0.17)	8.29(0.79)
	β_a	0.32(0.10)	0.28(0.02)	0.33(0.10)
	ρ	0.16(0.05)	0.14(0.01)	0.16(0.05)

where d_i is the dose administered to the ith cluster. Note that this is the same parameterization as was used before for the Bahadur model in Section 7.2.3. Table 16.3 shows the results for the three NTP studies, and for the four different outcomes.

For the sake of comparison, we will focus on the outcome 'External malformations' in the DEHP study. Table 16.4 summarizes the results from analyses based on marginal models (Chapters 7 and 8) conditional models (Chapters 11 and 12), and random-effects models (Chapters 14 and 16). As has been indicated in Section 11.4, estimates for the conditional models are typically considerably smaller than their marginal counterparts, due to the fundamental difference in interpretation. Indeed, conditional-model parameters describe the conditional logit and log odds ratios of outcomes, given other outcomes, whereas in marginal models no such conditioning takes place. A similar argument explains the differences between marginal and random-effects models (Section 16.3).

The results from conditional models are very similar, whatever estimation method is used (maximum likelihood or pseudo-likelihood). The various marginal modeling approaches (Bahadur, various forms of GEE, ALR) provide very similar inferences as well, even though some subtle differ-

TABLE 16.4. *NTP Data. External malformations in the DEHP study. Parameter estimates (standard errors) from analyses based on marginal models (Chapters 7 and 8), conditional models (Chapters 11 and 12), and random-effects models (Chapters 14 and 16). β_0 and β_d are the intercept and dose effect, respectively; the association parameter varies between models.*

Model	β_0	β_d	Association	
Conditional models				
Quadr. loglin. (ML)	-2.81(0.58)	3.07(0.65)	LOG OR	0.18(0.04)
Quadr. loglin. (PL)	-2.85(0.53)	3.24(0.60)	LOG OR	0.18(0.04)
Marginal models				
Lik. Bahadur	-4.93(0.39)	5.15(0.56)	β_a	0.11(0.03)
St. GEE1 (exch)	-4.98(0.37)	5.33(0.55)	ρ	0.11
St. GEE1 (ind)	-5.06(0.38)	5.31(0.57)		
Prent. GEE1 (exch)	-4.99(0.37)	5.32(0.55)	ρ	0.11 (0.04)
Prent. GEE1 (ind)	-5.06(0.38)	5.31(0.57)		
Lin. based (exch)	-5.00(0.37)	5.32(0.55)	ρ	0.06
Lin. based (ind)	-5.06(0.38)	5.31(0.57)		
GEE2	-4.98(0.37)	5.29(0.55)	β_a	0.15(0.05)
ALR	-.516(0.35)	5.64(0.52)	β_a	0.96(0.30)
Random-effects models				
Beta-binomial	-4.91(0.42)	5.20(0.59)	β_a	0.21(0.09)
GLLM (MQL)	-5.18(0.40)	5.70(0.66)	Int. var τ^2	1.20(0.53)
GLMM (PQL)	-5.32(0.40)	5.73(0.65)	Int. var τ^2	0.95(0.40)
GLMM (QUAD)	-5.97(0.57)	6.45(0.84)	Int. var τ^2	1.27(0.62)

ences exist, as was explained throughout the various analyses conducted in Chapter 8. More severe discrepancies are observed when the various random-effects analyses are compared. The differences between MQL, PQL and Gaussian quadrature have been observed and explained before in Section 16.4. However, note how the results from the beta-binomial model are closer to those from the marginal models than to those from the GLMM model under Gaussian quadrature. This can be explained as follows. It follows from (13.4) and (13.5) that the parameters π_i and ρ_i modeled in (16.4) and (16.5) have marginal interpretations. Hence, although the beta-binomial model has a random-effects genesis, the regression coefficients need to be interpreted marginally.

Part V

Case Studies and Extensions

17
The Analgesic Trial

17.1 Introduction

Marginal models, fitted to the analgesic trial, introduced in Section 2.2, more specifically to the binary 'general satisfaction assessment' outcome ('GSABIN,' denoted by Y_{ij}), will be studied in Section 17.2. Section 17.3 describes subject-specific models fitted to the GSABIN outcome. A comparison between both methods is offered in Section 17.4. Some key programs are presented in Section 17.5. We should keep in mind that the actual outcome, GSA, is measured on a five-point ordinal scale. Ordinal outcomes is the topic of Chapter 18, and there also, a number of analyses of the analgesic trial will be offered.

Another issue deserves mention at this point. As is to be expected in patients with severe chronic pain, a good number drops out before the end of the study. Unless the very strong assumption of missingness completely at random (MCAR) is made, GEE is strictly speaking not valid in this case. MCAR is violated as soon as the reason for missingness is outcome related, even when the dependence is on observed outcomes. The missing data concepts are outlined in Chapter 26. Ways to extend GEE to overcome this problem are presented in Chapter 27, where these data will be considered again.

17.2 Marginal Analyses of the Analgesic Trial

The analgesic trial has been introduced in Section 2.2. The primary outcome in this one-armed trial is ordinally scored global satisfaction assessment (GSA). For the purpose of our analysis, we will consider a dichotomized version of (2.1):

$$\text{GSABIN} = \begin{cases} 1 \text{ if GSA} \leq 3 \text{ ('Very Good' to 'Moderate')}, \\ 0 \text{ otherwise.} \end{cases} \quad (17.1)$$

Preliminary analyses have indicated that, among a set of potential covariates, the linear and square effects of time t_{ij}, as well as the effect of baseline pain control assessment ('PCA0,' denoted X_i) are of importance. The marginal regression model so obtained is

$$\text{logit}[P(Y_{ij} = 1 | t_{ij}, X_i)] = \beta_0 + \beta_1 t_{ij} + \beta_2 t_{ij}^2 + \beta_3 X_i. \quad (17.2)$$

Because there are four equally-spaced follow-up measurements, not only independence and exchangeable, but also autoregressive and unstructured working assumptions are consistent with the design of the study. Table 17.1 displays parameter estimates and standard errors for standard GEE (Section 8.2), under a variety of working assumptions. Table 17.2 presents the results for alternating logistic regression (Section 8.6). Table 17.3 summarizes analyses from Tables 17.1 and 17.2 that are based on exchangeable working assumptions, and supplements them with the corresponding fits obtained from ordinary logistic regression, Prentice's method (Section 8.4) and the linearization method (Section 8.8). It is clear from Table 17.1 that all analyses agree closely in terms of parameter estimates and standard errors. Even between the empirically corrected and model-based standard errors, there is little difference. This may be due to the fact that the correlation is relatively small. However, given the size of the dataset, it is likely that the correlation is significantly different from zero. Exploring the correlation in a little more detail, we find for the three non-trivial correlation matrices:

$$R_{\text{EXCH}} = \begin{pmatrix} 1 & 0.22 & 0.22 & 0.22 \\ & 1 & 0.22 & 0.22 \\ & & 1 & 0.22 \\ & & & 1 \end{pmatrix},$$

$$R_{\text{AR}} = \begin{pmatrix} 1 & 0.25 & 0.06 & 0.02 \\ & 1 & 0.25 & 0.06 \\ & & 1 & 0.25 \\ & & & 1 \end{pmatrix},$$

17.2 Marginal Analyses of the Analgesic Trial   311

TABLE 17.1. *Analgesic Trial. Parameter estimates (model-based standard errors; empirically corrected standard errors) for standard GEE under a variety of working assumptions: IND (independence), EXCH (exchangeable), AR (autoregressive), UN (unstructured).*

Effect	Parameter	IND	EXCH
Intercept	β_1	2.80(0.49;0.47)	2.92(0.49;0.46)
Time	β_2	−0.79(0.39;0.34)	−0.83(0.34;0.33)
Time^2	β_3	0.18(0.08;0.07)	0.18(0.07;0.07)
Basel. PCA	β_4	−0.21(0.09;0.10)	−0.23(0.10;0.10)
Correlation	ρ	—	0.22

Effect	Parameter	AR	UN
Intercept	β_1	2.94(0.49;0.47)	2.87(0.48;0.46)
Time	β_2	−0.90(0.35;0.33)	−0.78(0.33;0.32)
Time^2	β_3	0.20(0.07;0.07)	0.17(0.07;0.07)
Basel. PCA	β_4	−0.22(0.10;0.10)	−0.23(0.10;0.10)
Correlation	ρ	0.25	—
Correlation (1,2)	ρ_{12}		0.18
Correlation (1,3)	ρ_{13}		0.25
Correlation (1,4)	ρ_{14}		0.20
Correlation (2,3)	ρ_{23}		0.18
Correlation (2,4)	ρ_{24}		0.18
Correlation (3,4)	ρ_{34}		0.46

and

$$R_{\rm UN} = \begin{pmatrix} 1 & 0.18 & 0.25 & 0.20 \\ & 1 & 0.18 & 0.18 \\ & & 1 & 0.46 \\ & & & 1 \end{pmatrix},$$

with obvious notation. Inspecting $R_{\rm UN}$, it is clear that AR may be a working assumption, different from the true structure. EXCH looks more promising as a simplification to UN, even though it looks like ρ_{34} is higher than the others, while the others might well be equal to one another. Two remarks are in place. First, the above reasoning is irrelevant for the validity of GEE since the working assumptions are allowed to be incorrect, the only aspect that might be jeopardized being efficiency. This is clearly not the case in this analysis. Second, if one were interested in the correlation structure as such, there is no means within the standard GEE framework to make formal inferences about the correlation structure.

To overcome this, let us study the results for ALR in Table 17.2. Apart from exchangeability, an unstructured odds ratio model is assumed (termed

TABLE 17.2. *Analgesic Trial. Parameter estimates and empirically corrected standard errors for ALR under a variety of log odds ratio structure: EXCH (exchangeable), FULLCLUST (unstructured), and ZREP (a user-defined design).*

Effect	Parameter	EXCH	FULLCLUST	ZREP
Intercept	β_1	2.98(0.46)	2.92(0.46)	2.92(0.46)
Time	β_2	-0.87(0.32)	-0.80(0.32)	-0.80(0.32)
Time^2	β_3	0.18(0.07)	0.17(0.06)	0.17(0.07)
Basel. PCA	β_4	-0.23(0.22)	-0.24(0.10)	-0.24(0.10)
Log OR	α	1.43(0.22)		
Log OR(1,2)	α_{12}		1.13(0.33)	
Log OR(1,3)	α_{13}		1.56(0.39)	
Log OR(1,4)	α_{14}		1.60(0.42)	
Log OR(2,3)	α_{23}		1.19(0.37)	
Log OR(2,4)	α_{24}		0.93(0.42)	
Log OR(3,4)	α_{34}		2.44(0.48)	
Log OR par.	α_0			1.26(0.23)
Log OR par.	α_1			1.17(0.47)

'fullclust' in the SAS procedure GENMOD). As stated earlier, the odds ratios now have a standard error associated to them. It is clear that some of our conjectures, based on the correlations in Table 17.1 are confirmed straightaway. For example, the exchangeable log odds ratio is significantly different from zero, and so are all the odds ratios in the unstructured model. There is also a hint that α_{34} is different from the others, with all others being equal. To confirm this, a formal test is necessary. An easy approach is to consider a Wald test for the null hypothesis

$$H_0: \alpha_{12} = \alpha_{13} = \alpha_{14} = \alpha_{23} = \alpha_{24}.$$

A Wald test statistic for this null hypothesis would assume the form

$$W = (C\boldsymbol{\alpha})'(CVC')^{-1}(C\boldsymbol{\alpha})', \qquad (17.3)$$

where $\boldsymbol{\alpha} = (\alpha_{12}, \alpha_{13}, \alpha_{14}, \alpha_{23}, \alpha_{24}, \alpha_{34})'$, C is an appropriate contrast matrix:

$$C = \begin{pmatrix} 1 & -1 & 0 & 0 & 0 & 0 \\ 0 & 1 & -1 & 0 & 0 & 0 \\ 0 & 0 & 1 & -1 & 0 & 0 \\ 0 & 0 & 0 & 1 & -1 & 0 \end{pmatrix}, \qquad (17.4)$$

and V is the asymptotic covariance matrix of the log odds ratio parameters. An estimate for the matrix V is given in the SAS output by way of the

17.2 Marginal Analyses of the Analgesic Trial

'covb' option in the REPEATED statement and equals:

$$\widehat{V} = \begin{pmatrix} 0.107 & 0.023 & 0.023 & 0.030 & 0.033 & 0.008 \\ 0.023 & 0.149 & 0.068 & 0.016 & 0.012 & 0.026 \\ 0.023 & 0.068 & 0.176 & 0.012 & 0.033 & 0.054 \\ 0.030 & 0.016 & 0.012 & 0.135 & 0.074 & 0.032 \\ 0.033 & 0.012 & 0.033 & 0.074 & 0.178 & 0.069 \\ 0.008 & 0.026 & 0.054 & 0.032 & 0.069 & 0.231 \end{pmatrix}. \qquad (17.5)$$

Computing the Wald test statistic (17.3), using the estimated $\alpha_{j_1 j_2}$ parameters, yields $W = 2.04$ (4 d.f., $p = 0.7284$). Hence, the first five log odds ratio parameters can be considered equal. Given this, it is of interest to see whether these common parameters differ from the remaining one, α_{34}. A convenient null hypothesis then is

$$H_0 : \frac{1}{5}(\alpha_{12} + \alpha_{13} + \alpha_{14} + \alpha_{23} + \alpha_{24}) = \alpha_{34}.$$

A corresponding contrast matrix is

$$C = (1, 1, 1, 1, 1, -5). \qquad (17.6)$$

The corresponding Wald test statistic equals $W = 6.35$ (1 d.f., $p = 0.0117$) and hence we can conclude that there is a pair of distinct odds ratios: a common one for the first five, and then the sixth one. Should one test the null hypothesis whether the exchangeable model is a tolerable simplification of the unstructured one, then C in (17.4) would be augmented with an additional row $(0, 0, 0, 0, 1, -1)$ and the corresponding 6 d.f. Wald test statistic equals 8.93 ($p = 0.1119$). This need not be considered a contradiction: the 6 d.f. dilutes the power associated with the single degree of freedom contrast (17.6), by combining it with 5 non-significant contrasts, given by (17.4).

The so-obtained final model is presented in the column labeled 'ZREP' in Table 17.2, where now:

$$\alpha_{12} = \alpha_{13} = \alpha_{14} = \alpha_{23} = \alpha_{24} = \alpha_0,$$
$$\alpha_{34} = \alpha_0 + \alpha_1.$$

At the odds ratio level:

$$\widehat{\psi}_{12} = \widehat{\psi}_{13} = \widehat{\psi}_{14} = \widehat{\psi}_{23} = \widehat{\psi}_{24} = \widehat{\psi}_0 = 3.53,$$
$$\widehat{\psi}_{34} = \widehat{\psi}_0 \cdot \widehat{\psi}_1 = 11.36.$$

Note that the Z-statistic associated with α_0 is highly significant ($p < 0.0001$), even though the estimated value may seem moderate. The Z test for α_1 produces a p-value of $p = 0.0119$, in perfect agreement with the corresponding Wald test, obtained above.

Although not commonly done, we could present the "odds ratio matrices" based on the models in Table 17.2:

$$\Psi_{\text{EXCH}} = \left\{ \begin{array}{cccc} 1 & 4.18 & 4.18 & 4.18 \\ & 1 & 4.18 & 4.18 \\ & & 1 & 4.18 \\ & & & 1 \end{array} \right\},$$

$$\Psi_{\text{UN}} = \left\{ \begin{array}{cccc} 1 & 3.10 & 4.76 & 4.95 \\ & 1 & 3.29 & 2.53 \\ & & 1 & 11.47 \\ & & & 1 \end{array} \right\},$$

and

$$\Psi_{\text{ZREP}} = \left\{ \begin{array}{cccc} 1 & 3.53 & 3.53 & 3.53 \\ & 1 & 3.53 & 3.53 \\ & & 1 & 11.36 \\ & & & 1 \end{array} \right\}.$$

Curly braces are used rather than parentheses, to avoid confusion with a correlation or covariance matrix. In summary, the 'ZREP' structure is adequate for the odds ratios, it is not necessary to spend 6 unstructured parameters. Although exchangeability is off, the discrepancy is not very large, and there certainly is no strong impact on the marginal model parameter estimates.

Clearly, the various GEE methods provide virtually the same fit. Not only the empirically corrected standard errors, but also the model-based ones (not shown here, except for logistic regression), virtually coincide.

17.3 Random-effects Analyses of the Analgesic Trial

In this section, we will consider the random-effects counterparts of (17.2) from Section 17.2:

$$Y_{ij}|b_i \sim \text{Bernoulli}(\pi_{ij}),$$
$$\text{logit}(\pi_{ij}) = \beta_0 + b_i + \beta_1 t_{ij} + \beta_2 t_{ij}^2 + \beta_3 X_i, \qquad (17.7)$$

where notation is used as in Section 14.7, i.e.,

$$\pi_{ij} = \text{logit} P(Y_{ij} = 1|b_i, t_{ij}, X_i).$$

Thus, a random intercept has been added to the linear predictor (17.2), producing a random-intercept logistic regression model. Apart from the

TABLE 17.3. *Analgesic Trial. Parameter estimates (empirically corrected standard errors) for ordinary logistic regression, standard GEE, Prentice's GEE, the linearization-based method, and ALR under exchangeable working assumptions. (The standard errors for logistic regression are the usual, uncorrected ones.)*

Effect	Parameter	Log. regr.	Standard	Prentice
Intercept	β_1	2.80(0.49)	2.92(0.46)	2.94(0.46)
Time	β_2	-0.79(0.39)	-0.83(0.33)	-0.84(0.33)
Time^2	β_3	0.18(0.08)	0.18(0.07)	0.18(0.07)
Basel. PCA	β_4	-0.21(0.09)	-0.23(0.10)	-0.23(0.10)
Correlation	ρ		0.21	0.26(0.05)
Effect	Parameter	Lineariz.	ALR	
Intercept	β_1	2.94(0.46)	2.98(0.46)	
Time	β_2	-0.84(0.33)	-0.87(0.32)	
Time^2	β_3	0.18(0.07)	0.18(0.07)	
Basel. PCA	β_4	-0.23(0.10)	-0.23(0.10)	
Corr.	ρ	0.26(0.04)		
Log OR	α		1.43(0.22)	

NTP data in Section 14.7, similar models were considered for the toenail data in Section 14.8. For the random effect b_i we assume that $b_i \sim N(0, \tau^2)$.

Model (17.7) was fitted to the analgesic trial data using MQL and PQL, combined with REML, by means of the SAS procedure GLIMMIX. Using the SAS procedure NLMIXED, numerical integration was employed, using both non-adaptive and adaptive quadrature, in both cases with 10 and 20 quadrature points. Results are summarized in Table 17.4. The parameter τ, the standard deviation of the random intercept, was included directly into the numerical integration based NLMIXED programs. Its square and associated precision, the variance of the random intercept, was obtained through the delta method. Of course, it is very easy to obtain it by an additional run of the NLMIXED procedure, upon a slight change of the program code. In addition to the SAS-based analyses, we fitted model (17.7) using the MIXOR package and the MLwiN package. The MIXOR program is in the public domain and can be downloaded from

http://www.uic.edu/ hedeker/mixreg.html.

It is developed for mixed-effects ordinal regression analysis, and hence in particular in the binary case, and has been documented extensively in Hedeker and Gibbons (1993, 1994, 1996). It performs numerical integration (Gaussian quadrature) and uses the Newton-Raphson algorithm to maximize the marginal likelihood. Technically, MIXOR is most directly comparable to NLMIXED. This is reflected in the parameter estimates but

TABLE 17.4. *Analgesic Trial. Parameter estimates (standard errors) for generalized linear mixed models, under MQL and PQL (combined with REML) in SAS, PQL1 and PQL2 in MLwiN, as well as with numerical integration, in SAS (I: non-adaptive with 10 quadrature points; II: non-adaptive with 20 quadrature points and adaptive with both 10 and 20 quadrature points) and using MIXOR.*

| | | Integrand approximation | | | |
| | | SAS GLIMMIX | | MLwiN | |
Effect	Par.	MQL	PQL1	PQL1	PQL2
Intercept	β_1	2.91(0.53)	3.03(0.55)	3.02(0.55)	4.07(0.70)
Time	β_2	-0.83(0.39)	-0.87(0.41)	-0.87(0.41)	-1.17(0.48)
Time^2	β_3	0.18(0.08)	0.19(0.08)	0.19(0.08)	0.25(0.10)
Basel. PCA	β_4	-0.22(0.11)	-0.22(0.11)	-0.22(0.11)	-0.31(0.15)
Rand. int s.d.	τ	1.06(0.25)	1.04(0.23)	1.01(0.12)	1.61(0.15)
Rand. int var.	τ^2	1.12(0.53)	1.08(0.48)	1.02(0.25)	2.59(0.47)

| | | Numerical integration | | |
| | | SAS NLMIXED | | |
Effect	Par.	I	II	MIXOR
Intercept	β_1	4.07(0.71)	4.05(0.71)	4.05(0.55)
Time	β_2	-1.16(0.47)	-1.16(0.47)	-1.16(0.45)
Time^2	β_3	0.25(0.09)	0.24(0.09)	0.24(0.10)
Basel. PCA	β_4	-0.30(0.14)	-0.30(0.14)	-0.30(0.15)
Rand. int s.d.	τ	1.60(0.22)	1.59(0.21)	1.59(0.21)
Rand. int var.	τ^2	2.56(0.70)	2.53(0.68)	2.53(0.67)

not entirely in the standard errors, because MIXOR uses an approximation to the (empirical) information matrix, whereas NLMIXED uses numerical derivatives. MLwiN is the successor of an earlier DOS incarnation MLN, and is the implementation of the *multilevel modeling* approach, proposed in Bryk and Raudenbush (1992), Longford (1993), and Goldstein (1995). Kreft and de Leeuw (1998) provide a more informal and introductory approach to the subject. This modeling approach for hierarchical data (and hence in particular longitudinal data) is primarily used and known in the social sciences environment. While the language typically used to describe the model is somewhat different from the linear and generalized linear mixed model formalisms, it is very similar and a wide class of mixed models can be considered within the multilevel paradigm as well.

The MLwiN and MIXOR results are shown in Table 17.4 as well. Note that the MQL approximation is particularly bad in this case, and the parameter estimates are virtually the same as those obtained under GEE (Table 17.3). These results are more extreme than the ones obtained for the NTP data (Table 16.4). The main reason is that in the analgesic trial the number of binary measurements per subject is small, such that the approximations on which MQL and PQL are based do not work particularly well. For more details, see Section 14.4. The results for PQL are a bit better. This phenomenon is generally observed, although the difference between them is often larger. Recall that MQL linearizes the link function around the expected linear predictor, thus effectively bringing the model for the pseudo-data closer to a marginal one than PQL. Between the two PQL1 based estimates, there hardly is a difference. An important difference is seen when switching from PQL1 to PQL2 (see Section 14.3 for details), effectively bringing the results in line with the numerical integration based ones. It is fair to say that even in a case like this, where the number of measurements per subjects is relatively small, PQL2 tends to produce good approximations.

Among the numerical integration based ones, there is little or no difference. First, even though Table 17.4 presents only three columns for this class of methods, six analyses were done. From the four analyses based on the SAS procedure NLMIXED, three coincide within the reported precision, with only non-adaptive quadrature and 10 quadrature points giving a slightly different result. The MIXOR based estimates are identical, within the reported precision, to the ones form SAS, group II. The only difference is seen in the standard errors: whereas SAS bases its estimates upon Fisher's information matrix, MIXOR uses an approximation. For more details, see the MIXOR website.

17.4 Comparing Marginal and Random-effects Analyses

In Section 17.2, we presented several marginal analyses and offered a comparison among them. The key message is that the results are very similar. In Section 17.3, random effects analyses were offered, based on the corresponding model. The numerical integration based methods are virtually identical, and so are the PQL2 based ones. MQL and PQL1 produce relatively poor approximations in this case.

When comparing marginal with random effects analyses, the discussion offered in Chapter 16 should be kept in mind. A key warning is that the two model families are rather different, and that the parameters have to be interpreted differently. This was exemplified in Sections 16.4 and 16.5. Nevertheless, for a random-intercept logistic regression, like the one considered here, (16.3) can be used to calculate an approximation to the ratio between the two sets of parameters. Using standard GEE1 from Table 17.3 and the integration based estimates from Table 17.4, the approximate factor from (16.3) is 1.37, the ratios between the two sets of parameter estimates are

318   17. The Analgesic Trial

(1.39, 1.40, 1.33, 1.30), and the corresponding ratios between the standard errors are (1.54, 1.42, 1.29, 1.40), providing good agreement between both.

17.5 Programs for the Analgesic Trial

In this section, we will present a few key programs for the analgesic trial.

17.5.1 Marginal Models with SAS

A standard GEE1 program, with unstructured working assumptions, linear and quadratic effects of time as well as an effect of baseline pain control assessment, is given by:

```
proc genmod data=m.gsa descending;
  class patid timecls;
  model gsabin = time|time pca0 / dist=b;
  repeated subject=patid / withinsubject=timecls
                  type=un covb corrw modelse;
run;
```

The corresponding ALR program would change the repeated statement to

```
repeated subject=patid / withinsubject=timecls
                logor=fullclust covb corrw modelse;
```

The empirically corrected estimates for the latter case are

Analysis Of GEE Parameter Estimates
Empirical Standard Error Estimates

Parameter	Estimate	Standard Error	95% Confidence Limits		Z	Pr > |Z|
Intercept	2.9219	0.4583	2.0237	3.8201	6.38	<.0001
TIME	-0.7980	0.3207	-1.4266	-0.1694	-2.49	0.0128
TIME*TIME	0.1683	0.0648	0.0412	0.2953	2.60	0.0094
pca0	-0.2359	0.0960	-0.4241	-0.0478	-2.46	0.0140
Alpha1	1.1280	0.3278	0.4856	1.7705	3.44	0.0006
Alpha2	1.5631	0.3865	0.8056	2.3206	4.04	<.0001
Alpha3	1.6035	0.4192	0.7819	2.4251	3.83	0.0001
Alpha4	1.1864	0.3680	0.4652	1.9077	3.22	0.0013
Alpha5	0.9265	0.4218	0.0997	1.7533	2.20	0.0281
Alpha6	2.4387	0.4805	1.4970	3.3805	5.08	<.0001

Note, again, that a single panel contains both the marginal regression β parameters and the log odds ratio α parameters. The asymptotic covariance matrix panel (not shown) can be used directly to construct Wald tests. Note that, while there is a CONTRAST statement in the GENMOD procedure, it does not support the use of the α parameters, even though it does support typical linear contrasts of β parameters, whether in the cross-sectional case, GEE, or ALR.

In Table 17.2, a user-defined log odds ratio structure was considered, where all of them where set equal to each other, except α_{34}, which was allowed to have an excess. The REPEATED statement for this case is

```
repeated subject=patid / withinsubject=timecls
                  logor=zrep(
                        (1 2) 1 0,
                        (1 3) 1 0,
                        (2 3) 1 0,
                        (2 4) 1 0,
                        (3 4) 1 1
                        )
                  covb modelse;
```

The 'logor=zrep( )' option allows a flexible linear structure on the α parameters, producing a large number of covariance structures and providing flexibility to choose the most convenient one from among equivalent parameterizations. For example, changing the last line to (3 4) 0 1 would specify α_2 to be the log odds ratio for the last pair, rather than the difference between that one and the earlier ones. A serial structure can be mimicked by means of this option. For example,

```
logor=zrep((1 2) 1,
           (1 3) 0.5,
           (1 4) 0.3333,
           (2 3) 1,
           (2 4) 0.5,
           (3 4) 1)
```

would produce odds ratios of the form

$$\psi_{j_1 j_2} = e^{\frac{1}{j_2-j_1}\alpha} = \psi^{\frac{1}{j_2-j_1}},$$

and these diminish as the time interval between measurements increases, when $\psi > 1$.

Returning to the earlier program, the corresponding estimates are

```
              Analysis Of GEE Parameter Estimates
                Empirical Standard Error Estimates

                        Standard    95% Confidence
Parameter  Estimate     Error        Limits              Z Pr > |Z|
```

Intercept	2.9215	0.4607	2.0186	3.8244	6.34	<.0001
TIME	-0.8021	0.3215	-1.4323	-0.1720	-2.49	0.0126
TIME*TIME	0.1701	0.0650	0.0427	0.2975	2.62	0.0089
pca0	-0.2351	0.0958	-0.4229	-0.0474	-2.46	0.0141
Alpha1	1.2640	0.2309	0.8115	1.7166	5.47	<.0001
Alpha2	1.1719	0.4660	0.2584	2.0853	2.51	0.0119

We see at a glance that both α parameters are significant.

For completeness, let us present a program for the linearization-based method (Section 8.8), using the GLIMMIX macro,

```
%glimmix(data=gsa, procopt=%str(method=ml noclprint),
    stmts=%str(
        class patid timecls;
        model gsabin = time|time pca0 / solution;
        repeated timecls / sub=patid type=un rcorr=3;
    ),
    error=binomial,
    link=logit);
```

The option 'rcorr=3' is added to the REPEATED statement, and not 'rcorr,' since the first two subjects have incomplete follow-up, and hence only a particular upper left block of the entire working correlation matrix would be given. The GLIMMIX procedure counterpart is

```
proc glimmix data=gsa method=RSPL empirical;
class patid timecls;
model gsabin (event='1') = time|time pca0
                        / dist=binary solution;
random _residual_ / subject=patid type=un;
run;
```

17.5.2 Random-effects Models with SAS

Shifting attention to the random-effects models, the MQL analysis is obtained using the GLIMMIX procedure code:

```
proc glimmix data=m.gsa method=RMPL;
class patid timecls;
model gsabin (event='1') = time|time pca0
                        / dist=binary solution;
random intercept / subject=patid type=un;
run;
```

Clearly, changing the method via 'method=RSPL' produces the PQL version. The integration-based methods are obtained using code of the form:

```
proc nlmixed data=m.gsa qpoints=10 noad;
```

17.5 Programs for the Analgesic Trial

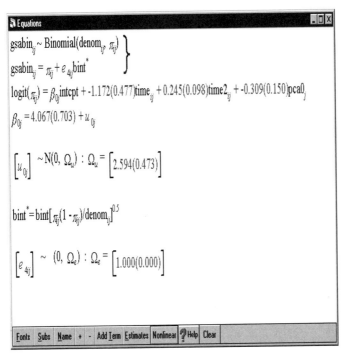

FIGURE 17.1. *Analgesic Trial. MLwIN Program for PQL2 without overdispersion parameter.*

```
parms beta0=4 beta1=-1 beta2=0.25 beta3=-0.25 tau=1.5;
theta = beta0 + b + beta1*time + beta2*time2 + beta3*pca0;
exptheta = exp(theta);
p = exptheta/(1+exptheta);
model gsabin ~ binary(p);
random b ~ normal(0,tau**2) subject=patid;
run;
```

Again, changing the 'qpoints=' option in the PROC NLMIXED statement, combined with inclusion or omission of the 'noad' option in the same statements, produces all of the analyses discussed in Section 17.3. When a probit rather than a logit link is desired, one merely adds the option 'link=probit' to the GENMOD and GLIMMIX programs. Here, however, one should remove the 'exptheta=' programming statement and replace the definition of p by 'p = probnorm(theta).'

17.5.3 MIXOR

A small portion of the output, obtained when calling MIXOR, is:

```
MIXOR - The program for mixed-effects ordinal regression analysis
          (version 2)

Global Satisfaction Assessment
Response function: logistic
Random-effects distribution: normal

------------------------------------------------------------
* Final Results - Maximum Marginal Likelihood Estimates *
------------------------------------------------------------

Total Iterations    =   10
Quad Pts per Dim    =   20
Log Likelihood      =   -506.275
Deviance (-2logL)   =   1012.549
Ridge               =   0.000

Variable       Estimate    Stand. Error          Z           p-value
--------       --------    ------------       --------      ----------
intcpt          4.04741       0.71278          5.67835      0.00000  (2)
Time           -1.16003       0.47453         -2.44457      0.01450  (2)
Time2           0.24449       0.09678          2.52624      0.01153  (2)
PCA0           -0.29971       0.15375         -1.94932      0.05126  (2)

Random effect variance term (standard deviation)
intcpt          1.59139       0.20578          7.73355      0.00000  (1)

note: (1) = 1-tailed p-value
      (2) = 2-tailed p-value
```

At the end, an estimate of an approximate intracluster correlation is presented, based on both the random-intercept variance and the variance of the standard logistic density ($\pi^2/3$).

```
Calculation of the intracluster correlation
-------------------------------------------
residual variance = pi*pi / 3 (assumed)
cluster  variance = (1.591 * 1.591) =  2.533

intracluster correlation =  2.533 / ( 2.533 + (pi*pi/3)) = 0.435
```

However, the basis for this calculation is not very strong and caution is needed with its use (Laenen et al 2004). These authors suggested it is better to calculate an intraclass correlation coefficient based on the observed outcomes, rather than in terms of the latent variable. However, in most cases no constant would be obtained, not even when there is a random intercept only.

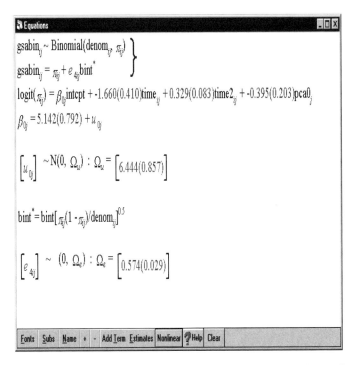

FIGURE 17.2. *Analgesic Trial. MLwiN Program for PQL2 with overdispersion parameter.*

17.5.4 MLwiN

MLwiN is a windows-driven program. The model is constructed in algebraic format, whereafter the unknown parameters are estimated. A random-intercepts logistic model would be called a two-level model within this setting, where the levels refer to the subject level on the one hand and the measurement within subject level on the other hand. There is a wide variety of options available for such aspects as the estimation method, the presence or absence of overdispersion, etc. Two example programs are provided in Figures 17.1–17.2.

18
Ordinal Data

Ordinal data are a specific form of categorical data, where the order of the response categories is of importance. Examples are levels of satisfaction, such as in the 'global satisfaction assessment' (GSA) outcome of the analgesic trial, introduced in Section 2.2 and analyzed in Chapter 17. However, Chapter 17 restricted attention to the binary outcome GSABIN, obtained by collapsing GSA as in (17.1). Another example of ordinal outcomes is found in the fluvoxamine trial (Section 2.4) and analyzed, among other places, in Chapter 6. In fact, Chapter 6 introduced conditional and marginal models for repeated ordinal outcomes, as was the case in Chapter 7, with in particular the multivariate probit model (Section 7.6) and the multivariate Dale model (Section 7.7). These models were then studied in particular for binary data.

In Chapter 8, generalized estimating equations were introduced and applied in particular to repeated binary outcomes. The same was true for the generalized linear mixed models of Chapter 14. Most of the methodology introduced can be used in a variety of settings, in particular if the corresponding univariate versions can be put within the generalized linear model framework (Chapter 3).

Although, as stated earlier, ordinal outcomes can be seen as an extension of binary outcomes, and although models do extend, there are a number of issues specific to the ordinal data case. Some of these will be reviewed in Section 18.1. Section 18.2 discusses marginal models, by referring back to Chapters 6 and 7 where full likelihood methods for ordinal data have been discussed already, and by then putting some emphasis on generalized estimating equations. Random-effects models are the subject of Section 18.3.

Both marginal and random-effects models, fitted to the original version of the 'global satisfaction assessment' outcome of the analgesic trial (Chapter 17), are presented in Section 18.4. A brief overview of the corresponding SAS programs is provided in Section 18.5.

18.1 Regression Models for Ordinal Data

Regression models for binary data have been extended to nominal and ordinal categorical outcomes (Agresti 2002). Let us concentrate on ordinal outcomes. Later on, we will briefly consider nominal data too. Assume that the binary variable $Y_i \in \{0, 1\}$ is replaced by an ordinal one taking values $Y_i \in \{1, 2, \ldots, c\}$. Consider the case of a single covariate x_i. A predictor, linear in the covariate, would take the following form in the binary case:

$$\text{logit}[P(Y_i = 1|x_i)] = \alpha + \beta x_i. \tag{18.1}$$

A commonly used extension of logistic regression to this case is so-called *proportional odds* logistic regression:

$$\text{logit}[P(Y_i \leq k|x_i)] = \alpha_k + \beta x_i, \quad k = 1, \ldots, c-1. \tag{18.2}$$

In (18.2), the probability of observing a lower response *versus* a higher one is modeled. The term *proportional odds* derives from the fact that the odds for a unit increase in an element of x_i are equal to $\exp(\beta)$, irrespective of the cutoff, yielding nice interpretational properties and elegance *provided the model is correctly specified*. The latter is important and fundamentally different from logistic regression. To see this, consider a logistic regression as in (18.1) with x_i binary and taking values 0 or 1. For each of the two levels of x_i, there is then one parameter, the probability of success given x_i. Because (18.1) contains two free parameters, the model is saturated and, in this case, logistic regression is merely a convenient way to model the two probabilities and the difference between them, thereby assuring that for all values of α and β valid (i.e., within the unit interval) probabilities are obtained. Of course, when several covariates, of various types are considered, logistic regression for binary data is based on assumptions too and there is a risk to misspecify the model.

In case of (18.2), there are $2c - 2$ free probabilities, implying that the c free parameters impose model constraints. An obvious extension would be to allow for category dependent effects β_k ($k = 1, \ldots, c-1$). This model is saturated and can be used as a starting point for model simplification, in this simple contingency table setting.

With continuous covariates, the situation is different. Assuming x_i is continuous, and the fit of model (18.2) is inadequate (assessed, for example, using a score test, as is routinely done in the SAS procedure GENMOD),

18.1 Regression Models for Ordinal Data

one could, in principle, let the covariate effects be category dependent. However, the consequence is that there always exist regions in the covariate space, for any combination of the parameters, where non-valid probabilities would be obtained. Indeed, it is easy to see that the conditions for valid probabilities

$$\alpha_k + \beta_k x_i \leq \alpha_{k+1} + \beta_{k+1} x_i, \qquad k = 1, \ldots, c-1,$$

impose $c-1$ linear inequality constraints. Depending on the signs of $\beta_{k+1} - \beta_k$, the resulting allowable space can be a finite or infinite interval. The only way in which to remove the constraints is by setting the β_k parameters equal, i.e., proportional odds regression.

In case the resulting allowable interval for x_i, for a given set of parameters, corresponds to a scientifically plausible range, the model could still be used. Thus, in general, it is important to realize that there ought to be a careful discussion, when using ordinal data logistic regression, considering the pros and cons in terms of plausibility, flexibility, and constraints.

Of course, (18.2) is not the only ordinal logistic regression type model. Alternatively, one can consider the multigroup logistic model (Albert and Lesaffre 1986), where each category is referred to the baseline category. Such a model is mathematically more convenient because it avoids parameter space violations and fits within the exponential family framework, but it does not exploit the ordinal nature of the data, having been conceived for nominal data. It may lead to less parsimonious models and, more importantly, to difficulties in extracting relevant conclusions from the data.

Another approach is to consider *continuation-ratio models*:

$$\text{logit}[P(Y_i > k | Y_i \geq k, x_i)] = \alpha_k + \beta_k x_i, \qquad k = 1, \ldots, c-1. \qquad (18.3)$$

This model has been given some attention in the literature (Agresti 2002). Such a model might be convenient and useful for subjects that gradually go through a number of states, where no return is possible (e.g., cancer stages). Fitting the model is easy because (18.3) consists of $c - 1$ separate logistic regressions; only a straightforward expansion of the data is necessary to prepare them for standard calls to logistic regression software.

Nevertheless, while this model might be a convenient option for *directionally* ordered categorical data, it is *not* so when the direction of the ordering is immaterial. This is the case, for example, when a 5-point scale, ranging from 'very bad' to 'very good' can just as well be reversed: 'very good' to 'very bad.' Reversing the coding in such a case merely changes the signs of the parameters involved in the case of proportional odds logistic regression, but it fundamentally changes the model in the continuation-ratio case. Not only is there no simple transformation between the parameters, significance may change as well and the likelihood at maximum can be different. This is one of the most dramatic instances, in the case of univariate logistic regression for ordinal data, where consideration of a particular model is not just open to criticism, but actually totally meaningless in a number of cases.

TABLE 18.1. *Fluvoxamine Trial. Proportional odds (PO) and continuation-ratio logistic regression models fitted to side effects at the first follow-up visit, with covariates duration and severity.*

Effect	Parameter	PO	Continuation-ratio	
		Side effects coded $1 \longrightarrow 4$		
Intercepts	α_1	-1.63(0.73)	-1.36(0.62)	-1.38(0.80)
	α_2	0.53(0.73)	0.12(0.62)	-0.36(1.11)
	α_3	1.69(0.75)	-0.29(0.66)	0.98(1.75)
Duration	β	0.016(0.005)	0.013(0.004)	
	β_1			0.016(0.006)
	β_2			-0.25(0.16)
	β_3			0.011(0.006)
Severity	γ	-0.29(0.14)	-0.24(0.12)	
	γ_1			-0.33(0.22)
	γ_2			0.0096(0.0109)
	γ_3			0.037(0.349)
		Side effects coded $4 \longrightarrow 1$		
Intercepts	α_1	-1.69(0.75)	-1.79(0.70)	-1.56(1.65)
	α_2	-0.53(0.73)	-1.07(0.69)	-0.34(1.25)
	α_3	1.63(0.73)	1.24(0.69)	0.82(0.88)
Duration	β	-0.016(0.005)	-0.014(0.004)	
	β_1			-0.020(0.008)
	β_2			0.34(0.33)
	β_3			-0.013(0.007)
Severity	γ	0.29(0.14)	0.27(0.13)	
	γ_1			0.41(0.25)
	γ_2			-0.012(0.007)
	γ_3			0.18(0.17)

18.1.1 The Fluvoxamine Trial

We will illustrate the points made about logistic regression for ordinal data, using the outcome side effects at the first follow-up visit from the fluvoxamine trial. For the sake of illustration, we will consider two covariates: prior duration of the disease and initial severity. Table 18.1 displays the results from one proportional odds logistic regression model and two continuation-ratio models. In the first model, the covariate effects are independent from the cutpoints, in the second case they do depend upon it. For all three models, the ordinal outcome severity is coded in two ways: from no side effect to the most severe level and vice versa.

The proportional odds logistic regression has been fitted using the SAS procedure LOGISTIC, while, using the NLMIXED procedure in SAS, the various continuation-ratio models have been coded upward. As stated earlier, the proportional odds parameters are coding invariant up to the sign, while the continuation-ratio models, irrespective of whether the covariate effects are assumed either common to the cutpoint or rather cutpoint-specific, produce parameters that depend in a non-trivial way on whether the outcome is coded upward or downward. This would be a problem in most situations. A noteworthy exception is when a subject or unit evolves through the categories in only one of the two senses. For example, in oncology, there are situations where cancer type would evolve from milder to more severe categories, but not the other way around. Thus, more than ever, when this model is going to be used, careful reflection on its sense is necessary.

18.2 Marginal Models for Repeated Ordinal Data

Likelihood-based marginal models have been introduced in Chapters 6 and 7. For several of these fully likelihood-based models, the general categorical case has been considered, such as for the probit (Section 7.6) and Dale models (Section 7.7), then producing the models for binary outcomes as a general case. In fact, the same holds true for the Goodman model (Section 6.2), which is a conditionally oriented model.

For the likelihood-based models for ordinal data, it is clear that the association structure can, in principle, be modeled in a more versatile way than with binary data. For example, the correlation structure, underlying the multivariate probit model, as well as the global odds ratio structure of the Dale model and the local odds ratio structure of Goodman's model, can be modeled in terms of covariates on the one hand, but also in terms of row and column effects, when the association is between two outcomes, or higher-order cell effects in case of higher-order association. In Section 7.6.1, such elaborate association modeling for longitudinal ordinal data were exemplified using the BIRNH study.

Chapter 8 was devoted to generalized estimating equations, an important non fully likelihood based method for the analysis of repeated or otherwise correlated measurements. In fact, the methodology was introduced, not just for binary data, but in fact in its full generality. This means that all generalized linear model settings are encompassed, including normal, binary, categorical, and count data.

Because the theory has been introduced in the most general form, the question might arise as to why it is necessary to study the ordinal case in particular. The specificity comes from the fact that it is not adequate to model directly an ordinal outcome Y_{ij} for subject $i = 1, \ldots, N$ at measurement occasion $j = 1,\ldots,n_i$, and taking values $k = 1,\ldots,c$. Rather, one has to pass to the binary or dummy variables (6.1), which we will denote here Z_{ijk}, with i, j, and k as before. This allows us to model $P(Y_{ij} \leq k|X_i) = E(Z_{ijk}|X_i)$. Since in a set of dummy variables there is always a redundant one, in this cumulative case $Z_{ijc} \equiv 1$, we need only $c-1$ rather than c. Of course, in the binary case, $c-1 = 2-1 = 1$, and hence in this special case Y_{ij} can just as well be used directly, which is what we did in Chapter 8. Thus, in the general case, the vector $\boldsymbol{Y}_i$ contains n_i components, but the vector $\boldsymbol{Z}_i$ made up of all non-redundant Z_{ijk} will contain $(c-1)\cdot n_i$ components. Obviously, we assume that c is constant across repeated outcomes. While in principle we can consider c_j rather than c categories, useful for multivariate outcomes, we will assume, without loss of generality, that the number of categories is constant across measurement occasions. This is natural in the case of longitudinal data, where typically the same response variable is measured repeatedly over time.

Thus, in the light of the discussion in Section 18.1, the proportional odds model (18.2) is a sensible choice for the repeated outcomes. In the spirit of standard GEE (Section 8.2), a specification of the working correlation structure is needed. Since GEE1 requires the specification of the pairwise correlation structure only, this means between all pairs $(Z_{ijk}, Z_{ij'k'})$, with $j \neq j'$ and/or $k \neq k'$. Unlike in the binary case, some correlations follow directly from the marginal mean vectors: the correlation between different indicators for the same measurement occasions is determined from the mean structure. Let us start from the well-known fact that:

$$\text{Cov}(\boldsymbol{Z}^*_{ij}) = \text{diag}(\boldsymbol{\mu}^*_{ij}) - \boldsymbol{\mu}^*_{ij}(\boldsymbol{\mu}^*_{ij})',$$

where $\boldsymbol{Z}^*_{ij} = (Z^*_{ij1},\ldots,Z^*_{ijc})$. Now, given the linear relationship between $\boldsymbol{Z}^*_{ij}$ and $\boldsymbol{Z}_{ij}$, in the sense that

$$\boldsymbol{Z}_{ij} = \mathcal{J}\boldsymbol{Z}^*_{ij}$$

with

$$\mathcal{J} = \begin{pmatrix} 1 & 0 & 0 & \cdots & 0 \\ 1 & 1 & 0 & \cdots & 0 \\ 1 & 1 & 1 & \cdots & 0 \\ \vdots & \vdots & \vdots & \ddots & \vdots \\ 1 & 1 & 1 & \cdots & 1 \end{pmatrix}.$$

Thus,

$$\text{Cov}(\boldsymbol{Z}_{ij}) = \mathcal{J}\left[\text{diag}(\boldsymbol{\mu}^*_{ij}) - \boldsymbol{\mu}^*_{ij}(\boldsymbol{\mu}^*_{ij})'\right]\mathcal{J}',$$

producing

$$\text{Cov}(\boldsymbol{Z}_{ij}) = \mathcal{M}_{ij} - \boldsymbol{\mu}_{ij}\boldsymbol{\mu}'_{ij},$$

with $\mathcal{M}_{ij,k\ell} = \mu_{i,j,\min(k,\ell)}$, i.e., a bordered matrix with the kth border equal to μ_{ijk}:

$$\mathcal{M}_{ij} = \begin{pmatrix} \mu_{ij1} & \mu_{ij1} & \mu_{ij1} & \cdots & \mu_{ij1} \\ \mu_{ij1} & \mu_{ij2} & \mu_{ij2} & \cdots & \mu_{ij2} \\ \mu_{ij1} & \mu_{ij2} & \mu_{ij3} & \cdots & \mu_{ij3} \\ \vdots & \vdots & \vdots & \ddots & \vdots \\ \mu_{ij1} & \mu_{ij2} & \mu_{ij3} & \cdots & \mu_{ijc} \end{pmatrix}.$$

For the others, working assumptions have to be made. Clearly, such structures will be more involved than in the binary case. Kenward, Lesaffre, and Molenberghs (1994) describe some particular structures. An easy choice is, of course, working independence, and this is the only structure available in the GENMOD procedure in SAS Version 9.1.

18.3 Random-effects Models for Repeated Ordinal Data

In agreement with the marginal-model version of the previous section, random-effects models can be formulated for the ordinal case too. For example, a random-effects version of the proportional-odds model (18.2) would take the form:

$$\text{logit}[P(Y_{ij} \leq k | X_i, Z_i)] = \alpha_k + x'_{ij}\boldsymbol{\beta} + z'_{ij}\boldsymbol{b}_i, \qquad k = 1, \ldots, c-1, \quad (18.4)$$

where X_i and Z_i are the usual design matrices for the fixed effects and random effects, respectively, x_{ij} and z_{ij} are the rows corresponding to the jth measurement occasion, and $\boldsymbol{\beta}$ and $\boldsymbol{b}_i$ are the usual vectors of fixed and random parameters. The only difference is that we have singled out the fixed intercepts, which are category (i.e., cutpoint) dependent. This choice implies that there are no intercept parameters in the vector $\boldsymbol{\beta}$. It would not be a problem to integrate them into the fixed-effects design matrix X_i, ensuring there is no difference between a random-effects model for ordinal data and a general one, such as described in Chapter 14. The most convenient way to represent a model of this type would be by stacking all cumulative indicators Z_{ijk} into a vector $\boldsymbol{Z}_i$ and then write

$$\text{logit}[E(\boldsymbol{Z}_i|X_i, Z_i, \boldsymbol{\beta}, \boldsymbol{b}_i)] = X_i\boldsymbol{\beta} + Z_i\boldsymbol{b}_i. \qquad (18.5)$$

Of course, a proportional odds model follows as a special case of (18.5), by ensuring all covariate effects are common for a given measurement occasion j, independent of the cutpoint k.

18.4 Ordinal Analysis of the Analgesic Trial

The original outcome in the analgesic trial, of which a binary version was analyzed in Chapter 17, is on a five-point ordinal scale:

$$GSA = \begin{cases} 1 & : \text{Very Good} \\ 2 & : \text{Good} \\ 3 & : \text{Moderate} \\ 4 & : \text{Bad} \\ 5 & : \text{Very Bad} \end{cases} \qquad (18.6)$$

Cross-sectional, i.e., classical, ordinal logistic regression (Section 18.1), generalized estimating equations (Section 18.2), and generalized linear mixed models (Section 18.3) can be fitted without any difficulty to the ordinal outcome (18.6), for example using the SAS procedures GENMOD, GLIMMIX, and NLMIXED. The ordinal marginal equivalent to (17.2) would be

$$\text{logit}[P(Y_{ij} \leq k|t_{ij}, X_i)] = \alpha_k + \beta_2 t_{ij} + \beta_3 t_{ij}^2 + \beta_4 X_i, \qquad (18.7)$$

($k = 1, \ldots, 4$), while a random-intercepts counterpart is given by:

$$\text{logit}[P(Y_{ij} \leq k|t_{ij}, X_i, b_i)] = \alpha_k + b_i + \beta_2 t_{ij} + \beta_3 t_{ij}^2 + \beta_4 X_i, \qquad (18.8)$$

($k = 1, \ldots, 4$).

Results of fitting ordinary logistic regression (i.e., as if data were cross-sectional), standard GEE, and generalized linear mixed models are presented in Table 18.2. Whereas Tables 17.1–17.4 contain a single intercept parameter β_1, there now are four cutpoint-specific intercepts $\alpha_1, \ldots, \alpha_4$. The remaining regression parameters are still labeled β_2, β_3, and β_4, to stress the correspondence to their binary counterparts in Tables 17.1–17.4. As in the binary case, the parameters from the random-intercepts model are larger, in absolute value, than their marginal counterparts. Strictly speaking, relationship (16.3) has been derived for the random-intercept binary logistic regression setting only. However, because a proportional odds logistic regression collapses, at every cutpoint, to a binary logistic regression, the relationship can be applied here as well. Applying (16.3) to the numerical integration based variance yields 1.59. The empirical ratios between the numerical integration based and standard GEE parameters are (1.56, 1.98, 1.68, 1.53, 2.70, 2.20, 1.52). Although these values lie around 1.59, there is much more variability in the ratios than was the case for the binary outcome. One of the reasons might be that the proportional odds assumption is not properly verified. Indeed, comparing parameter estimates in Tables 17.1–17.4 with their counterparts in Table 18.2, it is clear that substantial differences are seen. In cases where the proportional odds assumptions is verified, the binary models are submodels of the ordinal one, implying that parameters corresponding to regression effects such as the

TABLE 18.2. *Analgesic Trial. Parameter estimates (standard errors) for marginal models [ordinary logistic regression (OLR), and standard GEE) and random-effects models (using MQL, PQL, and numerical integration (N.Int.)]. For GEE, model-based and empirically corrected standard errors are given.*

		Marginal models	
Effect	Parameter	OLR	GEE
Intercept 1	α_1	-1.00(0.34)	-1.00(0.34;0.35)
Intercept 2	α_2	0.52(0.34)	0.52(0.34;0.36)
Intercept 3	α_3	2.32(0.35)	2.32(0.34;0.37)
Intercept 4	α_4	4.05(0.38)	4.05(0.37;0.39)
Time	β_2	-0.20(0.27)	-0.20(0.27;0.20)
Time^2	β_3	0.05(0.05)	0.05(0.05;0.04)
Basel. PCA	β_4	-0.21(0.06)	-0.21(0.06;0.09)

		Random-effects models		
Effect	Parameter	MQL	PQL	N.Int.
Intercept 1	α_1	-0.93(0.40)	-1.44(0.50)	-1.56(0.55)
Intercept 2	α_2	0.60(0.39)	0.51(0.50)	1.03(0.54)
Intercept 3	α_3	2.39(0.40)	3.47(0.51)	3.89(0.56)
Intercept 4	α_4	4.13(0.42)	5.63(0.54)	6.21(0.60)
Time	β_2	-0.30(0.28)	-0.48(0.30)	0.54(0.31)
Time^2	β_3	0.06(0.06)	0.10(0.06)	-0.11(0.06)
Basel. PCA	β_4	-0.21(0.09)	-0.28(0.12)	0.32(0.14)
Rand. int s.d.	τ	1.06(0.08)	1.88(0.11)	2.11(0.14)
Rand. int var.	τ^2	1.13(0.16)	3.53(0.42)	4.44(0.60)

linear and quadratic effects of time, and the effect of baseline pain control assessment, would roughly be the same. Obviously, this is not the case here. The random-effects variance τ^2 is estimated to be quite a bit larger than in the binary case, pointing in the direction of a non-valid proportional odds assumption. Relaxing the proportional odds assumption is relatively easy with, for example, the procedure NLMIXED.

Once again, note that the MQL parameters are very close to their marginal counterparts, underscoring the poor quality of the approximation. PQL performs a lot better than MQL and results are close to the numerical integration counterparts. Regarding numerical integration, adaptive Gaussian quadrature was used with 20 quadrature points. Results were the same, up to four decimal places, when only 10 quadrature points were used. For as few as 3 quadrature points, only small differences were observed.

18.5 Programs for the Analgesic Trial

In accordance with Section 17.5, we will now briefly review the corresponding SAS programs. Standard logistic regression is easy enough to conduct with the SAS procedure GENMOD:

```
proc genmod data=m.gsa;
  class patid timecls;
  model gsa = time|time pca0
             / dist=multinomial link=cumlogit;
run;
```

Indeed, we only need to change the distribution and the link function to 'dist=multinomial' and 'link=cumlogit' for a general multinomial model with cumulative logit link. As before, GEE is obtained by adding the REPEATED statement to the program:

```
proc genmod data=m.gsa;
  class patid timecls;
  model gsa = time|time pca0
             / dist=multinomial link=cumlogit;
  repeated subject=patid
             / type=ind covb within=timecls modelse;
run;
```

A restriction is that only 'type=ind' is allowed with the multinomial distribution, i.e., independence working assumption. Given that the parameter estimates and empirically corrected standard errors are valid, regardless of the working assumptions chosen, this is not a strong restriction. The output and the interpretation thereof is similar to the output described in Section 10.3. The linearization based method cannot be fitted with the SAS procedure GLIMMIX. This would need so-called R-side effects, which are not supported for the cumulative link functions. However, ordinal random-effects models, using PQL and MQL, can be fitted with this procedure, as exemplified in the following program:

```
proc glimmix data=m.gsa2 method=RSPL;
  class patid timecls;
  nloptions  maxiter=50;
  model gsa = time|time pca0
             / dist=multinomial link=cumlogit solution;
  random intercept / subject=patid type=un;
run;
```

The multinomial distribution, which would typically be chosen for ordinal data, can be combined with the cumulative logit link, but also with the cumulative complementary log-log, log-log, and probit links, using the 'link=cumcll,' 'link=cumloglog,' and 'link=cumprobit' options, respectively.

In case nominal data rather than ordinal ones are to be analyzed, the generalized logit link, using the 'link=genlogit' option, can be used instead. Because in our case the program failed to converge within the default 20 iterations, we increased the number of iterations by the NLOPTIONS statement.

A numerical integration based approach can be conducted using the SAS procedure NLMIXED. Perhaps here lies the largest difference with the binary counterpart. Indeed, the distributions supported by default are the normal, binary, binomial, negative binomial, gamma, and Poisson ones, excluding the multinomial. However, an extremely convenient and flexible feature is that a so-called general likelihood can be specified, using the 'general(·)' model specification. The entire responsibility for specifying the likelihood then lies with the user. An example program is given by:

```
proc nlmixed data=m.gsa2 qpoints=20;
 parms int1=-1.5585 int2=1.0292 int3=3.8916 int4=6.2144
       beta1=0.5410 beta2=-0.1123 beta3=0.3173 d=2.1082;
 eta = beta1*time + beta2*time*time + beta3*pca0 + b1;
 if gsa=1 then lik = 1/(1+exp(-(int1-eta)));
 else if gsa=2 then
   lik = 1/(1+exp(-(int2-eta))) - 1/(1+exp(-(int1-eta)));
 else if gsa=3 then
   lik = 1/(1+exp(-(int3-eta))) - 1/(1+exp(-(int2-eta)));
 else if gsa=4 then
   lik = 1/(1+exp(-(int4-eta))) - 1/(1+exp(-(int3-eta)));
 else lik = 1 - 1/(1+exp(-(int4-eta)));
 lik=log(lik);
 model gsa ~ general(lik);
 random b1 ~ normal(0,d*d) subject=patid;
 estimate 'var(b1)' d*d;
run;
```

In this program, the intercept-independent part of the linear predictor has been specified by means of 'eta.' Then, the probability to belong to a specific category can be written as the difference between two logistic-regression type expressions, based on the same linear predictor but with a different intercept. The only exceptions are the first one, where nothing needs to be subtracted, and the last one, where the difference needs to be made with one. The expression called 'lik' then represents the likelihood. After specifying the likelihood, the NLMIXED procedure takes responsibility over the optimization process, properly including the random-effects distribution. The general likelihood provides a great amount of flexibility, but the responsibility for correctly specifying the function resides, of course, with the user. When no random effects would be specified, a very flexible family of cross-sectional models would be specified as well.

19
The Epilepsy Data

19.1 Introduction

In this chapter, a marginal and a random-effects approach toward modelling repeated counts will be illustrated based on the Epilepsy data, introduced in Section 2.5. We will fit a marginal GEE model (Section 19.2) as well as a generalized linear mixed model (Section 19.3), and we will extensively compare the results in Section 19.4.

Throughout this chapter, Y_{ij} represents the number of epileptic seizures patient i experiences during week j of the follow-up period. Further, as before, let t_{ij} be the time-point at which Y_{ij} has been measured, $t_{ij} = 1, 2, \ldots$ until at most 27.

19.2 A Marginal GEE Analysis

We will first perform a GEE1 analysis (Section 8.2), assuming a marginal Poisson model, with logarithmic natural link function, and with linear, treatment-specific, time-effects. More specifically, it will be assumed that

$$Y_{ij} \sim \text{Poisson}(\lambda_{ij}),$$
$$\log(\lambda_{ij}) = \begin{cases} \beta_0 + \beta_1 t_{ij} & \text{if placebo} \\ \beta_0 + \beta_2 t_{ij} & \text{if treated.} \end{cases} \quad (19.1)$$

We assume a common intercept for both treatment groups in order to incorporate our prior belief that, due to the randomization, there is no sys-

TABLE 19.1. *Epilepsy Study. Parameter estimates and standard errors (empirically corrected; model-based) for the regression coefficients in Model (19.1), obtained from a GEE1 analysis with AR(1) working correlation matrix.*

Effect	Parameter	Estimate (s.e.)
Common intercept	β_0	1.3140 (0.1435; 0.1601)
Slope placebo	β_1	-0.0142 (0.0234; 0.0185)
Slope treatment	β_2	-0.0192 (0.0178; 0.0174)

tematic difference between both groups at the start of the study. Given the high number of repeated measurements (up to 27), an unstructured working correlation would require estimation of many correlation parameters. Further, the long observation period makes the assumption of an exchangeable correlation structure quite unrealistic. We therefore use the AR(1) working correlation structure, which is meaningful because we have equally spaced time points at which measurements have been taken.

Prior to the fitting of the model in (19.1), an extended model was fitted including quadratic time-evolutions, but these turned out not to be significantly different from zero ($p = 0.5239$). Therefore, from now on, we will restrict to models with linear time-effects. The analysis has been performed using the SAS procedure GENMOD. Without going into any more detail, the SAS program used for the GEE analysis for Model (19.1) is given by

```
proc genmod data=test;
class id timeclss trt;
model nseizw =  trt*time / dist=poisson;
repeated subject=id / withinsubject=timeclss
                type=AR(1) corrw modelse;
estimate 'diff slopes' trt*time 1 -1 ;
run;
```

and we refer to Section 10.3 for more details on fitting GEE models within the SAS system.

The results of the analysis are shown in Table 19.1. The auto-correlation coefficient has been estimated as 0.5963, i.e., two measurements from the same subject one week apart have correlation equal to 0.5963. For measurements two weeks apart, the correlation is estimated to be $0.5963^2 = 0.3556$, and so on. Note that the small differences between the model-based and the empirically corrected standard errors do not lead to different conclusions with respect to hypothesis testing. None of the average time effects is significantly different from zero (empirically corrected p-values equal to 0.5429 and 0.2795 for the placebo and the treated group, respectively), nor are they significantly different from each other ($p = 0.8721$, obtained by the

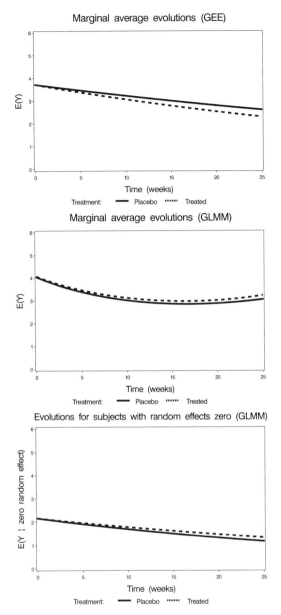

FIGURE 19.1. *Epilepsy Study. Treatment-arm specific evolutions. (a) Marginal evolutions as obtained from a marginal (GEE) model, (b) marginal evolutions as obtained from integrating out a GLMM, and (c) evolutions for an "average" subject from a GLMM, i.e., with $\boldsymbol{b}_i = 0$.*

ESTIMATE statement in the above program). Finally, the fitted average evolutions are shown in panel (a) of Figure 19.1.

19.3 A Generalized Linear Mixed Model

An alternative analysis could be based on a random-effects approach towards modeling the association structure. We then assume that, conditionally on random effects, the Y_{ij} are independent Poisson distributed random variables. As before, a logarithmic link function is used, with linear, treatment-specific, time trends. As random effects, we include random intercepts as well as random time effects. More specific, the model is given by

$$Y_{ij}|\boldsymbol{b}_i \sim \text{Poisson}(\lambda_{ij}),$$
$$\log(\lambda_{ij}) = \begin{cases} (\beta_0 + b_{i1}) + (\beta_1 + b_{i2})t_{ij} & \text{if placebo} \\ (\beta_0 + b_{i1}) + (\beta_2 + b_{i2})t_{ij} & \text{if treated,} \end{cases} \quad (19.2)$$

where the random effects $\boldsymbol{b}_i = (b_{i1}, b_{i2})'$ are assumed to be normally distributed with mean vector $\boldsymbol{0}$ and 2×2 covariance matrix D. As in the marginal model, we assume the same fixed intercept for the two groups. This reflects our prior belief that, due to the randomization, the initial values are equally distributed in both treatment groups.

The analysis has been performed using the SAS procedures GLIMMIX and NLMIXED. First, PQL and MQL have been applied, with REML estimation for the linear mixed models for the pseudo data (Section 15.2). Afterwards, we used adaptive Gaussian quadrature with 1 and with 10 quadrature points. Note that the adaptive Gaussian quadrature with one quadrature point is equivalent to applying the Laplace approximation to the integrals in the marginal likelihood function (Section 14.5.2).

The SAS programs are given by

```
proc glimmix data=test method=RSPL;
class id trt;
model nseizw =  trt*time / dist=poisson solution;
random intercept time / type=UNR subject=id;
estimate 'diff slopes' trt*time 1 -1;
run;

proc nlmixed data=test qpoints=1;
parms beta0=1 beta1=-0.1 beta2=-0.1
      d11=1 rho=0 d22=0.1;
if (trt = 0) then eta = beta0 + b1
                + beta1*time + b2*time;
else if (trt = 1) then eta = beta0 + b1
```

19.3 A Generalized Linear Mixed Model

TABLE 19.2. *Epilepsy Study. Parameter estimates and standard errors for the regression coefficients in Model (19.2), obtained from an MQL and PQL analysis, from an analysis based on the Laplace approximation, and from an analysis based on adaptive Gaussian quadrature with 10 quadrature points (QUAD).*

		MQL	PQL
Effect	Parameter	Estimate (s.e.)	Estimate (s.e.)
Common intercept	β_0	1.3525 (0.1492)	0.8079 (0.1261)
Slope placebo	β_1	−0.0180 (0.0144)	−0.0242 (0.0094)
Slope treatment	β_2	−0.0151 (0.0144)	−0.0191 (0.0094)
Variance of intercepts	d_{11}	1.9017 (0.2986)	1.2510 (0.2155)
Variance of slopes	d_{22}	0.0084 (0.0014)	0.0024 (0.0006)
Correlation rand.eff.	ρ	−0.3268 (0.1039)	−0.3394 (0.1294)
		Laplace	QUAD
Effect	Parameter	Estimate (s.e.)	Estimate (s.e.)
Common intercept	β_0	0.7740 (0.1291)	0.7739 (0.1293)
Slope placebo	β_1	−0.0244 (0.0096)	−0.0245 (0.0096)
Slope treatment	β_2	−0.0193 (0.0096)	−0.0193 (0.0097)
Variance of intercepts	d_{11}	1.2814 (0.2220)	1.2859 (0.2231)
Variance of slopes	d_{22}	0.0024 (0.0006)	0.0024 (0.0006)
Correlation rand.eff.	ρ	−0.3347 (0.1317)	−0.3349 (0.1318)

```
            + beta2*time + b2*time;
    lambda = exp(eta);
    model nseizw ~ poisson(lambda);
    random b1 b2 ~ normal([0, 0],
          [d11, rho*sqrt(d11)*sqrt(d22), d22])
          subject = id;
    estimate 'diff slopes' beta1-beta2;
    run;
```

We refer to the Sections 15.2 and 15.4 for more details on the SAS procedures GLIMMIX and NLMIXED, respectively.

The results of our analyses are summarized in Table 19.2. We find substantial differences between the MQL and PQL methods. For example, the difference in estimates for the intercepts equals $1.3525 - 0.8079 = 0.5785$, which is large when compared to the estimated standard errors. A similar remark holds for the random-intercepts variance d_{11}. Note also the similarity of the fixed-effects estimates obtained from the MQL method and those reported in Table 19.1, obtained from fitting a marginal GEE method. This phenomenon was already observed earlier in the context of the toenail dataset (Section 16.4). Further, we find very little differences between the results from the Laplace approximation and the results from the adaptive Gaussian quadrature with 10 quadrature points. Hence, in contrast

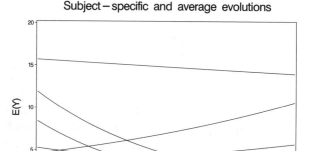

FIGURE 19.2. *Epilepsy Study. Sampled predicted profiles for 20 subjects in the placebo group (thin lines), and the resulting marginal evolution obtained from averaging over the 20 subjects (bold line).*

to earlier examples, the number of quadrature points used in the adaptive Gaussian quadrature approximation has negligable effect on the results. As was indicated in Section 14.3, this will typically be the case in datasets with many repeated measurements per subject, as in the present example. As was also observed earlier (Section 16.4), the results obtained from the PQL approach are closer to those obtained from adaptive Gaussian quadrature than those resulting from the MQL approach. Finally, in contrast to our earlier results based on the marginal GEE model, we now obtain slopes that are significantly different from zero (all p-values smaller than 0.05), unless under the MQL approach, but none of the four analyses revealed a significant difference between the slopes β_1 and β_2 (all p-values larger than 0.6).

19.4 Marginalizing the Mixed Model

As explained in Chapter 16, the regression coefficients in (19.2) need to be interpreted conditionally on the random effects $\boldsymbol{b}_i$, i.e., the parameters have a subject-specific interpretation. In case the population-averaged, marginal, evolutions are of interest, additional computations are needed. For example, the marginal expectation of the outcome Y_{ij}, measured at time-point t_{ij}, in the placebo group, is given by

$$\begin{aligned} E[Y_{ij}] &= E[E[Y_{ij}|\boldsymbol{b}_i]] \\ &= E\left[\exp[(\beta_0 + b_{i1}) + (\beta_1 + b_{i2})t_{ij}]\right] \end{aligned} \quad (19.3)$$

19.4 Marginalizing the Mixed Model

$$\neq \exp[\beta_0 + \beta_1 t_{ij}]$$

with an expression similar to (19.3) for the expected evolution in the treated group. Calculation of (19.3) requires integrating out the random effects over their fitted distribution. As explained in Section 16.3, this can be done based on numerical integration techniques or based on numerical averaging. Here, we will follow the latter procedure, with 1000 draws for each treatment group.

As an example, let us consider the placebo group, and let the model be fitted using adaptive Gaussian quadrature with 10 quadrature points. We start by randomly drawing 1000 realized values for the random effects b_i, taken from a bivariate normal distribution with mean vector zero, and with covariance matrix equal to the fitted random-effects covariance matrix (see Table 19.2)

$$D = \begin{pmatrix} 1.2859 & -0.0185 \\ -0.0185 & 0.0024 \end{pmatrix}.$$

The Cholesky decomposition of D, defined as the upper triangular matrix L such that $L'L = D$, and needed in the SAS code for drawing the 1000 random vectors b_i is given by

$$L = \begin{pmatrix} 1.1340 & -0.0163 \\ 0 & 0.0462 \end{pmatrix}.$$

For each of the 1000 realized random vectors b_i, and for a fine grid of time points t, the conditional expectation $\exp[(\beta_0+b_{i1})+(\beta_1+b_{i2})t]$ is calculated, with the fixed effects β_0 and β_1 replaced by their fitted values 0.7739 and -0.0245, respectively (see Table 19.2). An estimate for the unconditional mean at a given point t in time is then obtained from averaging the 1000 conditional means, i.e.,

$$\widehat{E}[Y(t)] = \frac{1}{1000} \sum_{i=1}^{1000} \exp[(0.7739 + b_{i1}) + (-0.0245 + b_{i2})t].$$

A graphical representation of the average evolution for the placebo group is then obtained by plotting this estimate for a sufficiently fine grid of t-values. A graphical representation of this procedure is given in Figure 19.2, for 20 placebo subjects randomly drawn from the fitted model (rather than the 1000 actually used in the calculations).

The SAS code needed for the implemenation of the above procedure is given by:

```
data h;
do treat=0 to 1 by 1;
  do subject=1 to 1000 by 1;
    b1=rannor(-1);b2=rannor(-1);
```

```
      ranint=1.1340*b1; ranslope=-0.0163*b1 + 0.0462*b2;
      do t=0 to 27 by 0.1;
          if treat=0 then y=exp(0.7739+ranint
                                  +(-0.0245+ranslope)*t);
          else y=exp(0.7739+ranint +(-0.0193+ranslope)*t);
          output;
      end;
   end;
end;

proc sort data=h;
by t treat;
run;

proc means data=h;
var y;
by t treat;
output out=out;
run;

proc gplot data=out;
plot y*t=treat  / haxis=axis1 vaxis=axis2 legend=legend1;
axis1 label=(h=2.5 'Time (weeks)') value=(h=1.5)
      order=(0 to 25 by 5)  minor=none;
axis2 label=(h=2.5 A=90 'E(Y)') value=(h=1.5)
      order=(0 to 6 by 1)  minor=none;
legend1 label=(h=2 'Treatment: ')
         value=(h=2 'Placebo' 'Treated');
title h=3 'Marginal average evolutions (GLMM)';
symbol1 c=black i=join w=5 l=1 mode=include;
symbol2 c=black i=join w=5 l=2 mode=include;
where _stat_='MEAN';
run;
```

The result is shown in panel (b) of Figure 19.1. Note the difference between the estimated average profiles obtained from this generalized linear mixed model and those obtained earlier from a marginal GEE analysis [shown in panel (a) of the same figure]. First, the GLMM results show clear curvature in the fitted average profiles and even suggest a small increase in average number of epileptic seizures toward the end of the study. This is completely absent in the GEE profiles. A possible explanation is that the GEE model (19.1) restricts the fitted averages to be monotone functions over time. The GLMM model can accomodate non-monotonicity, through the random effects, even though the linear predictor in (19.2) is linear in time. Further, the GEE approach slightly favors the treatment group, while the GLMM results tend to favor the placebo group (although none of the differences where found to be statistically significant). A possible explanation can be found in the fact that, as has been explained in Section 2.5, many patients leave the study after week 16. When those patients are compared to those who are still in the study at week 17, one can observe that, in the placebo group, the worst patients continue, while the opposite is true for the treated group. Hence, the two treatment groups are different with respect to the type of subjects that continue past week 16. As will be explained in Section 27.5, the GEE approach does not correct for this which may yield possibly over-optimistic conclusions about the treated group.

Finally, panel (c) in Figure 19.1 also shows the fitted evolution in both treatment groups, for 'average' patients, i.e., patients with random-effects values equal to zero. This again illustrates that the non-linearity of the link function implies that the average evolution cannot be obtained from setting the random effects in the generalized linear mixed model equal to zero, which is in contrast to the linear mixed model (Chapter 4).

20
Non-linear Models

20.1 Introduction

Chapter 3 introduced the generalized linear model as a flexible yet mathematically tractable and elegant framework for univariate outcomes of a Gaussian but primarily non-Gaussian type. It thus extends the classical linear model, of which linear regression and ANOVA are the best known forms of appearance. The linear model, producing the powerful linear mixed-effects model when extended to longitudinal data (Chapter 4), is too restrictive when outcomes are binary, categorical, or counts, for example. Thus, in turn, the generalized linear model has been extended to models for longitudinal or otherwise correlated data, and a key message has been that careful distinction needs to be made between the marginal, conditional, and random-effects model families (Chapter 5), and each of these received considerable attention in Parts II, III, and IV, respectively.

Yet, in spite of the tremendous amount of flexibility offered by, say, generalized estimating equations and the generalized linear mixed model, and their strictly speaking not being linear, they are subject to constraints. This stems from the fact that, in spite of the earlier statement, exhibit a specific form of linearity, at the level of the link function. Focusing for clarity on binary outcomes, a typical GLM specification writes the success probability as a non-linear function of covariates, but in a very controlled way: a non-linear link function transforms the probability onto, say, a logit or a probit, which is then written as a linear function of covariates, i.e., set equal to a linear predictor. In other words, non-linearity is confined to a non-linear but 1-1 transformation between the original scale (e.g., probability or mean count) and a scale natural from a mathematical point of view, such as the logit and probit scales for binary data and the log mean count scale for counts.

The advantage of this approach is that a large number of results, known for linear models, carry over. Especially in the univariate case, properties of the generalized linear model and the associated exponential family are almost as well described as those for the linear model and the associated normal distribution, although the latter is the champion of theoretical knowledge surrounding it, of course. Also their numerical properties are well understood, rendering univariate GLM is easy to fit, even though for most no closed-form solution exists. In particular, the existence of natural parameters and natural links makes the exponential family and the GLM framework extremely handy in practice.

Of course, some properties of the normal case are lost in passing to GLM. This is emanated through the strict separation between conditional, marginal, and random-effects families. For example, the entire Chapter 16 was devoted to the study of the relationship between marginal and random-effects models.

But, while appropriate transformations of responses and/or covariates, or the use of fractional polynomials (Royston and Altman 1994, see Section 12.4.2), can produce sufficiently adequate models to be of great practical value in many situations, some problems are too intrinsically non-linear to be tackled by models that are entirely or partly linear, such as the linear mixed model, generalized estimating equations, or the generalized linear mixed model. It is then time to switch to fully non-linear models. Such situations include growth phenomena over sufficiently extended periods, especially when the observational period includes both growth spurts and asymptotic behavior of growth toward maturation. Dose-response modeling, pharmacokinetic, and pharmacodynamic applications often demand non-linear models. as well.

In Section 20.2, the extension of generalized linear models to non-linear models for univariate data is briefly sketched and applied to pharmacokinetic data from the indomethacin study (Section 20.3). These models are extended to the longitudinal setting in Section 20.4, with emphasis on the mixed-models family in Section 20.5. Non-linear mixed models are illustrated using the orange tree example (Section 20.6). The specific case of pharmacokinetic and pharmacodynamic data is studied in Section 20.7, where the indomethacin study is now given a fully hierarchical analysis (Section 20.7.1). The classic theophylline data are analyzed in Section 20.7.2 and some remarks on the pharmacodynamic case are offered in Section 20.7.3. A worked case study on data from a songbird experiment is presented in Section 20.8. Although all analyses in this chapter, up to that point, are in continuous data, Section 20.9 emphasizes in particular the non-Gaussian setting. Some remarks on inferential problems that can occur in the non-linear setting, unlike in the linear and generalized linear settings, are given in Section 20.10. Finally, some brief comments on semi-parametric extensions are made in Section 20.11.

Unlike in other chapters, we put strong emphasis on the continuous case. One of the reasons is that, from a methodological point of view (estimation, inference, numerical optimization routines, etc.), even for continuous outcomes, non-linear models are closer to generalized linear models for discrete data, than they are to linear models for continuous data. This is the main reason why the non-linear models were absent in Verbeke and Molenberghs (2000). Moreover, the continuous non-linear case, together with the generalized linear model based approach of earlier chapters, provides a good basis for the non-Gaussian situation. A key reference in the area of non-linear models for repeated measures is the book by Davidian and Giltinan (1995).

20.2 Univariate Non-linear Models

As stated in the introduction, not only linear models, also generalized linear models enjoy a certain amount of linearity, even though there are important differences between both. Whereas linear models are primarily used for Gaussian or, more generally, continuous data, the generalized linear model family encompasses a wide variety of outcomes. Also as said before, there are situations, whether for Gaussian or non-Gaussian data, whether for cross-sectional or for repeated measures data, where more intrinsically non-linear models are needed, such as in growth curves modeling, pharmacokinetic and pharmacodynamic modeling, and dose-response modeling.

Starting from moment assumptions, a linear model for an outcome Y_i, conditional on a vector of covariates $\bm{x}_i$, takes the form:

$$E(Y_i|\bm{x}_i, \bm{\beta}) = \bm{x}_i'\bm{\beta}, \qquad (20.1)$$

where $\bm{\beta}$ is the usual vector of regression parameters. In generalized linear models (Chapter 3), expression (20.1) is updated by means of a link function $g(\cdot)$:

$$g\left[E(Y_i|\bm{x}_i, \bm{\beta})\right] = \bm{x}_i'\bm{\beta}, \qquad (20.2)$$

or, equivalently, using the inverse link function $h(\cdot) = g^{-1}(\cdot)$:

$$E(Y_i|\bm{x}_i, \bm{\beta}) = h(\bm{x}_i'\bm{\beta}). \qquad (20.3)$$

Thus, the linear predictor $\eta_i = \bm{x}_i'\bm{\beta}$ is preserved at an appropriately transformed scale. For logistic regression, not the success probability is a linear function of the covariates, but the logit is. In a non-linear model, one abandons the concept of linear predictors altogether, and replace (20.2) or (20.3) with

$$E(Y_i|\bm{x}_i, \bm{\beta}) = h(\bm{x}_i, \bm{\beta}), \qquad (20.4)$$

where now $h(\cdot)$ is an arbitrary function of covariates and parameters. A simple dose-response oriented example would be:

$$\text{logit}[E(Y_i|d_i,\boldsymbol{\beta})] = \beta_0 + \beta_1 d_i^\gamma, \tag{20.5}$$

where β_1 is the classical dose parameter that would be present in a standard logistic model too and γ is a power parameter, modifying the shape of the dose-response curve. Note that this model is non-linear due to the presence of the logit link on the left hand side of (20.5) *and* the non-linear predictor on the right hand side. The h function in (20.4) now equals:

$$h(d_i,\beta_0,\beta_1,\gamma) = \frac{\exp(\beta_0 + \beta_1 d_i^\gamma)}{1 + \exp(\beta_0 + \beta_1 d_i^\gamma)},$$

with d_i the dose level applied to unit i. Thus, the non-linear link function and the non-linear predictor can be integrated into a single function, or kept separately, whichever is convenient for modeling, numerical optimization, etc.

A version of (20.5) for continuous outcomes would be:

$$E(Y_i|d_i,\boldsymbol{\beta}) = \beta_0 + \beta_1 d_i^\gamma. \tag{20.6}$$

Thus, while the link function is linear, the predictor function is not, preserving the non-linear nature of the model.

The above models can be cast into a fully parametric framework, following the nature of the outcomes. For example, (20.6) can be seen as describing the mean of a normal outcome:

$$Y_i \sim N(\beta_0 + \beta_1 d_i^\gamma, \sigma^2), \tag{20.7}$$

or, equivalently: $Y_i = \mu_i + \varepsilon_i$ with $\varepsilon_i \sim N(0,\sigma^2)$. If necessary, the variance can be modeled in a non-constant fashion as well, as will be seen in Section 20.3. Similarly to the normal case, (20.5) can be seen as defining the probability structure of a parametric binomial model.

Fitting linear and generalized linear models is reasonably straightforward. For linear models, closed-form expressions exist and for generalized linear models, exponential family theory ensures the log-likelihood function has a unique maximum. When the natural link is used, Fisher scoring and Newton-Raphson iteration are equivalent, as the observed and expected information matrices coincide. The key reason is that the log-likelihood function is linear in the sufficient statistics. This property no longer holds with non-linear models. Newton-Raphson iteration replaces the value of the parameter $\boldsymbol{\beta}$ after t iterations, $\boldsymbol{\beta}^{(t)}$ say, by

$$\boldsymbol{\beta}^{(t+1)} = \boldsymbol{\beta}^{(t)} - H(\boldsymbol{\beta}^{(t)})^{-1} S(\boldsymbol{\beta}^{(t)}), \tag{20.8}$$

where $S(\boldsymbol{\beta})$ is the score function, i.e., the first-order derivative of the log-likelihood with respect to the parameters, and $H(\boldsymbol{\beta})$ is the Hessian matrix or matrix of second-order derivatives. In Fisher scoring, $H(\boldsymbol{\beta})$ is replaced by its expectation, producing:

$$\boldsymbol{\beta}^{(t+1)} = \boldsymbol{\beta}^{(t)} - \mathcal{H}(\boldsymbol{\beta}^{(t)})^{-1} S(\boldsymbol{\beta}^{(t)}). \tag{20.9}$$

A popular family of methods are so-called quasi-Newton methods, i.e., any method for which $H(\boldsymbol{\beta})$ is replaced by a certain alternative $\widetilde{H}(\boldsymbol{\beta})$. Some of these include steepest descent, Gauss-Newton, and Marquardt optimization. A thorough treatment on non-linear models and associated optimization issues is offered in Seber and Wild (2003). See also Dennis and Schnabel (1983), Lange (1999), and Nocedal and Wright (1999). Calculating the first, and in particular the second-order derivatives in (20.8), (20.9), or any other quasi-Newton method can be involved. Therefore, analytical derivation is often replaced by numerical derivation, i.e., finite differences with a very small step size.

The key message is that fitting non-linear models, i.e., optimizing non-linear functions, is involved and very sensitive to starting values and choice of optimization procedure. This is why most optimizers, whether generic or for a specific family of models, allow for a variety of optimization methods, each one having a good number of tuning parameters such as, for example, step size determination. One such implementation is to be found in the SAS procedure NLIN. Also, the SAS procedure NLMIXED, designed to handle non-linear mixed-effects models, offers great flexibility. It handles generalized linear mixed models (Chapters 15 and 17, for example) and univariate non-linear models as two special cases. For univariate non-linear models, in the absence of random effects, no numerical integration is necessary. The procedure then still offers a variety of Newton-Raphson, quasi-Newton, and gradient methods, among others. It even allows for the use of the Nelder-Mead (Nelder and Mead 1965) simplex algorithm, which can be slow but is considered to be stable.

Next, we will illustrate these ideas using data from a pharmacokinetics study.

20.3 The Indomethacin Study: Non-hierarchical Analysis

The data come from a pharmacokinetics study of indomethacin (Kwan *et al* 1976, Davidian and Giltinan 1995), following bolus intravenous injection of the same dose in six human volunteers. For each subject, plasma concentrations of indomethacin were measured at 11 time points ranging from 15 minutes to 8 hours post-injection. The individual profiles are shown in Figure 20.1 and displayed in Table 20.1. The measurement 2.72 of subject 3 at 0.25 hours is deemed outlying and deleted from analysis.

20. Non-linear Models

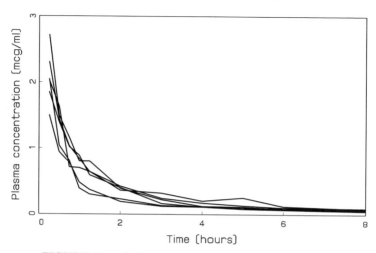

FIGURE 20.1. *Indomethacin Study. Individual profiles.*

To understand absorption and elimination of the drug, in an individual subject as well as in the population, is the goal of pharmacokinetics. Usually, the body is represented as a system of compartments, and it is then assumed that the rate of transfer between compartments follows first-order or linear kinetics. This leads to differential equations, the solution of which generally leads to non-linear relationships between drug concentration and time. For example, a two-compartment model to describe kinetics following intravenous injection leads to the so-called bi-exponential model (Davidian and Giltinan 1995):

$$C_i(t_{ij}) = Y_{ij} = \widetilde{\beta}_{i1} \exp(-\widetilde{\beta}_{i2} t_{ij}) + \widetilde{\beta}_{i3} \exp(-\widetilde{\beta}_{i4} t_{ij}) + \varepsilon_{ij}, \qquad (20.10)$$

under the restriction that $\beta_{i1}, \beta_{i2}, \beta_{i3}, \beta_{i4} > 0$. $C_i(t_{ij})$ is the drug plasma concentration. Here, we will fit the model to each subject separately. In Section 20.7.1, a fully hierarchical approach, using a non-linear mixed-effects model, will be employed.

The bi-exponential model (20.10) is easier to handle using a reparameterization

$$C_i(t_{ij}) = Y_{ij} = e^{\beta_{i1}} \exp\left(-e^{\beta_{i2}} t_{ij}\right) + e^{\beta_{i3}} \exp\left(-e^{\beta_{i4}} t_{ij}\right) + \varepsilon_{ij}. \qquad (20.11)$$

Here, e^{β_2} and e^{β_4} are the rate constants corresponding to the two apparent exponential phases of drug disposition. The half-life of the terminal phase of drug disposition is given by

$$a(\boldsymbol{\beta}) = \frac{\ln 2}{e^{\beta_4}},$$

TABLE 20.1. *Indomethacin Study. Measurements for six individuals over an eight hour period.*

Time	Subject					
(hours)	1	2	3	4	5	6
0.25	1.50	2.03	(2.72)	1.85	2.05	2.31
0.50	0.94	1.63	1.49	1.39	1.04	1.44
0.75	0.78	0.71	1.16	1.02	0.81	1.03
1.00	0.48	0.70	0.80	0.89	0.39	0.84
1.25	0.37	0.64	0.80	0.59	0.30	0.64
2.00	0.19	0.36	0.39	0.40	0.23	0.42
3.00	0.12	0.32	0.22	0.16	0.13	0.24
4.00	0.11	0.20	0.12	0.11	0.11	0.17
5.00	0.08	0.25	0.11	0.10	0.08	0.13
6.00	0.07	0.12	0.08	0.07	0.10	0.10
8.00	0.05	0.08	0.08	0.07	0.06	0.09

where it is understood that $\beta_4 < \beta_2$.

Because we defer a fully hierarchical model until later, now focusing on each of the profiles separately, we could in principle drop the index i for the time being. However, it will be retained for ease of reference to Section 20.7.1. Parameter estimates and standard errors, obtained from fitting model (20.11) to the indomethacin data, with constant variance, are displayed in Table 20.2.

Our model is non-linear in its mean structure, but assumes a classical homoscedastic error term, i.e., normally distributed with zero mean and constant variance σ^2. In many growth curve examples, and in particular in a pharmacokinetic context, such an assumption is frequently deemed unrealistic. It may be plausible to assume the error is constant in relative terms, i.e., having constant coefficient of variation. This makes the error proportional to the mean and hence the variance proportional to the mean-squared:

$$\varepsilon_{ij} \sim N(0, \sigma^2 \mu_{ij}^2). \tag{20.12}$$

Recall that we have chosen to retain both indices i and j, for clarity. Results from fitting the bi-exponential model (20.11) with variance structure (20.12) are presented in Table 20.3. The extension from a homoscedastic to a heteroscedastic structure is by no means the only one. Note that both models, while different, have the same number of parameters and hence are non-nested. A general formulation for the variance is provided by:

$$\text{Var}(y_{ij}) = \sigma^2 \gamma^2(\mu_{ij}, \boldsymbol{\theta}), \tag{20.13}$$

TABLE 20.2. *Indomethacin Study. Bi-exponential model fitted to each subject separately. Homoscedastic model. ('Variance' refers to the between-subject variability in a particular parameter.)*

Subject	β_1	β_2	β_3	β_4	σ^2
	\multicolumn{5}{c}{Parameter estimates}				
1	0.708	0.579	-1.653	-1.788	0.033
2	1.039	0.801	-0.695	-1.635	0.114
3	0.816	0.149	-1.481	-1.839	0.043
4	0.788	0.242	-1.368	-1.603	0.036
5	1.271	1.041	-1.233	-1.507	0.054
6	1.099	1.088	-0.032	-0.873	0.028
Mean	0.954	0.650	-1.077	-1.541	
Variance	0.047	0.158	0.368	0.122	
	\multicolumn{5}{c}{Standard errors}				
1	0.043	0.101	0.467	0.635	0.007
2	0.122	0.238	0.486	0.644	0.024
3	0.083	0.212	1.167	1.347	0.010
4	0.080	0.139	0.852	0.864	0.008
5	0.067	0.126	0.424	0.555	0.012
6	0.044	0.113	0.134	0.120	0.006

where $\gamma(\cdot)$ is a function of the mean, additional variance parameters, and perhaps other covariates. For example, the power model reads

$$\varepsilon_{ij} \sim N(0, \sigma^2 \mu_{ij}^{2\theta}). \tag{20.14}$$

The power model is similar to the constant variation-coefficient model, with now an additional parameter θ, and the heteroscedastic model (20.12) is retrieved for $\theta = 1$. Table 20.4 presents the results of fitting the bi-exponential model to the indomethacin data, with power variance structure. Note that we now have an additional parameter, compared to Table 20.3. Model comparison can be done by means of the likelihood ratio test statistic, for example, comparing twice the sum of the six individual log-likelihoods from Table 20.4 to those under Table 20.3. This is a standard exercise, asymptotically valid when the number of measurements per subjects is sufficiently large, and establishes that the power model is an improvement over the heteroscedastic one.

Figure 20.2 shows the observed profile for the first subject, together with the fit of the homoscedastic, heteroscedastic, and power models. For this subject (and also for the others), the non-homoscedastic models are clearly the best. The parameter estimates for the σ^2 parameter are relatively close to each other, with the same holding for the θ parameter. One might then

TABLE 20.3. *Indomethacin Study. Bi-exponential model fitted to each subject separately. Heteroscedastic model. ('Variance' refers to the between-subject variability in a particular parameter.)*

Subject	β_1	β_2	β_3	β_4	σ^2
	\multicolumn{5}{c}{Parameter estimates}				
1	0.731	0.604	-1.629	-1.764	0.055
2	1.145	1.050	-0.408	-1.355	0.170
3	0.771	-0.043	-2.409	-3.964	0.074
4	0.780	0.061	-2.316	-3.061	0.084
5	1.192	0.944	-1.440	-1.756	0.137
6	0.895	0.317	-1.202	-1.824	0.087
Mean	0.919	0.489	-1.567	-2.287	
Variance	0.041	0.206	0.553	1.010	
	\multicolumn{5}{c}{Standard errors}				
1	0.067	0.056	0.087	0.090	0.012
2	0.359	0.293	0.192	0.148	0.037
3	0.071	0.083	0.349	2.535	0.017
4	0.066	0.074	0.294	0.915	0.018
5	0.205	0.150	0.174	0.182	0.030
6	0.089	0.127	0.224	0.213	0.019

be inclined to set them equal to each other across subjects. This, however, suggests to analyze the profiles jointly, using hierarchical modeling ideas. Such an approach would be desirable for an important other reason as well. By analyzing the profiles individually, it was assumed that the measurements on a subject were independent, which is not correct if the subject-specific models are the purpose of inference. Of course, we essentially combined the results of each of the six subjects into summaries (mean and variance), thus yielding a two-stage analysis. The advantage of a longitudinal analysis is that it allows for correctly taking the intra-subject correlation into account. Therefore, Section 20.4 is devoted to non-linear models for repeated measurements.

20.4 Non-linear Models for Longitudinal Data

In Section 20.2, generic linear, generalized linear, and non-linear models for univariate outcomes were presented. Extensions to the longitudinal setting are straightforward. The longitudinal counterpart to (20.1) is the linear mixed model (4.3). We extended generalized linear model (20.2) in differ-

TABLE 20.4. *Indomethacin Study. Bi-exponential model fitted to each subject separately. Power variance model. ('Variance' refers to the between-subject variability in a particular parameter.)*

Subject	β_1	β_2	β_3	β_4	σ^2	θ
			Parameter estimates			
1	0.745	0.619	-1.615	-1.753	0.070	1.183
2	1.129	1.017	-0.431	-1.369	0.153	0.889
3	0.772	-0.043	-2.407	-3.948	0.073	0.990
4	0.789	0.070	-2.292	-2.983	0.068	0.826
5	1.226	0.964	-1.420	-1.728	0.105	0.817
6	0.681	-0.032	-1.800	-2.527	0.138	1.550
Mean	0.890	0.433	-1.661	-2.385		
Variance	0.052	0.246	0.509	0.937		
			Standard errors			
1	0.087	0.064	0.073	0.072	0.027	0.223
2	0.302	0.278	0.209	0.167	0.047	0.252
3	0.072	0.085	0.355	2.538	0.025	0.219
4	0.054	0.074	0.344	1.017	0.023	0.243
5	0.149	0.119	0.181	0.200	0.042	0.251
6	0.180	0.231	0.480	0.766	0.060	0.376

ent directions, to the marginal, conditional, and random-effects models of Parts II, III, and IV, respectively.

Now, all three families can be extended to non-linear models as well, by considering the marginal, conditional, and subject-specific counterparts of (20.4) or, looked at it in a different way, non-linear extensions of (5.1), (5.4), and (5.2), respectively. A marginal non-linear model would take the form:

$$E(Y_{ij}|\boldsymbol{x}_{ij}) = h(\boldsymbol{x}_{ij}, \boldsymbol{\beta}). \qquad (20.15)$$

As we know from Chapter 7, (20.15) does not specify the full joint distribution. The association structure needs to be specified as well and this can be done in a linear or non-linear fashion as well. We can then, just as before, consider full likelihood approaches or non-likelihood alternatives, such as generalized estimating equations. Such models have been given relatively little attention in the literature.

A conditional non-linear model would in addition allow $\overline{\boldsymbol{Y}}_{ij}$, the set of all outcomes except the one modeled, as an argument of h:

$$E(Y_{ij}|Y_{ik,k\neq j}, \boldsymbol{x}_{ij}) = h(\boldsymbol{x}_{ij}, \boldsymbol{\beta}, \overline{\boldsymbol{Y}}_{ij}, \boldsymbol{\alpha}). \qquad (20.16)$$

However, whereas a log-linear model produces a conditional specification as in (5.4), considering (20.16) in general is not guaranteed to produce a

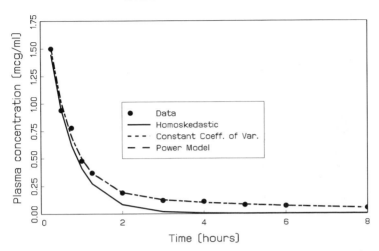

FIGURE 20.2. *Indomethacin Study. Observed and fitted profiles for the first subject.*

valid joint model. Just as (5.3), a non-linear version of a transition model is easier to handle.

Finally, the random-effects version is

$$E(Y_{ij}|\boldsymbol{b}_i, \boldsymbol{x}_{ij}, \boldsymbol{z}_{ij}) = h(\boldsymbol{x}_{ij}, \boldsymbol{\beta}, \boldsymbol{z}_{ij}, \boldsymbol{b}_i). \tag{20.17}$$

In the next section, we will concentrate on non-linear mixed-effects models, and then study both continuous as well as discrete versions of the model.

20.5 Non-linear Mixed Models

In the previous section, we allowed non-linear predictors in each of the three model families. In this section, we will consider the non-linear mixed-effects model in more detail, thereby extending both Chapter 14 and Section 20.5.

In a non-linear mixed-effects model, we assume that the conditional distribution of Y_{ij}, given $\boldsymbol{b}_i$ belongs to the exponential family, encompassing both normally distributed and non-normal outcomes. Precisely, the mean structure is specified by (20.17). In agreement with generalized linear mixed models, it is customary to assume normally distributed random effects with mean $\boldsymbol{0}$ and covariance matrix D, even though other distributions are possible in principle as well.

In agreement with the developments in Chapter 14, we write the conditional density of Y_{ij} given $\boldsymbol{b}_i$ as $f_{ij}(y_{ij}|\boldsymbol{b}_i, \boldsymbol{\beta}, \phi)$ and let $f(\boldsymbol{b}_i|D)$ be the density of the $N(\boldsymbol{0}, D)$ distribution. Then, expression (14.2) clearly applies here as well, provided it is again assumed that measurements Y_{ij} are

TABLE 20.5. *Orange Tree Data. Measurements in mm of trunk circumference.*

Day	Trunk circumference				
	Tree 1	Tree 2	Tree 3	Tree 4	Tree 5
118	30	33	30	32	30
484	58	69	51	62	49
664	87	111	75	112	81
1004	115	156	108	167	125
1231	120	172	115	179	142
1372	142	203	139	209	174
1582	145	203	140	214	177

independent conditionally on b_i. This implies that the same approaches can be used to parameter estimation, as were developed in Chapter 14 for generalized linear mixed models.

There are important differences, primarily of an interpretational type. We have stated that the marginal model, derived from a hierarchically formulated linear mixed model is easy to derive. The same is explicitly not true for the generalized linear mixed model. The differences in parameter values, already at population level, and their interpretation, carries over to the non-linear model, even when outcomes are continuous and the outcome distribution is assumed to be normal, as soon as the random effects enter the conditional expectation in a non-linear fashion. This means that obtaining the marginal mean, variance, and correlation functions are not straightforward.

20.6 The Orange Tree Data

We consider an experiment in which the trunk circumference (in mm) is measured for 5 orange trees, on 7 different occasions, over roughly a four-year period of growth. The data are presented in Table 20.5. Profiles are plotted in Figure 20.3.

The following non-linear mixed model has been proposed in the statistical literature (Pinheiro and Bates 2000):

$$Y_{ij} = \frac{\beta_1 + b_i}{1 + \exp[-(t_{ij} - \beta_2)/\beta_3]} + \varepsilon_{ij},$$

$$b_i \sim N(0, \sigma_b^2),$$

$$\varepsilon_{ij} \sim N(0, \sigma^2).$$

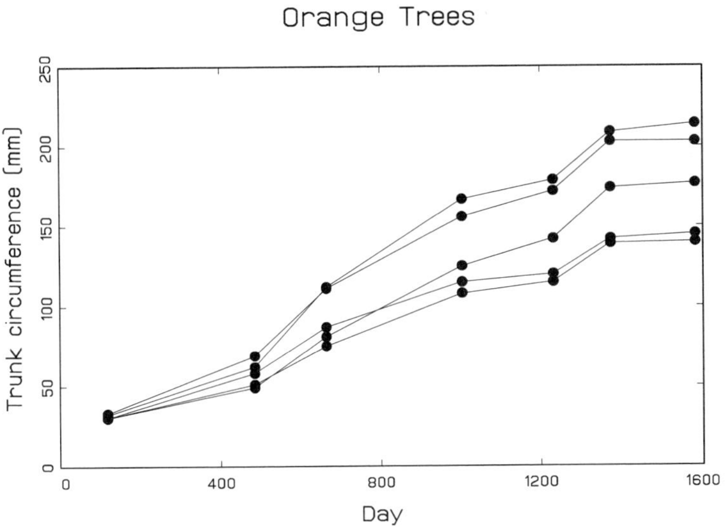

Orange Trees

FIGURE 20.3. *Orange Tree Data. Growth curves of trunk circumference for each of the five trees.*

Note that this model is non-linear in the fixed-effect parameters, but linear in the random effect b_i, simplifying the calculation of the marginal mean over the random-effects distribution. Thus, the conditional mean is

$$E(Y_{ij}|b_i) = \frac{\beta_1 + b_i}{1 + \exp[-(t_{ij} - \beta_2)/\beta_3]} \qquad (20.18)$$

while its marginal counterpart is

$$E(Y_{ij}) = \frac{\beta_1}{1 + \exp[-(t_{ij} - \beta_2)/\beta_3]}.$$

Such a simple situation will not occur in neither the analysis of the songbird data (Section 20.8) nor in the hierarchical analyses of the indomethacin data (Section 20.7.1) and the theophylline data (Section 20.7.2). A graphical representation of the model, with the meaning of the parameters associated to it, is given in Figure 20.4. Parameter estimates and standard errors are given in Table 20.6.

Empirical Bayes predictions are graphed in Figure 20.5. The model fit seems acceptable and a set of three population-level parameters, having a clear interpretable meaning, result.

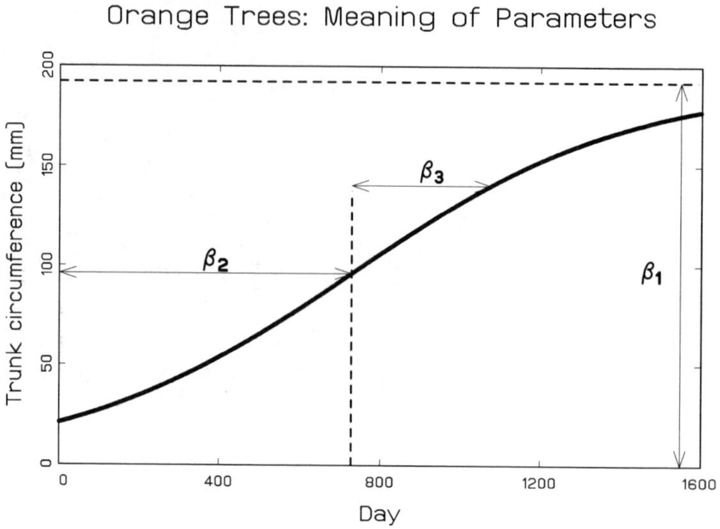

FIGURE 20.4. *Orange Tree Data. Interpretation of model parameters.*

TABLE 20.6. *Orange Tree Data. Parameter estimates and standard errors for model (20.18).*

Parameter	Estimate (s.e.)
β_1	192.05 (15.66)
β_2	727.91 (35.25)
β_3	348.07 (27.08)
σ_b	31.65 (10.26)
σ	7.84 (1.01)

20.7 Pharmacokinetic and Pharmacodynamic Models

In Section 20.3, a univariate non-linear analysis of the indomethacin data was presented, using the bi-exponential or two-compartment model. In the meantime, non-linear mixed-effects models have been introduced, and fitted to the orange tree data (Section 20.6) as well as to the songbird data (Section 20.8). We now consider the hierarchical version of this model for the indomethacin study. This will be done in Section 20.7.1. Section 20.7.2 will present a different pharmacokinetic model to a different set of data: the theophylline study. In Section 20.7.3, some remarks will be offered on pharmacodynamic models.

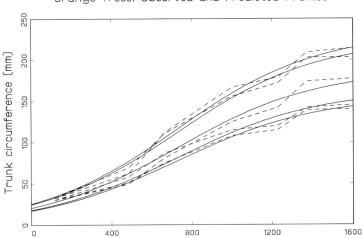

FIGURE 20.5. *Orange Tree Data. Observed profiles are presented with dashed lines, predicted ones by means of solid lines.*

20.7.1 Hierarchical Analysis of the Indomethacin Study

In Section 20.3, the bi-exponential or two-compartment model was fitted to the individual profiles of the indomethacin study, giving every subject its own set of parameters. Another extreme would be to assume that every subject can be described by exactly the same β's. From Section 20.5, illustrated using the orange data in Section 20.6, it is clear that a hierarchical non-linear analysis is possible, using the non-linear mixed-effects model, which can be seen as a theoretically well founded middle ground in between both extreme fixed effects views (parameters entirely different between subjects *versus* parameters identical). Hence, it is natural to introduce random effects into the bi-exponential model (20.11):

$$\begin{aligned}Y_{ij} = C_i(t_{ij}) &= e^{(\beta_1+b_{i1})}\exp\left(-e^{(\beta_2+b_{i2})}t_{ij}\right)\\ &\quad + e^{(\beta_3+b_{i3})}\exp\left(-e^{(\beta_4+b_{i4})}t_{ij}\right) + \varepsilon_{ij}.\end{aligned} \quad (20.19)$$

In line with standard practice, we will assume the random effects

$$(b_{i1}, b_{i2}, b_{i3}, b_{i4})'$$

to assume a four-variate normal distribution with zero mean vector and variance-covariance matrix D. To obtain an initial idea about D, the empirical variance-covariance matrix of the homoscedastic, heteroscedastic, or power model parameters, obtained in Section 20.3, and presented in Tables 20.2, 20.3, and 20.4, respectively, can be computed. For the power model, we obtain:

$$\widehat{D}_{\text{power}} = \begin{pmatrix} 0.052 & 0.096 & 0.110 & 0.130 \\ 0.096 & 0.246 & 0.301 & 0.417 \\ 0.110 & 0.301 & 0.509 & 0.600 \\ 0.130 & 0.417 & 0.600 & 0.937 \end{pmatrix}$$

with corresponding correlation matrix

$$\widehat{D}_{\text{power, corr}} = \begin{pmatrix} 1.000 & 0.852 & 0.677 & 0.588 \\ 0.852 & 1.000 & 0.848 & 0.868 \\ 0.677 & 0.848 & 1.000 & 0.869 \\ 0.588 & 0.868 & 0.869 & 1.000 \end{pmatrix}. \qquad (20.20)$$

From (20.20) it is clear that the random effects will be highly correlated. Thus, with in addition only a limited amount of data available, fitting a full 4×4 covariance matrix D with $4 + 6 = 10$ free parameters may be beyond reach. There are two alternatives. First, we might want to conduct a two-stage analysis based upon the results from Section 20.3, where the individual-specific regressions, obtained at the first occasion, are analyzed further at the second stage, providing averages (corresponding to fixed-effects), and variances (corresponding to D). Such an approach was reported in Tables 20.2–20.4. Second, a restricted hierarchical model could be fitted, i.e., one where the matrix D is subject to simplifying restrictions. For example, the four random effects could be assumed independent, even though the evidence in (20.20) points to the contrary. Parameter estimates and standard errors are presented in Table 20.7. Note that the fixed-effect parameters differ quite a bit from the marginal means, given in Table 20.4, due to the same phenomenon described in Chapter 16, governing the relationship between a generalized linear mixed model and the marginal model derived thereof. The variance of b_{i1} moved to the boundary of the parameter space. This can have a number of reasons, not only that it is truly equal to zero. For example, it can be an effect of misspecification (ignoring the covariances), or the true variance component could be negative, which is not allowed in the current NLMIXED procedure. We do notice from the two-stage analysis in Table 20.4 that the variability in β_{1i} is relatively small, even though the magnitude of the parameter is rather large. This suggests omitting the parameter may be sensible. Alternatively, both d_{11} and d_{44} could be removed, the latter based on using a $\chi^2_{0:1}$ p-value. SAS users should be warned that SAS output is incorrectly based on a χ^2_1 distribution. In summary, given the size of the dataset, it is better to restrict attention to two-stage analyses. Studies like this one are often used to get a first idea of the shape of the plasma concentration curve. More precise statistical inference is then based on larger, purposefully designed studies. The situation with the orange tree data was different, as only one

TABLE 20.7. *Indomethacin Study. Mixed bi-exponential model, with power variance model and independent random effects.*

Parameter	Estimate (s.e.)
Fixed effects:	
β_1	0.884 (0.061)
β_2	0.181 (0.062)
β_3	-1.752 (0.141)
β_4	-1.423 (0.083)
Residual variance:	
σ	0.125 (0.017)
θ	0.886 (0.087)
Random-effect (co-)variances:	
d_{11}	0.000 (0.000)
d_{22}	0.086 (0.016)
d_{33}	0.452 (0.103)
d_{44}	0.136 (0.076)

random-effect was assumed, entering linearly in the otherwise non-linear mean function.

20.7.2 *Pharmacokinetic Modeling and the Theophylline Data*

Theophylline is a well-known anti-asthmatic agent, administered orally (Boeckmann, Sheiner, and Beal 1992, Davidian and Giltinan 1995). Twelve subjects are given oral dose at time 0, whereafter blood samples are taken at 10 time points over the following 25 hours. The blood samples are then assayed for theophylline concentration. Individual profiles are presented in Figure 20.6. A common model for the kinetics of theophylline after oral administration is the so-called one-compartment open model with first-order absorption and elimination, as stated by Davidian and Giltinan (1995):

$$Y_{ij} = C_i(t_{ij}) = \frac{k_{ai}k_{ei}d_i}{C\ell_i(k_{ai} - k_{ei})}$$
$$\times [\exp(-k_{ei}t_{ij}) - \exp(-k_{ai}t_{ij})] + \varepsilon_{ij}, \quad (20.21)$$

where $C_i(t_{ij})$ is the observed concentration on subject i at occasion j (time t_{ij}), d_i is dose, administered to subject i, k_{ai} is the fractional absorption rate constant for subject i, k_{ei} is the fractional elimination rate constant for subject i, and $C\ell_i$ is the clearance for subject i.

Theophylline Data

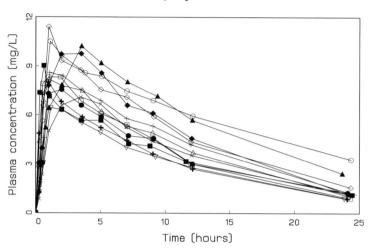

FIGURE 20.6. *Theophylline Data. Individual profiles.*

There are noteworthy differences with the indomethacin data (Sections 20.3 and 20.7.1). Not only is a different model used, based on different substantive theory, also the data exhibit a different structure in the sense that a larger set of data is used, with further variable measurement times across subjects.

Let us first model the individual profiles separately, in line with the initial indomethacin analysis (Section 20.3). To facilitate model fitting, we rewrite:

$$Cl = \exp(\beta_1), \qquad (20.22)$$
$$k_a = \exp(\beta_2), \qquad (20.23)$$
$$k_e = \exp(\beta_3). \qquad (20.24)$$

Results of the model fit are presented in Table 20.8. The variance-covariance of the β parameters in Table 20.9 is equal to:

$$\widehat{D} = \begin{pmatrix} 0.079 & -0.023 & 0.047 \\ -0.023 & 0.547 & -0.012 \\ 0.047 & -0.012 & 0.035 \end{pmatrix} \qquad (20.25)$$

with corresponding correlation matrix

$$\widehat{D}_{\text{corr}} = \begin{pmatrix} 1.000 & -0.109 & 0.904 \\ -0.109 & 1.000 & -0.089 \\ 0.904 & -0.089 & 1.000 \end{pmatrix}. \qquad (20.26)$$

It is clear that there is substantial correlation between the clearance and fractional elimination rate parameters. This suggests including correlated

20.7 Pharmacokinetic and Pharmacodynamic Models

TABLE 20.8. *Theophylline Data. One-compartment open model fitted to each subject separately.*

Subject	β_1	β_2	β_3	σ^2
	\multicolumn{4}{c}{Parameter estimates}			
1	-3.916	0.575	-2.920	0.390
2	-3.106	0.664	-2.286	0.813
3	-3.230	0.898	-2.508	0.040
4	-3.286	0.158	-2.436	0.521
5	-3.133	0.386	-2.425	1.224
6	-2.973	0.152	-2.307	0.222
7	-2.964	-0.386	-2.280	0.091
8	-3.069	0.319	-2.386	0.335
9	-3.421	2.182	-2.446	0.226
10	-3.428	-0.363	-2.604	0.123
11	-2.860	1.348	-2.322	0.039
12	-3.170	-0.183	-2.248	0.255
Mean	-3.213	0.479	-2.431	
Variance	0.079	0.547	0.035	
	\multicolumn{4}{c}{Standard errors}			
1	0.109	0.129	0.144	0.166
2	0.139	0.222	0.205	0.347
3	0.033	0.059	0.047	0.017
4	0.121	0.174	0.184	0.222
5	0.154	0.217	0.227	0.522
6	0.103	0.159	0.163	0.095
7	0.062	0.107	0.114	0.039
8	0.108	0.168	0.166	0.143
9	0.085	0.321	0.108	0.096
10	0.057	0.086	0.094	0.052
11	0.034	0.065	0.047	0.017
12	0.069	0.120	0.122	0.109

random effects into the model to achieve a hierarchical analysis. To this end, (20.22)–(20.24) are rewritten as:

$$Cl_i = \exp(\beta_1 + b_{i1}),$$
$$k_{a,i} = \exp(\beta_2 + b_{i2}),$$
$$k_{e,i} = \exp(\beta_3 + b_{i3}).$$

TABLE 20.9. *Theophylline Data. Mixed one-compartment open model with correlated random effects.*

Parameter	Estimate (s.e.)
Fixed effects:	
β_1	-3.277 (0.046)
β_2	0.537 (0.063)
β_3	-2.454 (0.064)
Residual variance:	
σ^2	0.623 (0.083)
Random-effect variances:	
d_{11}	0.057 (0.022)
d_{12}	-0.012 (0.018)
d_{22}	0.264 (0.054)
d_{13}	0.030 (0.020)
d_{23}	-0.025 (0.017)
d_{33}	0.035 (0.017)

The two-stage analysis provides useful starting values for fitting the hierarchical model. Because the model is forced to go through 0 when time is equal to 0, the corresponding measurement is removed prior to conducting the hierarchical analysis, as it may otherwise adversely affect the variance component and induce fitting problems. Parameter estimates and standard errors for fixed effects, residual variance, and variance-covariance parameters of the random-effects structure are presented in Table 20.9. The variance components can be assembled into

$$\widehat{D} = \begin{pmatrix} 0.057 & -0.012 & 0.030 \\ -0.012 & 0.263 & -0.025 \\ 0.030 & -0.025 & 0.035 \end{pmatrix} \qquad (20.27)$$

Note the effect of shrinkage, when compared to (20.25), obtained from the two-stage analysis. The correlation matrix, derived from (20.27) equals:

$$\widehat{D}_{\text{corr}} = \begin{pmatrix} 1.000 & -0.098 & 0.672 \\ -0.098 & 1.000 & -0.261 \\ 0.672 & -0.261 & 1.000 \end{pmatrix},$$

with correlations somewhat less extreme than those in (20.26), obtained from the two-stage analysis. A graphical comparison of fitted and observed profiles, presented in Figure 20.7, shows the fit is acceptable.

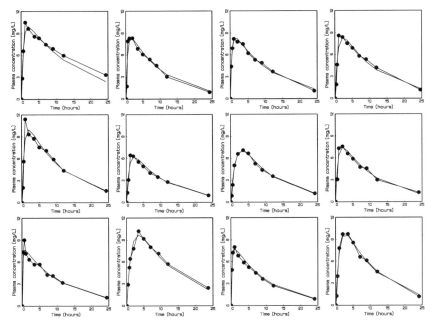

FIGURE 20.7. *Theophylline Data. Comparison of observed profiles with those obtained from fitting the one-compartment open model.*

Although the fit here is acceptable, it is useful to point out an alternative route. Because the correlation between clearance and fractional elimination rate is very high in (20.26), one might want to assume they are described by *the same* random effect, rather than two (highly) correlated ones. Then, b_{i3} would not be a separate random effect anymore, but merely a copy of b_{i1} or, more sensibly, a fixed multiple $b_{i3} = \lambda b_{i1}$, with λ a fixed variance inflation parameter, to be estimated along with the other fixed effects.

20.7.3 Pharmacodynamic Data

Pharmacokinetic (PK) data provide full profiles of response to drug administration, usually based on measuring a few subjects over an extended period of time. The exposure is the amount of drug administered, i.e., the dose level. The so-obtained information may be imprecise due to inter-subject variability. One reason for this is that for the same dose level administered, different subjects can absorb different amounts, whence the amount of drug available at the site of action is different.

Pharmacodynamic (PD) research aims to study the physiologic response by relating the drug response to the concentration available *at the site of action*. One issue is that the site of action in the body may not be accessible for examination, and then plasma or serum concentration can be used instead. Doing so reduces the effects of inter-kinetic variability, since the drug (seemingly) acts differently in different subjects, because absorption and elimination are different. Some have advocated that, ideally, this type of investigation ought to be done for all medicinal products, but doing so would make the logistics almost impossible. For a thorough discussion, see Davidian and Giltinan (1995). Usually, a relatively large number of subjects is measured repeatedly, both for drug concentration as well as for outcome. Because concentration may not vary too widely within a patient, a good range across patients should be ensured.

Unlike in PK modeling, one often does not have strong theory available, from which differential equations and ultimately models can be derived. Modeling therefore proceeds rather empirically, in line with practice in a vast number of substantive fields. A commonly used (empirical) functional form is:

$$Y = E_0 + \frac{E_{\max} - E_0}{1 + EC_{50}/C_e}, \tag{20.28}$$

where E_0 is the response at zero concentration, $E_{\max}$ is the maximal response, EC_{50} is the concentration eliciting a response halfway between E_0 and $E_{\max}$, and C_e is concentration of the drug at the effect site. Fitting a model like (20.28), using repeated measures data, is straightforward using non-linear mixed-effects methodology, such as developed in this chapter. The general model would then be written as:

$$Y_{ij} = E_{0i} + \frac{E_{\max,i} - E_{0i}}{1 + EC_{50,i}/C_{ij}} + \varepsilon_{ij},$$

with Y_{ij} the jth repeated measurement for subject i.

20.8 The Songbird Data

20.8.1 Introduction

Van der Linden et al (2002) and Van Meir et al (2004) established a novel in vivo magnetic resonance imaging (MRI) approach to discern the functional characteristics of specific neuronal populations in a strongly connected brain circuitry, the so-called song control system in the songbird brain. The high vocal center (HVC), one of the major nuclei in this circuit, contains interneurons and two distinct types of neurons projecting respectively to the so-called nucleus robustus arcopallii (RA) or to area X. This is graphically represented in Figure 20.8.

These authors analyzed the effect of testosterone on the dynamics of Mn^{2+} accumulation in RA and area X of female starling in individual birds injected with manganese in their HVC. The authors used relatively straightforward curve fitting techniques, combined with analysis of variance ideas. Although simple in nature, such techniques ignore dependencies

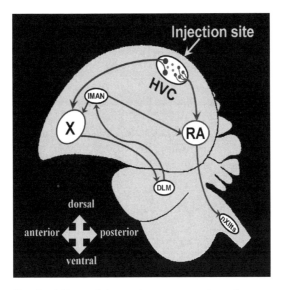

FIGURE 20.8. *Songbird Data. Schematic representation of song control nuclei in the songbird brain.*

in measurements in the same bird and may therefore be sub-optimal. To improve upon this approach, non-linear mixed-effects models prove to be useful. Using this more refined way of analysis Serroyen *et al* (2005) were able to detect testosterone effects that previously had gone unnoticed.

The outcomes analyzed are SI of RA, area X, and HVC. For the former two responses reasonably well accepted non-linear functional forms exist, but these have been used without taking the within-bird correlation into account. The same is not true for HVC. From graphically inspecting the data, it is clear that conventional linear models may be insufficient. We explore two possible routes: fractional polynomials that extend the collection of classical polynomial shapes (Royston and Altman 1994, Verbeke and Molenberghs 2000, Chapter 24, see also Section 12.4.2) and the two-compartment model known from pharmacokinetics and described in Section 20.3, to which the HVC problem is related.

Turning to the data, ten first-year female starlings were caught in the wild during the winter before February and housed in two indoor cages on a stable 10–14 hour light-dark light cycle, selected to maintain birds in a durable state of photosensitivity. All birds were studied by MRI for the first time between March 15 and April 30, 2001. One or two days after the first MRI measurement, the five treated birds were implanted with a capsule of crystalline testosterone subcutaneously in the neck region. The capsule was left empty for the five control birds. Birds were studied by MRI again five to six weeks after the treatment.

Previously, Van der Linden et al (2002) have employed the following parametric shape for a bird's profile:

$$SI_{ij}(RA) = \frac{(\phi_{0i} + \phi_{1i}G_i)t_{ij}^{\eta_{0i}+\eta_{1i}G_i}}{(\tau_{0i} + \tau_{1i}G_i)^{\eta_{0i}+\eta_{1i}G_i} + t_{ij}^{\eta_{0i}+\eta_{1i}G_i}} + \gamma_{0i} + \gamma_1 G_{1i} + \varepsilon_{ij}. \quad (20.29)$$

Here, $SI_{ij}(RA)$ is the measurement at time j for bird i, G_i is an indicator for group membership (1 for testosterone treated birds and 0 otherwise), and t_{ij} is the measurement time. The maximal signal intensity, sometimes termed SI_{max}, is denoted by ϕ_{0i} for an untreated bird and $\phi_{0i} + \phi_{1i}$ for a treated one. The time required to reach 50% of this maximum (T_{50}) is τ_{0i} and $\tau_{0i} + \tau_{1i}$, respectively. The shape of the curve is governed by the parameters η_{0i} and $\eta_{0i} + \eta_{1i}$. Finally, ε_{ij} is a measurement error term, typically assumed to follow a normal distribution. The genesis of this model is rooted in knowledge about Mn axonal transport and changes induced in the bird's brain caused by testosterone treatment. More details can be found in Brenowitz et al (1997), Van der Linden et al (2002), and Van Meir et al (2004).

Van der Linden et al (2002) fitted Model (20.29) to each of the birds under study, and then applied ANOVA to the estimated parameters. Such an approach rests on the assumption that the measurements within a bird are uncorrelated, similarly to the assumption made in Section 20.3 for the indomethacin data. To properly account for such correlation, we place this model within a mixed-effects framework, where the parameters of the above model are appropriately split into fixed and random effects.

20.8.2 A Non-linear Mixed-effects Model

Let us introduce random effects into model (20.29). In this model, all parameters (ϕ_{0i}, ϕ_{1i},...) were assumed to be different from songbird to songbird, since the non-linear model was fitted to each bird separately. We now are able to analyze all data together, separating out averaged (fixed) effects from bird-specific (random) effects, using the following replacements:

$$\phi_{0i} + \phi_{1i}G_i \rightarrow \phi_0 + \phi_1 G_i + f_i, \quad (20.30)$$
$$\eta_{0i} + \eta_{1i}G_i \rightarrow \eta_0 + \eta_1 G_i + h_i, \quad (20.31)$$
$$\tau_{0i} + \tau_{1i}G_i \rightarrow \tau_0 + \tau_1 G_i + t_i. \quad (20.32)$$

Thus, the ϕ, η, and τ parameters are fixed effects, whereas the vector (f_i, h_i, t_i) is a bird-specific vector of random effects, assumed to follow a trivariate normal distribution with mean $\mathbf{0}$ and covariance matrix D. Combining model (20.29) with replacements (20.30)–(20.32), we obtain:

$$SI_{ij}(RA) = \frac{(\phi_0 + \phi_1 G_i + f_i)t_{ij}^{\eta_0+\eta_1 G_i+h_i}}{(\tau_0 + \tau_1 G_i + t_i)^{\eta_0+\eta_1 G_i+h_i} + t_{ij}^{\eta_0+\eta_1 G_i+h_i}}$$

TABLE 20.10. *Songbird Data. Parameter estimates (standard errors) for the final model, fitted to* $SI_{ij}(RA)$ *at the first and second periods.*

Effect	Parameter	Estimate (s.e.) First	Second
	ϕ_0	0.4749 (0.0451)	0.4526 (0.0478)
	η_0	2.5608 (0.1375)	2.1826 (0.0802)
	η_1		0.4285 (0.1060)
	τ_0	3.1737 (0.1658)	2.8480 (0.1761)
$\text{Var}(f_i)$	d_{11}	0.0198 (0.0091)	0.0225 (0.0101)
$\text{Var}(t_i)$	d_{22}	0.2438 (0.1179)	0.2881 (0.1338)
$\text{Var}(h_i)$	d_{33}	0.1457 (0.0787)	
$\text{Cov}(f_i, t_i)$	d_{12}	0.0587 (0.0306)	
$\text{Var}(\varepsilon_{ij})$	σ^2	2.2E-04 (2.0E-05)	1.9E-04 (1.7E-05)

$$+\gamma_0 + \gamma_1 G_i + \varepsilon_{ij}. \tag{20.33}$$

The parameters retain the meaning they had in (20.29).

Regarding the residual error terms ε_{ij}, we assume them to be mutually independent and independent from the random effects, and to be drawn from a $N(0, \sigma^2)$ distribution.

20.8.3 *Analysis of SI at RA*

We will build a model for the second period, where treatment has been applied. We will also devote some comments to the first period, where measurements are taken prior to the application of treatment and consequently no treatment effect would be expected.

Let us discuss the model for the second, and more interesting, period. We will use Model (20.33) to analyze these data of which the general form has 8 fixed-effects parameters and 7 variance components (3 variances in D, 3 covariances in D, and σ^2). The model is fitted using the SAS procedure NLMIXED, using adaptive Gaussian quadrature. Backward selection led to the model:

$$SI_{ij}(RA) = \frac{(\phi_0 + f_i) t_{ij}^{\eta_0 + \eta_1 G_i}}{(\tau_0 + t_i)^{\eta_0 + \eta_1 G_i} + t_{ij}^{\eta_0 + \eta_1 G_i}} + \varepsilon_{ij}. \tag{20.34}$$

Fitted curves, for each bird separately, are displayed in Figure 20.9. A joint representation of these as well as the group specific averages, are given in Figure 20.10. These curves support our model selection procedure and confirm the final model is a parsimonious and adequate description of the data.

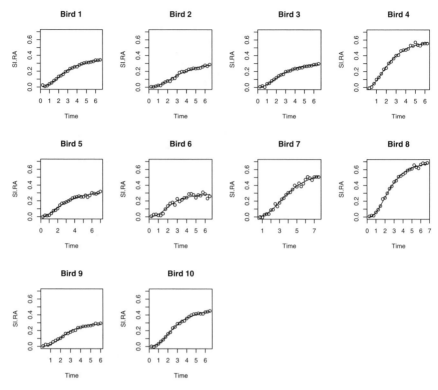

FIGURE 20.9. *Songbird Data. Fitted curves for $SI_{ij}(RA)$ at the second period, for each individual bird separately.*

It is worth to note that, in contrast to previous analyses, we do find a difference between both groups, in the sense that the shape parameter η is different between them. Further, there is substantial between-bird variability: there is a bird-specific component in the maximum change in relative signal intensity as well as in the time required to reach 50% of the maximum.

A similar model building exercise led to a model for the first period as well (Table 20.10). Here, in line with expectation, no effect of treatment was detected, as the treatment was applied after the first treatment.

20.8.4 Model Strategies for HVC

As stated before, there is a clear view on the hierarchical model needed to analyze RA and area X, rooted in the non-linear model used in the literature and previewed in the previous section. This is less the case for HVC. Therefore, it seems prudent to consider at least two different modeling

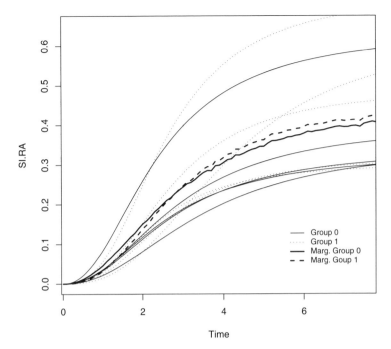

FIGURE 20.10. *Songbird Data. Individual and marginal fitted curves for $SI_{ij}(RA)$ at the second period.*

strategies: (1) fractional polynomials and (2) the bi-exponential pharmacokinetic model (20.19) already used in Section 20.7.1.

Let us briefly expand on fractional polynomials. As stated in, for example, Section 12.4.2, fractional polynomials allow a wide variety of parametric shapes by considering not only integer powers of a key covariate (e.g., time), but also fractional powers. This is handy whenever no clear prior view on the model is available. As soon as non-integer powers are allowed for, the number of potential models is virtually endless, and therefore it is wise to consider, a priori, a sensible model building strategy. This has been provided by Royston and Altman (1994).

Formally, Royston and Altman (1994) define a fractional polynomial as any function of the form

$$f(u) = \phi_0 + \sum_{k=1}^{m} \phi_k x^{(p_k)},$$

where the degree m is a positive integer, where $p_1 > \ldots > p_m$ are real-valued prespecified powers, and where ϕ_0 and $\phi_1, \ldots, \phi_m$ are real-valued unknown regression coefficients. Finally, $x^{(p_k)}$ is defined as

$$x^{(p_k)} = \begin{cases} x^{p_k} & \text{if } p_k \neq 0 \\ \ln(x) & \text{if } p_k = 0. \end{cases} \quad (20.35)$$

Thus, not only the conventional powers x, x^2,... are allowable, also $\ln(x)$, $\sqrt{x}$ (for $p_k = 0.5$), $1/x$ (for $p_k = -1$), etc.

In the context of linear and logistic regression analyses, Royston and Altman (1994) have shown that the family of fractional polynomials is very flexible and that models with degree m larger than 2 are rarely required. In practice, several values for the powers $p_1, \ldots, p_m$ can be tried, and the model with the best fit is then selected. Using a fractional polynomial within a linear or a non-linear mixed-effects model, is reasonably straightforward. One is merely required to construct the necessary covariate powers, logarithms, and interactions thereof, as a set of covariates in the dataset to be analyzed. In our case, fractional polynomials will be applied to the time covariate. Of course, given the relative complexity of the non-linear mixed effects model, we propose to keep the degree m of the polynomials relatively small. One can then fit several models with a variety of powers $p_1, \ldots, p_m$.

Although the fractional polynomial approach is flexible, it is also empirical in nature, allowing on the one hand a wide variety of parametric shapes, useful for a variety of applications, but not offering immediate biological insight into the meaning of the parameters and their estimated values. Arguably, their value lies in confirming or questioning other models, i.e., by way of sensitivity analysis, and to test treatment or other effects. In the next section, we will propose a different model that follows from pharmacokinetic principles.

20.8.5 Analysis of SI at HVC

Let us first consider the fractional polynomial approach. These were fitted with a range of power combinations. The combination associated with the highest likelihood value consists of ln(time) and $\sqrt{\text{time}}$. This leads to the following initial model:

$$SI_{ij}(\text{HVC}) = (\alpha_0 + \alpha_1 G_i + a_i) + (\lambda_0 + \lambda_1 G_i + l_i)\ln(t_{ij})$$
$$+ (\delta_0 + \delta_1 G_i + d_i)t_{ij}^{0.5} + \varepsilon_{ij}. \quad (20.36)$$

Parameter estimates and standard errors for the final model, obtained using backward selection, are presented in Table 20.11. Note that no significant group differences were found. The final model equals:

$$SI_{ij}(\text{HVC}) = (\alpha_0 + a_i) + (\lambda_0 + l_i)\ln(t_{ij}) + (\delta_0 + d_i)t_{ij}^{0.5} + \varepsilon_{ij}. \quad (20.37)$$

A graphical inspection (not shown) revealed the fit to be acceptable.

TABLE 20.11. *Songbird Data. Parameter estimates (standard errors) for the final fractional polynomial model, fitted to $SI_{ij}(HVC)$ at the first and second period.*

Effect	Parameter	Estimate (s.e.) First	Estimate (s.e.) Second
	α_0	3.4277 (0.2190)	2.9382 (0.3732)
	α_1	-1.3765 (0.3080)	
	λ_0	1.3278 (0.2354)	0.4140 (0.1277)
	λ_1	-1.0455 (0.3286)	
	δ_0	-1.7436 (0.1897)	-0.8395 (0.1247)
	δ_1	1.1783 (0.2631)	
Var(a_i)	d_{11}	0.2091 (0.1052)	1.3857 (0.6227)
Var(l_i)	d_{22}	0.2502 (0.1205)	0.1597 (0.0748)
Var(d_i)	d_{33}	0.1432 (0.0633)	0.1493 (0.0532)
Cov(a_i, d_i)	d_{13}	-0.0632 (0.0351)	-0.2675 (0.1271)
Cov(l_i, d_i)	d_{23}	-0.1743 (0.0858)	-0.1192 (0.0583)
Var(ε_{ij})	σ^2	0.0076 (0.0007)	0.0022 (0.0002)

Let us now turn to the pharmacokinetic two-compartment model (20.19). The HVC problem is strongly connected to pharmacokinetic theory, which studies the dispersion of a compound through a living organism. Because the HVC region can be regarded as the *central compartment* from which manganese is dispersed to area X and SA, a two-compartment model seems a reasonable choice. Let us consider a 'mixed-effects' way of representing (20.19):

$$Y_{ij} = \exp(\beta_{i1}) \exp[-\exp(-\beta_{i2} \, t_{ij})] \\ - \exp(\beta_{i3}) \exp(-\exp[-\beta_{i4} \, t_{ij})] + \varepsilon_{ij}. \quad (20.38)$$

Decomposing the β's into fixed and random effects, thereby including a group effect as well, we obtain:

$$Y_{ij} = e^{(\beta_1 + \gamma_1 G_i + b_{1i})} \exp[-e^{(-\beta_2 + \gamma_2 G_i + b_{2i}) \, t_{ij}}] \\ - e^{(\beta_3 + \gamma_3 G_i + b_{3i})} \exp[-e^{(-\beta_4 + \gamma_4 G_i + b_{4i}) \, t_{ij}}] + \varepsilon_{ij}. \quad (20.39)$$

Parameter estimates and standard errors, obtained after backward model selection, are presented in Table 20.12. The final model equals:

$$Y_{ij} = e^{(\beta_1 + b_{1i})} \exp[-e^{(-\beta_2 + b_{2i}) \, t_{ij}}] \\ - e^{(\beta_3 + b_{3i})} \exp[-e^{(-\beta_4 + b_{4i}) \, t_{ij}}] + \varepsilon_{ij}. \quad (20.40)$$

It is important to note that, while the fractional polynomial and two-compartment modeling strategies are rather different in nature, both coincide in the conclusions that (1) there is no treatment effect at the second

TABLE 20.12. *Songbird Data. Parameter estimates (standard errors) for the final two-compartment model, fitted to $SI_{ij}(HVC)$ at the first and second periods.*

Effect	Parameter	Estimate (s.e.) First	Second
	β_1	0.8306 (0.0921)	0.7964 (0.1330)
	γ_1	-0.3596 (0.1305)	
	β_2	-2.7425 (0.1974)	-2.7088 (0.0627)
	γ_2	0.2500 (0.2879)	
	β_3	1.2516 (0.6802)	-0.5711 (0.6436)
	γ_3	-2.5839 (1.0243)	
	β_4	0.9094 (0.1846)	1.2311 (0.4906)
	γ_4	0.0051 (0.4076)	
$\text{Var}(b_{1i})$	d_{11}	0.0416 (0.0191)	0.1744 (0.0792)
$\text{Var}(b_{2i})$	d_{22}	0.1810 (0.1045)	0.0241 (0.0157)
$\text{Var}(b_{3i})$	d_{33}	2.0659 (1.2933)	1.5106 (1.1534)
$\text{Var}(b_{4i})$	d_{44}	0.0690 (0.1086)	1.3865 (1.1047)
$\text{Var}(\varepsilon_{ij})$	σ^2	0.0050 (4.7E-04)	1.4E-03 (1.4E-04)

period and (2) there is a strong indication, by way of random effects, for between-bird variability.

Models for the first period were built as well. The results are reported in Tables 20.11 and 20.12. Again, both final models exhibit an excellent fit (details not shown) and in both cases, treatment effects are found.

20.9 Discrete Outcomes

In Section 20.4, a general framework was developed for non-linear longitudinal models, building on generalized linear models, linear mixed-effects models, generalized linear mixed models, etc. In Section 20.5, we zoomed in on a random-effects specification, producing so-called non-linear mixed models. A very general mean specification, conditional upon random effects, is then given by (20.17). This formulation is general enough to encompass non-linear random-effects models for both Gaussian and non-Gaussian outcomes. All examples analyzed so far have been of a Gaussian type. Of course, differences between the two settings will show up when (20.17) is made part of a full model specification. In the continuous examples, it could be thought of as specifying the mean of a normal distribution, whereas for a binary outcome it will lead to the probability in a Bernoulli model. In the latter case, the right hand side of (20.17) has to be chosen such that a valid probability is obtained. In generalized linear models, this is done via the choice of an appropriate link function. Now, the link function has been integrated into the $h(\cdot)$ function, but it might be convenient to separate them:

$$g^{-1}\left[E(Y_{ij}|\boldsymbol{b}_i, \boldsymbol{x}_{ij}, \boldsymbol{z}_{ij})\right] = \widetilde{h}(\boldsymbol{x}_{ij}, \boldsymbol{\beta}, \boldsymbol{z}'_{ij}\boldsymbol{b}_i), \tag{20.41}$$

where obviously $h(\cdot) \equiv g[\widetilde{h}(\cdot)]$. Here again, $g(\cdot)$ is a link function and $\widetilde{h}(\cdot)$ is said to be the non-linear predictor function. Although this decomposition is convenient for the modeler, to ensure a valid conditional mean model structure be obtained, it is strictly speaking not necessary for estimation. In other words, the theory developed in Section 20.5, which itself goes back to the theory developed for the generalized linear mixed model in Chapter 14, applies here without the need for modification.

20.9.1 Analysis of the NTP Data

The NTP data, introduced in Section 2.7, have been analyzed before in Sections 7.2.3, 8.9, 9.6, 11.4, 12.4, 14.7, and 16.5. In Section 16.5, a generalized linear mixed model was fitted to the external outcome of the DEHP study. Often, a simple linear dose model, either directly describing the mean in continuous outcomes or transformed by means of a suitably chosen link function for non-Gaussian outcomes, fails to capture the true dose-response relationship. A flexible yet simple extension is by means of including a power parameter, such as in Faes *et al* (2004). This implies that generalized linear mixed model (14.11) would change to

$$\begin{aligned} Y_{ij}|b_i &\sim \text{Bernoulli}(\pi_{ij}), \\ \text{logit}(\pi_{ij}) &= \beta_0 + b_i + \beta_d(d_i + 0.01)^\gamma, \end{aligned} \tag{20.42}$$

with γ a power dose effect, next to the usual linear dose effect β_d. We have added 0.01 to the dose, to avoid problems at dose level zero, i.e., to stay away from raising the value zero to a power. The so-obtained null model of linear dose effect only is equivalent to the one obtained without the offset 0.01. The g function in (20.41) is the logit link and $\widetilde{h}$ is the right hand side of (20.42).

Of course, many other dose-response curves can be tried in the absence of substantive knowledge such as, for example, in the pharmacokinetic data analyzed in Sections 20.3, 20.7.1, and 20.7.2, and, to a lesser extent, in the songbird data (Section 20.8). Model (20.42), although a simple and straightforward extension of (14.11), carries an intrinsic complexity. Testing the null hypothesis of no dose effects involves the parameters β_d and γ at the same time, in a non-trivial way. This point is briefly discussed in Section 20.10. It is in contrast to testing the null hypothesis of a linear dose trend, which comes down to testing for $H_0 : \gamma = 1$, a standard problem.

Parameter estimates, obtained using adaptive Gaussian quadrature with an algorithm-defined number of quadrature points, are presented in Table 20.13. We used Newton-Raphson as an updating algorithm, for its

TABLE 20.13. *NTP Data. Parameter estimates (standard errors) for a non-linear mixed-effects model with logit link. β_0, β_d, and γ are the marginal intercept, linear and power dose effects, respectively; τ^2 is the variance of the random intercept.*

Outcome	Parameter	DEHP	EG	DYME
External	β_0	-11.36(8.96)		-7.71(1.75)
	β_d	11.37(8.78)		8.60(1.81)
	γ	0.34(0.36)		1.26(0.50)
	τ	1.09(0.27)		1.19(0.36)
	τ^2	1.18(0.59)		1.41(0.85)
Visceral	β_0	-5.19(0.62)		-7.22(1.14)
	β_d	5.36(0.76)		5.50(1.17)
	γ	1.15(0.31)		2.10(1.26)
	τ	1.21(0.26)		1.52(0.45)
	τ^2	1.47(0.64)		2.30(1.37)
Skeletal	β_0	-6.07(0.82)	-10.58(5.36)	-6.74(0.98)
	β_d	6.06(0.95)	11.03(5.28)	9.20(1.15)
	γ	1.07(0.29)	0.24(0.15)	0.97(0.21)
	τ	1.43(0.30)	1.40(0.20)	1.64(0.28)
	τ^2	2.06(0.88)	1.95(0.56)	2.68(0.92)
Collapsed	β_0	-4.64(0.51)	-11.25(6.21)	-5.73(0.70)
	β_d	7.38(0.84)	11.82(6.13)	9.42(0.96)
	γ	1.28(0.25)	0.22(0.15)	1.19(0.20)
	τ	1.34(0.23)	1.39(0.20)	1.34(0.24)
	τ^2	1.80(0.62)	1.94(0.56)	1.80(0.65)

quadratic convergence properties near the maximum. For non-linear problems of this type, the convergence of quasi-Newton methods close to the maximum can be painstakingly slow.

The power parameter is not significant for the external outcome in the DEHP study and for the visceral outcome in the DYME study. For all other DEHP and DYME study outcomes, it is significant. The case of the EG data is a little problematic, in the sense that convergence to a plausible value for the external and visceral outcomes is hard or impossible to reach. This is not surprising, as the number of events is extremely small in these cases: 23 out of 1028 (2.24%) and 11 out of 1028 (1.07%), respectively. In contrast, for the skeletal outcome this number is 237 out of 1028 (23%). The number of events for the DEHP study are 69, 72, and 66 out of 1082 (149 for the collapsed outcome), and 99, 31, and 177 out of 1191 (207 for the collapsed outcome) for the DYME study. In other words, Model (20.42) is overly complex for the external and visceral outcomes in the EG study, and a linear-logistic specification, as in (14.11), would be sufficient.

20.10 Hypothesis Testing and Non-linear Models

Power models such as the dose-response model (20.42) allow for flexible modeling of the dose-response relationship, as illustrated in Section 20.9.1. However, as studied by Faes et al (2004), the use of power models leads to some critical statistical issues in the context of hypothesis testing. Indeed, the case of no effect of dose d_i can be formulated as either $\beta_d = 0$ or $\gamma = 0$. This corresponds to the union of two planes in the parameter space of $(\beta_0, \beta_d, \gamma)$, i.e., the planes with equation $\beta_d = 0$ and $\gamma = 0$, respectively. Furthermore, the condition that $\beta_d = 0$ or $\gamma = 0$ is equivalent to $\beta_d \gamma = 0$. The null model is then maximized, not in a single point, but in the union of two axes. This model is non-standard and hence classical asymptotic testing theory cannot be invoked.

Further, note that the regression parameters are not identifiable under the null hypothesis of no dose effect. Thus, we are confronted with (nuisance) parameters vanishing under the null hypothesis. This problem has received considerable attention lately (Conniffe 2001, Davies 2002, Severini 2004), is related to but different from the problem of null hypotheses on the boundary of the parameter space (Hall and Præstgaard 2001, Verbeke and Molenberghs 2003), and is one of the issues that can arise when non-linear predictors are used (Davidian and Giltinan 1995, Seber and Wild 2003).

For convenience, let us rewrite the right hand side of (20.42) as

$$\eta = \widetilde{h}(d_i, \beta_0, \beta_d, \gamma, b_i) = \beta_0 + b_i + \beta_d d_i^{\gamma}, \qquad (20.43)$$

where, if necessary, d_i can again be replaced by $d_i + 0.01$. The parameter γ is not identifiable if $\beta_d = 0$, since η then reduces to β_0. If $\gamma = 0$, the model simplifies to $\beta_0 + \beta_d$. In this case, one cannot identify β_0 and β_d separately, although their sum is identifiable. When conducting a test of no dose effect from a frequentist point of view, there are severe complications due to this non-identifiability issue. Consider, for example, the likelihood ratio test statistic. Assume the maximum under the null is reached for some value η^*. Then, all triplets $(\beta_0 = \eta^*, \beta_d = 0, \gamma)$ reach the maximum, as well as all triplets $(\beta_0, \beta_d = \eta^* - \beta_0, \gamma = 0)$. As a consequence, under the hypothesis of no dose effect, the likelihood is maximized at any parameter combination on two intersecting lines. Faes et al (2004) proposed a Bayesian route to deal with this non-standard problem.

20.11 Flexible Functions

Analyses such as those of the orange tree, songbird, indomethacin, theophylline, and NTP data underscore the tremendous flexibility and generality of the non-linear mixed model (20.41). It encompasses both continuous and non-Gaussian data, when a particular functional form is available as well as when a more empirical approach to model formulation is necessary. For example, the models for both the indomethacin and the theophylline data are based on pharmacokinetic theory, the parametric models deriving from an appropriate set of differential equations. One of these models, the bi-exponential model (20.11), could be used for the songbird data as well. The model for the NTP data was a simple power model extension of the linear model used before. For the orange tree growth data, the selected model has a more pragmatic background.

In spite of this flexibility, we should not loose from sight that the model is fully parametric, based on full distributional assumptions, with parametrically specified mean, variance, and association structure. For continuous outcomes (Chapter 4), the outcome is usually assumed to be normally distributed, whereas for non-Gaussian outcomes one assumes the distribution to be Bernoulli, binomial, multinomial (Chapter 18), Poisson (Chapter 19), etc. In the random-effects case, one usually complements these assumptions with normally distributed random effects in order to specify the association structure.

Sometimes, it may be desirable to increases one's distance from fully parametrically specified models. There are many ways in which a model can be non-parametric or semi-parametric. First, one may prefer not to fully specify the outcome distribution. When the specification is restricted to a few moments only, generalized estimating equations (Chapter 8) or pseudo-likelihood (Chapter 9) come into view. Considerable attention has gone to non-parametric specification of the random-effects distribution, for which so-called non-parametric maximum likelihood (NPML, Section 13.3.3, see also Böhning 1999, McLachlan and Peel 2000) has been developed. The random-effects distribution is then discrete with finite support. In other words, a finite mixture distribution is obtained as marginal model for the responses. Intermediate forms have been developed as well, such as assuming the random-effects distribution is a finite mixture of normal distributions (Verbeke and Molenberghs 2000, Chapter 12, see also Chapter 23 in this volume).

Although parametric in nature, the fractional polynomials described in Section 20.8.4 are very flexible, and they can be considered as going a long way toward non-parametric models. Another versatile approach is by means of splines (Ruppert, Wand, and Carroll 2003). Various forms of splines have been used in the literature, first in conventional regression problems and then also in the context of longitudinal and correlated data. The essence of a spline approach is the joining of smooth functions, usually polynomials, in a finite number of knots, where the transition from one base function to the other is made in a continuous way. Although splines can be used in the fixed-effects regression function, several authors have employed this idea at the random-effects level as well, providing a very flexible tool to capture subject-specific structure, and thus association. A seminal paper in this respect was written by Verbyla *et al* (1999), and a similar method is reported in Ruppert, Wand, and Carroll (2003). Although formulating random-effects by means of splines is in itself a nice idea, the beauty lies in the fact that such a model can be written in such a way that standard linear mixed-effects model theory applies, in other words, that the parameters can be estimated essentially by solving an appropriate set of mixed-model equations, where a particular spline-based model translates into a particular choice for the random-effects design matrix Z_i. Of course, this result holds by virtue of linearity and hence holds for the linear mixed-effects model. However, thanks to the linearization-based methodology, employed in Section 8.8 and in particular also in Section 14.4, the same concepts can be applied to generalized linear mixed models and in fact to non-linear mixed models as well. A version of this methodology has been implemented in the SAS procedure GLIMMIX.

In Section 20.11.1, we will provide a brief introduction to smoothing splines for random effects and then illustrate these ideas using the ordinal analgesic trial outcomes in Section 20.11.2, building upon the analysis presented in Section 18.4.

20.11.1 Random Smoothing Splines

As an alternative to consider the fully general, non-linear but parametric model (20.41), we might want to consider a version where the random effects structure contains a spline part. Ruppert, Wand, and Carroll (2003, Sections 13.4–13.5), in analogy with Verbyla *et al* (1999), considered approximate low rank thin plate splines, and employ the analogy with mixed-model fitting to arrive at efficient updating algorithms. This method is employed in the SAS procedure GLIMMIX as well (SAS Institute Inc. 2004, p. 107). The key result is the similarity between the penalized spline fitting criterion and the minimization problem that yields the mixed-model equations. There is a difference with classical spline fitting since in this approach the spline coefficients are random effects, whereas they are fixed effects in a classical approach.

Consider a classical linear mixed model formulation for an outcome vector Y_i or, using data approximations as in Section 14.4.1, for an approximate outcome vector Y_i^*. For convenience, stack all outcome vectors for all subjects $i = 1, \ldots N$ on top of each other, with similar conventions for random vectors, and design matrices ordered in a block-diagonal fashion:

$$Y = X\beta + Zb + \varepsilon. \tag{20.44}$$

The above model is replaced by an appropriate expression for Y^* in the generalized linear case, as in (14.7). Mixed-model equations are derived from maximizing the joint density $f(b, \varepsilon)$ with respect to β and b. Even though b is not a vector of outcomes, and hence this approach looks at odds with genuine likelihood inference, it is well-known to work (Henderson

1984). Thus, if we assume that var(ε^*) = $\sigma^2 I$ and var(b) = $\tau^2 I$, then maximization of this joint density is equivalent to minimization of

$$Q(\beta, b) = \frac{1}{\sigma^2}(Y^* - X\beta - Zb)'(Y^* - X\beta - Zb) + \frac{1}{\tau^2}b'b. \qquad (20.45)$$

Next, consider a linear spline, as in Ruppert, Wand, and Carroll (2003, p. 108). For example,

$$f(x) = \beta_0 + \beta_1 x + \sum_{k=1}^{K} \gamma_k (x - t_k)_+. \qquad (20.46)$$

The coefficients γ_k in (20.46) are the spline coefficients and the t_k are the knots. Upon incorporating the intercept and covariate effect x into the design matrix X and the truncated line functions $(x - t_k)_+$ into the design matrix Z, spline fitting is equivalent to the minimization of:

$$Q^*(\beta, \gamma) = (Y^* - X\beta - Z\gamma)'(Y^* - X\beta - Z\gamma) + \lambda^2 \gamma'\gamma. \qquad (20.47)$$

Note that γ in (20.47) plays the role of the random effects b in (20.45). Since minimization of (20.47) is equivalent to the minimization of $Q^*(\beta, \gamma)/\sigma^2$, it is clear that both problems (20.45) and (20.47) are equivalent and the smoothing parameter is

$$\lambda = \frac{\sigma}{\tau}.$$

Clearly, the smoothing parameter is selected automatically and derives from a single additional variance component, similar to a random-intercept variance parameter.

In a generalized linear setting, i.e., with non-normal outcomes and link function different from the identify, the variance of ε for the working variate Y^* is typically structured as

$$\text{var}(\varepsilon) = \sigma^2 \Delta^{-1} A \Delta^{-1}, \qquad (20.48)$$

where A is made up of variance functions and Δ is an appropriate model derivative. This leads to a slight update of (20.47):

$$Q^*(\beta, \gamma) = \frac{1}{\sigma^2}(Y^* - X\beta - Z\gamma)' \Delta A^{-1} \Delta (Y^* - X\beta - Z\gamma) + \frac{\lambda^2}{\sigma^2}\gamma'\gamma. \qquad (20.49)$$

The SAS procedure GLIMMIX uses radial base functions and transforms them to approximate a thin-plate spline.

We will illustrate this method using the ordinal global satisfaction assessment outcome in the analgesic trial in Section 20.11.2, together with the algorithm used to drive the knots, which is based on a so-called k-d tree (Friedman, Bentley, and Finkel 1977, Cleveland and Grosse 1991). Example SAS procedure GLIMMIX code is presented and discussed, along with the output, in Section 20.12.6.

20.11.2 Analysis of the Analgesic Trial

In Section 18.4, we fitted a marginal (GEE) model and a random-intercept logistic regression model (18.8) to the five-point ordinal GSA outcome in the analgesic trial. Results were presented in Table 18.2. We will now consider the model:

$$\text{logit} P(Y_{ij} \leq k | t_{ij}, X_i) = \alpha_k + \text{spl}_i(t_{ij}) + \beta_2 t_{ij} + \beta_3 t_{ij}^2 + \beta_4 X_i, \quad (20.50)$$

($k = 1, \ldots, 4$), where $\text{spl}_i(t_{ij})$ is a random smoothing spline in time, instead of a random intercept b_i. Clearly, association is induced by the inclusion of such random splines, in analogy with the inclusion of conventional random effects.

Results of fitting these models, using the SAS procedure GLIMMIX, are presented in Table 20.14. Apart from the fully parametric random-intercept model as in Table 18.2 (PQL column), a fully parametric model with random intercept and random slope in time is considered as well:

$$\text{logit} P(Y_{ij} \leq k | t_{ij}, X_i, b_i) = \alpha_k + b_{1i} + (\beta_2 + b_{2i}) t_{ij} + \beta_3 t_{ij}^2 + \beta_4 X_i, \quad (20.51)$$

($k = 1, \ldots, 4$). Clearly, there is very little evidence for the need of additional random effects. The fixed-effects parameters are virtually unaffected. The main part of the table concerns the results of the random spline based estimation. A key factor in the specification of the spline-based method is the so-called bucket size, a tool to determine the knots. Larger bucket sizes implies less knots, and vice versa. A discussion of the bucket size concept is given in Section 20.12.6. We considered bucket sizes of 100, 200, 1000, 2000, and 5000. Because knots occur at data points only, and we have only four time points (1, 2, 3, 4), it is not surprising to see the five different bucket sizes give rise to three different fits only: 100 and 200 produce two knots, 1000 leads to three knots, and all four possible knots are obtained for bucket sizes 100 and 200. These results illustrate that the number of knots decreases with bucket size. Between the different random smoothing splines analyses, results are not very different and, while a difference in parameter estimates with the fully parametric fits is noticeable, they are not overwhelming. It is noteworthy that the standard errors in the smoothing based models are smaller, illustrating that a more refined association structure had led to increased precision. Of course, simply omitting association might reduce standard errors as well, but such an assumption would typically be incorrect. The variance of the random spline coefficients is relatively small, but highly significant nevertheless, underscoring the point that a considerable improvement of model fit is obtained in this way. Example SAS code to fit this type of models is presented in Section 20.12.6. Using selected output, it is illustrated how the k-d tree splitting process operates in practice.

TABLE 20.14. *Analgesic Trial. Parameter estimates (standard errors) for generalized linear mixed models (using PQL) with random smoothing splines in time.*

		Fully parametric models	
Effect	Par.	R.I.	R.I.+R.S.
Intercept 1	α_1	-1.45(0.50)	-1.44(0.50)
Intercept 2	α_2	0.90(0.50)	0.51(0.50)
Intercept 3	α_3	3.47(0.51)	3.47(0.51)
Intercept 4	α_4	5.62(0.54)	5.63(0.54)
Time	β_2	-0.48(0.30)	-0.48(0.30)
Time^2	β_3	0.10(0.06)	0.10(0.06)
Basel. PCA	β_4	-0.28(0.13)	-0.28(0.12)
Var(b_{1i})	d_{11}	3.53(0.42)	3.28(0.74)
Cov(b_{1i}, b_{2i})	d_{12}		0.05(0.21)
Var(b_{2i})	d_{22}		0.01(0.07)

		Smoothing-based models		
		Bucket size		
Effect	Par.	5000/2000	1000	200/100
Intercept 1	α_1	-1.15(0.41)	-1.19(0.42)	-1.17(0.41)
Intercept 2	α_2	0.68(0.41)	0.70(0.42)	0.67(0.41)
Intercept 3	α_3	2.78(0.41)	2.86(0.42)	2.79(0.42)
Intercept 4	α_4	4.70(0.44)	4.82(0.45)	4.71(0.44)
Time	β_2	-0.27(0.30)	-0.29(0.31)	-0.27(0.31)
Time^2	β_3	0.06(0.06)	0.07(0.06)	0.06(0.06)
Basel. PCA	β_4	-0.26(0.08)	0.27(0.08)	-0.26(0.08)
Var. R. Sp.	τ^2	0.093(0.0013)	0.108(0.015)	0.093(0.013)
Knots		1,4	1,2,4	1,2,3,4

20.12 Using SAS for Non-linear Mixed-effects Models

In this section we will present typical SAS programs used for the analysis of the various examples analyzed in this chapter. We will concentrate on the programs and not on the output, which is in line with output obtained for generalized linear mixed models, as in Chapter 15.

20.12.1 SAS Program for the Orange Tree Data Analysis

The model was fitted, using the SAS procedure NLMIXED. Code to this effect is

20.12 Using SAS for Non-linear Mixed-effects Models

```
proc nlmixed data=tree;
 parms beta1=190 beta2=700 beta3=350
       sigmab=10 sigma=10;
 num = b + beta1;
 ex = exp(-(day-beta2)/beta3);
 den = 1 + ex;
 ratio = num/den;
 model y ~ normal(ratio,sigma**2);
 random b ~ normal(0,sigmab**2) subject=tree out=eb;
 predict ratio out=ratio;
run;
```

Clearly, the ability to use program statements ensures very general model formulations can be obtained. Because we are assuming a normal distribution, a residual variance σ^2 needs to be included. The actual parameter is σ, in an effort of defensive programming. Note that the 'out=eb' option in the RANDOM statement produces empirical Bayes estimates of the random effects. In addition, the PREDICT statement ensures that the quantity 'ratio' is predicted, needed for plotting the fitted conditional profiles, shown in Figure 20.5.

20.12.2 SAS Programs for the Indomethacin Analyses

The models presented in Section 20.3 can be fitted most easily using the SAS procedure NLMIXED. Code for the homoscedastic model is

```
proc nlmixed data=indo01 qpoints=3;
 parms beta1=1.27 beta2=1.04 beta3=-1.23 beta4=-1.51
       sigma=0.1;
 aver = exp(beta1)*exp(-exp(beta2)*time)
        + exp(beta3)*exp(-exp(beta4)*time);
 model plasma ~ normal(aver, sigma**2);
 by subject;
run;
```

Clearly, the procedure NLMIXED, used without the RANDOM statement, becomes a module for standard non-linear regression. The use of the BY statement ensures that every subject is modeled separately. Parameters have the same meaning as in Section 20.3. Switching to the heteroscedastic model is done by replacing the MODEL statement with:

```
model plasma ~ normal(aver, (aver**2) * (sigma**2));
```

Finally, the power model is obtained by means of:

```
model plasma ~ normal(aver,(aver**(2*theta)) * (sigma**2));
```

with appropriate modification to the PARMS statement as well, so as to provide a starting value for the θ parameter.

Switching to the hierarchical model, the BY statement is removed and the RANDOM statement added. SAS code to fit this model is

```
proc nlmixed data=indo01 noad qpoints=3;
  parms beta1=0.89 beta2=0.43 beta3=-1.66 beta4=-2.39 sigma=0.1
        theta=1.043 d11=0.052 d22=0.246 d33=0.509 d44=0.937;
  aver = exp(beta1+b1)*exp(-exp(beta2+b2)*time)
         + exp(beta3+b3)*exp(-exp(beta4+b4)*time);
  model plasma ~ normal(aver,(aver**(2*theta)) * (sigma**2));
  random b1 b2 b3 b4 ~
         normal([0,0,0,0],[d11,0,d22,0,0,d33,0,0,0,d44])
         subject=subject;
  predict aver out=m.aver;
run;
```

For ease of convergence with a relatively extensive random-effects structure, non-adaptive Gaussian quadrature with 3 quadrature points was used. Adaptive Gaussian quadrature and/or more quadrature points can be considered to check stability and numerical convergence of the fit.

20.12.3 SAS Programs for the Theophylline Analyses

In line with Section 20.12.2, we first consider a program for the analysis of the profiles individually:

```
proc nlmixed data=theoph;
  parms beta1=-3.22 beta2=0.47 beta3=-2.45 s2=0.5;
  cl = exp(beta1);
  ka = exp(beta2);
  ke = exp(beta3);
  pred = dose*ke*ka*(exp(-ke*time)-exp(-ka*time))/cl/(ka-ke);
  model conc ~ normal(pred,s2);
  by subject;
  ods output parameterestimates=theopar;
run;
```

When switching to the hierarchical analysis, it is important to remove the structural zeros at baseline:

```
data help;
set theoph;
if time=0 then delete;
run;
```

The program then becomes:

```
proc nlmixed data=help noad qpoints=3;
  parms beta1=-3.22 beta2=0.47 beta3=-2.45
```

```
        d11=0.03 d12=0 d22=0.4 d13=0 d23=0 d33=0.03
        s2=0.5;
 cl = exp(beta1 + b1);
 ka = exp(beta2 + b2);
 ke = exp(beta3 + b3);
 pred = dose*ke*ka*(exp(-ke*time)-exp(-ka*time))/cl/(ka-ke);
 model conc ~ normal(pred,s2);
 random b1 b2 b3 ~ normal([0,0,0],[d11,d12,d22,d13,d23,d33])
                   subject=subject;
 predict pred out=theopred;
run;
```

The predicted values can be used, among others, to easily graph the empirical Bayes predictions of the individual profiles, as in Figure 20.7. Because the random-effects structure is extensive, it is best not to use too many quadrature points, and also adaptive quadrature may be prohibitive. At the same time, choosing decent starting values is of the utmost importance.

20.12.4 SAS Program for the Songbird Data

An example program for the songbird data, for the outcome SI at area X, which is not reported in Section 20.8, is given by:

```
proc nlmixed data=help2 qpoints=3;
 parms phim=0.1124 phimdiff=0.1200
       eta=2.4158 etadiff=-0.1582
       tau=3.8297 taudiff=-0.05259
       gamma=-0.00187 gdiff=0.002502
       sigma2=0.000156
       d11=0.002667 d22=0.2793 d33=0.08505 d12=0 d13=0 d23=0;
 num = (phim + phimdiff * group + vm)
       * (time ** (eta + etadiff * group + n));
 den = ((tau + taudiff * group + t)
       ** (eta + etadiff * group + n))
       + (time ** (eta + etadiff * group +n ));
 aver = num/den + gamma + gdiff * group;
 model si_area_X ~ normal(aver,sigma2);
 random vm t n ~
        normal([0, 0, 0],[d11, d12, d22, d13, d23, d33])
        subject=bird out=eb2;
run;
```

Also here, the random-effects structure is rather elaborate. A cautious model fitting practice is to start with a fixed-effects model, i.e., one without random effects, analyzing the birds either jointly or separately. Then, random effects can be added one by one, assuming independence between them at first and then gradually including covariances as well. At each stage, the parameters from the previous, slightly less elaborate model can be used as starting values. This is merely a 'step up' procedure to attain convergence of the initial, most elaborate model. Once such model has been fitted, one can then undertake model simplification through, for example, backward selection, based on formal testing procedures. Alternatively one could consider forward selection, which is computationally easier, but there are important drawbacks associated to this, as one would determine a fixed-effects structure without a general random-effects structure and hence based on improper residuals. This can severely affect the quality of the model built.

20.12.5 SAS Program for the NTP Data

We now present a SAS program used to fit the non-linear dose-response model (20.42) in Section 20.9.1:

```
proc nlmixed data=dehp33 technique=newrap;
  parms beta0=-5.97 betad=4.45 gamma=1.0 tau=1.27;
  eta = beta0 + b + betad*(dose+0.01)**gamma;
  expeta = exp(eta);
  p = expeta/(1+expeta);
  model external ~ binary(p);
  random b ~ normal(0,tau**2) subject=litter;
  estimate 'RI variance tau^2' (tau*tau);
run;
```

Due to the binary nature of the outcome and the non-linear predictor fuction, it is ever so important to use good starting values. We have chosen them from the linear equivalent of the model, i.e., the model with the γ parameter removed. Further, it may be safer to use Newton-Raphson, close to the maximum, than a quasi-Newton technique. The latter may take a long time to converge or even keep jumping around in the neighborhood of the maximum, without ever converging.

The additional ESTIMATE statement conveniently provides us with an estimate and standard error for the random-intercept variance τ^2, even though τ is the model parameter and not τ^2 itself, for reasons of defensive programming.

20.12.6 SAS Program for the Random Smoothing Spline Model: The Analgesic Trial

In Section 20.11.2, a random smoothing spline based approach was fitted to the analgesic trial, using the experimental SAS procedure GLIMMIX. Examples of how to use this procedure with continuous outcomes are presented in the manual for the procedure (SAS Institute Inc. 2004). Possible code to fit model (20.50) is:

```
proc glimmix data=gsa2 method=RSPL;
 class patid;
 nloptions  maxiter=250 technique=newrap;
 model gsa = time|time pca0
             / dist=multinomial link=cumlogit
               solution ddfm=satterth;
 random time / subject=patid type=rsmooth
               knotmethod=kdtree(bucket=1000
               knotinfo treeinfo);
run;
```

The random smoothing splines are invoked by calling the RANDOM statement, with 'time' as the random effect and then the 'type=rsmooth' option. This option is defining for the random smoothing spline structure and with it come a number of fine tuning options. The 'knotmethod=kdtree' option specifies the use of the so-called 'k-d tree' method (Friedman, Bentley, and Finkel 1977, Cleveland and Grosse 1991). The method can be usefully employed to find the nearest neighbors of a point. The process starts from a hypercube, encompassing the values of the random effects. Then, recursive splitting takes place as long as there are cells that contain more than a pre-specified number of bucket points. The bucket size can be specified by means of the 'bucket=' argument to the 'knotmethod=kdtree' option. Further, info on the tree splitting process and on the resulting knots can be obtained by adding the 'treeinfo' and 'knotinfo' arguments, respectively, to the option.

Fitting models of this type, especially with non-continuous data, can be involved, and some precautionary and fine tuning measures to the updating algorithm can be in place. For example, we increased the number of iterations to 250 and chose Newton-Raphson as the updating algorithm. In problems of this type, quasi-Newton methods, due to their super-linear but sub-quadratic convergence, may fail to reach the maximum, but rather get trapped in a small number of points close to the maximum, between which the algorithm keeps jumping around.

The 'ddfm=satterth' option is added to the MODEL statement, to ensure that Satterthwaite degrees of freedom are computed. The containment method is problematic, because the random spline structure is added to the Z matrix, which might seemingly reduce and even eliminate the available degrees of freedom for conducting hypothesis testing about fixed effects.

The algorithm works rather efficiently thanks to profiling the fixed-effects out from the resulting likelihood, effectively reducing the iterative process to the variance components.

Let us now discuss some elements of the output. A large number of output panels is exactly equal to their counterparts in fully parametric applications of the procedure, as described in Sections 10.5.3 and 15.2. These include the model information, solutions for fixed effects, and standard type III tests of fixed effects panels. Due to profiling of fixed-effects, only one parameter remains in the optimization, i.e., the variance of the random spline coefficients:

Covariance Parameter Estimates

Cov Parm	Subject	Estimate	Standard Error
Var[RSmooth(TIME)]	PATID	0.1083	0.01459

In the dimensions panel (not shown), the number of columns for the Z matrix is listed as three. This is because three knots are retained in this case. The final knots are presented as follows:

Radial Smoother
  Knots for
RSmooth(TIME)

Knot Number	TIME
1	1.0000
2	2.0000
3	4.0000

The tree splitting process is represented in the following panel:

kd-Tree for RSmooth(TIME)

Node Number	Left Child	Right Child	Split Direction	Split Value
0	1	2	TIME	2.0000
1			TERMINAL	
2			TERMINAL	

Thus, a single split takes place, at $t_{ij} = 2$, whereafter only terminal nodes are obtained. Assembling the first (1), the last (4), and the split values produces the knots 1, 2, and 4, as listed in Table 20.14. Should we consider a bucket of size 100, then a much more elaborate tree splitting process ensues:

kd-Tree for RSmooth(TIME)

| Node | Left | Right | Split | Split |

20.12 Using SAS for Non-linear Mixed-effects Models 391

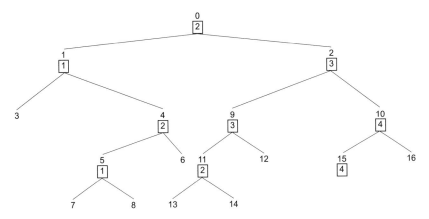

FIGURE 20.11. *Analgesic Trial. Representation of the k-d tree for random smoothing spline based model (20.50), with a bucket size of 100.*

Number	Child	Child	Direction	Value
0	1	2	TIME	2.0000
1	3	4	TIME	1.0000
2	9	10	TIME	3.0000
3			TERMINAL	
4	5	6	TIME	2.0000
5	7	8	TIME	1.0000
6			TERMINAL	
7			TERMINAL	
8			TERMINAL	
9	11	12	TIME	3.0000
10	15	16	TIME	4.0000
11	13	14	TIME	2.0000
12			TERMINAL	
13			TERMINAL	
14			TERMINAL	
15	17	18	TIME	4.0000
16			TERMINAL	
17			TERMINAL	
18			TERMINAL	

The tree structure can nicely be reconstructed from this panel, and is depicted in Figure 20.11. Should we, on the other hand, switch to a large bucket size of 2000, which is almost twice as large as the number 1137 of observations available for analysis, then the tree splitting process stops instantaneously:

```
kd-Tree for RSmooth(TIME)
```

Node Number	Left Child	Right Child	Split Direction	Split Value
0			TERMINAL	

and hence the trivial tree is obtained, with knots at the first (1) and last (4) observation time.

21
Pseudo-Likelihood for a Hierarchical Model

21.1 Introduction

Pseudo-likelihood methodology for marginal models has been introduced in Chapter 9. Chapter 12 was devoted to pseudo-likelihood ideas applied to the conditional modeling family. In this chapter, we will introduce how the concept of pseudo-likelihood can be usefully used when the model under consideration is of a subject-specific or multilevel (Goldstein 1995) nature.

It has been made clear in Chapter 14 that the marginal likelihood function of a generalized linear mixed model (GLMM), obtained after integrating over random effects, nearly always involves intractable integrals. The chapter introduced two main approaches to parameter estimation. The first one was based on numerical integration methods (Section 14.3, see also Anderson and Aitkin 1985), a technique suffering from the curse of dimensionality when several random effects are considered at the same time. A second approach consisted of approximations to the data (Section 14.4), with such techniques as penalized quasi-likelihood (PQL) and marginal quasi-likelihood (MQL). Based on simulated data, Rodríguez and Goldman (1995) demonstrate that the latter procedures may be seriously biased when applied to binary response data. Their simulations reveal that both fixed effects and variance components may suffer from substantial, if not severe, attenuation bias under certain circumstances. Goldstein and Rasbash (1996) show that including a second-order term in the PQL expansion (PQL2) essentially eliminates biases described by Rodríguez and Goldman. The analyses of our case studies (Section 14.7, Chapter 17) confirm these findings. Other authors have advised the introduction of bias-correction terms (Lin and Breslow 1995). It should be emphasized, however, that the PQL approximate estimation procedure exhibits many numerical problems and it is not so uncommon that it fails to converge in practical applications. This situation tends to worsen when second-order terms are added or when the model becomes more complicated (Renard *et al* 2004). Alternative solutions to find ML estimates can be based on Monte Carlo methods such as the Monte Carlo EM algorithm (McCulloch 1994, 1997). Monte Carlo methods are highly computer-intensive in general.

In this chapter, a pseudo-likelihood (PL, Chapter 9) approach will be explored to fit hierarchical models for binary responses with probit link specification. One could, for example, consider only pairwise likelihoods within the same cluster instead of the full contribution of an independent unit to the likelihood. Marginal model applications can be found in Chapter 9, while PL applications to conditional models are the subject of Chapter 12. Other applications can be found in le Cessie and Van Houwelingen (1994), who present a marginal application, and in Heagerty and Lele (1998) who applied a pairwise likelihood approach, which they termed composite likelihood after Lindsay (1988), to model binary spatial data using a hierarchical generalized linear model.

Section 21.2 presents the PL methodology for this context. In Section 21.3, the specific case of two binary outcomes, as encountered in the evaluation of surrogate endpoints in randomized clinical trials is presented. An illustration based on a meta-analysis in schizophrenia is presented in Section 21.4. Simulations to assess the performance of the method are reported in Renard, Molenberghs, and Geys (2004). See also Burzykowski, Molenberghs, and Buyse (2005).

Similar ideas will be used in the next chapter and in Chapter 25.

21.2 Pseudo-Likelihood Estimation

A simple model that captures the essence of the problem is one where level 1 units, e.g., repeated measurements in a longitudinal study or members of a household in a two-stage survey, are nested within level 2 units, that is, subjects in the longitudinal context or households in a survey. The procedure described hereafter can be applied to higher-order hierarchies, as will be illustrated in Sections 21.3 and 21.4. The methodology presented here hinges on the use of the probit link because then both the marginal as well as the hierarchical model are of a multivariate probit type. Although the commonly used logit link has an advantage with respect to parameter interpretation, both tend to provide similar model fit in practice, therefore we do not see this as a strong limitation.

21.2 Pseudo-Likelihood Estimation

To make matters concrete, consider the following two-level probit model:

$$\Phi^{-1}(P[Y_{ij} = 1|b_i]) = x'_{ij}\boldsymbol{\beta} + z'_{ij}\boldsymbol{b}_i, \tag{21.1}$$

for the probability that a response is observed for the jth observation in the ith subject ($i = 1, \ldots, N$). See also Section 13.4.3. As usual, x_{ij} represents a set of fixed covariates (in the following, dependence on x_{ij} is ignored in the notation), and z_{ij} denotes the random-effects covariates. For the vector of random effects, assume that $\boldsymbol{b}_i \sim N(0, D)$. In case where we assume there is a random intercept only, i.e., $z_{ij} = 1$ for all i and j, then we write τ^2 for D.

For ease of development, we posit the existence of an unobservable latent variable $\widetilde{Y}_{ij}$ that is continuously distributed and related to the actual response Y_{ij} through the threshold concept. This assumption is commonly made in ordinal regression models in which a series of thresholds are employed (Chapter 18). For binary data only one threshold is necessary and its value, assuming that an intercept term is included in (21.1), can be chosen to be 0 without loss of generality. We therefore suppose that a positive response is recorded ($Y_{ij} = 1$) if $\widetilde{Y}_{ij} > 0$ and a negative response ($Y_{ij} = 0$) otherwise. If we further assume that $\widetilde{Y}_{ij}$ is normally distributed, then the model for the latent variable corresponding to (21.1) can be written as:

$$\widetilde{Y}_{ij} = x'_{ij}\boldsymbol{\beta} + z'_{ij}\boldsymbol{b}_i + \widetilde{\varepsilon}_{ij}, \tag{21.2}$$

with the residual error term $\widetilde{\varepsilon}_{ij}$ being $N(0, \sigma^2)$. Since the variable $\widetilde{\varepsilon}_{ij}$ is unobservable, making the parameter σ^2 non-identifiable, its value can be fixed arbitrarily. Without loss of generality we set $\sigma^2 \equiv 1$.

Likelihood estimation proceeds by maximizing the marginal distribution obtained by integrating over the random effects. More formally, the contribution for the ith subject to the likelihood function for this model can be written as:

$$\ell_i(\boldsymbol{\beta}, D) = \int_{-\infty}^{+\infty} \prod_{j=1}^{n_i} P[Y_{ij} = 1|\boldsymbol{b}_i] \phi(\boldsymbol{b}_i; D) d\boldsymbol{b}_i,$$

where $\phi(\boldsymbol{b}_i, D)$ denotes the density function of the multivariate normal distribution with mean $\boldsymbol{0}$ and covariance matrix D. In this case, numerical integration using Gaussian quadrature is easily accomplished to evaluate the above expression, but would become more and more laborious as the number of random effects increases.

In general, when maximization of the likelihood is awkward, an alternative is to replace the joint likelihood by a function that is easier to evaluate and hence to maximize. For this purpose, any suitable product of conditional or marginal densities involving some of the variables could be appropriate. We refer to Sections 9.2 and 9.3 for a general introduction and to Section 9.4 for an application to marginal models, including the technique of pairwise likelihood, which will be used here as well in a for random-effects models appropriate version.

The basic contribution of the ith individual to the log PL can be written:

$$p\ell_i(\boldsymbol{\beta}, D) = \sum_{j=1}^{n_i} \sum_{k=j+1}^{n_i} \sum_{\ell,m=0}^{1} \delta_{ijk\ell m} \log P[Y_{ij} = \ell, Y_{ik} = m], \qquad (21.3)$$

with

$$\delta_{ijk\ell m} = \begin{cases} 1 & \text{if } Y_{ij} = \ell \text{ and } Y_{ik} = m, \\ 0 & \text{otherwise.} \end{cases} \qquad (21.4)$$

Note how marginal pairwise probabilities emerge in (21.3). These can be calculated in terms of univariate and bivariate probits. For example, the probability that $Y_{ij} = 0$ and $Y_{ik} = 0$ can be written, using (21.2):

$$P[Y_{ij} = 0, Y_{ik} = 0]$$
$$= P[\widetilde{Y}_{ij} < 0, \widetilde{Y}_{ik} < 0]$$
$$= \int_{-\infty}^{-x'_{ij}\boldsymbol{\beta}/\text{var}\widetilde{Y}_{ij}} \int_{-\infty}^{-x'_{ik}\boldsymbol{\beta}/\text{var}\widetilde{Y}_{ik}} \phi_2(y_1, y_2; \rho_{ijk}) dy_1 dy_2$$
$$= \Phi_2\left(\frac{-x'_{ij}\boldsymbol{\beta}}{\text{var}[\widetilde{Y}_{ij}]}, \frac{-x'_{ik}\boldsymbol{\beta}}{\text{var}[\widetilde{Y}_{ik}]}; \rho_{ijk}\right).$$

In this expression, $\text{var}(\widetilde{Y}_{ij})$, $\text{var}(\widetilde{Y}_{ik})$ and $\rho_{ijk} = \text{corr}(Y_{ij}, Y_{ik})$ are obtained by selecting the appropriate 2×2 submatrix of the covariance matrix $V_i = Z_i D Z'_i + I_{n_i}$. The function $\phi_2(x, y; \rho)$ denotes the standardized bivariate normal distribution function with correlation coefficient ρ.

The PL estimators $(\widetilde{\boldsymbol{\beta}}, \widetilde{D})$ are obtained by maximizing the function

$$p\ell(\boldsymbol{\beta}, D) = \sum_{i=1}^{N} p\ell_i(\boldsymbol{\beta}, D). \qquad (21.5)$$

General results on the consistency and asymptotic normality of PL estimators can be derived along the lines of classical proofs for maximum likelihood estimators (Section 9.3). The asymptotic covariance matrix of the PL estimators $(\widetilde{\boldsymbol{\beta}}, \widetilde{D})$ can be approximated by the 'sandwich estimator' (9.4). As can be anticipated, the PL estimator will generally be less efficient than the maximum likelihood estimator because it relies on a limited amount of information. Therefore, with this approach a compromise between computational ease and loss of efficiency is sought.

Note that in (21.3), each response Y_{ij} occurs $(n_i - 1)$ times in the ith contribution to the log PL. Thus, information about an observation will tend to be over-used in larger clusters and this can be counter-balanced by weighting each contribution from a cluster to the PL by a factor inversely proportional to $(n_i - 1)$. This leads to the (non-equivalent) specification:

$$p\ell^*(\boldsymbol{\beta}, D) = \sum_{i=1}^{N} \frac{p\ell_i(\boldsymbol{\beta}, D)}{n_i - 1}, \qquad (21.6)$$

in line with the marginal developments (Section 9.4), where it was shown that $p\ell^*$ is much more efficient than $p\ell$ for estimating fixed effects. However, if main interest lies in the estimation of association parameters, the advice was to use of $p\ell$. If interest is combined, and one type of analysis should be chosen, $p\ell$ might be preferable as well. Distinguishing between both versions is particularly important when the number of measurements n_i is itself informative for some parameters. For example, in a clustered toxicological experiment, higher doses may negatively influence the number of viable foetuses.

21.3 Two Binary Endpoints

In a meta-analytic surrogate endpoint approach, a surrogate endpoint S_{ij} is measured along with the true endpoint T_{ij}, for each subject $j = 1, \ldots, n_i$ in a number of trials $i = 1, \ldots, N$. Let the binary treatment indicator be denoted by X_{ij}. Buyse et al (2000) presented a hierarchical formulation for the case of normally distributed endpoints S_{ij} and T_{ij}:

$$\begin{cases} S_{ij} &= \mu_S + m_{S_i} + (\alpha + a_i)X_{ij} + \varepsilon_{S_{ij}}, \\ T_{ij} &= \mu_T + m_{T_i} + (\beta + b_i)X_{ij} + \varepsilon_{T_{ij}}, \end{cases} \qquad (21.7)$$

where μ_{S_i} and μ_{T_i} are trial-specific intercepts, and α_i and β_i are trial-specific effects of treatment X on the two endpoints in trial $i = 1, \ldots, N$. Finally, $\varepsilon_{S_{ij}}$ and $\varepsilon_{T_{ij}}$ are correlated error terms, assumed to be mean-zero normally distributed with covariance matrix

$$\Sigma = \begin{pmatrix} \sigma_{SS} & \sigma_{ST} \\ \sigma_{ST} & \sigma_{TT} \end{pmatrix}. \qquad (21.8)$$

Regarding the random effects, we assume that they are zero-mean normally distributed with covariance matrix

$$D = \begin{pmatrix} d_{SS} & d_{ST} & d_{Sa} & d_{Sb} \\ d_{ST} & d_{TT} & d_{Ta} & d_{Tb} \\ d_{Sa} & d_{Ta} & d_{aa} & d_{ab} \\ d_{Sb} & d_{Tb} & d_{ab} & d_{bb} \end{pmatrix}. \qquad (21.9)$$

Buyse et al (2000) discussed estimation methods and showed how this model can be used to quantify surrogacy both at the trial level and at the individual level. See also Burzykowski, Molenberghs, and Buyse (2005).

To adapt this model to the case of two binary hierarchical endpoints, we will now posit the existence of a pair of continuously distributed latent variables $(\widetilde{S}_{ij}, \widetilde{T}_{ij})$ which produce the actual binary values (S_{ij}, T_{ij}). These unobservable variables are assumed to have a joint normal distribution and the realized value of S_{ij} (resp. T_{ij}) equals 1 if $\widetilde{S}_{ij} > 0$ (resp. $\widetilde{T}_{ij} > 0$), and 0 otherwise.

We are now in a position to adopt the modeling strategy outlined in Section 9.4. Consider the following random-effects model on the latent variable scale:

$$\begin{cases} \widetilde{S}_{ij} &= \mu_S + m_{S_i} + (\alpha + a_i)X_{ij} + \widetilde{\varepsilon}_{S_{ij}}, \\ \widetilde{T}_{ij} &= \mu_T + m_{T_i} + (\beta + b_i)X_{ij} + \widetilde{\varepsilon}_{T_{ij}}. \end{cases} \quad (21.10)$$

The sole difference here is that variances at the individual level (σ_{SS} and σ_{TT}) are non-identifiable parameters and can be fixed, arbitrarily and without loss of generality, to one, as in (21.2). The Σ matrix defined in (21.8) can therefore be replaced by

$$\Sigma = \begin{pmatrix} 1 & \rho_{ST} \\ \rho_{ST} & 1 \end{pmatrix}. \quad (21.11)$$

This formulation is attractive because the coefficients of determination defined in the previous section can readily be employed without any modification, although formally, their interpretation is bound to the postulated latent variables generating the observed binary responses. Model (21.10) leads to the following models:

$$\Phi^{-1}(P[S_{ij} = 1 | X_{ij}, m_{S_i}, a_i, m_{T_i}, b_i])$$
$$= \mu_S + m_{S_i} + (\alpha + a_i)X_{ij}, \quad (21.12)$$

$$\Phi^{-1}(P[T_{ij} = 1 | X_{ij}, m_{S_i}, a_i, m_{T_i}, b_i])$$
$$= \mu_T + m_{T_i} + (\beta + b_i)X_{ij}. \quad (21.13)$$

This model can be considered either a three-level model or a bivariate two-level model for binary response data. The contribution of the ith trial to the likelihood function for the parameters $\boldsymbol{\beta} = (\mu_S, \alpha, \mu_T, \beta)'$, D and ρ_{ST}, conditionally on $\boldsymbol{b}_i = (m_{S_i}, a_i, m_{T_i}, b_i)'$, is

$$\ell_i(\boldsymbol{\beta}, D, \rho_{ST} \mid \boldsymbol{b}_i) = \prod_{j=1}^{n_i} \prod_{k=0}^{1} \prod_{\ell=0}^{1} P[S_{ij} = k, T_{ij} = \ell \mid \boldsymbol{b}_i]^{\delta_{ijk\ell}}, \quad (21.14)$$

where $\delta_{ijk\ell}$ is as in (21.4).

21.3 Two Binary Endpoints

Maximum likelihood estimates for the unknown parameters can be obtained by maximizing the integrated likelihood function, of which the ith contribution is given by

$$\ell_i(\boldsymbol{\beta}, D, \rho_{ST}) = \int \ell_i(\boldsymbol{\beta}, D, \rho_{ST} \mid \boldsymbol{b}_i) \phi_4(\boldsymbol{b}_i; D) d\boldsymbol{b}_i, \qquad (21.15)$$

where $\phi_4(\boldsymbol{b}_i; D)$ denotes the joint density function of the normal distribution with mean $\boldsymbol{0}$ and covariance matrix D. We can now apply pseudo-likelihood ideas, just as in Section 21.2. The contribution of the ith trial to the log PL can be written

$$p\ell_i = \sum_{j=1}^{2n_i} \sum_{k=1}^{j-1} \ell_{jk}, \qquad (21.16)$$

where ℓ_{jk} is the likelihood of the pair (Y_{ij}, Y_{ik}), with

$$\boldsymbol{Y}_i = (S_{i1}, \ldots, S_{in_i}, T_{i1}, \ldots, T_{in_i}),$$

that is:

$$\ell_{jk} = Y_{jk}^{(11)} \log p_{jk}^{(11)} + Y_{jk}^{(10)} \log p_{jk}^{(10)} + Y_{jk}^{(01)} \log p_{jk}^{(01)} + Y_{jk}^{(00)} \log p_{jk}^{(00)},$$

where

$$p_{jk}^{(\ell m)} = P[Y_{ij} = \ell, Y_{ik} = m \mid Z_{ij}, Z_{ik}]$$

and

$$Y_{ij}^{(lm)} = \begin{cases} 1 & \text{if } Y_{ij} = l \text{ and } Y_{ik} = m, \\ 0 & \text{otherwise.} \end{cases}$$

The different terms in (21.16) reflect four different types of association, as illustrated in Figure 21.1:

(i) the association between the surrogate and true endpoints measured on the same individual;

(ii) the association between the surrogate endpoints measured on two distinct individuals;

(iii) the association between the true endpoints measured on two distinct individuals;

(iv) the association between the surrogate and true endpoints measured on two distinct individuals.

Each of these pairwise contributions can be written in terms of univariate and bivariate probits. For example, the probability that both S and T be

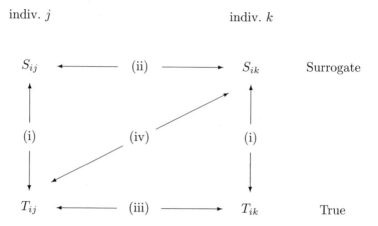

FIGURE 21.1. *Association structure for the surrogate and true endpoints in two distinct individuals j and k.*

zero for subject j in trial i can be written as:

$$P[S_{ij} = 0, T_{ij} = 0 | Z_{ij}]$$
$$= P[\widetilde{S}_{ij} < 0, \widetilde{T}_{ij} < 0 | Z_{ij}]$$
$$= \Phi_2 \left(-\frac{\mu_S + \alpha Z_{ij}}{\sqrt{\mathrm{var}(\widetilde{S}_{ij})}}, -\frac{\mu_T + \beta Z_{ij}}{\sqrt{\mathrm{var}(\widetilde{T}_{ij})}}; \rho_{ij} \right). \qquad (21.17)$$

In (21.17), $\mathrm{var}(\widetilde{S}_{ij})$, $\mathrm{var}(\widetilde{T}_{ij})$ and ρ_{ij} are obtained by selecting the appropriate 2×2 submatrix of the covariance matrix $V_i = Z_i D Z_i' + \Sigma_i$, where Z_i is a suitable design matrix and R_i is a block-diagonal matrix with blocks equal to D.

Estimates of $\boldsymbol{\beta}$, D, and ρ_{ST} can be obtained by maximizing the log PL function

$$p\ell = \sum_{i=1}^{N} p\ell_i^* = \sum_{i=1}^{N} p\ell_i / (2n_i - 1),$$

which is similar to (21.6). Precision estimation proceeds once more by using the sandwich estimator.

21.4 A Meta-analysis of Trials in Schizophrenic Subjects

To illustrate the methodology, we use data from five clinical trials comparing the effects of risperidone to conventional antipsychotic agents (or placebo) for the treatment of chronic schizophrenia. Only subjects who received optimal doses of risperidone (4–6 mg/day) or an active control (haloperidol, perphenazine, zuclopenthixol) were included in this analysis. Depending on the trial, treatment was administered for a duration of 4 to 8 weeks and data at endpoint are analyzed here.

Even though this is not a standard situation for surrogate validation due to the lack of a 'gold standard' scale, we consider as our primary measure (true endpoint) the 'Clinical Global Impression' (CGI) overall change versus baseline. This scale ranges from 1 ='very much improved' to 7 ='very much worsened' and is used by the treating physician to assess a subject's overall clinical improvement compared to baseline. We define a response in CGI as an improvement since baseline (CGI grade of 1 to 3) and a non-response otherwise (worsening). As a surrogate measure for global improvement, we consider clinical response defined as a 20% or higher reduction in the 'Positive and Negative Symptoms Scale' (PANSS) score from baseline to endpoint. This corresponds to a commonly accepted criterion for defining a clinical response (Kay et al 1988). Therefore, we try to quantify the extent to which a response in PANSS, a measure of psychiatric disorder, can predict clinical improvement as observed by the physician.

Pooled data from the five trials are presented in Table 21.1. It can be seen that the relationship between S and T is very strong ($OR_{ST} = 31.5$, $\chi^2 = 261.4$, $P < 0.0001$), as can be expected. Note that patients were rated by the same treating physicians on PANSS and CGI, thereby bringing some possible contamination bias. Table 21.2 shows parameter estimates and their standard errors for Model (21.12)–(21.13). This model was fitted using the PQL2 procedure implemented in the MLwiN software package (Goldstein et al 1998) as well as using the PL approach. Because the number of trials is too small in this example, centers were treated as grouping units. Thus, 176 units were available for the analysis.

Based on the fitted variance components, Buyse et al (2000) consider two measures to assess the quality of surrogacy. First, a measure to assess the quality of a surrogate at the trial level is given by the coefficient of determination:

$$R^2_{\text{trial(f)}} = \frac{\begin{pmatrix} d_{sb} \\ d_{ab} \end{pmatrix}' \begin{pmatrix} d_{ss} & d_{sa} \\ d_{sa} & d_{aa} \end{pmatrix}^{-1} \begin{pmatrix} d_{sb} \\ d_{ab} \end{pmatrix}}{d_{bb}}. \qquad (21.18)$$

This coefficient measures how precisely the effect of treatment on the true endpoint can be predicted when the treatment effect on the surrogate end-

TABLE 21.1. *Meta-analysis in Schizophrenia. Pooled data for the schizophrenia example: surrogate endpoint (S) = response in PANSS score (1=response), true endpoint (T) = improvement in CGI overall change versus baseline (1=improved). X indicates treatment allocation.*

			T	
X		S	0	1
Active control		0	151 (72)†	58 (28)
		1	15 (6)	220 (94)
Risperidone		0	91 (71)	37 (29)
		1	20 (9)	213 (91)

† Frequency (row percentage)

point has been observed in a new trial ($i = 0$). It is unitless and ranges in the unit interval if the corresponding variance-covariance matrix D is positive-definite, two desirable features for its interpretation. Second, the association between the surrogate and final endpoints is captured by the coefficient of determination

$$R^2_{\text{indiv}} = \frac{\sigma^2_{ST}}{\sigma_{SS}\sigma_{TT}}, \qquad (21.19)$$

which simply is the squared correlation between S and T after accounting for trial and treatment effects.

As can be seen in Table 21.2, the PL procedure leads to an estimated D matrix that is positive-definite. With PQL2, on the other hand, some elements of D were *a priori* constrained to be zero and as a result, the value of the coefficient $R^2_{\text{trial(f)}}$ cannot even be calculated. This underscores the potential advantage of PL in a case like this. This aside, fixed-effects parameter estimates are quite similar and their anticipated loss in efficiency is moderate (less than 15%). Also, the parameter ρ_{ST} exhibits both a much higher point estimate and a much larger standard error.

Interestingly, the estimated value of $R^2_{\text{trial(f)}}$ is really low (0.006), whereas the estimated value of R^2_{indiv} is rather high (0.924). The latter confirms the strong association between S and T (at the individual level) which was seen in Table 21.1 and suggests that they both capture overlapping components of a subject's psychotic status. The very low estimated value for $R^2_{\text{trial(f)}}$, on the other hand, shows that S provides very bad predictions for treatment effects on T (at the center level), thereby making of clinical response a rather poor surrogate for clinical improvement according to our criterion. We see here one advantage of this approach in that individual and trial (center in this example) level components of association can be

TABLE 21.2. *Meta-analysis in Schizophrenia. Results for the schizophrenia example: PQL2 and pseudo-likelihood (PL) estimation procedures. Parameter estimates (standard errors) are presented.*

	PQL2	PL
μ_S	0.227 (0.056)	0.233 (0.062)
α†	0.166 (0.046)	0.161 (0.049)
μ_T	0.441 (0.054)	0.445 (0.062)
β†	0.100 (0.050)	0.109 (0.057)
d_{SS}	0.126 (0.050)	0.121 (0.057)
d_{ST}	0.088 (0.042)	0.091 (0.055)
d_{TT}	0.083 (0.045)	0.076 (0.063)
d_{Sa}	—	-0.005 (0.054)
d_{Ta}	—	-0.004 (0.040)
d_{aa}	—	0.001 (0.005)
d_{Sb}	-0.007 (0.024)	0.006 (0.046)
d_{Tb}	0.001 (0.022)	0.024 (0.041)
d_{ab}	—	-0.001 (0.002)
d_{bb}	0.029 (0.023)	0.059 (0.045)
ρ_{ST}	0.679 (0.018)	0.961 (0.027)
$R^2_{\text{trial(f)}}$	—	0.006 (0.082)
R^2_{indiv}	0.461 (0.024)	0.924 (0.052)

† Treatment coding: -1 = active control
$+1$ = risperidone.

completely disentangled. In an example like this, this is important because both are indeed very different. In the next chapter, an extension to allow for autocorrelation in addition to random effects is offered. There, also a connection to a generalized linear mixed model with autocorrelation will be presented (Section 22.4). The programs to fit such models (Section 22.6) also encompasses models without autocorrelation, i.e., the ones presented here.

21.5 Concluding Remarks

In general, numerical integration based methods, combined with such methods as PQL, MQL, or their second-order versions, provide a versatile toolkit to tackle estimation problems in many generalized linear mixed-effects model. However, there are situations where numerical integration may become prohibitive and where methods based on the approximation of the data may break down or provide an extremely poor approximation, especially for binary outcomes. It is in such settings that pseudo-likelihood methodology, as presented and illustrated in this chapter, can be of practical use.

Simulations done by Renard et al (2002) confirm the numerical stability of PL, a clear advantage of the method over ML and PQL2. It is not so uncommon that the PQL algorithm fails to converge in practical applications, and the problem tends to worsen as more complicated models are fitted. The PQL2 algorithm also turns out to be sensitive to extreme response probabilities, that is, response probabilities that are either very small (close to 0) or high (close to 1).

The other main advantage of PL compared to ML estimation stands at the computation time level because it involves evaluation of univariate and bivariate probits only. Therefore, its use will not be appealing when the number of random effects is small because ML estimation could be effectively employed instead. The computational cost to evaluate the marginal likelihood using quadrature increases exponentially with the number of quadrature nodes. With PL, on the other hand, the complexity increases roughly linearly with the number of parameters and as a quadratic function of the number of measurements.

As discussed in Section 21.2, contributions from a unit to the PL function can be inversely weighted by the number of repeated measurements. In marginal models, considerations about whether to use weighted or unweighted PL are driven primarily by whether interest lies in the fixed or in the association parameters, respectively (Geys, Molenberghs, and Lipsitz 1998; see also Section 9.4). The unweighted PL estimator was also investigated in the simulation study by Renard et al (2002), and their conclusions were that it is slightly less efficient than the weighted estimator, regardless of the type of parameter (fixed or random). It is not clear that this will uniformly be the case, but weighted PL seems to be the preferred estimator in multilevel models.

This chapter has dealt exclusively with models specified via a probit link. Although a logit link specification would be straightforward by assuming a standard logistic rather than normal distribution for $\widetilde{\varepsilon}_{ij}$ in (21.2), this leads to intractable integrals for pairwise likelihoods. Therefore, PL cannot be applied to claim computational gains in models with logit link specification. An way to circumvent this issue while maintaining a logit link is presented in Chapter 25, with an example in Section 25.4.

22
Random-effects Models with Serial Correlation

22.1 Introduction

In the previous chapter, we presented a random-effects based probit model and applied pseudo-likelihood ideas for parameter estimation. The model was generated from a multivariate normally distributed latent variable. This means that the latent variable follows a linear mixed model. An obvious extension is the inclusion of serial correlation, or autocorrelation, as can be done for the standard linear mixed-effects model. The extension proposed by Renard, Molenberghs, and Geys (2004) is the basis for this chapter. The model presented in Section 21.3 exhibits residual correlation between the surrogate and true endpoints on the same subject, in addition to the correlation induced by the random effects. The approach formulated in this chapter can be seen as a general version of this.

Barbosa and Goldstein (2000) propose to extend the standard multi-level model for binary outcomes, and hence the standard generalized linear mixed model, by allowing the residuals at the individual level to be correlated. These authors wrote the covariance between residuals for individual i at occasions j and k as

$$\sqrt{\pi_{ij}(1-\pi_{ij})\pi_{ik}(1-\pi_{ik})}f(|t_{ij}-t_{ik}|),$$

where the conditional mean, given random effects $\bm{b}_i$, $\pi_{ij} = E(y_{ij}|\bm{b}_i)$ is modeled as usual and $f(u)$ is a function of u, the time lag between measurement times t_{ij} and t_{ik}, i.e., $|t_{ij}-t_{ik}|$. For example, Barbosa and Goldstein

(2000) proposed the form:

$$f(u) = \alpha + \exp[-\kappa(u)], \tag{22.1}$$

for some function κ of the time lag, and they used the PQL algorithm to estimate parameters. In what follows, we will propose different parametric shapes for autocorrelation functions. A drawback of this approach, common with other PQL applications, especially with binary data, is the severe bias that can result. Also, the correction described above is *ad hoc* and falls outside the likelihood framework.

We first propose a full probabilistic model, starting from a general probit model, based on an underlying latent linear mixed model with serial correlation. The model is proposed in Section 22.2. Full likelihood estimation of this model is computationally demanding, however, and we therefore propose to use pairwise likelihood for estimation purposes in Section 22.3, building on the methodology presented in Chapter 21. In Section 22.4, a generalized linear mixed models augmented with autocorrelation is presented. The psychiatric study, analyzed before in Section 21.4, will be analyzed again in Section 22.5, using both autocorrelation methods. Whereas the analysis in Section 21.4 considered the specific context of surrogate marker evaluation, here we focus on the CGI outcome only. In Section 22.6, SAS code to fit the random-effects multivariate probit model, with or without serial correlation, as well as the generalized linear mixed model with serial correlation, is presented.

22.2 A Multilevel Probit Model with Autocorrelation

The model we propose for repeated binary data extends model (21.2), i.e., it extends the standard hierarchical or multilevel probit model. It is related to the model discussed in Heagerty and Lele (1998), which deals with binary spatial data. We will focus on a two-level hierarchy, or two-level model with, using multilevel terminology, subjects at the second level and measurements within subjects at the first level.

As in Section 21.2, we will introduce the model from a latent variable perspective. As usual, let $\boldsymbol{Y}_i = (Y_{i1}, \ldots, Y_{in_i})'$ denote the vector of binary measurements on subject i ($i = 1, \ldots N$). We posit the existence of an unobserved continuous variable $\widetilde{Y}_{ij}$ and assume that the observed binary response is obtained by dichotomizing $\widetilde{Y}_{ij}$ based on a certain threshold or cut-off value. This threshold can be chosen to be 0 without loss of generality, provided an intercept term is included in the model. In other words, it is assumed that a positive response, $Y_{ij} = 1$, is recorded if $\widetilde{Y}_{ij} > 0$ and a negative response ($Y_{ij} = 0$) otherwise. On the latent variable scale the model, generalizing (21.2), can be written as:

$$\widetilde{Y}_{ij} = x'_{ij}\beta + z'_{ij}b_i + \widetilde{\varepsilon}_{ij}. \tag{22.2}$$

The standard multilevel probit model is obtained by assuming that the random effects b_i and residual error terms $\widetilde{\varepsilon}_{ij}$ are normally distributed. An additional assumption is that of conditional independence among responses, that is, conditionally on b_i, the $\widetilde{Y}_{ij}$'s are independent. This implies that $b_i \sim N(0, D)$ and, for reasons of identification, that $\widetilde{Y}_{ij} \sim N(0, 1)$. Whereas this assumption was made in Chapter 21, we relax it here by assuming instead that the $\widetilde{Y}_{ij}$'s are realizations from a stationary unit-variance Gaussian process $\widetilde{\varepsilon}(t)$ with autocorrelation function

$$\mathrm{corr}[\widetilde{\varepsilon}(t), \widetilde{\varepsilon}(t')] = \rho(|t' - t|), \tag{22.3}$$

which is similar in spirit to (22.1). Indeed, following Goldstein, Healy, and Rasbash (1994), we assume that $\rho(u) = \exp[-\kappa(u)]$, where $\kappa(u)$ is a positive increasing function, not necessarily linear. Obvious choices include

$$\kappa(u) = \alpha u,$$

the exponential decay model,

$$\kappa(u) = \alpha u^2,$$

the Gaussian decay model, or, more generally,

$$\kappa(u) = \sum_{k=1}^{K} \alpha_k u^k$$

for any (fractional) polynomial constrained to take on positive values on $[0, +\infty[$. As pointed out by Goldstein, Healy, and Rasbash (1994), a difficulty when $\kappa(u)$ is a polynomial is that successive powers tend to be highly correlated and this may cause estimation difficulties. Another possible choice is then to add an inverse polynomial term such as in

$$\kappa(u) = \alpha_1 u + \alpha_2 u^{-1},$$

which avoids the high correlations associated with ordinary polynomial functions. One could even consider fractional polynomials within the κ function. Verbeke and Molenberghs (2000, Section 10.3) provide examples of serial correlation functions with fractional polynomials. Another useful extension is to make the parameters α_k explicitly dependent on explanatory variables. As to the choice of the κ function, Goldstein, Healy, and Rasbash (1994) state that it should "contain as few parameters as necessary to be flexible enough to describe real data. (...) There seems to be little substantive guidance on choice, and it is likely that different functional forms will be appropriate for different kinds of data." Especially when covariates are allowed in the autocorrelation function, options for $\kappa(u)$ and hence for $\rho(u)$ in (22.3) are virtually unlimited.

As a result, $\widetilde{\boldsymbol{Y}}_i$ is a normally distributed vector with variance-covariance matrix $\Sigma_i = R(\boldsymbol{t}_i) = R_i$, since the variances are kept equal to unity, and for reasons of model identification. The matrix $R(\boldsymbol{t}_i)$ has its (j,k)th element equal to $\rho(|t_{ij} - t_{ik}|)$, where t_{ij} is the time at which the jth measurement on subject i is made.

22.3 Parameter Estimation for the Multilevel Probit Model

The log-likelihood for the observed (binary) data can be written

$$\ell = \sum_{i=1}^{N} \sum_{a_{i1},\ldots,a_{in_i}=0}^{1} \delta_{a_{i1},\ldots,a_{in_i}}$$

$$\times \ln \int P(Y_{i1} = a_{i1}, \ldots, Y_{in_i} = a_{in_i}|\boldsymbol{b}_i)\phi(\boldsymbol{b}_i)d\boldsymbol{b}_i, \qquad (22.4)$$

with

$$\delta_{a_{i1},\ldots,a_{in_i}} = \begin{cases} 1 & \text{if } Y_{i1} = a_{i1},\ldots,Y_{in_i} = a_{in_i}, \\ 0 & \text{otherwise.} \end{cases}$$

Exactly as in Chapter 21, this expression entails the evaluation of multivariate normal probabilities. For instance, we have

$$P(Y_{i1} = 1, \ldots, Y_{in_i} = 1|\boldsymbol{b}_i)$$
$$= P(\widetilde{Y}_{i1} > 0, \ldots, \widetilde{Y}_{in_i} > 0|\boldsymbol{b}_i)$$
$$= \int_{-\infty}^{\xi_{i1}} \cdots \int_{-\infty}^{\xi_{in_i}} \phi[x_1,\ldots,x_{n_i}; R(\boldsymbol{t}_i)]dx_1 \ldots dx_{n_i}, \qquad (22.5)$$

where we define

$$\xi_{ij} = \boldsymbol{x}'_{ij}\boldsymbol{\beta} + \boldsymbol{z}'_{ij}\boldsymbol{b}_i,$$

$\phi(\boldsymbol{x}; R)$ denotes the standardized multivariate normal density function, in the sense of having unit variances, with correlation matrix R.

As in Section 21.2, we propose the use of maximum pairwise likelihood (PL) to overcome the computational burden of full likelihood. In this case, we assemble all possible pairwise probabilities $P(Y_{ij} = \ell, Y_{ik} = m)$ $(\ell, k = 0, 1)$ within the ith unit. For the present model, these marginal bivariate probabilities can all be expressed in terms of univariate and bivariate probits that are computationally inexpensive to evaluate. For instance,

we have
$$P(Y_{ij}=1, Y_{ik}=1) = \Phi_2\left(\xi_{ij}, \xi_{ik}; \rho_{ijk}\right), \qquad (22.6)$$
with
$$\xi_{ij} = \frac{x'_{ij}\beta}{\sqrt{\text{var}(\widetilde{Y}_{ij})}} \qquad (22.7)$$

and overall correlations, induced in part by the random-effects structure and in part by the autocorrelation,

$$\widetilde{\rho}_{ijk} = \frac{z'_{ij}Dz_{ik} + \rho(|t_{ij}-t_{ik}|)}{\sqrt{1+z'_{ij}Dz_{ij}}\sqrt{1+z'_{ik}Dz_{ik}}}, \qquad (22.8)$$

where D denotes the variance-covariance matrix of b_i, the function Φ_2 denotes the standard bivariate Gaussian distribution function, and $\text{var}(\widetilde{Y}_{ij})$, $\text{var}(\widetilde{Y}_{i'j})$ and $\rho_{ii'j}$ are obtained by selecting the appropriate 2×2 submatrix of the (marginal) covariance matrix of $\widetilde{Y}_i$,

$$V_i = Z_i D Z'_i + R(t_i).$$

Parameter estimation and inference follows from the methodology described in Section 21.2, built upon estimation and inferential tools laid out in Sections 9.2 and 9.3. In particular, the sandwich estimation ought to be used for precision estimation, and hypothesis testing can proceed using the test statistics laid out in Section 9.3.

A SAS macro was written to implement the methodology in the case of a model with random intercept and autocorrelation function $\rho(u) = \exp(-\alpha u^k)$. The algorithm was implemented in SAS IML (SAS Institute Inc. 1995) and maximization of the log PL performed using the NLPDD (Double-Dogleg) optimization routine (SAS Institute Inc. 1995). This optimization procedure requires only function and gradient calls that are less expensive to evaluate than second-order derivatives. To avoid constrained optimization, a Cholesky decomposition for D was used and the parameter α was log transformed. To estimate the covariance matrix of the PL estimator by way of the sandwich estimator, it should be observed that (9.6) requires only gradient calls, whereas (9.5) can be computed using numerical second-order derivatives (e.g., by forward difference approximation).

Renard, Molenberghs, and Geys (2004) assessed the proposed methodology by means of a simulation study. Their simulations indicate that the mean and dependence parameters are strongly biased with a small number of subjects ($N = 100$). Increasing the number of measurements somewhat reduces the extent of bias. With a medium number of subjects ($N = 500$), parameters are still largely biased when the number of measurement occasions is small ($n_i = 5$) but the bias falls within more acceptable limits with an increased number of measurement occasions per subject. The autocorrelation parameter is noticeably biased, though. With a large number of subjects ($N = 1000$), the bias for the mean parameters and the random-effect variance parameter becomes small but for the autocorrelation parameter it is still sizeable with datasets containing as many as $N = 20,000$ observations. Regarding precision estimation, the estimated standard errors somewhat overestimate the sampling variability, especially for the random-effect variance. These authors also reported on various convergence problems. This is not surprising for complicated models of this nature. Already for the general linear random-effects model, involving fixed effects, random effects, and serial correlation, convergence can be very involved. Here, the model additionally has a non-linear link structure and further binary data carry way less information than continuous outcomes. Model fitting for models this complex should therefore proceed with caution.

22.4 A Generalized Linear Mixed Model with Autocorrelation

In Section 8.8, marginal models based on linearization were considered, based on the concept of data approximation which later was employed in Section 14.4. In the first case, dependence among repeated measures is introduced by means of a residual covariance matrix, Σ_i in (8.36). In the second case, random effects are introduced. In both cases, the SAS procedure GLIMMIX could be used for parameter estimation, using PQL or MQL approximation.

The basis for this model development is the decomposition, in line with (14.6):

$$\boldsymbol{Y}_i = \boldsymbol{\mu}_i + \boldsymbol{\varepsilon}_i, \qquad (22.9)$$

where $\boldsymbol{\mu}_i$ is specified by means of a GLMM and $\boldsymbol{\varepsilon}_i$ is the residual error structure. In a standard GLMM, $\boldsymbol{\varepsilon}_i$ is assumed to be uncorrelated and hence does not lead to additional parameters, as the variances follow from the mean-variance link. In the linearization based method of Section 8.8, $\boldsymbol{\mu}_i$ does not contain random effects, but $\boldsymbol{\varepsilon}_i$ is assumed to be correlated. One can choose an autocorrelation model to determine the variance of $\boldsymbol{\varepsilon}_i$ in (22.9), i.e., the matrix Σ_i in (8.36). Obvious choices include spatial exponential or spatial Gaussian models, an AR(1) structure if measurements are equally spaced, or any autocorrelation structure described in Section 22.2.

Combining both ideas produces a generalized linear mixed model with autocorrelation, just as the model in Section 22.2. The main difference is that (22.2) specifies a linear mixed model with autocorrelation in terms of the latent outcome underlying the multivariate probit model, whereas here the random effects are introduced at the level of the linear predictor

22.4 A Generalized Linear Mixed Model with Autocorrelation

TABLE 22.1. *Meta-analysis in Schizophrenia. Maximum pseudo-likelihood parameter estimates (standard errors) for the probit random-intercept model with and without autocorrelation. The exponential and Gaussian models were taken for the autocorrelation structure. Coding for 'Treat': 0 = standard, 1 = experimental.*

Effect	Random intercept	Random intercept + autocorrelation	
		Expon.	Gaussian
Intercept	-0.27 (0.16)	-0.18 (0.12)	-0.22 (0.14)
Week 1	-1.88 (0.18)	-1.34 (0.20)	-1.62 (0.17)
Week 2	-1.17 (0.17)	-0.88 (0.16)	-1.08 (0.15)
Week 4	-0.70 (0.16)	-0.52 (0.13)	-0.62 (0.15)
Week 6	-0.21 (0.14)	-0.16 (0.11)	-0.18 (0.13)
Treat×Week 1	0.29 (0.21)	0.19 (0.15)	0.23 (0.18)
Treat×Week 2	0.58 (0.21)	0.43 (0.16)	0.52 (0.18)
Treat×Week 4	0.54 (0.21)	0.39 (0.16)	0.47 (0.19)
Treat×Week 6	0.33 (0.22)	0.24 (0.16)	0.29 (0.19)
Treat×Week 8	0.20 (0.22)	0.14 (0.17)	0.17 (0.20)
R.I. s.d. τ	1.83 (0.11)	1.12 (0.23)	1.53 (0.12)
R.I. var. τ^2	3.53 (0.40)	1.25 (0.52)	2.34 (0.37)
Autocorr. par. $\ln \phi$		-1.34 (0.33)	-1.21 (0.17)
Autocorr. $\rho = \rho(u=1)$		0.27 (0.03)	0.26 (0.02)
log PL	-1727.0	-1722.2	-1726.3

describing μ_i after application of the link function, whereas the autocorrelation structure is introduced at the level of ε_i. In other words, whereas the random effects and autocorrelation structures sit 'side by side' in (22.2), this is not the case here. To illustrate this, consider a logit-based model with autocorrelation function:

$$Y_i = \frac{e^{X_i\beta+Z_ib_i}}{1+e^{X_i\beta+Z_ib_i}} + \varepsilon_i \qquad (22.10)$$

where ε_i is assumed to exhibit residual correlation, entering the covariance expression as in (20.48). Both structures enter the pseudo data as in (14.7) and it may appear that then the random effects and the residual error are side by side. However, the residual error of the pseudo data (14.7) is now a transformed version of the original error ε_i.

TABLE 22.2. *Meta-analysis in Schizophrenia. PQL parameter estimates (model-based standard errors) for a linearization-based marginal model with autoregressive autocorrelation structure, random-intercept model, and random-intercept model with autoregressive autocorrelation structure. Logit link. Estimates obtained using the SAS procedure GLIMMIX. Coding for 'Treat': 0 = standard, 1 = experimental.*

Effect	Auto-correlation	Random intercept	R.I. + Autocorr.
Intercept	-0.22 (0.13)	-0.15 (0.20)	-0.13 (0.19)
Week 1	-1.58 (0.18)	-2.33 (0.24)	-2.89 (0.21)
Week 2	-0.95 (0.16)	-1.42 (0.23)	-1.80 (0.20)
Week 4	-0.54 (0.15)	-0.86 (0.22)	-1.12 (0.19)
Week 6	-0.15 (0.13)	-0.28 (0.22)	-0.37 (0.18)
Treat×Week 1	0.30 (0.20)	0.28 (0.27)	0.22 (0.27)
Treat×Week 2	0.51 (0.16)	0.63 (0.25)	0.76 (0.25)
Treat×Week 4	0.44 (0.16)	0.59 (0.25)	0.76 (0.25)
Treat×Week 6	0.26 (0.17)	0.37 (0.26)	0.48 (0.26)
Treat×Week 8	0.17 (0.18)	0.21 (0.28)	0.28 (0.28)
R.I. var. τ^2		3.54 (0.30)	5.92 (0.49)
Autocorr. par. θ	3.00 (0.14)		0.77 (0.10)
Autocorr. $\rho = \rho(u=1)$	0.72 (0.01)		0.27 (0.04)
Autocorr. var. σ^2	1.02 (0.03)		0.55 (0.02)

22.5 A Meta-analysis of Trials in Schizophrenic Subjects

We consider the same meta-analysis based on five trials as in Section 21.4, and focus on the CGI ('Clinician's Global Impression') outcome. This is somewhat different from Section 21.4, where PANSS and CGI were analyzed jointly, in the context of surrogate marker evaluation. More specifically, the CGI overall change versus baseline is considered. Dichotomization was obtained by defining a success ($Y_{ij} = 1$) as clinical improvement since baseline (i.e., CGI grade equal to 1 or 2) and a failure otherwise.

We will first consider the multilevel probit models of Section 22.2 and then turn to generalized linear mixed models with serial correlation in Section 22.4.

The parameterization includes a saturated treatment by time model for the mean structure and include a random intercept in the model. For the autocorrelation structure, we assumed that $\kappa(u) = \alpha u^\gamma$ and tried several values of $\gamma = -1, 0.5, 1, 2$. The exponential model ($\gamma = 1$) provided the best fit in terms of (pseudo-)likelihood value at maximum. Both $\gamma = 1$ and

22.5 A Meta-analysis of Trials in Schizophrenic Subjects

$\gamma = 2$ are reported in Table 22.1. We also fitted a model with

$$\kappa(u) = \alpha_1 u + \alpha_2 u^{-1},$$

but a boundary solution was obtained.

The parameter α was rewritten as $\alpha = \exp(\phi)$. This implies that the overall autocorrelation function, for $\gamma = 1$, is

$$\rho(u) = \exp[-\kappa(u)] = \exp[-\exp(\phi)u], \qquad (22.11)$$

and hence the correlation between, for example, two measurements one time unit apart is

$$\rho = \rho(1) = \exp[-\kappa(1)] = \exp[-\exp(\phi)]. \qquad (22.12)$$

In Table 22.1, parameter estimates and standard errors are reported for the random-intercept model with and without exponential autocorrelation structure. Apart from the autocorrelation parameter ϕ, we also present ρ as in (22.12), for ease of reference and interpretation. As can be seen, parameter estimates for the model with exponential autocorrelation are all reduced in magnitude by an amount of roughly 30%. This is essentially due to the fact that the error terms in (22.2) are assumed to be autocorrelated; hence the autocorrelation explains a certain amount of variability that is otherwise captured in the residual variance. This residual variance itself depends on the regression parameters, which is why they are affected by such a change. The $\log PL$ value shows an improvement in the fit of the model. Formal testing needs to be done based on the method laid out in Section 9.3. As stated earlier, Gaussian autocorrelation fits the data less well than exponential autocorrelation. This also explains why the regression parameters in the Gaussian decay case change less.

Let us now switch to the generalized linear mixed models with autocorrelation. The autocorrelation function can be modeled using model (22.11). However, we will use a slightly reparameterized form, in agreement with the parameterization used by SAS, for convenience:

$$\rho(u) = \exp\left(-\frac{1}{\theta}u^\gamma\right)$$

and thus the correlation between two measurements one time unit apart is:

$$\rho = \rho(1) = \exp\left(-\frac{1}{\theta}\right). \qquad (22.13)$$

Table 22.2 presents three models, with the same fixed-effects structure as in Table 22.1. Apart from the autocorrelation parameter θ, we also present the correlation ρ as in (22.13).

The first model exhibits an exponential autocorrelation structure only, and no random effects. The second model is the random-intercepts model, and the third model combines both features. Observe that the correlation parameter ρ for the latter model is very similar to the one obtained in Table 22.1, which is not surprising. Fixed-effects parameter estimates are different, due to two causes. First, we use the logit link in Table 22.2 *versus* the probit link in Table 22.1. Second, PQL estimation in the GLMM case is known to lead to parameter attenuation, as reported in several instances (Tables 14.1 and 17.4).

To separate both issues, the same three models as in Table 22.2, but now with probit link, are presented in Table 22.3. Now, compare the second model in Table 22.3 to the first model in Table 22.1. Both are random-intercepts models, without serial correlation and with probit link. The attenuation in the PQL case is then clear, suggesting the use of integration based methods (Section 14.3) for pure random-effects GLMM, or of the pseudo-likelihood method when autocorrelation is additionally present. At least, this comparison issues caution regarding the use of PQL for generalized linear mixed models with autocorrelation, just as care is needed in the absence of autocorrelation.

The fixed effects in the first columns of Tables 22.2 and 22.3 are somewhat smaller than in the corresponding second and third columns. This is to be expected since these models are marginal, whereas the other two are random-effects based (Chapter 16). Recall the approximate relationship between a random-intercepts model and the corresponding marginal model, given by (16.3). In fact, the discrepancy is not as large as it could be, due to the attenuation of the PQL based methods.

Another comparison is between the fixed-effects parameter estimates in Table 22.3 and their counterparts in Table 22.2. This reveals, once more, the relationship between probit based parameters and their logit counterparts, the approximate conversion factor being $\pi/\sqrt{3}$, as explained in Section 3.4.

In both Tables 22.2 and 22.3, the autocorrelation in the first model is considerably larger than in the third model. This is to be expected, as in the third model a part of the autocorrelation is captured by the random intercept, whereas all correlation is accounted for by the autocorrelation process in the first model. In the first model in both tables, the autocorrelation variance σ^2 plays the role of an overdispersion parameter, indicating no evidence for overdispersion in this case. The same cannot be said for the third models, as the variance is captured by both the random-intercept variance and the serial variance, and the relationship between both is not straightforward because non-linear, as is clear from the position of the random effects *versus* the residual association in (22.10).

TABLE 22.3. *Meta-analysis in Schizophrenia. PQL parameter estimates (model-based standard errors) for a linearization-based marginal model with autoregressive autocorrelation structure, random-intercept model, and random-intercept model with autoregressive autocorrelation structure. Probit link. Estimates obtained using the SAS procedure GLIMMIX. Coding for 'Treat': 0 = standard, 1 = experimental.*

Effect	Auto-correlation	Random intercept	R.I. + Autocorr.
Intercept	-0.14 (0.08)	-0.11 (0.11)	-0.11 (0.11)
Week 1	-0.94 (0.11)	-1.38 (0.14)	-1.68 (0.12)
Week 2	-0.58 (0.10)	-0.84 (0.13)	-1.05 (0.11)
Week 4	-0.34 (0.09)	-0.51 (0.13)	-0.66 (0.10)
Week 6	-0.10 (0.08)	-0.16 (0.13)	-0.21 (0.10)
Treat×Week 1	0.17 (0.11)	0.17 (0.16)	0.15 (0.15)
Treat×Week 2	0.30 (0.10)	0.38 (0.14)	0.44 (0.14)
Treat×Week 4	0.27 (0.10)	0.37 (0.14)	0.45 (0.14)
Treat×Week 6	0.17 (0.10)	0.23 (0.15)	0.28 (0.15)
Treat×Week 8	0.11 (0.11)	0.13 (0.16)	0.17 (0.16)
R.I. var. τ^2		1.25 (0.10)	2.08 (0.15)
Autocorr. par. θ	3.00 (0.14)		0.75 (0.10)
Autocorr. $\rho = \rho(u=1)$	0.72 (0.01)		0.26 (0.05)
Autocorr. var. σ^2	1.02 (0.03)		0.51 (0.02)

22.6 SAS Code for Random-effects Models with Autocorrelation

The method presented in Section 22.2 has been implemented, for the case of a random-intercept probit model with autocorrelation, by Didier Renard (Renard, Molenberghs, and Geys 2004) in a SAS macro, available from the authors upon request. A call to the macro to fit the random-intercept only model in Table 22.1 is:

```
%plrint_corr(dataset=cgi, y=cgi_bin, x=weekcls treat*weekcls,
             classvar=weekcls, id=id, varinit=, weight=1,
             info=0, scorrtim=, scorrinit=, scorrpow=);
```

Most of the arguments to the macro are self-evident and in agreement with standard SAS statements. These include 'y' and 'x' for the response and independent variables, respectively, 'classvar' for the independent variables that need to be treated as class variables, and 'id' to indicate the levels of independent replication. Pseudo-likelihood is requested by 'weight=1,' whereas 'weight=0' refers to full maximum likelihood. Convergence in gradient terms is governed by 'conv,' with a default value of 10^{-4}, and 'maxiter' controls the maximum number of iterations, with a default value of 100. The user can control whether the information matrix is calculated using first-order derivatives ('info=0') or rather numerically calculatead second-order derivatives ('info=1'). An initial value for the random-intercept variance can be passed on by way of 'varinit.' The remaining options control the autocorrelation process. The time variable used in the autocorrelation process is passed on through 'scorrtim.' If this argument is left empty, then no autocorrelation is included and hence a standard random-intercept probit model is obtained. The power p of the exponential process $\exp[-\alpha(t_{ij} - t_{ik})^k]$ is specified via 'scorrpow,' with a (default) value of 1 for exponential decay and $k = 2$ for Gaussian decay. The parameter α can be initialized using 'scorrinit.'

The use of these options implies that for the model with random intercept and exponential autocorrelation, the call changes to:

```
%plrint_corr(dataset=cgi, y=cgi_bin, x=weekcls treat*weekcls,
            classvar=weekcls, id=id, varinit=%str(1.117),
            weight=1, info=0, scorrtim=weekcls,
            scorrinit=%str(0.5), scorrpow=1);
```

Turning attention to the generalized linear mixed model with autocorrelation, the following code can be used:

```
proc glimmix data=m.cgi method=RSPL;
  class id weekcls;
  nloptions maxiter=50 technique=newrap absftol=1e-4;
  model cgi_bin (event='1') = weekcls treat*weekcls
                            / dist=binary link=probit solution;
  random intercept / subject=id type=un;
  random _residual_ / subject=id type=sp(exp)(timecls);
run;
```

The RANDOM statement with 'intercept' argument produces the random intercept model, whereas the serial process is invoked by means of the RANDOM statement with '_residual_' argument. The 'type=sp(exp)' requests exponential decay. Removing the first RANDOM statement produces a marginal model with autocorrelation process only. Removing the second one yields the classical random-intercept model. Removing the 'link=probit' option from the MODEL statement yields the logit link equivalents to these models. Since convergence can be challenging, it might be necessary to try several NLOPTIONS arguments to control updating, convergence criteria, etc. In our case, it has been necessary to switch the updating algorithm to Newton-Rahpson with the 'technique=newrap' option because quasi-Newton methods tend to get trapped in an infinite cycling between two or more values. Moreover, the number of iterations needs to be increased since for some analyses the default number of 20 was exceeded. Finally, the convergence criterion was relaxed, either in terms of the function itself, using the 'absftol=' option, or in terms of the gradient, using the 'absgtol=' option.

22.7 Concluding Remarks

We have presented two approaches to deal with hierarchical generalized linear models, with both random effects and serial correlations. The first one is based on a probit model, overlaying a linear mixed model. The second one is based on the generalized linear mixed model framework, where the residual error terms are allowed to be correlated.

Both approaches have advantages and disadvantages. The hierarchical probit model is simple and appealing because the various effects enter the latent variable in a way very similar to the linear mixed model. On the other hand, the approach is restricted to a probit specification. Even though extensions could start from other fully specified marginal models, the properties and simplicity of an underlying multivariate normal are important factors rendering the probit specification unique. Although this seems to imply a restriction to binary data at the same time, the multilevel probit approach could in fact be applied to ordinal data, as in Section 7.6. Pseudo-likelihood provides a convenient estimation method. Renard, Molenberghs, and Geys (2004) reported good computational properties, but a loss in efficiency. A large sample size might be necessary for the asymptotic properties of the PL estimator to hold and the autocorrelation parameter may be subject to substantial bias in samples of small to moderate size. Nevertheless, in the analysis of our example, the autocorrelation parameter was estimated very similarly between the multilevel probit model and the GLMM-based approach.

Although the PL estimation procedure can, in principle, be applied to hierarchies with more than two levels, practical limitations on the number of levels will arise. For instance, in a three-level model all possible pairs within and between level 2 units pertaining to the same level 3 unit should be considered. This will become computationally prohibitive as the number of levels and the number of replicates per level increase.

The GLMM-based approach is very general and applies to all link functions. Nevertheless, because the random effects and the autocorrelation structure enter at different places into the model, irrespective of whether one consider the direct outcomes or the pseudo data derived from them, the model is somewhat less transparent and, for example, calculation of the overall variance or the overall correlation is far from straightforward. Although PQL is convenient, it suffers from potentially severe attenuation bias in the fixed efects parameter estimates, the estimates of the variance components, as well as in all standard errors. This phenomenon has been reported before and switching from PQL to MQL would make things worse.

Finally, convergence difficulties should be anticipated to occur quite frequently in applications, regardless of which of the two routes were chosen. Even in linear mixed models, convergence failures are relatively common when modeling of the covariance structure involves joint specification of random effects, serial correlation, and measurement error, simply because these components of variability cannot easily be disentangled. An example in the context of the linear mixed model can be found in Verbeke and Molenberghs (2000, Section 9.4). Not surprisingly, this phenomenon amplifies with binary data, which contain less information than their continuous counterparts.

23
Non-Gaussian Random Effects

23.1 Introduction

The mixed models discussed so far all assume that the random effects are normally distributed. This assumption has been carried over from the linear mixed models, where it has proven to be mathematically very convenient in the sense that the marginal likelihood can easily be calculated analytically (Chapter 4). In non-linear mixed models, as well as in generalized linear mixed models, this normality assumption has been the cause of many computational difficulties because the marginal likelihood can no longer be computed analytically, which has resulted in many proposals in the statistical literature about how to approximate the likelihood to be maximized (see Chapter 14 for an overview).

For linear mixed models, it has been shown (Verbeke and Lesaffre 1996, 1997) that deviations from this normality assumption have very little impact on the estimation of the parameters in the marginal model, but much more on the empirical Bayes estimates for the random effects. For non-linear and generalized linear mixed models, misspecification of the random-effects distribution can lead to biased estimates for the parameters in the marginal model, including the fixed effects that are usually of primary interest. We refer to Neuhaus, Hauck, and Kalbfleisch (1992), Butler and Louis (1992), Pfeiffer *et al* (2003), Heagerty and Zeger (2000), and Litiére *et al* (2005) for more details on the effect of misspecifications of random-effects distributions in generalized linear mixed models.

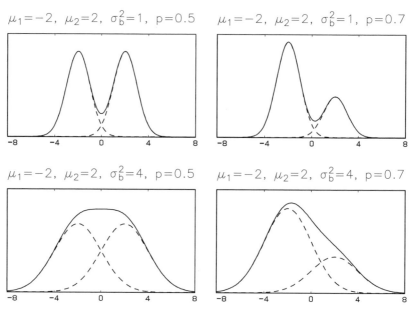

FIGURE 23.1. *Density functions of mixtures $pN(\mu_1, \sigma_b^2) + (1-p)N(\mu_2, \sigma_b^2)$ of two normal distributions, for varying values for p and σ_b^2. The dashed lines represents the densities of the normal components; the solid line represents the density of the mixture.*

This calls for methods to check the normality of the random effects and for models that relax the distributional assumptions. In the context of linear mixed models, it has been shown (Verbeke and Molenberghs 2000 Section 7.8) that the empirical Bayes estimates for the random effects, obtained under normality, cannot be used to check normality because the prior belief of normality often forces the estimates to satisfy this assumption such that non-normality of the random effects may not be reflected in their empirical Bayes estimates. Therefore, Verbeke and Lesaffre (1996), Magder and Zeger (1996), and Verbeke and Molenberghs (2000, Chapter 12) have extended the linear mixed model with mixtures of normals as random-effects distribution. This particular extension has several advantages. First, as shown in Figure 23.1, the class of finite mixtures of normal distributions is a very flexible class of distributions: unimodal as well as multimodal, symmetric as well as very skewed. Second, mixtures can be used to model unobserved heterogeneity in the random-effects distribution. Third, the fact that the mixture components are still normally distributed allows the implementation to take advantage of algorithms and software already available for fitting the models with normally distributed random effects. Finally, the mixture models can be used for classification purposes, which makes them particularly useful in contexts of discriminant analysis or cluster analysis, based on longitudinal profiles.

In this chapter, we will present and illustrate the mixture approach in the context of generalized linear, or non-linear, mixed models. In Section 23.2, the model will be introduced. In Section 23.3, estimation and inference will be discussed. Section 23.4 briefly explains how random effects can be estimated under the mixture assumption and shows how the mixture models can be used for classification purposes. Finally, an example will be worked out in Section 23.5. More details on the model, as well as on the related estimation and inference can be found in Fieuws, Spiessens, and Draney (2004) or in Muthén and Shedden (1999).

23.2 The Heterogeneity Model

As before, let Y_i be the n_i-dimensional vector of all measurements available for cluster $i = 1, \ldots, N$, and let $f_i(y_i|b_i)$ be the corresponding density, conditional on a q-dimensional vector b_i of random effects. We hereby do not explicitly denote possible dependence of $f_i(y_i|b_i)$ on unknown parameters such as fixed effects. In the mixed models considered so far, the random effects b_i were always assumed to be sampled from a normal distribution with mean vector zero and a covariance matrix D, i.e., $b_i \sim N(0, D)$. This assumption reflects the prior believe that the random effects are drawn from one homogeneous population of random effects. From now on, the so-obtained mixed model will be termed 'homogeneity' model.

The 'heterogeneity' model is obtained by replacing the normality assumption for the random effects by a mixture of g q-dimensional normal distributions with mean vectors μ_r and covariance matrices D_r, i.e.,

$$b_i \sim \sum_{r=1}^{g} p_r N(\mu_r, D_r), \qquad (23.1)$$

with $\sum_{r=1}^{g} p_r = 1$. The population under study can then be interpreted as a combination of g sub-populations, each representing a fraction p_r of the total population. In the rth sub-population, the random effects are normally distributed with mean μ_r, and covariance D_r. Clearly, model (23.1) reflects prior belief of presence of unobserved heterogeneity. Therefore, the resulting mixed model is called 'heterogeneity' model.

We now define $z_{ir} = 1$ if b_i is sampled from the rth component in the mixture, and 0 otherwise, $r = 1, \ldots, g$. We then have that $P(z_{ir} = 1) = E(z_{ir}) = p_r$ and that

$$E(b_i) = E\left[E(b_i \mid z_{i1}, \ldots, z_{ig})\right] = E\left(\sum_{r=1}^{g} \mu_r \, z_{ir}\right) = \sum_{r=1}^{g} p_r \, \mu_r.$$

Therefore, the additional constraint $\sum_{r=1}^{g} p_r \mu_r = 0$ is needed to ensure that the random effects still have mean zero. Further, we have that the overall covariance matrix of the b_i is given by

$$\begin{aligned}
D^* &= \text{var}\left[E(b_i \mid z_{i1}, \ldots, z_{ig})\right] + E\left[\text{var}(b_i \mid z_{i1}, \ldots, z_{ig})\right] \\
&= \text{var}\left(\sum_{r=1}^{g} \mu_r \, z_{ir}\right) + E\left(\sum_{r=1}^{g} D_r \, z_{ir}\right) \\
&= \sum_{r=1}^{g} p_r \mu_r \mu_r' + \sum_{r=1}^{g} p_r D_r.
\end{aligned} \qquad (23.2)$$

The first term represents variability between the mixture components, and the second term is the average within-component variability. Hence, (23.2) can be interpreted as a decomposition of variability in the random effects in terms of variability between and variability within the sub-populations. Finally, denoting the density within the rth mixture component by $f_r(b_i)$, we have that the density function corresponding to (23.1) is given by

$$\begin{aligned}
f(b_i) &= \sum_{r=1}^{g} p_r f_r(b_i) \\
&= \sum_{r=1}^{g} p_r \, (2\pi)^{-q/2} \, |D_r|^{-1/2} \\
&\quad \times \exp\left\{-\frac{1}{2}(b_i - \mu_r)' D_r^{-1}(b_i - \mu_r)\right\}. \qquad (23.3)
\end{aligned}$$

It should be emphasized that we consider the number of components g in (23.1) to be known. In practice, several models can be fitted, with increasing values for g, leading to a series of nested models, and testing procedures such as the likelihood ratio test could be used for the comparison of these models. However, as discussed by Ghosh and Sen (1985), testing for the number of components in a finite mixture is seriously complicated by boundary problems similar to the ones discussed in Section 14.6 in the context of tests for variance components. In order to briefly highlight the main problems, we consider testing $H_0 : g = 1$ versus $H_A : g = 2$. The null hypothesis can then be expressed as $H_0 : \mu_1 = \mu_2$. However, the same hypothesis is obtained by setting $H_0 : p_1 = 0$ or $H_0 : p_2 = 0$, which clearly illustrates that H_0 is on the boundary of the parameter space, and hence also that the usual regularity conditions for application of the classical maximum likelihood theory are violated. Therefore, simulations are needed to derive the correct null distribution of the LR test statistic. We refer to Verbeke (1995, Section 4.6) for an example in the context of linear mixed models, and to McLachlan and Basford (1988, Section 1.10) for an extensive overview of the literature on the use of the LR test in finite mixture problems. In practice it is often sufficient to fit several heterogeneity models and to explore how increasing g affects the inference for the parameters of interest.

In the context of linear mixed models, Magder and Zeger (1996) also considered mixtures of normal distributions as random-effects distribution, but they treated the number g of components as an unknown parameter, to be estimated from the data. In order to avoid that non-smooth mixture distributions, with many components, would be obtained, they pre-specify a lower boundary h for the within-component variability measured by the determinants $|D_r|$ of the within-component covariance matrices. In practice, very little difference is expected from models that pre-specify the number of mixture components. Indeed, when a very smooth mixing distribution is required, a large value of h can be specified, which will yield a mixture of a relatively small number of normal distributions.

23.3 Estimation and Inference

Estimation and inference for the heterogeneity model will be based on maximum likelihood (ML) principles for the marginal likelihood of the data. The marginal distribution of $\boldsymbol{Y}_i$, obtained from integrating out the random effects, is given by

$$\begin{aligned} f_i(\boldsymbol{y}_i) &= \int f_i(\boldsymbol{y}_i|\boldsymbol{b}_i) \, f(\boldsymbol{b}_i) \, d\boldsymbol{b}_i \\ &= \sum_{r=1}^{g} p_r \int f_i(\boldsymbol{y}_i|\boldsymbol{b}_i) \, f_r(\boldsymbol{b}_i) \, d\boldsymbol{b}_i \\ &= \sum_{r=1}^{g} p_r f_{ir}(\boldsymbol{y}_i) \end{aligned} \qquad (23.4)$$

in which $f_{ir}(\boldsymbol{y}_i)$ is the marginal density corresponding to a mixed model with random effects that are normally distributed with mean $\boldsymbol{\mu}_r$ and covariance D_r. Hence, the marginal density of $\boldsymbol{Y}_i$ is again a g-component finite mixture, with the same mixing proportions p_r, and where the component-specific densities are marginal mixed model densities within the specific sub-population. This specific feature will simplify implementation considerably because it will be possible to build on existing software for generalized linear and/or non-linear mixed models.

Maximization of the marginal likelihood resulting from (23.4) will be based on the so-called Expectation-Maximization (EM) algorithm, see Laird (1978). See also Section 28.3 for a general introduction of the algorithm in the context of missing data. The EM algorithm is particularly useful for mixture problems because it often happens that a model is fitted with too many components (g too large), leading to a likelihood that is maximal anywhere on a ridge. As shown by Dempster, Laird, and Rubin (1977), the EM algorithm is capable of converging to some particular point on that ridge. Titterington, Smith, and Makov (1985, pp. 88–89) compare the EM algorithm with the Newton-Raphson (NR) algorithm. Their conclusions can be summarized as follows:

- EM is usually simple to apply and satisfies the appealing monotonic property in that it increases the objective function at each iteration step. NR is more complicated, and there is no guarantee of monotonicity.

- If NR converges, it is of second order (i.e., fast), whereas EM is often painfully slow. However, if the separation between the components in the mixture is poor, even the numerical performance of NR can be disappointing. Simulations have shown that, in such cases, NR can fail to converge in up to half the simulations, even when the algorithm was started from the true parameter values.

- Convergence is not guaranteed with any of the techniques because EM, even with the monotonicity property, can converge to a local maximum of the likelihood surface.

Böhning and Lindsay (1988) have considered maximization of log-likelihoods for which the quadratic approximation based on the Taylor series is "flatter" than the objective function, thereby sending the solution too far at the next step. They conclude that, in a mixture framework, flat log-likelihoods often occur. It is known that this often leads to problems in convergence and to instabilities for the Newton-Raphson algorithm.

Note also that because the random effects are assumed to follow a mixture of distributions of the same parametric family, the vector of all parameters in the marginal model is, strictly speaking, not identifiable. Indeed, the log-likelihood is invariant under the $g!$ possible permutations of the mean vectors $\boldsymbol{\mu}_r$, the covariances D_r, and the corresponding component probabilities p_r. Therefore, the likelihood will have at least $g!$ local maxima with the same likelihood value. However, this lack of identifiability is of no concern in practice, as it can easily be overcome by imposing some constraint on the parameters. For example, Aitkin and Rubin (1985) use the constraint that

$$p_1 \geq p_2 \geq \ldots \geq p_g. \tag{23.5}$$

The likelihood is then maximized without the restriction, and the component labels are permuted afterwards to achieve (23.5).

The EM algorithm is frequently used for the calculation of maximum likelihood estimates for missing data problems (Section 28.3). Strictly speaking, we do not necessarily have missingness in our context. However, it will prove extremely convenient to treat the component membership indicators

z_{ir}, $i = 1, \ldots, N$, $r = 1, \ldots, g$ as missing. We now give a brief introduction on the EM algorithm in the context of the heterogeneity model, and we refer to McLachlan and Basford (1988, Section 1.6) for an application of the EM algorithm in a simpler mixture context, where it is assumed that the available data are all drawn from the same mixture distribution (no different dimensions, no covariates).

Let $\boldsymbol{\pi}$ be the vector of component probabilities [i.e., $\boldsymbol{\pi}' = (p_1, \ldots, p_g)$] and let $\boldsymbol{\gamma}$ be the vector containing the remaining parameters, i.e., the parameters in the conditional densities $f_i(\boldsymbol{y}_i|\boldsymbol{b}_i)$ as well as in all $\boldsymbol{\mu}_r$ and all D_r. Further, $\boldsymbol{\theta}' = (\boldsymbol{\pi}', \boldsymbol{\gamma}')$ denotes the vector of all parameters in the marginal heterogeneity model (23.4). Further, we now explicitly denote dependence of the within-component marginal densities $f_{ir}(\boldsymbol{y}_i)$ on $\boldsymbol{\gamma}$ by $f_{ir}(\boldsymbol{y}_i|\boldsymbol{\gamma})$. The marginal likelihood function is then given by

$$L(\boldsymbol{\theta}|\boldsymbol{y}) = \prod_{i=1}^{N} \left[\sum_{r=1}^{g} p_r \, f_{ir}(\boldsymbol{y}_i \mid \boldsymbol{\gamma}) \right], \tag{23.6}$$

where $\boldsymbol{y}' = (\boldsymbol{y_1}', \ldots, \boldsymbol{y_N}')$ is the vector containing all observed response values.

Let z_{ir} be as defined before in Section 23.2. The prior probability for an individual to belong to component r is then $P(z_{ir} = 1) = p_r$, the mixture proportion for that component. The log-likelihood function for the observed measurements $\boldsymbol{y}$ and for the vector $\boldsymbol{z}$ of all unobserved z_{ir} is then

$$\ell(\boldsymbol{\theta}|\boldsymbol{y}, \boldsymbol{z}) = \sum_{i=1}^{N} \sum_{r=1}^{g} z_{ir} \left[\ln p_r + \ln f_{ir}(\boldsymbol{y}_i|\boldsymbol{\gamma}) \right],$$

which is easier to maximize than the log-likelihood function corresponding to the likelihood (23.6) of the observed data vector $\boldsymbol{y}$ only. On the other hand, maximizing $\ell(\boldsymbol{\theta}|\boldsymbol{y}, \boldsymbol{z})$ with respect to $\boldsymbol{\theta}$ yields estimates which depend on the unobserved ("missing") indicators z_{ir}. A compromise is obtained with the EM algorithm, where the expected value of $\ell(\boldsymbol{\theta}|\boldsymbol{y}, \boldsymbol{z})$, rather than $\ell(\boldsymbol{\theta}|\boldsymbol{y}, \boldsymbol{z})$ itself, is maximized with respect to $\boldsymbol{\theta}$, where the expectation is taken over all the unobserved z_{ir}. In the E step (expectation step), the conditional expectation of $\ell(\boldsymbol{\theta}|\boldsymbol{y}, \boldsymbol{z})$, given the observed data vector $\boldsymbol{y}$, is calculated. In the M step (maximization step), the so-obtained expected log-likelihood function is maximized with respect to $\boldsymbol{\theta}$, providing an updated estimate for $\boldsymbol{\theta}$. Finally, one keeps iterating between the E step and the M step until convergence is attained.

More specifically, let $\boldsymbol{\theta}^{(t)}$ be the current estimate for $\boldsymbol{\theta}$, and $\boldsymbol{\theta}^{(t+1)}$ stands for the updated estimate, obtained from one further iteration in the EM algorithm. We then have the following E and M steps in the estimation process for the heterogeneity model.

The E Step. The conditional expectation

$$Q(\boldsymbol{\theta}|\boldsymbol{\theta}^{(t)}) = E\left[\ell(\boldsymbol{\theta}|\boldsymbol{y}, \boldsymbol{z}) \mid \boldsymbol{y}, \boldsymbol{\theta}^{(t)}\right]$$

is given by

$$Q(\boldsymbol{\theta}|\boldsymbol{\theta}^{(t)}) = \sum_{i=1}^{N}\sum_{r=1}^{g} p_{ir}(\boldsymbol{\theta}^{(t)})\left[\ln p_r + \ln f_{ir}(\boldsymbol{y_i}|\boldsymbol{\gamma})\right], \quad (23.7)$$

where only the posterior probability for the ith individual to belong to the rth component of the mixture, given by

$$\begin{aligned} p_{ir}(\boldsymbol{\theta}^{(t)}) &= E(z_{ir} \mid \boldsymbol{y_i}, \boldsymbol{\theta}^{(t)}) = P(z_{ir} = 1 \mid \boldsymbol{y_i}, \boldsymbol{\theta}^{(t)}) \\ &= \left.\frac{p_r f_{ir}(\boldsymbol{y_i}|\boldsymbol{\gamma})}{\sum_{k=1}^{g} p_k f_{ik}(\boldsymbol{y_i}|\boldsymbol{\gamma})}\right|_{\hat{\pi}^{(t)},\hat{\gamma}^{(t)}} \end{aligned}$$

has to be calculated for each i and r.

The M Step. To get the updated estimate $\boldsymbol{\theta}^{(t+1)}$, we have to maximize expression (23.7) with respect to $\boldsymbol{\theta}$. We first maximize

$$\sum_{i=1}^{N}\sum_{r=1}^{g} p_{ir}(\boldsymbol{\theta}^{(t)}) \ln p_r$$

$$= \sum_{i=1}^{N}\sum_{r=1}^{g-1} p_{ir}(\boldsymbol{\theta}^{(t)}) \ln p_r + \sum_{i=1}^{N} p_{ig}(\boldsymbol{\theta}^{(t)}) \ln\left(1 - \sum_{r=1}^{g-1} p_r\right)$$

with respect to $p_1, \ldots, p_{g-1}$. Setting all first-order derivatives equal to zero establishes that the updated estimates satisfy

$$\frac{p_r^{(t+1)}}{p_g^{(t+1)}} = \frac{\sum_{i=1}^{N} p_{ir}(\boldsymbol{\theta}^{(t)})}{\sum_{i=1}^{N} p_{ig}(\boldsymbol{\theta}^{(t)})},$$

for all $r = 1, \ldots, g-1$. This also implies that

$$1 = \sum_{r=1}^{g} p_r^{(t+1)} = \frac{N \, p_g^{(t+1)}}{\sum_{i=1}^{N} p_{ig}(\boldsymbol{\theta}^{(t)})},$$

from which it follows that all estimates $p_r^{(t+1)}$ satisfy

$$p_r^{(t+1)} = \frac{1}{N}\sum_{i=1}^{N} p_{ir}(\boldsymbol{\theta}^{(t)}).$$

Unfortunately, the second part of (23.7) cannot be maximized analytically, and a numerical maximization procedure such as Newton-Raphson is needed to maximize

$$\sum_{i=1}^{N}\sum_{r=1}^{g} p_{ir}(\boldsymbol{\theta}^{(t)}) \ln f_{ir}(\boldsymbol{y_i}|\boldsymbol{\gamma}) \quad (23.8)$$

with respect to γ. Luckily, (23.8) can be interpreted as a weighted log-likelihood of a generalized linear or non-linear mixed model. Therefore, maximization of (23.8), can often be based on software procedures available for fitting generalized linear and non-linear mixed models, such as the SAS procedures GLIMMIX and NLMIXED (Chapter 15). We refer to Fieuws, Spiessens, and Draney (2004) for an implementation based on the NLMIXED procedure.

Often, numerical maximization algorithms are based on second-order derivatives of the log-likelihood function. This allows easy calculation of the observed Fisher information matrix and hence also of asymptotic standard errors for all ML estimates. This is not the case for the EM algorithm, which immediately highlights one of the main drawbacks of this algorithm. However, Louis (1982) has provided a procedure for approximating the observed information matrix with few additional calculations. The so-obtained standard errors can then be used to construct classical asymptotic Wald-type tests, based on the asymptotic normality of the ML estimators. Alternative inferences can be based on likelihood ratio principles as well.

23.4 Empirical Bayes Estimation and Classification

When the random effects b_i are of interest, empirical Bayes (EB) techniques can be used for their estimation. As explained in Section 14.2.4, it is customary to define the EB estimates as the posterior modes of the random effects b_i, i.e., as the value for b_i that maximizes the posterior density $f_i(b_i|y_i)$, in which all unknown parameters have been replaced by their estimates obtained from maximizing the marginal likelihood function. Under the heterogeneity model, the posterior density of b_i is given by

$$f_i(b_i \mid y_i, \theta) = \sum_{r=1}^{g} p_{ir}(\theta) f_{ir}(b_i \mid y_i, \gamma), \qquad (23.9)$$

where $f_{ir}(b_i|y_i, \gamma)$ is the posterior density function of b_i, conditional on $z_{ir} = 1$, i.e., conditional on the knowledge that b_i was sampled from the rth component in the mixture. Hence, the posterior distribution of b_i is a mixture of the posterior distributions of b_i within each component of the mixture, with the posterior probabilities $p_{ir}(\theta)$ as subject-specific mixture proportions. The possible multimodality of the posterior density of b_i implies that the posterior mode is not a good point estimate for b_i, in many applications. However, expression (23.9) suggests estimating the random effect b_i for cluster i by the weighted sum

$$\widehat{b_i} = \sum_{r=1}^{g} p_{ir}(\theta) \widehat{b_{ir}}(\gamma)$$

of the component-specific posterior modes $\widehat{b_{ir}}(\gamma)$, with weights equal to the posterior probabilities for that subject to belong to the different mixture components, and with the parameters θ and γ replaced by their ML estimates obtained from the EM algorithm. The resulting estimates will still be called empirical Bayes estimates.

Interest could also lie in the classification of the subjects into the different mixture components. It is natural in mixture models for such a classification to be based on the estimated posterior probabilities $p_{ir}(\widehat{\theta})$ (McLachlan and Basford 1988, Section 1.4). One then classifies the ith subject into the component for which it has the highest estimated posterior probability to belong to, that is, to the $r(i)$th component, where $r(i)$ is the index for which

$$p_{i,r(i)}(\widehat{\theta}) = \max_{1 \leq r \leq g} p_{ir}(\widehat{\theta}).$$

Note how this technique can be used for cluster analysis within the framework of non-linear or generalized linear mixed models: If the individual profiles are to be classified into g subgroups, fit a mixture model with g components and use the above rule for classification in either one of the g clusters. In the context of discriminant analysis, a mixed model can be fitted to each group separately, and a mixture model can be used for the classification of future clusters. Examples in the context of linear models for continuous data can be found in Verbeke and Lesaffre (1996), Tomasko, Helms, and Snapinn (1999), Verbeke and Molenberghs (2000, Chapter 12), and Brant et al (2003). An example in the context of non-linear mixed models can be found in Fieuws, Verbeke, and Brant (2005).

23.5 The Verbal Aggression Data

As an illustration of the mixture approach, we re-analyze the data of Vansteelandt (2000), which were also used by De Boeck and Wilson (2004), as key example throughout their whole book. The data are responses from 316 persons to questions (items) about verbal aggression. All items refer to verbally aggressive reactions in a frustrating situation. For example, one item is: 'A bus fails to stop for me. I would curse.' Possible responses are 'Yes,' or 'No.' Further, the experimental design has four factors, summarized in Table 23.1. The first one is the type of behavior, with possible values 'Curse,' 'Scold,' and 'Shout.' The second design factor is the behavior mode. A differentiation is made between actual doing (i.e., cursing, scolding, or shouting) and wanting to do (i.e., wanting to curse, wanting to scold, or wanting to shout). The third design factor is the situation type. This factor has two levels: situations in which someone else is to blame, and situations in which one is self to blame. Examples of other-to-blame situations are 'A bus fails to stop for me,' and 'I miss a train because a clerk gave me faulty information.' Examples of self-to-blame situations are 'The

23.5 The Verbal Aggression Data

TABLE 23.1. *Verbal Aggression Data. Summary of the 24 items. Two versions exist of each item. The version with 'want to' in the item formulation refers to items with behavior mode 'Want.' The version without 'want to' in the item formulation refers to items with behavior mode 'Do.'*

Items		Situation type	Behavior
1.	A bus fails to stop for me. I would (want to) curse.	Other to blame	Curse
2.	A bus fails to stop for me. I would (want to) scold.		Scold
3.	A bus fails to stop for me. I would (want to) shout.		Shout
4.	I miss a train because a clerk gave me faulty information. I would (want to) curse.		Curse
5.	I miss a train because a clerk gave me faulty information. I would (want to) scold.		Scold
6.	I miss a train because a clerk gave me faulty information. I would (want to) shout.		Shout
7.	The grocery store closes just as I am about to enter. I would (want to) curse.	Self to blame	Curse
8.	The grocery store closes just as I am about to enter. I would (want to) scold		Scold
9.	The grocery store closes just as I am about to enter. I would (want to) shout.		Shout
10.	The operator disconnects me when I had used up my last 10 cents for a call. I would (want to) curse.		Curse
11.	The operator disconnects me when I had used up my last 10 cents for a call. I would (want to) scold.		Scold
12.	The operator disconnects me when I had used up my last 10 cents for a call. I would (want to) shout.		Shout

operator disconnects me when I had used up my last 10 cents for a call,' and 'The grocery store closes just as I am about to enter.' The fourth factor, the specific situations that are asked about (2 of each-see Table 23.1), is nested within the third. This factor will not be used in the analyses here. In conclusion, the design is a 3 × 2 × 2 design with a fourth factor nested within the third, with 24 items in total.

Let Y_{ij} be the outcome for the jth item, measured on respondent i, $i = 1, \ldots, 316$, $j = 1, \ldots, 24$. Further, we define four dummy variables, as defined in Table 23.2. The definition of X_2 and X_3 is such that they characterize expression of frustration (X_2) and expression of blame (X_3). In our analyses, we will focuss on the effect of the factor 'Type of situation,' and more specifically, to the heterogeneity in the population with respect to the effect this factor has on the outcome. All our models will be of the

TABLE 23.2. *Verbal Aggression Data. Definition of the dummy variables for the design factors.*

Dummy	Design factor	Definition	
X_1:	Type of situation:	$X_1 = 1$	Other to blame
		$X_1 = 0$	Self to blame
X_2, X_3:	Type of behavior:	$X_2 = 1$	Cursing or shouting
		$X_2 = 0$	Scolding
		$X_3 = 1$	Cursing or scolding
		$X_3 = 0$	Shouting
X_4:	Mode of behavior:	$X_4 = 1$	Do mode
		$X_4 = 0$	Want mode

form

$$\begin{aligned} Y_{ij}|\boldsymbol{b}_i &\sim \text{Bernoulli}(\pi_{ir}), \\ \text{logit}(\pi_{ir}) &= (\beta_0 + b_{i0}) + (\beta_1 + b_{i1})X_{1i} \\ &\quad + \beta_2 X_{2i} + \beta_3 X_{3i} + \beta_4 X_{4i}, \end{aligned} \qquad (23.10)$$

in which $\boldsymbol{b}_i = (b_{i0}, b_{i1})'$ represents the vector of random (subject-specific) intercepts and random (subject-specific) effects of 'Others to blame' (X_1). It is assumed that the random effects $\boldsymbol{b}_i$ satisfy

$$\boldsymbol{b}_i \sim \sum_{r=1}^{g} p_r N(\boldsymbol{\mu_r}, D_r),$$

where, as before $\sum_r p_r \boldsymbol{\mu_r} = \boldsymbol{0}$. Here, we will only consider models with the same covariance matrix in all mixture components, i.e., with all D_r equal to D,

$$\boldsymbol{b}_i \sim \sum_{r=1}^{g} p_r N\left[\begin{pmatrix} \mu_{0j} \\ \mu_{1j} \end{pmatrix}, \begin{pmatrix} d_{11} & d_{12} \\ d_{21} & d_{22} \end{pmatrix}\right],$$

where $\boldsymbol{\mu_r} = (\mu_{0j}, \mu_{1j})'$.

Depending on the actual form of the $\boldsymbol{\mu_r}$ and of D, we get a variety of models all known in the psychometric literature. We refer to Fieuws, Spiessens, and Draney (2004) for a detailed discussion. A graphical representation of several of those models is given in Figure 23.2, in case of two mixture components, i.e., $g = 2$. For example, if the within-component covariance D is the 2×2 zero matrix, then no within-component variability is present, and Model (23.10) reduces to a so-called latent class model,

23.5 The Verbal Aggression Data

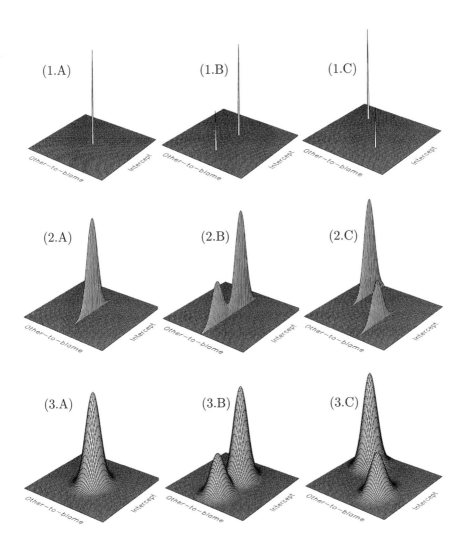

FIGURE 23.2. *Verbal Aggression Data. Graphical representation of different distributional assumptions for random effects.*
Classification according to amount of variability within the mixture components:
  Row 1: no variability
  Row 2: only variability for intercepts
  Row 3: variability for intercepts and effects of other to blame
Classification according to discrimination of the mixture components:
  Column A: no discrimination at all
  Column B: discrimination on intercepts only
  Column C: discrimination on intercepts and effects of other to blame

TABLE 23.3. *Verbal Aggression Data. Maximum likelihood estimates (standard errors) for a one-component and several two-component mixture models.*

Effect	Homogeneity	Heterogeneity models ($g = 2$)		
		Model A	Model B	Model C
β_0	−0.31 (0.096)			−0.32 (0.06)
$\beta_0 + \mu_{01}$		0.20 (0.10)	−0.17 (0.12)	
$\beta_0 + \mu_{02}$		−0.83 (0.11)	−0.41 (0.08)	
β_1	1.03 (0.06)	1.03 (0.05)		
$\beta_1 + \mu_{11}$			2.47 (0.15)	2.64 (0.16)
$\beta_1 + \mu_{12}$			0.50 (0.10)	0.50 (0.09)
β_2	0.70 (0.05)	0.70 (0.04)	0.72 (0.04)	0.72 (0.04)
β_3	1.36 (0.05)	1.36 (0.03)	1.41 (0.03)	1.41 (0.03)
β_4	−0.67 (0.06)	−0.67 (0.04)	−0.69 (0.04)	−0.69 (0.04)
d_{11}	1.86 (0.20)	1.53 (0.16)	1.30 (0.10)	1.35 (0.10)
p_1		0.52 (0.07)	0.30 (0.05)	0.27 (0.04)
p_2		0.48 (0.01)	0.70 (0.05)	0.73 (0.04)
Log-likelihood	−4116.05	−4115.39	−4079.07	−4079.84

which assumes that at most two different values are possible for the intercepts, as well as for the slopes (row 1 in Figure 23.2). Depending on the actual location of the mean parameters μ_1 and μ_2, the model further reduces to a one-component mixture (column A in Figure 23.2), or to a two-component mixture with discrimination in only one dimension or in both dimensions (columns B and C, respectively, in Figure 23.2). A similar column-classification is also possible in case one dimension of the random-effects distribution shows within-component variability (row 2 in Figure 23.2), or when within-component variability is present in both dimensions (row 3 in Figure 23.2).

As an example, several of these models have been fitted to the verbal aggression data, all assuming within-component variability for the intercepts (i.e., $d_{11} > 0$), but a latent class structure for the effect of the behavior mode (i.e., $d_{12} = d_{22} = 0$). Hence, all models are of the type as shown in row 2 of Figure 23.2. The results have been summarized in Table 23.3. First, the homogeneity model, i.e., a one-component model, was fitted ($g = 1$). Clearly, people tend to be more verbally aggressive when others are to blame and when the considered behavior is expressing blame or expressing frustration. Moreover, they want to be more aggressive than they say they would actually be.

23.5 The Verbal Aggression Data

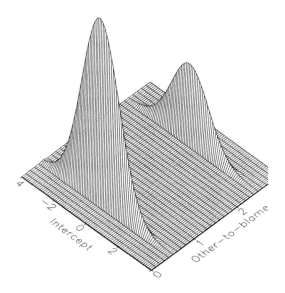

FIGURE 23.3. *Verbal Aggression Data. Fitted random-effects distribution based on the two-component mixture model, Model B.*

Our first two-component mixture model (Model A) assumes a two-component mixture for the intercepts, but still one common effect of the covariate X_1. More specifically, we assume that

$$\begin{pmatrix} b_{i0} \\ b_{i1} \end{pmatrix} \sim p_1\, N\left[\begin{pmatrix} \mu_{01} \\ 0 \end{pmatrix}, \begin{pmatrix} d_{11} & 0 \\ 0 & 0 \end{pmatrix}\right]$$
$$+\, p_2\, N\left[\begin{pmatrix} \mu_{02} \\ 0 \end{pmatrix}, \begin{pmatrix} d_{11} & 0 \\ 0 & 0 \end{pmatrix}\right],$$

which graphically corresponds to panel (2.B) in Figure 23.2. The two mixture components get estimated weights (prior probabilities) equal to 0.52 and 0.48. Note that the results in Table 23.3 are the component means μ_{01} and μ_{02}, with the fixed effect β_0 added, yielding the average intercept within each mixture component separately. In case β_0 would be of interest, the estimate immediately follows from the fact that

$$\beta_0 = p_1(\mu_{01} + \beta_0) + p_2(\mu_{02} + \beta_0),$$

because the random effects have been assumed to have prior mean equal to zero. In our example, this yields

$$\widehat{\beta_0} = 0.52 \times 0.20 - 0.48 \times 0.83 = -0.29,$$

relatively close to the overall intercept we obtained under the homogeneity model. Note also the reduction in within-component variability d_{11}. Finally, although classical likelihood ratio tests for the comparison of the one-component model with Model A are not valid (see Section 23.2), comparison of the log-likelihood values does yield very little evidence in favor of the two-component model.

Model A assumes the same effect of X_1 in both mixture components. In Model B, this is relaxed by assuming that

$$\begin{pmatrix} b_{i0} \\ b_{i1} \end{pmatrix} \sim p_1 \, N\left[\begin{pmatrix} \mu_{01} \\ \mu_{11} \end{pmatrix}, \begin{pmatrix} d_{11} & 0 \\ 0 & 0 \end{pmatrix}\right]$$
$$+ p_2 \, N\left[\begin{pmatrix} \mu_{02} \\ \mu_{12} \end{pmatrix}, \begin{pmatrix} d_{11} & 0 \\ 0 & 0 \end{pmatrix}\right],$$

graphically represented in panel (2.C) of Figure 23.2. Clearly, this model yields an improved fit, when compared to Model A. Figure 23.3 shows the fitted random-effects distribution. The smaller class represents approximately 30% of the population, the larger class 70%. Figure 23.3 clearly shows that a major distinction between the two mixture components is given by the effect of the 'other-to-blame' factor. Our homogeneity model showed that verbal aggression is higher when others are to blame, compared to situations in which one should blame oneself. In the smaller class this difference is much higher than in the larger class (2.474 *versus* 0.501). This means that there are two types of people: Those who do not differentiate very much between other-to-blame situations and self-to-blame situations and those who are clearly more verbally aggressive when others are to blame.

Figure 23.3 also suggests that there is very little differentiation between the mixture components with respect to the random intercepts: The average intercepts in the two components are estimated as -0.167 in the first component versus -0.414 in the second mixture component. Therefore, a two-component model, with a common average random intercept for both components has also been fitted (Model C). The random effects are then assumed to satisfy

$$\begin{pmatrix} b_{i0} \\ b_{i1} \end{pmatrix} \sim p_1 \, N\left[\begin{pmatrix} 0 \\ \mu_{11} \end{pmatrix}, \begin{pmatrix} d_{11} & 0 \\ 0 & 0 \end{pmatrix}\right]$$
$$+ p_2 \, N\left[\begin{pmatrix} 0 \\ \mu_{12} \end{pmatrix}, \begin{pmatrix} d_{11} & 0 \\ 0 & 0 \end{pmatrix}\right].$$

The maximized log-likelihood value is now -4079.84, which is only slightly smaller than what was obtained under Model B.

23.6 Concluding Remarks

In linear mixed models, inferences for the fixed effects and variance components are quite robust with respect to non-normality of the random effects. This no longer holds for non-linear or generalized linear mixed models. We have presented a flexible class of models with less strict distributional assumptions for the random effects, which includes the traditional mixed models based on Gaussian random effects, as special cases.

In the analysis of the verbal aggression data (Section 23.5), we have illustrated the flexibility of the models, in the context of a mixed logistic model for a binary outcome variable. However, the heterogeneity model can equally well be applied to non-linear mixed models (Section 20.5).

Note also that many further extensions of the models presented in the example in Section 23.5 would be possible. The number of mixture components could be further increased, class-specific variances could be assumed, within-component variability could be allowed for the effects of the type of situation, or other random effects could be included as well. Our purpose has been to illustrate the flexibility of the heterogeneity model, rather than to give a complete overview of all possible models that fit within this framework.

24
Joint Continuous and Discrete Responses

24.1 Introduction

Statistical problems where various outcomes of a mixed nature are observed have been around for about a half century and are rather common at present. Perhaps the most common situation, whether in psychometry, biometry, or other fields, is that of the joint occurrence of a continuous, often normally distributed, and a binary or ordinal outcome. Emphasis can be placed on the determination of the entire joint distribution of both outcomes, or on specific aspects, such as the association in general or correlation in particular between both outcomes.

For the problem sketched above, there broadly are three approaches. The first one postulates a marginal model for the binary outcome and then formulates a conditional model for the continuous outcome, given the categorical one. For the former, one can use logistic regression, whereas for the latter conditional normal models are a straightforward choice, i.e., a normal model with the categorical outcome used as a covariate (Tate 1954). The second family starts from the reverse factorization, combining a marginal model for the continuous outcome with a conditional one for the categorical outcome. Conditional models have been discussed by Cox and Wermuth (1992, 1994b), Krzanowski (1988), and Little and Schluchter (1985). Schafer (1997) presents a so-called *general location model* where a number of continuous and binary outcomes can be modeled together.

The third model family directly formulates a joint model for the two outcomes. In this context, one often starts from an bivariate continuous variable, one component of which is explicitly observed and the other one observed in dichotomized, or generally discretized, version only (Tate 1955). Molenberghs, Geys, and Buyse (2001) presented a model based on a Plackett-Dale approach, where a bivariate Plackett distribution is assumed, of which one margin is directly observed and the other one only after dichotomization. General multivariate exponential family based models have been proposed by Prentice and Zhao (1991), Zhao, Prentice, and Self (1992), and Sammel, Ryan, and Legler (1997).

Of course, these developments have not been limited to bivariate joint outcomes. One can obviously extend these ideas and families to a multivariate continuous outcome and/or a multivariate categorical outcome. For the first and second families, one then starts from conditional and marginal multivariate normal and appropriately chosen multinomial models. Such a model within the first family has been formulated by Olkin and Tate (1961). Within the third family, models were formulated by Hannan and Tate (1965) and Cox (1974) for a multivariate normal with a univariate bivariate or discrete variable.

Apart from an extension from the bivariate to the multivariate case, one can introduce other hierarchies as well. For example, each of the outcomes may be measured repeatedly over time, and there could even be several repeated outcomes in both the continuous and the categorical subgroup, and then some of the approaches described in Chapter 25 can be used. A very specific hierarchy stems from clustered data, where a continuous and a categorical, or several of each, are observed for each member of a family, a household, a cluster, etc. For the specific context of developmental toxicity studies, often conducted in rats and mice, a number of developments have been made. An overview of such methods, together with developments for probit-normal and Plackett-Dale based models, was presented in Regan and Catalano (2002). Catalano and Ryan (1992) and Fitzmaurice and Laird (1995) propose models for a combined continuous and discrete outcome, but differ in the choice of which outcome to condition on the other one. Both use generalized estimating equations to allow for clustering. Catalano (1997) extended the model by Catalano and Ryan (1992) to accommodate ordinal variables.

Regan and Catalano (1999a) proposed a probit-type model to accommodate joint continuous and binary outcomes in a clustered data context, thus extending the correlated probit model for binary outcomes (Ochi and Prentice 1984) to incorporate continuous outcomes. Geys et al (2001) used a Plackett latent variable to the same effect, extending the bivariate version proposed by Molenberghs, Geys, and Buyse (2001). Estimation in such hierarchical joint models can be challenging. Regan and Catalano (1999a) proposed maximum likelihood, but considered GEE as an option too (Regan and Catalano 1999b). Geys et al (2001) made use of pseudo-likelihood. Ordinal extensions have been proposed in Regan and Catalano (2000).

It is clear that the literature on joint modeling of outcomes of various natures is diverse and growing. A broad ranging review of hierarchical models for joint continuous and discrete models can be found in Regan and Catalano (2002). In this chapter, we will focus on a few methods. We will emphasize the case of a continuous and a binary outcome as a basic paradigm (Section 24.2). In particular, a probit-normal formulation will be developed (Section 24.2.1), a Plackett-Dale approach (Section 24.2.2), and a bivariate generalized linear mixed model of a joint nature (Section 24.2.3). Hierarchical versions will be discussed in Section 24.3. Using data from an opthalmology study, used in the context of surrogate marker validation and introduced in Section 2.9, a concept also discussed in Section 21.3, the methods presented will be illustrated.

24.2 A Continuous and a Binary Endpoint

In this section, we start of with the bivariate, non-hierarchical, setting. Extensions to the fully hierarchical case are the topic of Section 24.

Two modeling strategies can be considered to accommodate mixed binary–continuous endpoints. Indeed, the joint distribution of a mixed continuous–discrete outcome vector can always be expressed as the product of the marginal distribution of one of the responses and the conditional distribution of the remaining response given the former response. One can choose either the continuous or the discrete outcome for the marginal model. The main problem with such approaches is that no easy expressions for the association between both endpoints are obtained. Therefore, we opt for a more symmetric treatment of the two outcome variables. We treat the case where the surrogate is binary and the true endpoint is continuous. The reverse case is entirely similar.

Let $\widetilde{S}_i$ be a latent variable of which S_i is the dichotomized version. In Section 24.2.1 we will describe a bivariate normal model for $\widetilde{S}_i$ and T_i, resulting in a probit-linear model for S_i and T_i. Section 24.2.2 presents an alternative formulation based on the bivariate Plackett (1965) density and resulting in a Plackett-Dale model.

24.2.1 A Probit-normal Formulation

In this formulation, we assume the following model:

$$T_i = \mu_T + \beta X_i + \varepsilon_{Ti}, \qquad (24.1)$$
$$\widetilde{S}_i = \mu_S + \alpha X_i + \varepsilon_{Si}, \qquad (24.2)$$

where μ_S and μ_T are fixed intercepts and α and β are the fixed effects of the treatment X on the surrogate and true endpoints respectively. Further,

ε_{Si} and ε_{Ti} are correlated error terms, assumed to satisfy:

$$\begin{pmatrix} \varepsilon_{Ti} \\ \varepsilon_{Si} \end{pmatrix} \sim N\left[\begin{pmatrix} 0 \\ 0 \end{pmatrix}, \begin{pmatrix} \sigma^2 & \frac{\rho\sigma}{\sqrt{1-\rho^2}} \\ & \frac{1}{1-\rho^2} \end{pmatrix}\right]. \qquad (24.3)$$

Model (24.1)–(24.2) specifies a bivariate normal density. The variance of $\widetilde{S}_i$ is chosen for reasons that will be made clear in what follows. From this model, it is easily seen that the density of T_i is univariate normal with regression given in (24.1) and variance σ^2, implying that the parameters μ_T, β, and σ^2 can be estimated using linear regression software with response T_i and single covariate Z_i. Similarly, the conditional density of $\widetilde{S}_i$, given X_i and T_i is

$$\widetilde{S}_i \sim N\left[\left(\mu_S - \frac{\rho}{\sigma\sqrt{1-\rho^2}}\mu_T\right) + \left(\alpha - \frac{\rho}{\sigma\sqrt{1-\rho^2}}\beta\right)X_i \right.$$
$$\left. + \frac{\rho}{\sigma\sqrt{1-\rho^2}}T_i; 1\right], \qquad (24.4)$$

having unit variance and thus motivating our earlier choice for the covariance matrix of T_i and $\widetilde{S}_i$. Note that in Chapters 21 and 22 the marginal variances were set equal to one. In principle, these choices are equivalent, as long as no additional variance parameter for the latent variables is introduced. The corresponding probability

$$P(S_i = 1|T_i, X_i) = \Phi_1(\lambda_0 + \lambda_X X_i + \lambda_T T_i), \qquad (24.5)$$

where

$$\lambda_0 = \mu_S - \frac{\rho}{\sigma\sqrt{1-\rho^2}}\mu_T, \qquad (24.6)$$

$$\lambda_X = \alpha - \frac{\rho}{\sigma\sqrt{1-\rho^2}}\beta, \qquad (24.7)$$

$$\lambda_T = \frac{\rho}{\sigma\sqrt{1-\rho^2}}, \qquad (24.8)$$

and Φ_1 is the standard normal cumulative density function. Note that (24.5) implicitly defines the cutoff value for the dichotomized version. The λ parameters can be found by fitting model (24.5) to S_i with covariates X_i and T_i. This can be done with standard logistic regression software if it allows to specify the probit rather than the logit link, such as the LOGISTIC and GENMOD procedures in SAS. Given the parameters from the linear regression on T_i (μ_T, β, and σ^2) and the probit regression on S_i (λ_0, λ_X, and λ_T), the parameters from the linear regression on $\widetilde{S}_i$ can now be obtained from (24.6)–(24.8):

$$\mu_S = \lambda_0 + \lambda_T \mu_T, \tag{24.9}$$
$$\alpha = \lambda_Z + \lambda_X \beta, \tag{24.10}$$
$$\rho^2 = \frac{\lambda_T^2 \sigma^2}{1 + \lambda_T^2 \sigma^2}. \tag{24.11}$$

The asymptotic covariance matrix of the parameters (μ_T, β) can be found from standard linear regression output. The variance of $\widehat{\sigma}^2$ equals $2\sigma^4/N$. The asymptotic covariance of $(\widehat{\lambda}_0, \widehat{\lambda}_X, \widehat{\lambda}_T)$ follows from logistic (probit) regression output. These three statements yield the covariance matrix of the six parameters upon noting that it is block-diagonal. To derive the asymptotic covariance of (μ_S, α, ρ) it suffices to calculate the derivatives of (24.9)–(24.11) with respect to the six original parameters and apply the delta method. They are:

$$\frac{\partial(\mu_S, \alpha, \rho)}{\partial(\mu_T, \beta, \sigma^2, \lambda_0, \lambda_X, \lambda_T)} = \begin{pmatrix} \lambda_T & 0 & 0 & 1 & 0 & \mu_T \\ 0 & \lambda_T & 0 & 0 & 1 & \beta \\ 0 & 0 & h_1 & 0 & 0 & h_2 \end{pmatrix},$$

where

$$h_1 = \frac{1}{2\rho} \frac{\lambda_T^2}{(1 + \lambda_T^2 \sigma^2)^2},$$
$$h_2 = \frac{1}{2\rho} \frac{2\lambda_T \sigma^2}{(1 + \lambda_T^2 \sigma^2)^2}.$$

Molenberghs, Geys, and Buyse (2001) developed a program in GAUSS that performs the joint estimation directly by maximizing the likelihood based on contributions (24.1) and (24.5).

24.2.2 A Plackett-Dale Formulation

Assume that the cumulative distributions of S_i and T_i are given by F_{S_i} and F_{T_i}. The joint cumulative distribution of both these quantities has been studied by Plackett (1965) and is discussed for the bivariate binary and ordinal cases in Section 7.7:

$$F_{T_i, S_i} = \begin{cases} \dfrac{1 + (F_{T_i} + F_{S_i})(\psi_i - 1) - C(F_{T_i}, F_{S_i}, \psi_i)}{2(\psi_i - 1)} & \text{if } \psi_i \neq 1, \\ F_{T_i} F_{S_i} & \text{if } \psi_i = 1, \end{cases}$$

where ψ_i, $C(\cdot)$, F_{T_i}, and F_{S_i} take the roles of ψ, $S(\cdot)$, μ_{1+}, and μ_{+1} in (7.40), respectively.

We can now derive a bivariate Plackett "density" function $G_i(t,s)$ for mixed continuous- binary outcomes. Suppose the success probability for S_i is denoted by π_i, then we can define $G_i(t,s)$ by specifying $G_i(t,0)$ and $G_i(t,1)$ such that they sum to $f_{T_i}(t)$. If we define

$$G_i(t,0) = \frac{\partial F_{T_i,S_i}(t,0)}{\partial t},$$

then this leads to specifying G_i by:

$$G_i(t,0) = \begin{cases} \frac{f_{T_i}(t)}{2}\left(1 - \frac{1+F_{T_i}(t)(\psi_i-1)-F_{S_i}(s)(\psi_i+1)}{C(F_{T_i},1-\pi_i,\psi_i)}\right) & \text{if } \psi_i \neq 1, \\ f_{T_i}(t)(1-\pi_i) & \text{if } \psi_i = 1, \end{cases} \quad (24.12)$$

and

$$G_i(t,1) = f_{T_i}(t) - G_i(t,0). \quad (24.13)$$

In this formulation we assume $T_i \sim N(\mu_i, \sigma^2)$, with $\mu_i = \mu_T + \beta X_i$ and $\text{logit}(\pi_i) = \mu_S + \alpha X_i$ with similar notation as in the probit case. The global odds ratio is assumed to be constant, but this is obviously open to extension. If we write

$$\boldsymbol{\theta}_i = \begin{pmatrix} \mu_i \\ \sigma^2 \\ \pi_i \\ \psi \end{pmatrix} \quad \text{and} \quad \boldsymbol{\eta}_i = \begin{pmatrix} \mu_i \\ \ln(\sigma^2) \\ \text{logit}(\pi_i) \\ \ln(\psi) \end{pmatrix},$$

estimates of the regression parameters $\boldsymbol{\nu} = (\boldsymbol{\mu}, \boldsymbol{\beta}, \boldsymbol{\alpha}, \ln\sigma^2, \ln\psi)$ are easily obtained by solving the estimating equations $\boldsymbol{U}(\boldsymbol{\nu}) = \boldsymbol{0}$, using a Newton-Raphson iteration scheme, where $\boldsymbol{U}(\boldsymbol{\nu})$ is given by:

$$\sum_{i=1}^{n} \left(\frac{\partial \boldsymbol{\eta}_i}{\partial \boldsymbol{\nu}}\right)' \left\{\left(\frac{\partial \boldsymbol{\eta}_i}{\partial \boldsymbol{\theta}_i}\right)'\right\}^{-1} \left(\frac{\partial}{\partial \boldsymbol{\theta}_i} \ln G_i(t_i, s_i)\right).$$

24.2.3 A Generalized Linear Mixed Model Formulation

The developments in Section 8.8, where a linearization based marginal model has been presented, and in Chapter 14, where generalized linear mixed models have been introduced, can now be adapted to the present setting as well. In fact, it is useful to start from the formulation in Section 22.4, where both random effects and serial correlation have been allowed for. Expression (22.9) provides a general formulation, and (22.10) is specific for a random-effects logistic regression for repeated measures with serial, or residual, correlation. It is straightforward to consider this framework in situations where various outcomes of a different nature are observed. In general, we merely have to write, as before,

$$Y_i = \mu_i + \varepsilon_i, \qquad (24.14)$$

where

$$\mu_i = \mu_i(\eta_i) = h(X_i\beta + Z_i b_i). \qquad (24.15)$$

As usual, we assume $b_i \sim N(0, D)$. The key relaxing assumption is that the components of the inverse link functions h are allowed to change with the nature of the various outcomes in Y_i. The variance of ε_i depends on the mean-variance links of the various outcomes, and can contain, in addition, a correlation matrix $R_i(\alpha)$ and overdispersion parameters ϕ_i. When there are no random effects in (24.15) a marginal model is obtained, as in Section 8.8. We will refer to this as a *marginal generalized linear models* (MGLM) approach. Reversely, assuming there are no residual correlations in $R_i(\alpha)$, a conditional independence model or purely random effects model results, which is still denoted by GLMM.

Using straightforward derivations, a general first-order approximate expression for the variance-covariance matrix of Y_i is:

$$V_i = \text{Var}(Y_i) \simeq \Delta_i Z_i D Z_i' \Delta_i' + \Sigma_i. \qquad (24.16)$$

Here,

$$\Delta_i = \left.\left(\frac{\partial \mu_i}{\partial \eta_i}\right)\right|_{b_i=0},$$

and

$$\Sigma_i \simeq \Xi_i^{1/2} A_i^{1/2} R_i(\alpha) A_i^{1/2} \Xi_i^{1/2},$$

with A_i a diagonal matrix containing the variances following from the generalized linear model specification of Y_{ij} given the random effects $b_i = 0$, i.e., with diagonal elements $v(\mu_{ij}|b_i = 0)$. Likewise Ξ_i is a diagonal matrix with the overdispersion parameters along the diagonal. When an outcome component is normally distributed, the overdispersion parameter is σ_i^2 and the variance function is 1. For a binary outcome with logit link, we obtain

$$\mu_{ij}(b_i = 0)[1 - \mu_{ij}(b_i = 0)].$$

The evaluation under $b_i = 0$ derives from a Taylor series expansion of the mean components around $b_i = 0$.

When an exponential family specification is used for all components, with canonical link, $\Delta_i = A_i$ and we can write:

$$V_i = \text{Var}(Y_i) \simeq \Delta_i Z_i D Z_i' \Delta_i' + \Xi_i^{1/2} \Delta_i^{1/2} R_i(\alpha) \Delta_i^{1/2} \Xi_i^{1/2}. \qquad (24.17)$$

Under conditional independence R_i vanishes and

$$V_i = \text{Var}(Y_i) = \Delta_i Z_i D Z_i' \Delta_i' + \Xi_i^{1/2} \Delta_i \Xi_i^{1/2}. \qquad (24.18)$$

For the setting already considered in Sections 24.2.1 and 24.2.2, a suitable version of (24.14) is:

$$\begin{pmatrix} S_i \\ T_i \end{pmatrix} = \begin{pmatrix} \mu_S + \lambda b_i + \alpha X_i \\ \dfrac{\exp[\mu_T + b_i + \beta X_i]}{1 + \exp[\mu_T + b_i + \beta X_i]} \end{pmatrix} + \begin{pmatrix} \varepsilon_{Si} \\ \varepsilon_{Ti} \end{pmatrix}. \qquad (24.19)$$

Note that we have included a scale parameter λ in the continuous component of an otherwise random-intercept model, given the continuous and binary outcome are measured on different scales. In this case,

$$Z_i = \begin{pmatrix} \lambda \\ 1 \end{pmatrix}, \qquad \Delta_i = \begin{pmatrix} 1 & 0 \\ 0 & v_{i2} \end{pmatrix}, \qquad \Phi = \begin{pmatrix} \sigma^2 & 0 \\ 0 & 1 \end{pmatrix},$$

with $v_{i2} = \mu_{i2}(\boldsymbol{b}_i = \boldsymbol{0})[1 - \mu_{i2}(\boldsymbol{b}_i = \boldsymbol{0})]$. Further, let ρ be the correlation between ε_{Si} and ε_{Ti}. Note that Z_i is not a design matrix in the strict sense, since it contains an unknown parameter. Nevertheless, it is useful to consider this decomposition.

This implies that (24.16) becomes

$$\begin{aligned} V_i &= \begin{pmatrix} \lambda^2 & v_{i2}\lambda \\ v_{i2}\lambda & v_{i2}^2 \end{pmatrix} \tau^2 + \begin{pmatrix} \sigma^2 & \rho\sigma\sqrt{v_{i2}} \\ \rho\sigma\sqrt{v_{i2}} & v_{i2} \end{pmatrix} \\ &= \begin{pmatrix} \lambda^2\tau^2 + \sigma^2 & v_{i2}\lambda\tau^2 + \rho\sigma\sqrt{v_{i2}} \\ v_{i2}\lambda\tau^2 + \rho\sigma\sqrt{v_{i2}} & v_{i2}^2\tau^2 + v_{i2} \end{pmatrix}. \end{aligned} \qquad (24.20)$$

The approximate marginal correlation function derived thereof equals:

$$\rho(\boldsymbol{\beta}) = \frac{v_{i2}\lambda\tau^2 + \rho\sigma\sqrt{v_{i2}}}{\sqrt{\lambda^2\tau^2 + \sigma^2}\sqrt{v_{i2}^2\tau^2 + v_{i2}}}. \qquad (24.21)$$

Obviously, (24.21) depends on the fixed effects through v_{i2}. In the special case of no random effects, the model can be written as:

$$\begin{pmatrix} S_i \\ T_i \end{pmatrix} = \begin{pmatrix} \mu_S + \alpha X_i \\ \dfrac{\exp(\mu_T + \beta X_i)}{1 + \exp(\mu_T + \beta X_i)} \end{pmatrix} + \begin{pmatrix} \varepsilon_{Si} \\ \varepsilon_{Ti} \end{pmatrix}, \qquad (24.22)$$

and (24.21) simply reduces to ρ, by virtue of its fully marginal specification. Under conditional independence, ρ in (24.20) satisfies $\rho \equiv 0$ and (24.21) reduces to

$$\rho(\boldsymbol{\beta}) = \frac{v_{i2}\lambda\tau^2}{\sqrt{\lambda^2\tau^2 + \sigma^2}\sqrt{v_{i2}^2\tau^2 + v_{i2}}}, \qquad (24.23)$$

somewhat simpler but still a function of the fixed effects.

In case both endpoints are binary, the counterpart to (24.21) is

$$\rho(\boldsymbol{\beta}) = \frac{v_{i1}v_{i2}\tau^2 + \rho\sigma\sqrt{v_{i1}v_{i2}}}{\sqrt{v_{i1}^2\tau^2 + v_{i1}}\sqrt{v_{i2}^2\tau^2 + v_{i2}}}, \qquad (24.24)$$

with again a constant correlation ρ when there are no random effects and, when there is no residual correlation:

$$\rho(\boldsymbol{\beta}) = \frac{v_{i1}v_{i2}\tau^2}{\sqrt{v_{i1}^2\tau^2 + v_{i1}}\sqrt{v_{i2}^2\tau^2 + v_{i2}}}, \qquad (24.25)$$

Of course, the above calculations can be performed with ease for general random effects design matrices Z_i and for more than two components, of arbitrary nature and not just continuous and binary. This is useful, for example, for a fully hierarchical specification such as in Section 24.3.

In the general model, no full joint distribution needs to be specified, even when we assume the first one to be normally distributed, and the second one to be Bernoulli distributed. We still can leave the specification of the joint moments to the second one, by way of the marginal correlation. A full joint specification would need full bivariate model specification, conditional upon the random effects.

Under conditional independence, the specification of the outcome distributions conditional upon the random effects, together with the normality assumptions made about the random effects, fully specifies the joint distribution.

24.3 Hierarchical Joint Models

In the previous section, bivariate models have been discussed for the joint analysis of a continuous and a binary outcome. The focus was placed on a probit-normal and a Plackett-Dale formulation, next to the generalized linear mixed model framework, which can be used to flexibly derive marginal as well as random-effects models. Of course, joint outcomes can be measured repeatedly over time, or might be observed within a hierarchical context. In Section 24.3.1, a two-stage approach is presented, whereas Section 24.3.2 discusses fully hierarchical models.

24.3.1 Two-stage Analysis

In this section, we retain the setting of a binary and a continuous endpoint, measured within a hierarchical setting. Molenberghs, Geys, and Buyse (2001) used this approach in the context of surrogate marker evaluation. Let $\widetilde{S}_{ij}$ be a latent variable of which S_{ij} is a dichotomized version. One option is to consider a two-step analysis. Assume that subject j is measured within trial i. For repeated measures, j would refer to time and i to subject.

At the first step, we can assume the following model:

$$\widetilde{S}_{ij} = \mu_{S_i} + \alpha_i X_{ij} + \varepsilon_{S_{ij}},$$
$$T_{ij} = \mu_{T_i} + \beta_i X_{ij} + \varepsilon_{T_{ij}},$$

where α_i and β_i are study-specific effects of treatment X on the endpoints in trial i, μ_{S_i} and μ_{T_i} are trial-specific intercepts, and ε_{S_i} and ε_{T_i} are correlated error terms, assumed to be mean-zero normally distributed with covariance matrix

$$\Sigma = \begin{pmatrix} \frac{1}{(1-\rho^2)} & \frac{\rho\sigma}{\sqrt{1-\rho^2}} \\ \frac{\rho\sigma}{\sqrt{1-\rho^2}} & \sigma^2 \end{pmatrix}.$$

In short, we use the probit formulation, described in Section 24.2.1. Due to the replication at the study level, we can impose a distribution on the study-specific parameters. At the second stage we assume

$$\begin{pmatrix} \mu_{S_i} \\ \mu_{T_i} \\ \alpha_i \\ \beta_i \end{pmatrix} = \begin{pmatrix} \mu_S \\ \mu_T \\ \alpha \\ \beta \end{pmatrix} + \begin{pmatrix} m_{S_i} \\ m_{T_i} \\ a_i \\ b_i \end{pmatrix} \quad (24.26)$$

where the second term on the right hand side of (24.26) is assumed to follow a zero-mean normal distribution with dispersion matrix D.

24.3.2 Fully Hierarchical Modeling

We first indicate how the probit-normal and Plackett-Dale models can be generalized to the hierarchical setting. Ample detail can be found in Geys et al (2001) and Regan and Catalano (2002). Next, the generalized linear mixed model case will be considered.

24.3.2.1 A Probit-normal Formulation

The model of Section 24.2.1 can be seen as the basis for this model. Whereas Model (24.1)–(24.2) applies to one continuous and one binary outcome, we could equally well consider multiple copies of each and then assume that the resulting stochastic vector, composed of directly observed and latent outcomes, is normally distributed.

Although this approach is natural and appealing, the problem is the handling of potentially high dimensional probits, and several authors have considered this problem in detail. Regan and Catalano (1999a) introduced a mixed-outcome probit model that extends a correlated probit model for binary outcomes (Ochi and Prentice 1984) to incorporate continuous outcomes. These authors consider exchangeability among the continuous outcomes, among the binary outcomes, and between the continuous and binary outcomes.

Regan and Catalano (1999b) avoided fully specifying the joint distribution of the n_i bivariate outcomes on related subjects within unit i by specifying only the marginal distribution of the bivariate outcomes and applying generalized estimating equations to take correlation into account. Precisely, they fully model the bivariate outcomes for a subject and then apply GEE to accommodate for the correlations between subjects within unit i.

24.3.2.2 A Plackett-Dale Approach

Likewise, the Plackett-Dale model of Section 24.2.2 can be embedded in a hierarchical setting. Geys *et al* (2001) applied marginal pseudo-likelihood ideas (Chapter 9)

In Section 24.2.2, a bivariate density-distribution was defined for a joint continuous and binary outcome, by means of (24.12)–(24.13). In principle, a $2n_i$-dimensional Plackett-Dale model needs to be specified. Alternatively, progress can be made by solely specifying the bivariate outcomes, just as before, and assembling them into a (log) pseudo-likelihood function:

$$p\ell = \sum_{i=1}^{N} \sum_{j=1}^{n_i} \ln G_{ij}(t_{ij}, s_{ij}), \qquad (24.27)$$

where T_{ij} is the continuous outcomes for subject j within unit (study, trial, center,...) i and S_{ij} is the binary one. Thus, with this particular choice of pseudo-likelihood function, the longitudinal part of the correlation structure is left unspecified. Of course, alternative pseudo-likelihood functions can be used as well, depending on which parameters are needed to formulate answers to scientific questions. Sometimes, the correlation structure between outcomes on different subjects within the same unit can be of interest, calling for other types of pseudo-likelihood function. Parameter and precision estimation based on (24.27) is straightforward, given the developments in Chapter 9, in particular Section 9.4.

24.3.2.3 A Generalized Linear Mixed Model Formulation

The developments in Section 24.2.3 extend straightforwardly to the hierarchical case, including repeated measures, meta-analyses, clustered data, correlated data, etc. In fact, Model (24.14) is sufficiently general to generate marginal and random-effects models for such settings. The fixed and random effects structures can be formulated sufficiently generally so as to cover all of these settings. Of course, when parameters are shared between models for outcomes of different types, care has to be taken to ensure the models are meaningful. For example, inflation factors might have to be used to share random effects across binary and continuous outcomes, exactly as the parameter λ in (24.19).

Correlations follow in a straightforward fashion when purely marginal versions are used. When random effects are involved, correlation structures can be derived from (24.16) or specific forms derived thereof.

24.4 Age Related Macular Degeneration Trial

In the Age Related Macular Degeneration Study, introduced in Section 2.9, the mixed discrete-continuous case is encountered in data from a simple yet real situation. Indeed, visual acuity is assessed in terms of number of letters read, which can be treated as continuous. The dichotomization in terms of at least 2 or 3 lines of vision lost at 6 and 12 months, respectively, is a binary outcome.

In Section 24.4.1, a number of bivariate marginal analyses are presented, with bivariate random-effects analyses discussed in Section 24.4.2. Hierarchical analyses, based on including center as a hierarchy defining variable on the one hand, and repeated measures on each of the binary and continuous outcomes on the other hand, are presented in Section 24.4.3.

24.4.1 Bivariate Marginal Analyses

First, we consider dichotomized visual acuity at 6 months as the surrogate and (continuous) visual acuity at 12 months as the true endpoint. Dichotomization is achieved by setting a binary variable to 1 if visual acuity at 6 months is larger than the value at baseline and to 0 otherwise. We consider a probit-normal model as in Section 24.2.1, a Plackett-Dale model as in Section 24.2.2, and a GLM-based marginal model as in Section 24.2.3. Of course, the roles of S_i and T_i are reversed in the corresponding equations, as here the surrogate is assumed binary while the true outcome was binary in the earlier sections. For the latter model, both a logit as well as a probit link is considered for the MGLM. PQL is used as approximation method. For the Plackett-Dale model, a logit link is employed for the true endpoint. Parameter estimates (standard errors) are displayed in Table 24.1.

The correlation between both endpoints is estimated as $\widehat{\rho} = 0.74$ under the probit model. This parameter is of direct interest in surrogate marker evaluation since it captures the so-called adjusted association (Buyse and Molenberghs 1998) or individual-level association (Buyse et al 2000, Molenberghs, Geys, and Buyse 2001). It also justifies the use of a joint model for both endpoints, rather than considering them separately. This parameter is estimated very precisely and there is apparently a strong correlation between both endpoints. Now, the corresponding correlation under the GLM

TABLE 24.1. *Age Related Macular Degeneration Trial. Bivariate marginal analyses with a binary surrogate and a continuous true endpoint.*

Effect	Par.	probit-normal	Plackett-Dale	MGLM logit	MGLM probit
\multicolumn{6}{c}{Binary surrogate endpoint}					
Intercept	μ_S	0.64(0.20)	0.74(0.19)	1.25(0.24)	0.76(0.14)
Treatm. eff.	α	0.39(0.28)	0.45(0.30)	0.40(0.38)	0.23(0.21)
Overdis. par.	ϕ			1.01(0.10)	1.01(0.10)
\multicolumn{6}{c}{Continuous true endpoint}					
Intercept	μ_T	11.04(1.57)	10.89(1.56)	11.04(1.58)	11.04(1.58)
Treatm. eff.	β	4.12(2.32)	4.02(2.32)	4.12(2.33)	4.12(2.33)
Standard dev.	σ_T	15.95(0.82)	16.04(0.81)		
Variance	σ_T^2	254.4(26.2)	257.3(26.0)	257.0(26.5)	257.0(26.5)
\multicolumn{6}{c}{Association}					
Correlation	ρ	0.74(0.05)		0.62(0.05)	0.62(0.05)
Log odds r.	$\ln \psi$		2.85(0.37)		
Odds r.	ψ		17.29(6.40)		

is quite a bit lower. Although, due to the use of PQL, there typically is downward bias in the parameter estimates, a more important reason for the difference is that the probit model features the correlation between a pair of *latent* variables, whereas the GLM captures the correlation between the observable outcomes. The Plackett-Dale model, of course, is based on the use of the odds ratio rather than the correlation as association parameter. For the binary endpoint, the treatment effect parameters differ somewhat, with the differences in the intercepts a bit larger. The parameter estimates for the continuous endpoint agree much closer.

Let us now switch to the situation of continuous visual acuity at 6 months as a surrogate for the binary indicator for loss of at least 3 lines of vision lost at one year. The same models as in Table 24.1 are considered here too, with of course the roles of the continuous and binary endpoints reversed. Parameter estimates (standard errors) are given in Table 24.2. Qualitative conclusions agree very closely with their counterparts for the earlier analyses, although there are some quantitative differences. With the probit model, the correlation is $\widehat{\rho} = 0.81$, but again, for the GLM-based models they are quite a bit smaller, underscoring once more that the two correlation parameters are not really directly comparable, as the probit (and also Dale) versions are describing the correlation of the underlying bivariate latent variable. With the Plackett-Dale model, the odds ratio is estimated to be $\widehat{\psi} = 16.93$. As in Table 24.1, parameter estimates across models agree

TABLE 24.2. *Age Related Macular Degeneration Trial. Bivariate marginal analyses with a continuous surrogate and a binary true endpoint.*

Effect	Par.	Probit-normal	Plackett-Dale	MGLM logit	MGLM probit
		Continuous surrogate endpoint			
Intercept	μ_S	5.53(1.26)	5.89(1.24)	5.53(1.27)	5.53(1.27)
Treatm. eff.	α	2.83(1.87)	2.72(1.84)	2.83(1.87)	2.83(1.87)
Standard dev.	σ_S	12.80(0.66)	12.90(0.65)		
Variance	σ_S^2	163.8(16.9)	166.4(16.8)	165.7(17.1)	165.7(17.1)
		Binary true endpoint			
Intercept	μ_T	-0.36(0.21)	-0.36(0.19)	-0.50(0.20)	-0.31(0.13)
Treatm. eff.	β	0.60(0.30)	0.58(0.28)	0.66(0.30)	0.41(0.19)
Overdis. par.	ϕ			1.01(0.10)	1.01(0.10)
		Association			
Correlation	ρ	0.81(0.04)		0.62(0.04)	0.62(0.04)
Log odds r.	$\ln \psi$		2.83(0.29)		
Odds r.	ψ		16.93(4.91)		

fairly closely, but the agreement is better for the continuous endpoint than for the binary one.

Of course, one could also analyze both endpoints as binary, or both endpoints as continuous. Although not the theme of the chapter, it is useful to do so for the sake of comparison. In the first case, a standard probit or Dale model (Chapter 7) could be used. In the second case, a bivariate normal is the obvious choice. Let us first focus on the situation of two binary outcomes. Buyse and Molenberghs (1998) analyzed both binary endpoints using the Dale model with logit links and obtained an odds ratio of $\widehat{\psi} = 18.53$. Table 24.3 presents five different analyses of the pair of binary outcomes. First, the Dale model is fitted with both logit and probit links. Second, a marginal linearization based model with correlated error terms (Section 8.8 is considered, again with logit and probit links. Third, a bivariate probit model is fitted. Table 24.3 organizes the models by link functions, so that similarities and differences between parameter estimates become more apparent.

Even more so than in the heterogenous outcome cases, there is close agreement between the intercept and treatment effect parameter estimates for the logit and probit models, respectively. At the same time, there is agreement between the association measures as far as they are comparable, but once again the probit based correlation is quite a bit higher than the GLM-based correlation, for reasons explained above.

TABLE 24.3. *Age Related Macular Degeneration Trial. Bivariate marginal analyses with binary endpoints, based on the Dale model (probit and logit links), the bivariate probit model, and a marginal joint GLM (logit and probit links).*

		Logit links	
Effect	Parameter	Dale	MGLM
Surrogate endpoint			
Intercept	μ_S	-0.54(0.20)	-0.54(0.21)
Treatm. eff.	α	0.70(0.30)	0.70(0.30)
Overdis. par.	ϕ		1.01(0.10)
True endpoint			
Intercept	μ_T	-0.50(0.20)	-0.50(0.20)
Treatm. eff.	β	0.66(0.30)	0.66(0.30)
Overdis. par.	ϕ		1.01(0.10)
Association			
Correlation	ρ		0.62(0.05)
Log odds r.	$\ln\psi$	2.92(0.38)	
Odds r.	ψ	18.54(7.05)	

		Probit links		
Effect	Parameter	biv. probit	Dale	MGLM
Surrogate endpoint				
Intercept	μ_S	-0.34(0.13)	-0.33(0.13)	-0.33(0.13)
Treatm. eff.	α	0.44(0.18)	0.44(0.18)	0.44(0.19)
Overdis. par.	ϕ			1.01(0.10)
True endpoint				
Intercept	μ_T	-0.31(0.13)	-0.31(0.13)	-0.31(0.13)
Treatm. eff.	β	0.41(0.18)	0.41(0.18)	0.41(0.19)
Overdis. par.	ϕ			1.01(0.10)
Association				
Correlation	ρ	0.83(0.05)		0.62(0.05)
Log odds r.	$\ln\psi$		2.92(0.38)	
Odds r.	ψ		18.54(7.05)	

Finally, both outcomes can be considered continuous. Then, the counterparts of all models in Tables 24.1–24.3 collapse to a bivariate normal model, and so does the output obtained from virtually all relevant software tools, such as the SAS procedures MIXED, NLMIXED, and GLIMMIX. Results are presented in Table 24.4. The correlation obtained here is 0.75. Note that this is closer to the bivariate probit and probit-normal models than to the GLM one. Indeed, we now have a bivariate continuous outcome, which

TABLE 24.4. *Age Related Macular Degeneration Trial. Bivariate marginal analyses with continuous endpoints, using a bivariate normal model.*

Effect	Par.	Estimate (s.e.)
Surrogate endpoint		
Intercept	μ_S	5.53(1.27)
Treatm. eff.	α	2.83(1.87)
Standard dev.	σ_S	12.87(0.66)
Variance	σ_S^2	165.7(17.1)
True endpoint		
Intercept	μ_T	11.04(1.58)
Treatm. eff.	β	4.12(2.33)
Standard dev.	σ_T	16.03(0.83)
Variance	σ_T^2	257.0(26.5)
Association		
Correlation	ρ	0.75(0.03)

is more informative than a pair of binary outcomes or the joint occurrence of a binary and a continuous outcome. Nevertheless, in all situations do the probit and probit-normal models attempt to describe the association of the underlying pair of normal outcomes, whether or not they are directly observed.

Generally note that, when continuous or binary outcome results are compared across Tables 24.1–24.4, whether from a heterogeneous or homogenous model, there is reasonably close agreement, especially within a model family (probit-normal, Plackett-Dale, GLM based), and especially for treatment effects and association parameters.

24.4.2 Bivariate Random-effects Analyses

Although all models above are of a marginal type, we can also consider random-effects models. So far, we have considered marginal versions of (24.14), denoted by MGLM, but we will now switch to conditional independence model (24.19) with a scaled random intercept, for the case of a binary and a continuous outcome, a classical random-intercepts logistic regression model when both outcomes are binary, and a random-intercept linear mixed-effects model for continuous outcomes. Results are presented in Table 24.5.

Comparing the continuous-binary case with the results in Table 24.2, it is clear that fixed effects in the Gaussian model roughly remain the same, but the fixed effects for the binary outcome are larger, in agreement with the results in Chapter 16. A similar inflation is seen in the binary-binary case, at least when numerical integration is used. For PQL, the bias is severe and the parameter estimates are hardly larger than their marginal counterparts in Table 24.3. Given the estimate of the random-intercept variance ($\hat{\tau}^2 = 14.51$) and (16.3), the correspondence between the random-effects parameters and their marginal counterparts in Table 24.3 would be 2.45. Comparing the corresponding estimates yields factors of roughly 2.62. In line with general results about the linear mixed model (Chapter 4), the estimates in the last column are very close to those in Table 24.4, even though the assumption of a constant variance, made here, may be somewhat too simplistic, given the variances in Table 24.4 are quite a bit different.

As before, the correlation between both endpoints is of interest. With the exception of the continuous-continuous case, it is somewhat less straightforward to derive. For the continuous-binary case, we can make use of (24.23) and for the binary-binary case, (24.24) is the proper choice. Clearly, the correlation is different between both treatment arms now, given the dependence of the correlation function on the fixed effects. However, in this case, the difference is negligible. However, the poverty of the PQL approximation is shown, not only in the fixed effect and variance component estimates, but in the correlation parameters as well. For the others, irrespective on the nature of the outcomes, the results are very close to their marginal counterparts in Tables 24.1–24.4, which is reassuring.

It is worthwhile to note that the parameters in the continuous-binary case are identifiable, but due to the non-linearity of the model, induced by the factor λ, care has to be taken in monitoring the convergence process. Having said this, the effect is most clearly seen on the binary outcome fixed effects, and not quite as much on the continuous outcome parameters.

24.4.3 Hierarchical Analyses

Let us now switch attention to the hierarchical case. First, let us observe that the trial is of the multicenter type. It is natural to consider the center in which the patients were treated as the unit of analysis. A total of 36 centers were thus available for analysis, with a number of individual patients per center ranging from 2 to 18. We analyze the situation where dichotomized visual acuity at 6 months acts as surrogate for the continuous visual acuity at 12 months. A two-stage approach is followed. Table 24.6 shows the parameter estimates for the hierarchical probit model (Section 24.3.1). Two versions are considered, with trial-specific treatment effects on the one hand (reduced model) and with trial-specific intercepts and treatment effects on the other hand (full model). The correlation, obtained from the full model, is similar to the ones obtained from the bivariate analyses. When the reduced model is employed, the correlation is quite a bit smaller.

Of course, also fully hierarchical models can be fitted. For example, the hierarchical probit or Plackett-Dale models can be used. Applications of these models can be found in Regan and Catalano (2002). Also the joint

TABLE 24.5. *Age Related Macular Degeneration Trial. Bivariate joint generalized linear mixed model analyses. Some models lead to a treatment-arm dependent correlation estimate, denoted by 'stand' for the standard arm and 'exp' for the experimental arm.*

Surrogate endpoint:		cont.	binary	binary	cont.
True endpoint:		binary	binary	binary	cont.
Estimation method:		PQL	Num. int.	PQL	ML
Effect	Par.				
		Surrogate endpoint parameters			
Intercept	μ_S	5.53(1.26)	1.42(0.57)	-0.62(0.26)	5.53(1.42)
Treatm. eff.	α	2.83(1.86)	-1.84(0.82)	0.81(0.39)	2.83(2.11)
Standard dev.	σ_S	7.18(1.15)			
Variance	σ_S^2	51.59(16.55)			
Inflation	λ	-1.41(1.68)			
		True endpoint parameters			
Intercept	μ_T	1.63(1.94)	1.31(0.56)	-0.57(0.26)	11.04(1.42)
Treatm. eff.	β	-2.72(3.15)	-1.73(0.81)	0.76(0.39)	4.12(2.11)
		Common parameters, including association			
R.I. std.d.	τ	7.50(8.50)	3.81(0.69)	1.95(0.47)	12.41(0.76)
R.I. var.	τ^2	56.2(127.4)	14.51(5.28)	3.76(1.82)	154.0(18.8)
Res. st.d.	σ				7.43(0.38)
Res. var.	σ^2				55.1(15.7)
Correlation	ρ				0.74
Corr. (stand.)	$\rho[1]$	0.79	0.78	0.48	
Corr. (exp.)	$\rho[2]$	0.78	0.70	0.46	

generalized linear mixed effects model of Section 24.2.3 can be used for hierarchical analyses. Although we have focused so far on outcomes at 6 months and 1 year, we will now also consider the intermediate endpoints at 4 and 12 weeks as well. Thus, we have two repeated sequences of four components each, one binary, and one continuous. The binary outcomes are dichotomizations of the number of letters lost as negative *versus* non-negative. We consider on the one hand a marginal model, with fully unstructured 8×8 variance-covariance matrix and a conditional independence random-intercepts model on the other hand. Parameter estimates are presented in Table 24.7.

Once more, the relationship between the fixed effects is in line with expectation. For the continuous outcome sequence, they are virtually equal. For the binary outcome, the ratios vary between 1.55 and 1.98, with an average of 1.80, whereas (16.3) predicts a ratio of 1.80. Model parameters here are better identifiable than their counterparts from the bivariate models, even

TABLE 24.6. *Age Related Macular Degeneration Trial. Parameter estimates (standard errors) for the full and reduced two-stage fixed effects probit model.*

Effect	Parameter	Full	Reduced
Surrogate endpoint			
Intercept	μ_S	1.46(0.68)	0.67(0.15)
Treatm. eff.	α	1.10(0.98)	1.75(0.69)
True endpoint			
Intercept	μ_T	11.13(1.69)	11.82(1.00)
Treatm. eff.	β	4.40(2.94)	3.72(2.38)
Standard dev.	σ_T	11.43(0.60)	13.60(0.71)
Variance	σ_T^2	130.6(13.7)	185.0(19.3)
Association			
Correlation	ρ	0.75(0.05)	0.66(0.07)

though care is still needed when selecting starting values. Every possible pair of outcomes in the marginal model has its own correlation coefficient (not shown), whereas in the random-effects model, they follow from the fixed effects and variance components, as was illustrated in Section 24.4.2, based on such expressions as (24.21), (24.23), (24.24), and (24.25).

24.5 Joint Models in SAS

We will present a program and selected output for the joint analysis of a continuous and a binary outcome, by means of the generalized linear mixed model and using the SAS procedure GLIMMIX. To create the bivariate outcome vectors, out of the continuous outcomes measured at 6 months (24 weeks) and 12 months (52 weeks), 'diff24' and 'diff52,' and their binary counterparts 'bindif24' and 'bindif52,' the following code can be used:

```
data armd77;
set armd7;
array x (2) diff24 diff52;
array y (2) bindif24 bindif52;
array z (2) bindh24 diff52;
array w (2) diff24 bindif52;
do j=1 to 2;
   visual=x(j);
   bindif=y(j);
   bincont=z(j);
   contbin=w(j);
   time=j;
```

456   24. Joint Continuous and Discrete Responses

TABLE 24.7. *Age Related Macular Degeneration Trial. Hierarchical models for joint longitudinal continuous and binary visual acuity sequences. For the marginal model-based and empirically corrected standard errors are presented.*

Effect	Parameter	Marginal	Random Int.
Continuous sequence			
Intercept 4	β_{11}	-3.26(0.77;0.81)	-3.27(1.30)
Intercept 12	β_{21}	-4.62(1.14:1.07)	-4.62(1.29)
Intercept 24	β_{31}	-8.37(1.38;1.26)	-8.37(1.29)
Intercept 52	β_{41}	-15.16(1.72;1.64)	-15.16(1.29)
Treatment eff. 4	β_{12}	2.31(1.05;1.05)	2.38(1.76)
Treatment eff. 12	β_{22}	2.34(1.54;1.52)	2.34(1.76)
Treatment eff. 24	β_{32}	2.83(1.87;1.84)	2.83(1.76)
Treatment eff. 52	β_{42}	4.12(2.33;2.31)	4.12(1.76)
Res. st. deviation	σ		8.21(0.23)
Res. variance	σ^2		67.45(3.81)
Inflation	λ		-3.32(0.34)
Binary sequence			
Intercept 4	β_{11}	-1.02(0.24;0.24)	-2.02(0.46)
Intercept 12	β_{21}	-0.91(0.24;0.24)	-1.81(0.45)
Intercept 24	β_{31}	-1.15(0.25;0.25)	-2.24(0.47)
Intercept 52	β_{41}	-1.65(0.29;0.29)	-3.11(0.52)
Treatment eff. 4	β_{12}	0.40(0.32;0.32)	0.66(0.59)
Treatment eff. 12	β_{22}	0.54(0.31:0.31)	0.93(0.58)
Treatment eff. 24	β_{32}	0.52(0.33;0.32)	0.88(0.60)
Treatment eff. 52	β_{42}	0.40(0.38;0.38)	0.62(0.64)
Common parameters			
R.I. st. deviation	τ		2.66(0.29)
R.I. variance	τ^2		7.07(1.64)

```
    subject=_n_;
    output;
end;
run;
```

There are four new outcomes created, consisting of the two continuous outcomes ('visual'), the two binary outcomes ('bindif'), a binary surrogate followed by a continuous true outcome ('bincont'), and finally a continuous surrogate followed by a binary true outcome ('contbin').

Because we cannot uniformly specify the outcome distribution nor the link function, a special device has been created to this effect, i.e., the 'byobs=(·)' specification that can be used in both the 'link=' and the 'dist='

24.5 Joint Models in SAS

options. Practically, a variable needs to be created to specify the outcome distribution and link function for each observation in the set of data. For example, analyzing the ARMD data with a continuous, normally distributed, surrogate and a binary true endpoint, can be done by means of the 'dist=byobs(distcb)' option where 'distcb' is a variable denoting a Gaussian distribution for the first measurement of every subject and a Bernoulli one for the second. The procedure recognizes both a numerical indicator, with a proper map between distributions and numerical labels being provided in the manual (SAS Institute Inc. 2004), as well as a four-character label, by means of the first four characters of each distributions. All but the multinomial distribution can be used. The following code creates to distributional indicators, one for a continuous surrogate and a binary true endpoint ('distcb') and one for the reverse case ('distbc'). In addition, four link function indicators are created, referring to the identity link for the continuous outcome and then either a logit or a probit link for the binary outcome.

Code to create these indicators is

```
data armd77;
set armd77;
distcb='BINA';
if time=1 then distcb='GAUS';
distbc='BINA';
if time=2 then distbc='GAUS';
linkcb1='LOGI';
if time=1 then linkcb1='IDEN';
linkcb2='PROB';
if time=1 then linkcb2='IDEN';
linkbc1='LOGI';
if time=2 then linkbc1='IDEN';
linkbc2='PROB';
if time=2 then linkbc2='IDEN';
run;
```

The relevant variables for analysis, for the first 5 subjects, are

obs	subject	time	treat	visual	bin	cont	dist	distbin	distcont	distbc	distcb	linkcb1	linkcb2	linkbc1	linkbc2
1	1	1	1	0	0	1	0	GAUS	BINA	IDEN	IDEN	LOGI	PROB
2	1	2	1	-10	0	-10	0	BINA	GAUS	LOGI	PROB	IDEN	IDEN

```
 3   2  1  2   -3  0    0  -3  GAUS BINA IDEN IDEN LOGI PROB
 4   2  2  2    1  0    1   0  BINA GAUS LOGI PROB IDEN IDEN

 5   3  1  1   -6  1    1  -6  GAUS BINA IDEN IDEN LOGI PROB
 6   3  2  1  -17  1  -17   1  BINA GAUS LOGI PROB IDEN IDEN

 7   4  1  2    8  0    0   8  GAUS BINA IDEN IDEN LOGI PROB
 8   4  2  2    1  0    1   0  BINA GAUS LOGI PROB IDEN IDEN

 9   5  1  2   -2  0    1  -2  GAUS BINA IDEN IDEN LOGI PROB
10   5  2  2   -2  0   -2   0  BINA GAUS LOGI PROB IDEN IDEN
...
```

The variable 'contbin' is clearly made up of the first component of 'visual' and the second one of 'bindif.' For 'bincont,' a somewhat different definition is used for the surrogate, which is an indicator for whether letters are lost or gained, rather than an indicator for at least two lines lost. This definition was chosen in agreement with the choice made by Molenberghs, Geys, and Buyse (2001).

We can now use the program:

```
proc glimmix data=armd77 method=rspl;
class treat distcb subject;
nloptions maxiter=50 technique=newrap;
model contbin = distcb treat*distcb
              / noint dist=byobs(distcb) solution;
random _residual_ / subject=subject type=un r;
run;
```

Note that there is no link function specification in this program, implying that the default link is used. Equivalently, one could specify the option 'link=byobs(linkcb1),' which would produce exactly the same model. However, the advantage then is that the link functions chosen become very explicit. Changing the link variable to 'link=byobs(linkcb2),' the probit link would be chosen for the binary variable, while maintaining the identity link for the continuous variable. The variable 'distcb' is also used in the fixed-effects structure, through the MODEL statements. This means that a separate intercept (μ_S and μ_T, respectively) and a separate treatment effect (α and β, respectively) are included for each of the two outcomes. This could be done equally well by using the variable 'time' as a class variable, since both 'time' and 'distcb,' and in fact also the link function variables, contain the same information when used as class variable. The choice for 'distcb' is motivated by clarity of the output, where it will be made clear which parameters belong to the Gaussian outcome and which to the binary one.

Given that the outcomes are of a different nature, this is a very natural choice. By including 'noint' into the MODEL statement options, both intercepts are directly shown, rather than as a main effect and a difference between both, which would be less meaningful. The NLOPTIONS statement is included to control convergence. In examples like this, in agreement with the comments made in Section 22.6, convergence can be an issue and the user may need to change such aspects as the iterative technique, the maximum number of iterations, and the convergence tolerance.

Because the response and link functions depend on the outcome, the 'Model Information' panel does not specify them individually but rather gives a generic indication:

Model Information

Response Distribution	Multivariate
Link Function	Multiple
Variance Function	Default

Let us now turn to the estimates of the covariance parameters.

Covariance Parameter Estimates

Cov Parm	Subject	Estimate	Standard Error
UN(1,1)	subject	165.69	17.0897
UN(2,1)	subject	8.0235	1.1105
UN(2,2)	subject	1.0106	0.1042

The parameter 'UN(1,1)' is the variance of the Gaussian outcome, the parameter 'UN(2,2)' is the variance of the binary outcome and as such merely is an overdispersion parameter. Finally, 'UN(2,1)' is the covariance between both. In our example, the correlation is of interest more than the covariance. Because it can be calculated without problem from the three parameters, and the standard error could be calculated from the asymptotic covariance matrix of the variance parameters, it is actually easy to obtain it directly, but changing the structure option for the covariance matrix in the RANDOM statement to 'type=unr' rather than the 'type=un' structure used above. Obviously, both parameterizations are equivalent. The above panel then changes to:

Covariance Parameter Estimates

Cov Parm	Subject	Estimate	Standard Error
Corr(2,1)	subject	165.69	17.0897
Corr(3,1)	subject	1.0106	0.1042
Corr(3,2)	subject	0.6200	0.04489

Of course, the two variance parameters are the same as above, but the correlation estimate $\widehat{\rho} = 0.62$ is now presented directly. Two observations are worth making. First, the order of the parameters in both panels is different and, somewhat misleading, the double indices have changed from the intuitive (1,1), (2,1), and (2,2) coding to (2,1), (3,1), and (3,2). These would correspond to correlations in a 3×3 correlation matrix, but not to the situation we encounter. So we advise to be careful with these labels and cautiously map the 'type=unr' parameters to their counterparts coming from the 'type=un' structure, to avoid confusion.

Finally, the fixed effects parameters, presenting the two intercepts μ_T and μ_S, and treatment effects and β and α are presented.

Solutions for Fixed Effects

Effect	distcb	treat	Estimate	Standard Error	DF
distcb	BINA		0.4953	0.2042	186
distcb	GAUS		-5.5340	1.2683	186
treat*distcb	BINA	1	-0.6566	0.2974	186
treat*distcb	GAUS	1	-2.8338	1.8743	186
treat*distcb	BINA	2	0	.	.
treat*distcb	GAUS	2	0	.	.

While in the bivariate vector of outcomes per subject the Gaussian outcome measured at six months, preceded the binary outcomes measured at one year, here the binary parameters preceed their Gaussian counterparts. This is merely because the levels in the 'distcb' variable are ordered alphabetically. So again, some care is needed.

Let us now switch to the random-effects models. Focusing on fitting model (24.19) to the ARMD data, the non-linear parameter λ prohibits the use of the GLIMMIX procedure, whence the procedure NLMIXED can be used. It is instructive to first focus on the case of two continuous outcome. In this case, the following three programs produce exactly the same model fit:

/*First program*/

```
proc mixed data=armd77 method=ml;
class treat time subject;
model visual = time treat*time
      / noint solution ddfm=satterthwaite;
random intercept
        / subject=subject type=un g v vcorr;
run;
```

24.5 Joint Models in SAS

```
/* Second program */

proc nlmixed data=armd77 qpoints=20 maxiter=50;
if time=1 then  eta = beta11 + b + beta12*(2-treat);
else if time=2 then eta = beta21 + b + beta22*(2-treat);
model visual ~ normal(eta,sigma*sigma);
random b ~ normal(0,tau*tau) subject=subject;
estimate 'tau^2' tau*tau;
estimate 'sigma^2' sigma*sigma;
run;

/* Third program */

proc nlmixed data=armd77 qpoints=20 maxiter=50;
if time=1 then do;
   mean = beta11 + b + beta12*(2-treat);
   dens = -0.5*log(3.14159265358) - log(sigma)
          - 0.5*(visual-mean)**2/(sigma**2);
   ll = dens;
end;
else if time=2 then do;
   mean = beta21 + b + beta22*(2-treat);
   dens = -0.5*log(3.14159265358) - log(sigma)
          - 0.5*(visual-mean)**2/(sigma**2);
   ll = dens;
end;
model visual ~ general(ll);
random b ~ normal(0,tau*tau) subject=subject;
estimate 'tau^2' tau*tau;
estimate 'sigma^2' sigma*sigma;
run;
```

Although the programs increase in terms of complexity and, for normally distributed outcomes, the first one perfectly does the job, they also increase the flexibility, but only the last one generalizes to joint outcomes. Indeed, the second one still is based on the assumption of a common outcome distribution, albeit with a differently defined mean structure. In the third one, the general likelihood feature is used and hence a different one can be used for each outcome separately.

Thus, a program of a continuous first outcome, combined with a binary second one, is as follows:

```
proc nlmixed data=armd77 qpoints=20 maxiter=100
             maxfunc=2000 technique=newrap;
parms beta11=-5.53 beta12=-2.83 beta21=-0.50
      beta22=0.66 sigma=7 lambda=3 tau=3;
```

```
if time=1 then do;
   mean = beta11 + lambda*b + beta12*(2-treat);
   dens = -0.5*log(3.14159265358) - log(sigma)
          -0.5*(contbin-mean)**2/(sigma**2);
   ll = dens;
end;
else if time=2 then do;
   eta = beta21 + b + beta22*(2-treat);
   p = exp(eta)/(1+exp(eta));
   ll = contbin*log(p) + (1-contbin)*log(1-p);
end;
model contbin ~ general(ll);
random b ~ normal(0,tau*tau) subject=subject;
estimate 'tau^2' tau*tau;
estimate 'sigma^2' sigma*sigma;
run;
```

Reaching convergence is not straightforward, given the non-linear nature of the program, with the incorporation of λ, and a careful selection of starting values, and fine tuning using the convergence and updating method switches may be required.

Let us now turn attention to the MGLM and GLMM hierarchical models, presented in Section 24.4.3. The data need to be organized in a 'vertical' way, implying that the 4 continuous and 4 binary outcomes are stacked into a vector of length eight. An outprint for the first two patients:

Obs	subject	treat	repeat	time	dist	link	outcome
1	1	2	1	1	GAUS	IDEN	5
2	1	2	2	2	GAUS	IDEN	0
3	1	2	3	3	GAUS	IDEN	0
4	1	2	4	4	GAUS	IDEN	-10
5	1	2	5	1	BINA	LOGI	0
6	1	2	6	2	BINA	LOGI	1
7	1	2	7	3	BINA	LOGI	1
8	1	2	8	4	BINA	LOGI	1
9	2	1	1	1	GAUS	IDEN	-3
10	2	1	2	2	GAUS	IDEN	-3
11	2	1	3	3	GAUS	IDEN	-3
12	2	1	4	4	GAUS	IDEN	1
13	2	1	5	1	BINA	LOGI	1
14	2	1	6	2	BINA	LOGI	1
15	2	1	7	3	BINA	LOGI	1
16	2	1	8	4	BINA	LOGI	0

A program for the marginal model, using the GLIMMIX procedure, is

```
proc glimmix data=armd99 method=rspl empirical;
```

```
class time treat dist subject;
nloptions maxiter=50 technique=newrap;
model outcome = time*dist treat*time*dist
     / noint dist=byobs(dist) link=byobs(link) solution;
random _residual_ / subject=subject type=un r;
run;
```

which is a straightforward extension of the bivariate program.

Now, more work is needed to adapt the NLMIXED code for the conditional independence model:

```
proc nlmixed data=armd99 qpoints=20 maxiter=100
     maxfunc=2000 technique=newrap;
parms beta11=-1.55  beta12=1.00
      beta21=-2.93  beta22=1.02
  beta31=-6.68   beta32=1.52
  beta41=-13.47  beta42=2.81
  beta51=1.17    beta52=-0.22
  beta61=0.99    beta62=-0.47
  beta71=1.36    beta72=-0.41
  beta81=2.17    beta82=-0.11
  tau=1.77
  sigma=8.58
  lambda=-4.18
  ;
if repeat=1 then do;
   mean = beta11 + lambda*b + beta12*(2-treat);
   dens = -0.5*log(3.14159265358) - log(sigma)
          - 0.5*(outcome-mean)**2/(sigma**2);
   ll = dens;
end;
else if repeat=2 then do;
   mean = beta21 + lambda*b + beta22*(2-treat);
   dens = -0.5*log(3.14159265358) - log(sigma)
          - 0.5*(outcome-mean)**2/(sigma**2);
   ll = dens;
end;
else if repeat=3 then do;
   mean = beta31 + lambda*b + beta32*(2-treat);
   dens = -0.5*log(3.14159265358) - log(sigma)
          - 0.5*(outcome-mean)**2/(sigma**2);
   ll = dens;
end;
else if repeat=4 then do;
   mean = beta41 + lambda*b + beta42*(2-treat);
   dens = -0.5*log(3.14159265358) - log(sigma)
```

```
              - 0.5*(outcome-mean)**2/(sigma**2);
   ll = dens;
end;
else if repeat=5 then do;
   eta = beta51 + b + beta52*(2-treat);
   p = exp(eta)/(1+exp(eta));
   ll = outcome*log(p) + (1-outcome)*log(1-p);
end;
else if repeat=6 then do;
   eta = beta61 + b + beta62*(2-treat);
   p = exp(eta)/(1+exp(eta));
   ll = outcome*log(p) + (1-outcome)*log(1-p);
end;
else if repeat=7 then do;
   eta = beta71 + b + beta72*(2-treat);
   p = exp(eta)/(1+exp(eta));
   ll = outcome*log(p) + (1-outcome)*log(1-p);
end;
else if repeat=8 then do;
   eta = beta81 + b + beta82*(2-treat);
   p = exp(eta)/(1+exp(eta));
   ll = outcome*log(p) + (1-outcome)*log(1-p);
end;
model outcome ~ general(ll);
random b ~ normal(0,tau*tau) subject=subject;
estimate 'tau^2' tau*tau;
estimate 'sigma^2' sigma*sigma;
run;
```

Clearly, the code can be made a little more efficient in terms of programming code, but the advantage of the current program is clarity.

24.6 Concluding Remarks

We have discussed a number of methods to model correlated data when not all outcomes are of the same type. It is not uncommon to observe binary or otherwise categorical outcomes jointly with continuous outcomes, but also other combinations are perfectly possible. One might view such outcomes as multivariate. In addition, such a multivariate outcome of a heterogeneous nature can then be observed repeatedly over time, for various subjects within a trial, a cluster, or within other hierarchically organized units. Just as in the general case, we have distinguished between marginal, conditional, and random-effects models. A relatively large number of proposals have been made in the literature, many developed for specific applications.

24.6 Concluding Remarks

We have focused on three modeling approaches in particular. The probit-normal and Plackett-Dale models are of a marginal nature and within the generalized linear mixed-effects modeling framework both marginal models, random-effects models, and random-effects models with residual or serial correlation can be considered. Each of these apply to a simple multivariate setting as well as to a fully hierarchical setting. In the literature, the marginal models have been combined with GEE and pseudo-likelihood ideas to enable parameter estimation when the outcome vectors are relatively long. In the GLMM framework, PQL and MQL can be used, as well as fully numerical integration. The examples have shown that these are feasible routes, but PQL and MQL are not recommended for random-effects models, due to the well-known bias issue. Therefore, numerical integration, such as in the SAS procedure NLMIXED, is a viable route. The SAS procedure GLIMMIX is useful for the purely marginal versions that can be seen as a version of GEE as well (Section 8.8).

In conclusion, thanks to recent software developments, the joint modeling of repeated measures of various outcome types can be done with standard statistical software and is not confined any more to user defined programming tools.

25
High-dimensional Joint Models

25.1 Introduction

In Chapter 24, it has been discussed how multiple sequences of repeated measurements can be jointly analyzed. The examples given there all considered joint modeling of two (longitudinal) outcomes only. Here, we will extend this to (much) higher dimensions. The motivation for joint modeling will remain the same. In some cases, joint modeling is required because the association structure between the outcomes is of interest. For example, one may be interested in studying how the association between outcomes evolves over time or how outcome-specific evolutions are related to each other (Fieuws and Verbeke 2004). In other cases, joint modeling is needed in order to be able to draw joint inferences about the different outcomes. As examples, consider testing whether a set of outcomes shows the same average evolution, or testing for the effect of covariates on all outcomes simultaneously.

An example where joint modeling of many longitudinal outcomes has proven useful can be found in Fieuws and Verbeke (2005a), where longitudinally measured hearing thresholds were jointly analyzed, for the left ear and for the right ear, and for 11 different frequencies. This yielded a total of 22 longitudinal sequences per subject.

The possibly high dimension raises at least two additional problems, in addition to the issues discussed in Chapter 24. First, some of the models often used for the joint analysis of two longitudinal sequences are less applicable for higher dimensions. For example, when using conditional models

(Section 24.1), only two possibilities for the conditioning are possible in the case of two outcomes only: The first outcome can be modeled conditionally on the second, or vice versa. With (much) higher dimensions, (many) more possible conditioning strategies are possible, all yielding different models, of which parameters have different interpretations. Moreover, several of the research questions that require joint modeling are phrased in terms of the parameters in each of the univariate longitudinal models (i.e., longitudinal models for each repeated outcome separately), as was the case in the examples given earlier. Also, the models that are available for two outcomes often exploit the specific nature of those two outcomes, making extensions to higher dimensions far from straightforward. For example, the multivariate vector of responses may consist of outcomes of (many) different types, all requiring different models such as linear mixed models (Chapter 4), generalized linear mixed models (Chapter 14), as well as non-linear mixed models (Chapter 20). Second, even if a plausible joint model can be formulated, fitting of these high-dimensional models can become very cumbersome, unless under unrealistically strong assumptions.

In this chapter, we will focus on the random-effects approach, which can be viewed as an extension of the models discussed in Section 24.3. The model will be introduced in Section 25.2. Many applications of this type of joint models can be found in the statistical literature. For example, the approach has been used in a non-longitudinal setting to validate surrogate endpoints in meta-analyses (Buyse *et al* 2000, Burzykowski *et al* 2001) or to model multivariate clustered data (Thum 1997). Gueorguieva (2001) used the approach for the joint modeling of a continuous and a binary outcome measure in a developmental toxicity study on mice. Also in a longitudinal setting, Chakraborty *et al* (2003) obtained estimates of the correlation between blood and semen HIV-1 RNA by using a joint random-effects model. Other examples with longitudinal studies can be found in MacCallum *et al* (1997), Thiébaut *et al* (2002ab) and Shah *et al* (1997). All these examples refer to situations where the number of different outcomes is (very) low. Although the model formulation can be done irrespective of the number of outcomes to be modeled jointly, standard fitting procedures, such as maximum likelihood estimation, will only be feasible when the dimension in sufficiently low (typically dimension 2 or 3, at most). Therefore, Section 25.3 presents a model-fitting procedure which is applicable, irrespective of the dimensionality of the problem, and explains how inferences can be obtained for all parameters in the joint model. Finally, Section 25.4 applies the methodology for the joint analysis of 7 sets of questionnaires, each consisting of a number of binary outcomes. Other examples, simulation results, and more details on the models as well as on estimation and inference, can be found in Fieuws and Verbeke (2005ab).

In the remainder of this chapter, models for a single longitudinal outcome are called 'univariate' models, although they are, strictly speaking, multivariate models since they model a vector of repeated measurements, but all of the same outcome. Similarly, we will use the terminology 'bivariate' and 'multivariate' models to indicate joint longitudinal models for two or more outcomes, respectively.

25.2 Joint Mixed Model

A flexible joint model that meets the requirements discussed in Section 25.1 can be obtained by modeling each outcome separately using a mixed model (linear, generalized linear, or non-linear), by assuming that, conditionally on these random effects, the different outcomes are independent, and by imposing a joint multivariate distribution on the vector of all random effects. This approach has many advantages and is applicable in a wide variety of situations. First, the data can be highly unbalanced. For example, it is not necessary that all outcomes are measured at the same time points. Moreover, the approach is applicable for combining linear mixed models, non-linear mixed models, or generalized linear mixed models. The procedure also allows the combination of different types of mixed models, such as a generalized linear mixed model for a discrete outcome and a non-linear mixed model for a continuous outcome.

Let m be the dimension of the problem, i.e., the number of outcomes that need to be modeled jointly. Further, let Y_{rij} denote the jth measurement taken on the ith subject, for the rth outcome, $i = 1, \ldots, N$, $r = 1, \ldots, m$, and $j = 1, \ldots, n_{ri}$. Note that we do not assume that the same number of measurements is available for all subjects, nor for all outcomes. Let $\boldsymbol{Y_{ri}}$ be the vector of n_{ri} measurements taken on subject i, for outcome r. Our model assumes that each $\boldsymbol{Y_{ri}}$ satisfies a mixed model. Following our earlier notation of the Sections 13.2 and 20.5, let $f_{ri}(\boldsymbol{y_{ri}}|\boldsymbol{b_{ri}},\boldsymbol{\theta_r})$ be the density of $\boldsymbol{Y_{ri}}$, conditional on a q_r-dimensional vector $\boldsymbol{b_{ri}}$ of random effects for the rth outcome on subject i. The vector $\boldsymbol{\theta_r}$ contains all fixed effects and possibly also a scale parameter needed in the model for the rth outcome. Note that we do not assume the same type of model for all outcomes: A combination of linear, generalized linear, and non-linear mixed models is possible. It is also not assumed that the same number q_r of random effects is used for all m outcomes.

In most applications, it will be assumed that, conditionally on the random effects $\boldsymbol{b_{1i}}, \boldsymbol{b_{2i}}, \ldots, \boldsymbol{b_{mi}}$, the m outcomes $\boldsymbol{Y_{1i}}, \boldsymbol{Y_{2i}}, \ldots, \boldsymbol{Y_{mi}}$ are independent. Extensions of this assumption can be found in Section 24.3 in the context of surrogate markers, or in Fieuws and Verbeke (2005a) in the analysis of the 22 longitudinal sequences of hearing thresholds. Finally, the model is completed by assuming that the vector $\boldsymbol{b_i}$ of all random effects for subject i is multivariate normal with mean zero and covariance D, i.e.,

$$\boldsymbol{b}_i = \begin{pmatrix} \boldsymbol{b}_{1i} \\ \boldsymbol{b}_{2i} \\ \vdots \\ \boldsymbol{b}_{mi} \end{pmatrix} \sim N \left[\begin{pmatrix} 0 \\ 0 \\ \vdots \\ 0 \end{pmatrix}, \begin{pmatrix} D_{11} & D_{12} & \cdots & D_{1m} \\ D_{21} & D_{22} & \cdots & D_{2m} \\ \vdots & \vdots & \ddots & \vdots \\ D_{m1} & D_{m2} & \cdots & D_{mm} \end{pmatrix} \right].$$

The matrices D_{rs} represent the covariances between $\boldsymbol{b}_{ri}$ and $\boldsymbol{b}_{si}$, $r,s = 1,\ldots,m$. Finally, D is the matrix with blocks D_{rs} as entries.

A special case of the above model is the so-called shared-parameter model, which assumes the same set of random effects for all outcomes. An example of this is (24.19), where, in the context of surrogate marker evaluation, a random intercept b_i was used simultaneously in the model for the surrogate outcome as well as in the model for the true outcome. This clearly can be obtained as a special case of the above model by assuming perfect correlation between some of the random effects. The advantage of such shared-parameter models is the relatively low dimension of the random-effects distribution, when compared to the above model. The dimension of the random effects in shared parameter models does not increase with the number of outcomes to be modeled. In the above model, each new outcome added to the model introduces new random effects, thereby increasing the dimension of $\boldsymbol{b}_i$. Although the shared-parameter models can reasonably easy be fitted using standard software (Section 24.5), this is no longer the case for the model considered here. Estimation and inference under the above model will require specific procedures, which will be discussed in Section 25.3. A disadvantage of the shared-parameter model is that it is based on much stronger assumptions about the association between the outcomes, which may not be valid, especially in high-dimensional settings as considered in this chapter.

Note also that, joining valid univariate mixed models does not necessarily lead to a correct joint model. Fieuws and Verbeke (2004) illustrate this in the context of linear mixed models for two continuous outcomes. It is shown how the joint model may imply association structures between the two sets of longitudinal profiles that may strongly depend on the actual parameterization of the individual models and that are not necessarily valid.

As before, estimation and inference will be based on the marginal model for the vector $\boldsymbol{Y}_i$ of all measurements for subject i. Assuming independence of the outcomes conditionally on the vector $\boldsymbol{b}_i$ of random effects, the log-likelihood contribution for subject i equals

$$\ell_i(\boldsymbol{y}_{1i}, \boldsymbol{y}_{2i}, \ldots, \boldsymbol{y}_{mi} | \boldsymbol{\Psi}^*)$$
$$= \ln \int \prod_{r=1}^{m} f_{ri}(\boldsymbol{y}_{ri} | \boldsymbol{b}_{ri}, \boldsymbol{\theta}_r) f(\boldsymbol{b}_i | D) d\boldsymbol{b}_i, \qquad (25.1)$$

in which all parameters present in the joint model (fixed effects parameters as well as covariance parameters) have been combined into the vector $\boldsymbol{\Psi}^*$.

Clearly, expression (25.1) shows that the joint model can be interpreted as one mixed-effects model, with conditional density

$$f_i(\boldsymbol{y}_i|\boldsymbol{b}_i) = \prod_{r=1}^{m} f_{ri}(\boldsymbol{y}_{ri}|\boldsymbol{b}_{ri}, \boldsymbol{\theta}_r)$$

and with random effect $\boldsymbol{b}_i$. Hence, fitting of the model can, strictly speaking, be based on standard methods and standard software, available for fitting mixed models in general. However, computational problems will arise as the dimension of the random-effects vector $\boldsymbol{b}_i$ in the joint model increases. For example, re-consider the hearing thresholds mentioned earlier. If each of the 22 outcomes is modeled by way of a linear mixed model with random intercepts and random slopes for the time-evolution, then the resulting joint model contains $22 \times 2 = 44$ random effects, resulting in a 44-dimensional matrix D which contains 990 unknown parameters. Even in this case of linear models for continuous data, where the marginal likelihood can be calculated analytically, standard maximization algorithms are no longer sufficient to maximize this marginal likelihood with respect to this many parameters. Moreover, when approximation methods are needed in the calculation of the likelihood, as is the case for generalized or non-linear mixed models (Chapters 14 and 20), maximizing the joint likelihood becomes completely impossible using optimization techniques currently implemented for single outcomes. In Section 25.3, we will describe how estimates and inferences for all parameters can be obtained from pairwise fitting of the model, i.e., from separately fitting the implied joint model for each pair of outcomes.

25.3 Model Fitting and Inference

The general idea behind the pairwise fitting approach is straightforward. Instead of maximizing the likelihood of the full joint model presented in the previous section, all pairwise bivariate models will be fitted separately in a first step. Note the similarity between the pairwise approach used here and the pairwise pseudo-likelihood approach used in the Sections 9.4.1 and 21.3. In a second step, the parameters obtained by fitting the pairwise models will be combined to obtain one single estimate for each parameter in the full joint model.

25.3.1 Pairwise Fitting

The parameters in each univariate model can be estimated by fitting a model for that specific response only. Hence, the only parameters that cannot be estimated by fitting the univariate models are the parameters needed to model the association between the different outcomes. In the model introduced in Section 25.2, these are the parameters in the matrices D_{rs}, $r \neq s$. However, estimation of these parameters does not necessarily require fitting of the complete joint model for all outcomes, it is sufficient to fit all $m(m-1)/2$ bivariate models, i.e., all joint models for all possible pairs

$$(Y_1, Y_2), (Y_1, Y_3), \ldots, (Y_1, Y_m), (Y_2, Y_3), \ldots, (Y_2, Y_m), \ldots, (Y_{m-1}, Y_m)$$

of the outcomes $Y_1, Y_2, \ldots, Y_m$. Let the log-likelihood function corresponding to the pair (r, s) be denoted by $\ell(y_r, y_s | \Psi_{rs})$. The vector Ψ_{rs} contains all parameters in the bivariate model for pair (r, s), i.e., the parameters in each of the univariate models, as well as the parameters in D_{rs}.

Let Ψ now be the stacked vector combining all $m(m-1)/2$ pair-specific parameter vectors Ψ_{rs}. Estimates for the elements in Ψ are obtained by maximizing each of the $m(m-1)/2$ log-likelihoods $\ell(y_r, y_s | \Psi_{rs})$ separately. It is important to realize that the parameter vectors Ψ and Ψ^* are not equivalent. Indeed, some parameters in Ψ^* will have a single counterpart in Ψ, e.g., the parameters in D_{rs}, $r \neq s$, representing covariances between random effects from different outcomes. Other elements in Ψ^* will have multiple counterparts in Ψ, e.g., the parameters in D_{rr}, representing variances and covariances of random effects from the same outcome. In the latter case, a single estimate for the corresponding parameter in Ψ^* is obtained by averaging all corresponding pair-specific estimates in $\widehat{\Psi}$. Standard errors of the so-obtained estimates clearly cannot be obtained from averaging standard errors or variances. Indeed, the variability amongst the pair-specific estimates needs to be taken into account. Furthermore, two pair-specific estimates corresponding to two pairwise models with a common outcome are based on overlapping information and hence correlated. This correlation should also be accounted for in the sampling variability of the combined estimates in $\widehat{\Psi}^*$. In the remainder of this section, we will use pseudo-likelihood ideas to obtain standard errors for the estimates, first in $\widehat{\Psi}$, afterwards in $\widehat{\Psi}^*$.

25.3.2 Inference for Ψ

Fitting all bivariate models is equivalent to maximizing the function

$$\begin{aligned} p\ell(\Psi) &\equiv p\ell(y_{1i}, y_{2i}, \ldots, y_{mi} | \Psi) \\ &= \sum_{r<s} \ell(Y_r, Y_s | \Psi_{rs}), \end{aligned} \quad (25.2)$$

ignoring the fact that some of the vectors Ψ_{rs} have common elements, i.e., assuming that all vectors Ψ_{rs} are completely distinct. Obviously, (25.2), is of the form (9.3) and hence our pairwise fitting procedure fits within the general framework of pseudo-likelihood (Chapters 9 and 21). Our application of pseudo-likelihood methodology is different from most other applications in the sense that the same parameter vector is usually present in the different parts of the pseudo-likelihood function. Here, the set of parameters in $\boldsymbol{\Psi}_{rs}$ is treated pair-specific, which allows separate maximization of each term in the pseudo log-likelihood function (25.2). In Section 25.3.3, we will account for the fact that $\boldsymbol{\Psi}_{rs}$ and $\boldsymbol{\Psi}_{rs'}$, $s \neq s'$, are not completely distinct, as they share the parameters referring to the rth outcome.

Because the pairwise approach fits within the pseudo-likelihood framework, an asymptotic multivariate normal distribution for $\widehat{\boldsymbol{\Psi}}$ can be derived, using the general pseudo-likelihood theory presented in Section 9.2. More specifically, we have that $\widehat{\boldsymbol{\Psi}}$ asymptotically satisfies

$$\sqrt{N}(\widehat{\boldsymbol{\Psi}} - \boldsymbol{\Psi}) \approx N(\mathbf{0}, I_0^{-1} I_1 I_0^{-1})$$

in which $I_0^{-1} I_1 I_0^{-1}$ is a 'sandwich-type' robust variance estimator, and where I_0 and I_1 can be constructed using first- and second-order derivatives of the components in (25.2). Strictly speaking, I_0 and I_1 depend on the unknown parameters in $\boldsymbol{\Psi}$, but these are traditionally replaced by their estimates in $\widehat{\boldsymbol{\Psi}}$.

25.3.3 Combining Information: Inference for $\boldsymbol{\Psi}^*$

In a final step, estimates for the parameters in $\boldsymbol{\Psi}^*$ can be calculated, as suggested before, by taking averages of all the available estimates for that specific parameter. Obviously, this implies that $\widehat{\boldsymbol{\Psi}}^* = A'\widehat{\boldsymbol{\Psi}}$ for an appropriate weight matrix A. Hence, inference for the elements in $\widehat{\boldsymbol{\Psi}}^*$ will be based on

$$\begin{aligned}\sqrt{N}(\widehat{\boldsymbol{\Psi}}^* - \boldsymbol{\Psi}^*) &= \sqrt{N}(A'\widehat{\boldsymbol{\Psi}} - A'\boldsymbol{\Psi}) \\ &\approx N(\mathbf{0}, A' I_0^{-1} I_1 I_0^{-1} A).\end{aligned} \quad (25.3)$$

As explained in Section 9.2, pseudo-likelihood methods often are less efficient than full maximum likelihood. However, simulation results of Fieuws and Verbeke (2005ab) suggest that, in the present context, this loss of efficiency is negligible, if any.

25.4 A Study in Psycho-Cognitive Functioning

To illustrate the pairwise approach for fitting high-dimensional multivariate repeated measurements, we analyze data from an experiment in which 105 Dutch-speaking elderly participants (54 females and 51 males) were randomly assigned to one of two physical activity oriented exercise programs. The first is a classical fitness program consisting of 3 weekly visits

TABLE 25.1. *Psycho-Cognitive Functioning. Parameter estimates (standard errors) for the fixed effects in model (25.4) obtained by fitting 7 separate univariate models, as well as obtained by fitting the joint model with the pairwise fitting approach.*

	7 Univariate models	
	$\widehat{\beta}_{r0}$ (s.e.)	$\widehat{\beta}_{r1}$ (s.e.)
Physical well-being	1.63 (0.26)	−0.13 (0.37)
Psychological well-being	1.56 (0.30)	1.22 (0.61)
Self-esteem	1.69 (0.30)	0.43 (0.42)
Physical self-perception	−0.55 (0.14)	0.58 (0.24)
Degree of opposition	1.48 (0.17)	0.06 (0.24)
Self-efficacy	1.71 (0.25)	−0.24 (0.33)
Motivation	0.95 (0.11)	−0.35 (0.16)
	Joint model	
	$\widehat{\beta}_{r0}$ (s.e.)	$\widehat{\beta}_{r1}$ (s.e.)
Physical well-being	1.62 (0.25)	−0.12 (0.37)
Psychological well-being	1.71 (0.32)	1.00 (0.68)
Self-esteem	1.68 (0.32)	0.49 (0.39)
Physical self-perception	−0.52 (0.14)	0.52 (0.25)
Degree of opposition	1.47 (0.17)	0.07 (0.24)
Self-efficacy	1.70 (0.23)	−0.22 (0.33)
Motivation	0.94 (0.09)	−0.34 (0.16)

to the gym. The second is a distance coaching program with an emphasis on incorporating physical activities in daily life. One of the aims of the study was to investigate whether the two programs have different impacts on the psycho-cognitive functioning of the participants. Different aspects of psycho-cognitive functioning referring to subjective well-being, self-esteem, self-perception and motivation were considered. A set of questionnaires has been used to measure these different aspects. More specifically, 7 sets of questions (items) were used, originating from different questionnaires and each set consisting of a different number of items: 10 items measuring physical well-being, 14 items for psychological well-being, 10 items for self-esteem, 30 items for physical self-perception, 21 items measuring the degree of opposition to physical activities, 5 items for perceived self-efficacy toward physical activity, and 16 items for motivation for the intervention program. All item scores were dichotomized, with a score equal to one expressing positive psycho-cognitive functioning. All subjects filled in at least one item for each of the seven sets. 64 subjects had no missing information for the 106 items. 20 subjects had one item missing. The missing item scores for the other subjects ranged from 2 to 22. The mean age equals

25.4 A Study in Psycho-Cognitive Functioning

66.6 years (range 60–76 years) and the mean body mass index (BMI) is 27.0 kg/m^2 (range 20.7–38.0). Questionnaires considered in this analysis were completed by the participants, 6 months after the start of the study.

The aim of our analyses is to assess differences in efficacy between both exercise programs, as well as to study the strength of association between the 7 sets of questionnaires. Although not of a longitudinal nature, this data set clearly is an example of multivariate repeated measurements, of dimension 7, where a number of binary repeated measurements of psycho-cognitive functioning are available for each dimension. The random variable Y_{rij} now denotes the jth measurement (0 or 1), taken on the ith study participant, for the rth questionnaire, $i = 1, \ldots, 105$, $r = 1, \ldots, 7$, and $j = 1, \ldots, n_{ri}$. A score $Y_{rij} = 1$ reflects positive psycho-cognitive functioning, while $Y_{rij} = 0$ is an indication of negative psycho-cognitive functioning.

We will assume that each of the 7 questionnaires satisfy a random-intercepts logistic model, given by

$$\text{logit}[P(Y_{rij} = 1)] = \beta_{r0} + \beta_{r1}\text{DC}_i + b_{ri}, \tag{25.4}$$

in which DC$_i$ is an indicator variable equal to 1 for the participants in the distance coaching program, and zero otherwise. Hence, $\exp(\beta_{r1})$ represents the multiplicative effect of this program on the odds for positive psycho-cognitive functioning measured by the items in questionnaire r, with $r = 1, \ldots, 7$ (1=physical well-being, 2=psychological well-being, 3=self-esteem, 4=physical self-perception, 5=degree of opposition, 6=self-efficacy, and 7=motivation). Note that this model allows for questionnaire-specific intercepts as well as intervention effects. More parsimonious models could be obtained by assuming, for example, the same regression parameters for all questionnaires, or by assuming some random effects to be common to a subset of the questionnaires (i.e., some of the b_{ri} are equal). Correlation between the items of the same set is modeled through the inclusion of the random effects b_{ri}. Correlation between the items of the different questionnaires is implied by the joint distribution for the 7 random intercepts, i.e.,

$$\left(b_{1i}, b_{2i}, b_{3i}, b_{4i}, b_{5i}, b_{6i}, b_{7i} \right)' \sim N\left(\mathbf{0}, \mathbf{D}\right),$$

where $\mathbf{D}$ is now the 7×7 unstructured covariance matrix of the random intercepts.

Table 25.1 shows the results from fitting the 7 univariate models separately, as well as from fitting the joint model using the pairwise fitting approach. Very similar estimates as well as inferences are obtained. Using approximate Wald-type tests (Z-tests), the separate analyses show significant differences between both groups on 3 of the 7 questionnaires. The DC-group scores better on physical self-perception and on psychological well-being, but worse on motivation.

TABLE 25.2. *Psycho-Cognitive Functioning. Estimated correlation matrix for the random intercepts in Model (25.4).*

Physical well-being	1.00						
Psychological well-being	0.75	1.00					
Self-esteem	0.55	0.76	1.00				
Physical self-perception	0.66	0.46	0.53	1.00			
Degree of opposition	0.19	0.12	0.23	0.38	1.00		
Self-efficacy	0.29	0.24	0.25	0.36	0.23	1.00	
Motivation	0.42	0.31	0.28	0.40	0.47	0.30	1.00

Using the results from the joint model, an overall test can be constructed for the presence of any systematic difference between both exercise programs. Formally, this corresponds to testing the null-hypothesis

$$H_0 : \beta_{11} = \beta_{21} = \beta_{31} = \beta_{41} = \beta_{51} = \beta_{61} = \beta_{71} = 0$$

versus the alternative that at least one of these parameters differs from zero. Since this null hypothesis is of the general form $H_0 : L'\Psi^* = \mathbf{0}$ for the appropriate matrix L, a Wald-type test (χ^2-test) can easily be derived from the asymptotic distribution (25.3) for $\widehat{\Psi}^*$. This yields a test statistic value equal to 17.84, which is significant when compared to the χ_7^2 distribution ($p = 0.013$). Similarly, other hypotheses of interest can be tested as well.

An additional aim of our analyses was to study the strength of association between the 7 sets of questionnaires. Table 25.2 presents the correlations obtained from the fitted covariance matrix $\widehat{D}$. These correlations express the association between the different constructs underlying each of the seven scales. Performing a principal components analysis (PCA) on the 7×7 correlation matrix of the random effects reveals that the first principal component explains only 49% of the variability. One approach sometimes used to join multiple random-effects models in such a way that the joint model can still easily be fitted using standard software, assumes common random effects for all outcomes, leading to so-called shared-parameter models. An example in a slightly different context can be found in De Gruttola and Tu (1994). More specifically, it is then assumed that all $\boldsymbol{b}_{ri}$ equal $\boldsymbol{b}_i$. In our example, this would lead to univariate random intercepts common to all questionnaires. The advantage would be that this model can very easily be fitted because only one random effect is involved. However, the PCA results suggest that this would be a very unrealistic model for the data set at hand, which could result in biased inferences for the fixed effects of interest (Adams et al 1997, Folk and Green 1989).

Figure 25.1 plots the component loadings of the random intercepts for the seven questionnaires on the first two principal components, explaining 49% and 17.4% of the variation. In this reduced representation, we observe,

25.4 A Study in Psycho-Cognitive Functioning 477

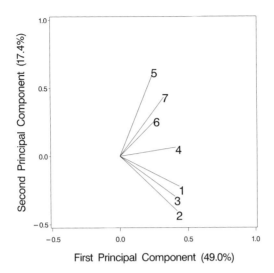

FIGURE 25.1. *Psycho-Cognitive Functioning. Component loadings for the seven questionnaires on the first two principal components for the 7×7 correlation matrix of the random intercepts in model (25.4).*
1: physical well-being; 2: psychological well-being; 3: self-esteem; 4: physical self-perception; 5: degree of opposition; 6: self-efficacy; 7: motivation.

not surprisingly, that the scales referring to well-being and self-esteem are strongly correlated with each other, as opposed to their relation with motivational oriented scales.

Part VI

Missing Data

26
Missing Data Concepts

26.1 Introduction

It is not unusual for some measurement sequences in a longitudinal study to terminate early for reasons outside the control of the investigator. Any unit so affected is called a dropout. In addition, intermediate scheduled measurements might be missed, which we term intermittent missing values. It might be necessary to accommodate missingness in general and dropout in particular into the modeling process.

Early work on missing values was largely concerned with algorithmic and computational solutions to the induced lack of balance or deviations from the intended study design (Afifi and Elashoff 1966, Hartley and Hocking 1971). Later, general algorithms such as expectation-maximization (EM) (Dempster, Laird, and Rubin 1977), and data imputation and augmentation procedures (Rubin 1987), combined with powerful computing have largely provided a solution to this aspect of the problem. There remains the tricky but important question of assessing the impact of missing data on subsequent statistical inference.

Many methods are formulated as *selection models* (Little and Rubin 1987, 2002) as opposed to *pattern-mixture modeling* (Little 1993, 1994a). A selection model factors the joint distribution of the measurement and non-response mechanisms into the marginal measurement distribution and the non-response distribution, conditional on the measurements. This is intuitively appealing because the marginal measurement distribution would be of interest also with complete data. Little and Rubin's taxonomy is most easily developed in the selection setting. Parameterizing and making inference about the effect of treatment and evolutions over time is straightforward in the selection model context.

Let us turn to the terminology of Rubin (1976) and Little and Rubin (1987, Chapter 6). Key concepts are: (1) *missing completely at random* (MCAR), if the missingness is independent of both unobserved and observed data, (2) *missing at random* (MAR) if, conditional on the observed data, the missingness is independent of the unobserved measurements, and (3) *missingness not at random* (MNAR), when neither MCAR nor MAR applies. In the context of likelihood or Bayesian inference, and when the parameters describing the measurement process are functionally independent of the parameters describing the missingness process, MCAR and MAR are *ignorable*, while a non-random process is non-ignorable. Ignorability means that inferences about the measurement mechanism can be made without explicitly addressing the missingness mechanism. With frequentist inference, the stronger MCAR generally provides a sufficient condition for ignorability.

This chapter sketches a general taxonomy within which incomplete data methods can be placed. The emphasis lies on longitudinal data, in line with the theme of the book. Subsequent chapters deal with simple methods and direct likelihood (Chapter 27), the EM algorithm and multiple imputation (Chapter 28) and MNAR, with attention for both selection models (Chapter 29) and pattern-mixture models (Chapter 30). In Chapter 31 selected sensitivity analysis tools are discussed and Chapter 32 explains how a number of key methods can be implemented using the SAS system.

26.2 A Formal Taxonomy

In this section, we build on the standard framework for missing data, which is largely due to Rubin (1976) and Little and Rubin (1987).

In line with our conventions in earlier parts of the book, we assume that for subject i in the study, a sequence of measurements Y_{ij} is *designed* to be measured at occasions $j = 1, \ldots, n_i$. As before, the outcomes are grouped into a vector $\boldsymbol{Y}_i = (Y_{i1}, \ldots, Y_{in_i})'$. In most, but not all, designed experiments where missingness is an issue, n_i might be a constant. Counterexamples are rotating panels or samples in which a subset of the subjects is designed to be measured more intensively than the rest of the sample, etc.

We now additionally define, for each occasion j, an indicator

$$R_{ij} = \begin{cases} 1 & \text{if } Y_{ij} \text{ is observed,} \\ 0 & \text{otherwise.} \end{cases}$$

The *missing data indicators* R_{ij} are grouped into a vector $\boldsymbol{R}_i$ which is, of course, of the same length as $\boldsymbol{Y}_i$. We then partition $\boldsymbol{Y}_i$ into two subvectors such that $\boldsymbol{Y}_i^o$ is the vector containing those Y_{ij} for which $R_{ij} = 1$ and $\boldsymbol{Y}_i^m$ contains the remaining components. These subvectors are referred to as the *observed* and *missing* components, respectively. Clearly, the partition is allowed to differ with subject, and $\boldsymbol{Y}_i^o$ can contain components which are measured later than occasions at which components of $\boldsymbol{Y}_i^m$ ought to have been measured.

The following terminology is adopted. *Complete data* refers to the vector $\boldsymbol{Y}_i$ of scheduled measurements. This is the outcome vector that would have been recorded if there were no missing data. The *missing data indicators* are assembled into the vector $\boldsymbol{R}_i$ and the process generating $\boldsymbol{R}_i$ is referred to as the *missing data process*. The *full data* $(\boldsymbol{Y}_i, \boldsymbol{R}_i)$ consist of the complete data, together with the missing data indicators. Note that, unless all components of $\boldsymbol{R}_i$ are equal to 1, the full data components are never all observed. Then, obviously, the *observed data* refer to $\boldsymbol{Y}_i^o$ and the *missing data* to $\boldsymbol{Y}_i^m$. Note that one observes the measurements $\boldsymbol{Y}_i^o$ together with the dropout indicators $\boldsymbol{R}_i$.

Some confusion might arise between the terms *complete data* introduced here and *complete case analysis*. Whereas the former refers to the (hypothetical) data set that would arise if there were no missing data, 'complete case analysis' refers to analyses based on first deleting all subjects for which at least one component is missing.

When missingness is restricted to dropout or attrition, we can replace the vector $\boldsymbol{R}_i$ by a scalar variable D_i, the *dropout indicator*. Indeed, in this case, each vector $\boldsymbol{R}_i$ is of the form $(1, \ldots, 1, 0, \ldots, 0)$ and we can define the scalar dropout indicator

$$D_i = 1 + \sum_{j=1}^{n_i} R_{ij}. \tag{26.1}$$

For an incomplete sequence, D_i denotes the occasion at which dropout occurs. For a complete sequence, $D_i = n_i + 1$. In both cases, D_i indicates 1+ the length of the measurement sequence, whether complete or incomplete.

Dropout or attrition is a particular *monotone* pattern of missingness. In order to have monotone missingness there has to exist a permutation of the measurement occasions such that a measurement earlier in the permuted sequence is observed for at least those subjects that are observed at later measurements. Note that, for this definition to be meaningful, we need to have a balanced design in the sense of a common set of measurement occasions. Other patterns are called *non-monotone*.

26.2.1 Missing Data Frameworks

We will first consider the so-called selection, pattern-mixture, and shared-parameter modeling frameworks. Then, Rubin's taxonomy encompassing MCAR, MAR, and MNAR will be developed.

When data are incomplete due to a stochastic mechanism one should start from the full data density

$$f(\boldsymbol{y}_i, \boldsymbol{r}_i | X_i, Z_i, W_i, \boldsymbol{\theta}, \boldsymbol{\psi}), \tag{26.2}$$

where X_i, Z_i, and W_i are design matrices for fixed effects, random effects (if applicable), and missing data process and where $\boldsymbol{\theta}$ and $\boldsymbol{\psi}$ are vectors that parameterize the joint distribution. We will use $\boldsymbol{\theta} = (\boldsymbol{\beta}', \boldsymbol{\alpha}')'$ and $\boldsymbol{\psi}$ to describe the measurement and missingness processes, respectively, where $\boldsymbol{\beta}$ is the fixed-effects parameter vector and $\boldsymbol{\alpha}$ assembles variance components and/or association parameters.

The *selection model* factorization equals

$$f(\boldsymbol{y}_i, \boldsymbol{r}_i | X_i, Z_i, W_i, \boldsymbol{\theta}, \boldsymbol{\psi}) = f(\boldsymbol{y}_i | X_i, Z_i, \boldsymbol{\theta}) f(\boldsymbol{r}_i | \boldsymbol{y}_i, W_i, \boldsymbol{\psi}), \tag{26.3}$$

where the first factor is the marginal density of the measurement process and the second one is the density of the missingness process, conditional on the outcomes. Factor $f(\boldsymbol{r}_i | \boldsymbol{y}_i, W_i, \boldsymbol{\psi})$ describes one's self-selection mechanism to either continue or leave the study.

The term selection model originates from the econometric literature (Heckman 1976) and it can be thought of that a subject's missing values are "selected" through the probability model, given their measurements, whether observed or not.

An alternative family can be built based on so-called *pattern-mixture models* (Little 1993, 1995, Molenberghs, Kenward and Lesaffre 1997). These are based on the factorization

$$f(\boldsymbol{y}_i, \boldsymbol{r}_i | X_i, Z_i, W_i, \boldsymbol{\theta}, \boldsymbol{\psi}) = f(\boldsymbol{y}_i | \boldsymbol{r}_i, X_i, Z_i, \boldsymbol{\theta}) f(\boldsymbol{r}_i | W_i, \boldsymbol{\psi}). \tag{26.4}$$

The pattern mixture model allows for a different response model for each pattern of missing values, the observed data being a mixture of these weighted by the probability of each missing value or dropout pattern. At first sight, such a model is less appealing in terms of probability mechanisms for generating the data, but it has other important advantages.

The third family is referred to as *shared-parameter models*:

$$f(\boldsymbol{y}_i, \boldsymbol{r}_i | X_i, Z_i, W_i, \boldsymbol{\theta}, \boldsymbol{\psi}, \boldsymbol{b}_i)$$
$$= f(\boldsymbol{y}_i | \boldsymbol{r}_i, X_i, Z_i, \boldsymbol{\theta}, \boldsymbol{b}_i) f(\boldsymbol{r}_i | Z_i, W_i, \boldsymbol{\psi}, \boldsymbol{b}_i), \tag{26.5}$$

where we now explicitly include a vector of random effects $\boldsymbol{b}_i$ of which one or more components are shared between both factors. This model family has been studied by Wu and Carroll (1988) and Wu and Bailey (1988, 1989). A sensible assumption is that $\boldsymbol{Y}_i$ and $\boldsymbol{R}_i$ are independent, given the random effects $\boldsymbol{b}_i$. The random effects $\boldsymbol{b}_i$ can be used to define a linear, generalized linear, or non-linear mixed effects model. The same vector can then be used to describe the missing data process. As such, the shared parameter $\boldsymbol{b}_i$ can be thought of as referring to a latent trait driving both the measurement and missingness processes. At first sight, this principle is related to the joint outcomes of Sections 24.2.3 and 24.3. The difference is that there all outcomes are assumed to be observed, whereas here the components $\boldsymbol{Y}_i^m$ are missing.

The natural parameters of selection models, pattern-mixture models, and shared-parameter models have a different meaning, and transforming one probability model into one of the other framework is in general not straightforward, not for normal measurement models but even less so in the general case.

26.2.2 Missing Data Mechanisms

Rubin's taxonomy (Rubin 1976, Little and Rubin 1987) of missing value processes is fundamental to modeling incomplete data. It is based on the second factor of (26.3), within the selection modeling framework:

$$f(\boldsymbol{r}_i|\boldsymbol{y}_i, W_i, \boldsymbol{\psi}) = f(\boldsymbol{r}_i|\boldsymbol{y}_i^o, \boldsymbol{y}_i^m, W_i, \boldsymbol{\psi}). \qquad (26.6)$$

Rubin's classification essentially distinguishes settings in which important simplifications of this process are possible.

Missing Completely at Random (MCAR). Under an MCAR mechanism, the probability of an observation being missing is independent of the responses:

$$f(\boldsymbol{r}_i|\boldsymbol{y}_i, W_i, \boldsymbol{\psi}) = f(\boldsymbol{r}_i|W_i, \boldsymbol{\psi}) \qquad (26.7)$$

and hence (26.3) simplifies to

$$f(\boldsymbol{y}_i, \boldsymbol{r}_i|X_i, Z_i, W_i, \boldsymbol{\theta}, \boldsymbol{\psi}) = f(\boldsymbol{y}_i|X_i, Z_i, \boldsymbol{\theta})f(\boldsymbol{r}_i|W_i, \boldsymbol{\psi}), \qquad (26.8)$$

implying that both components are independent. The implication is that the joint distribution of $\boldsymbol{y}_i^o$ and $\boldsymbol{r}_i$ becomes

$$f(\boldsymbol{y}_i^o, \boldsymbol{r}_i|X_i, Z_i, W_i, \boldsymbol{\theta}, \boldsymbol{\psi}) = f(\boldsymbol{y}_i^o|X_i, Z_i, \boldsymbol{\theta})f(\boldsymbol{r}_i|W_i, \boldsymbol{\psi}). \qquad (26.9)$$

Under MCAR the observed data can be analyzed as though the pattern of missing values were predetermined. In whatever way the data are analyzed, whether using a frequentist, likelihood, or Bayesian procedure, the process(es) generating the missing values can be ignored. For example, in this situation simple averages of the observed data at different times provide unbiased estimates of the underlying marginal profiles.

Note that this definition and the ones to follow are conditional on covariates. When covariates, assembled into X_i, Z_i, and W_i are removed, it is possible that the nature of a mechanism changes.

Missing at Random (MAR). Under an MAR mechanism, the probability of an observation being missing is *conditionally* independent of the unobserved data, given the values of the observed data:

$$f(\boldsymbol{r}_i|\boldsymbol{y}_i, W_i, \boldsymbol{\psi}) = f(\boldsymbol{r}_i|\boldsymbol{y}_i^o, W_i, \boldsymbol{\psi}). \tag{26.10}$$

and again the joint distribution of the observed data can be partitioned:

$$f(\boldsymbol{y}_i, \boldsymbol{r}_i|X_i, Z_i, W_i, \boldsymbol{\theta}, \boldsymbol{\psi}) = f(\boldsymbol{y}_i|X_i, Z_i, \boldsymbol{\theta})f(\boldsymbol{r}_i|\boldsymbol{y}_i^o, W_i, \boldsymbol{\psi}), \tag{26.11}$$

and hence at the observed data level:

$$f(\boldsymbol{y}_i^o, \boldsymbol{r}_i|X_i, Z_i, W_i, \boldsymbol{\theta}, \boldsymbol{\psi}) = f(\boldsymbol{y}_i^o|X_i, Z_i, \boldsymbol{\theta})f(\boldsymbol{r}_i|\boldsymbol{y}_i^o, W_i, \boldsymbol{\psi}). \tag{26.12}$$

Given the simplicity of (26.12), handling of MAR processes is much easier than handling MNAR.

Although the MAR assumption is particularly convenient in that it leads to considerable simplification in the issues surrounding the analysis of incomplete longitudinal data, it is rare in practice for an investigator to be able to justify its adoption, and so in many situations the final class of missing value mechanisms cannot be ruled out.

Missing Not at Random (MNAR). In this case, neither MCAR nor MAR hold. Under MNAR the probability of a measurement being missing depends on unobserved data. No simplification of the joint distribution is possible and the joint distribution of the observed measurements and the missingness process has to be written as:

$$f(\boldsymbol{y}_i^o, \boldsymbol{r}_i|X_i, Z_i, W_i, \boldsymbol{\theta}, \boldsymbol{\psi}) = \int f(\boldsymbol{y}_i|X_i, Z_i, \boldsymbol{\theta})f(\boldsymbol{r}_i|\boldsymbol{y}_i, W_i, \boldsymbol{\psi})d\boldsymbol{y}_i^m. \tag{26.13}$$

Inferences can only be made by making further assumptions, about which the observed data alone carry no information. Ideally, the choice of such assumptions should be guided by external information, but the degree to which this is possible in practice varies greatly. Such models can be formulated within each of the three main families: selection, pattern-mixture, and shared-parameter models. The differences between the families are especially important in the MNAR case, and lead to quite different, but complementary, views of the missing value problem. Little (1995), Hogan and Laird (1997), and Kenward and Molenberghs (1999) provide detailed reviews. See also Verbeke and Molenberghs (2000).

It has been shown, for dropout, how the Rubin classification can be applied in the pattern-mixture framework as well (Molenberghs, Michiels, Kenward, and Diggle 1998, Kenward, Molenberghs, and Thijs 2003).

It is important to note that the MCAR–MAR–MNAR terminology is independent of the statistical framework chosen to analyze the data. This is to be contrasted with the terms *ignorable* and *non-ignorable* missingness. The latter terms depend crucially on the inferential framework (Rubin 1976) and will be considered next.

26.2.3 Ignorability

One can see the importance of the MAR assumption from an intuitive viewpoint. Essentially it states that once appropriate account is taken of what we have observed, there remains no dependence on unobserved data, at least in terms of the probability model. We should as a consequence expect much of the missing value problem to disappear under the MAR mechanism and this is in fact the case. This can be shown more formally through consideration of the likelihood. The full data likelihood contribution for subject i assumes the form

$$L^*(\boldsymbol{\theta}, \boldsymbol{\psi} | X_i, Z_i, W_i, \boldsymbol{y}_i, \boldsymbol{r}_i) \propto f(\boldsymbol{y}_i, \boldsymbol{r}_i | X_i, Z_i, W_i, \boldsymbol{\theta}, \boldsymbol{\psi}).$$

Because inference has to be based on what is observed, the full data likelihood L^* has to be replaced by the observed data likelihood L:

$$L(\boldsymbol{\theta}, \boldsymbol{\psi} | X_i, Z_i, W_i, \boldsymbol{y}_i, \boldsymbol{r}_i) \propto f(\boldsymbol{y}_i^o, \boldsymbol{r}_i | X_i, Z_i, W_i, \boldsymbol{\theta}, \boldsymbol{\psi})$$

with

$$\begin{aligned} f(\boldsymbol{y}_i^o, \boldsymbol{r}_i | \boldsymbol{\theta}, \boldsymbol{\psi}) &= \int f(\boldsymbol{y}_i, \boldsymbol{r}_i | X_i, Z_i, W_i, \boldsymbol{\theta}, \boldsymbol{\psi}) d\boldsymbol{y}_i^m \\ &= \int f(\boldsymbol{y}_i^o, \boldsymbol{y}_i^m | X_i, Z_i, \boldsymbol{\theta}) f(\boldsymbol{r}_i | \boldsymbol{y}_i^o, \boldsymbol{y}_i^m, W_i, \boldsymbol{\psi}) d\boldsymbol{y}_i^m. \end{aligned}$$

Under an MAR process, we obtain

$$\begin{aligned} f(\boldsymbol{y}_i^o, \boldsymbol{r}_i | \boldsymbol{\theta}, \boldsymbol{\psi}) &= \int f(\boldsymbol{y}_i^o, \boldsymbol{y}_i^m | X_i, Z_i, \boldsymbol{\theta}) f(\boldsymbol{r}_i | \boldsymbol{y}_i^o, W_i, \boldsymbol{\psi}) d\boldsymbol{y}_i^m \\ &= f(\boldsymbol{y}_i^o | X_i, Z_i, \boldsymbol{\theta}) f(\boldsymbol{r}_i | \boldsymbol{y}_i^o, W_i, \boldsymbol{\psi}), \end{aligned} \quad (26.14)$$

i.e., the likelihood factors into two components of the same functional form as the general factorization (26.3) of the complete data, in agreement with (26.12). If further $\boldsymbol{\theta}$ and $\boldsymbol{\psi}$ are disjoint in the sense that the parameter space of the full vector $(\boldsymbol{\theta}', \boldsymbol{\psi}')'$ is the product of the individual parameter spaces, then inference can be based on the marginal observed data density only. This technical requirement is referred to as the separability condition.

In conclusion, when the separability condition is satisfied, *within the likelihood framework*, ignorability is equivalent to the union of MAR and MCAR. A formal derivation is given in Rubin (1976), where it is also shown that the same requirements hold for Bayesian inference, but that frequentist inference is ignorable only under MCAR. Of course, it is possible that at least part of the scientific interest is directed toward the missingness process. Although one would then not ignore the missing data process, it is still advantageous to dispose of the convenient factorization (26.14), allowing to consider the measurement and missingness processes in turn.

However, still some caution should be used when constructing precision estimators. Indeed, although the correct maximum likelihood estimates and likelihood ratio statistics will be generated by the use of (26.14), some care needs to be taken with the choice of appropriate sampling distribution in a frequentist analysis. For this aspect the missing value mechanism is *not* ignorable, even under MAR (Kenward and Molenberghs 1998). In practice though there is little reason for worry since this just means that estimates of precision should be based on the observed rather than the expected information matrix.

Classical examples of the more stringent MCAR condition needed for frequentist methods are ordinary least squares and the generalized estimating equations approach (Chapter 8). These define an unbiased estimator only under MCAR. More recently it has been shown how non-likelihood approaches can be developed for the MAR case (Robins, Rotnitzky, and Zhao 1995, Robins, Rotnitzky, and Scharfstein 1998, Fitzmaurice, Molenberghs, and Lipsitz 1995). See also Chapter 27.

27
Simple Methods, Direct Likelihood, and Weighted Generalized Estimating Equations

27.1 Introduction

Commonly used methods to analyze incomplete longitudinal data include complete case analysis (CC) and last observation carried forward (LOCF). However, such methods rest on strong assumptions, including missing completely at random (MCAR). Such assumptions are too strong to generally hold. Over the past decades, a number of full longitudinal data analysis methods have become available, such as the linear, generalized linear, and non-linear mixed modeling frameworks, and the likelihood-based models of Chapters 6 and 7, that are valid under the much weaker missing at random (MAR) assumption. Such methods are useful, even if the scientific question is in terms of a single time point, e.g., the last planned measurement occasion in a clinical trial. The validity of such a method rests on the use of maximum likelihood, under which the missing data mechanism is ignorable as soon as MAR applies. Specific attention needs to be devoted to generalized estimating equations, given their non-likelihood status.

In many clinical trial and other settings, the standard methodology used to analyze incomplete longitudinal data is based on such methods as *last observation carried forward* (LOCF), *complete case analysis* (CC), or simple forms of imputation. This is often done without questioning the possible influence of these assumptions on the final results, even though several authors have written about this topic. A relatively early account is given in Heyting, Tolboom, and Essers (1992). Mallinckrodt *et al* (2003ab) and Lavori, Dawson, and Shera (1995) propose direct-likelihood and multiple-imputation methods, respectively, to deal with incomplete longitudinal data. Siddiqui and Ali (1998) compare direct-likelihood and LOCF methods.

It is unfortunate that such a strong emphasis is placed on methods like LOCF and CC in clinical trial settings, as they are based on strong and unrealistic assumptions. Even the strong MCAR assumption does not suffice to guarantee that an LOCF analysis is valid. In contrast, under the less restrictive assumption of MAR, valid inference can be obtained through a likelihood-based analysis without modeling the dropout process. One can then use linear or generalized linear mixed models (Verbeke and Molenberghs 2000, see also Chapter 4 in this volume), without additional complication or effort. We will argue that such an analysis is more likely to be valid, and even easier to implement than LOCF and CC analyses.

In Section 27.2, the status of longitudinal and non-longitudinal data analysis is briefly discussed in the context of incomplete longitudinal sequences. Section 27.3 reviews simple methods, with emphasis on CC and LOCF, and then goes on to advocate direct likelihood as an important and viable alternative. The bias that occurs in CC and LOCF is studied analytically, in the context of a specific and simple model, is studied in Section 27.4. The specific situation of generalized estimating equations is the topic of Section 27.5. The concepts developed in this chapter are then exemplified using a depression clinical trial (Section 27.6), the Age Related Macular Degeneration study (Section 27.7), which was introduced in Section 2.9 and analyzed before in Section 24.4, and finally the analgesic trial (Section 27.8), which has been analyzed before in Chapter 17 and Section 18.4.

27.2 Longitudinal Analysis or Not?

In principle, one should start by considering the density of the full data (26.2), but by the very nature of the missing data problem, parts of the outcome vector $\boldsymbol{Y}_i$ may be left unobserved, and hence one has to focus on the observed data only, i.e., $\boldsymbol{Y}_i^o$ and $\boldsymbol{R}_i$. Of course, when ignorability applies (Section 26.2.3), one can further ignore the missing data itself. As stated in the introduction, one often sees much simpler analyses, which often overlook the important issues altogether.

Whatever the perspective taken, it usually belongs to one of two possible views for the measurement model on the one hand and a philosophy adopted for the missingness model on the other hand. We will describe these in turn.

Model for measurements. A choice has to be made regarding the modeling approach to the measurements. Several views are possible.

View 1. One can choose to analyze the entire longitudinal profile, irrespective of whether interest focuses on the entire profile (e.g., difference in slope between groups) or on a specific time point (e.g., the last planned occasion). In the latter case, one would make inferences about such an occasion using the posited model.

View 2. One states the scientific question in terms of the outcome at a well-defined point in time. Several choices are possible:

View 2a. The scientific question is defined in terms of the *last planned occasion*. In this case, one can either accept the dropout as it is or use one or other strategy (e.g., imputation) to incorporate the missing outcomes.

View 2b. One can choose to define the question and the corresponding analysis in terms of the *last observed measurement*.

Although Views 1 and 2a necessitate reflection on the missing data mechanism, View 2b avoids the missing data problem because the question is couched completely in terms of observed measurements. Thus, under View 2b, an LOCF analysis might be acceptable, provided it matched the scientific goals, but is then better described as a last observation analysis because nothing is carried forward. Such an analysis should properly be combined with an analysis of time to dropout, perhaps in a survival analysis framework. Of course, an investigator should reflect very carefully on whether View 2b represents a relevant and meaningful scientific question (Shih and Quan 1997).

Method for handling missingness. A choice has to be made regarding the modeling approach for the missingness process. Under certain assumptions this process can be ignored (e.g., a likelihood-based ignorable analysis). Some simple methods, such as a complete case analysis and LOCF, do not explicitly address the missingness process either.

The measurement model will depend on whether or not a full longitudinal analysis is done. When the focus is on the last observed measurement or on the last measurement occasion only, one typically opts for classical two- or multi-group comparisons (*t*-test, Wilcoxon, etc.). When a longitudinal analysis is deemed necessary, the choice depends on the nature of the outcome. Options include the linear and generalized linear mixed models, generalized estimating equations, etc.

27.3 Simple Methods

We will briefly review a number of relatively simple methods that still are commonly used. For the validity of many of these methods, MCAR is required. For others, such as LOCF, MCAR is necessary but not sufficient.

The focus will be on the complete case method, for which data are removed, and on imputation strategies, where data are filled in. Regarding imputation, one distinguishes between single and multiple imputation. In the first case, a single value is substituted for every 'hole' in the dataset and the resulting dataset is analyzed as if it represented the true complete data. Multiple imputation acknowledges the uncertainty stemming from filling in missing values rather than observing them (Rubin 1987, Schafer 1997). LOCF will be discussed within the context of imputation strategies, although LOCF can be placed in other frameworks as well.

A **complete case analysis** includes only those cases for which all measurements were recorded. This method has obvious advantages. It is simple to describe and almost any software can be used because there are no missing data. Unfortunately, the method suffers from severe drawbacks. First, there is nearly always a substantial loss of information. For example, suppose there are 20 measurements, with 10% of missing data on each measurement. Suppose, further, that missingness on the different measurements is independent; then, the estimated percentage of incomplete observations is as high as 87%. The impact on precision and power may be dramatic. Even though the reduction of the number of complete cases will be less severe in settings where the missingness indicators are correlated, this loss of information will usually militate against a complete case analysis. Second, severe bias can result when the missingness mechanism is MAR but not MCAR. Indeed, should an estimator be consistent in the complete data problem, then the derived complete case analysis is consistent only if the missingness process is MCAR. A CC analysis can be conducted when Views 1 and 2 of Section 27.2 are adopted. It is obviously not a reasonable choice with View 2b.

An alternative way to obtain a data set on which complete data methods can be used is to fill in rather than delete (Little and Rubin 1987). Concern has been raised regarding imputation strategies. Dempster and Rubin (1983) write: "The idea of imputation is both seductive and dangerous. It is seductive because it can lull the user into the pleasurable state of believing that the data are complete after all, and it is dangerous because it lumps together situations where the problem is sufficiently minor that it can be legitimately handled in this way and situations where standard estimators applied to the real and imputed data have substantial biases." For example, Little and Rubin (1987) show that the application of imputation could be considered acceptable in a linear model with one fixed effect and one error term, but that it is generally not acceptable for hierarchical models, split-plot designs, repeated measures with a complicated error structure, random-effects, and mixed-effects models.

Thus, the user of imputation strategies faces several dangers. First, the imputation model could be wrong and, hence, the point estimates biased. Second, even for a correct imputation model, the uncertainty resulting from missingness is ignored. Indeed, even when one is reasonably sure about the mean value the unknown observation *would have had*, the actual stochastic realization, depending on both the mean and error structures, is still unknown. In addition, most methods require the MCAR assumption to hold while some even require additional and often unrealistically strong assumptions.

A method that has received considerable attention (Siddiqui and Ali 1998, Mallinckrodt *et al* 2003ab) is **last observation carried forward** (LOCF). In the LOCF method, whenever a value is missing, the last observed value is substituted. The technique can be applied to both monotone and non-monotone missing data. It is typically applied in settings where incompleteness is due to attrition.

LOCF can, but not necessarily has to, be regarded as an imputation strategy, depending on which of the views of Section 27.2 is taken. The choice of viewpoint has a number of consequences. First, when the problem is approached from a missing data standpoint, one has to think it plausible that subjects' measurements do not change from the moment of dropout onwards (or during the period they are unobserved in the case of intermittent missingness). In a clinical trial setting, one might believe that the response profile *changes* as soon as a patient goes off treatment and even that it would flatten. However, the constant profile assumption is even stronger. Second, LOCF shares with other single imputation methods that it artificially increases the amount of information in the data, by treating imputed and actually observed values on an equal footing. This is especially true if a longitudinal view is taken. Verbeke and Molenberghs (1997, Chapter 5) have shown that all features of a linear mixed model (group difference, evolution over time, variance structure, correlation structure, random effects structure, ...) can be affected.

Thus, scientific questions with which LOCF is compatible will be those that are phrased in terms of the last obtained measurement (View 2b). Whether or not such questions are sensible should be the subject of scientific debate, which is quite different from a *post hoc* rationale behind the use of LOCF. Likewise, it can be of interest to model the complete cases separately and to make inferences about them. In such cases, a CC analysis is of course the only reasonable way forward. This is fundamentally different from treating a CC analysis as one that can answer questions about the randomized population as a whole.

We will briefly describe two other imputation methods. The idea behind **unconditional mean imputation** (Little and Rubin 1987) is to replace a missing value with the average of the observed values on the same variable over the other subjects. Thus, the term *unconditional* refers to the fact that one does not use (i.e., condition on) information on the subject for which an imputation is generated. It is clear that this method is developed primarily for continuous data and its application to binary outcomes would be problematic. Because values are imputed that are unrelated to a subject's other measurements, all aspects of a model, such as a linear mixed model, are typically distorted (Verbeke and Molenberghs 1997). In this sense, unconditional mean imputation can be as damaging as LOCF.

Buck's method or **conditional mean imputation** (Buck 1960, Little and Rubin 1987) is similar in complexity to mean imputation. Consider, for example, a single multivariate normal sample. The first step is to estimate the mean vector $\boldsymbol{\mu}$ and the covariance matrix $\boldsymbol{\Sigma}$ from the complete cases, assuming that $\boldsymbol{Y} \sim N(\boldsymbol{\mu}, \boldsymbol{\Sigma})$. For a subject with missing components, the regression of the missing components $(\boldsymbol{Y}_i^m)$ on the observed ones $(\boldsymbol{y}_i^o)$ is

$$\boldsymbol{Y}_i^m | \boldsymbol{y}_i^o \sim N(\boldsymbol{\mu}^m + \boldsymbol{\Sigma}^{mo}(\boldsymbol{\Sigma}^{oo})^{-1}(\boldsymbol{y}_i^o - \boldsymbol{\mu}_i^o), \boldsymbol{\Sigma}^{mm} - \boldsymbol{\Sigma}^{mo}(\boldsymbol{\Sigma}^{oo})^{-1}\boldsymbol{\Sigma}^{om}).$$

The second step calculates the conditional mean from the regression of the missing components on the observed components, and substitutes the conditional mean for the corresponding missing values. In this way, "vertical" information (estimates for $\boldsymbol{\mu}$ and $\boldsymbol{\Sigma}$) is combined with "horizontal" information $(\boldsymbol{y}_i^o)$. Buck (1960) showed that under mild conditions, the method is valid under MCAR mechanisms. Little and Rubin (1987) added that the method is also valid under certain MAR mechanisms. Even though the distribution of the observed components is allowed to differ between complete and incomplete observations, it is very important that the regression of the missing components on the observed ones is constant across missingness patterns. Again, this method shares with other single imputation strategies that, although point estimation may be consistent, the precision will be overestimated. There is a connection between *the concept* of conditional mean imputation and a likelihood-based ignorable analysis, in the sense that the latter analysis produces expectations for the missing observations that are formally equal to those obtained under conditional mean imputation. However, in likelihood-based ignorable analyses, no explicit imputation takes place, hence the amount of information in the data is not overestimated and important model elements, such as mean structure and variance components, are not distorted.

Historically, an important motivation behind the simpler methods was their simplicity. Currently, with the availability of commercial software tools such as, for example, the SAS procedures MIXED, GLIMMIX, and NLMIXED and the SPlus and R nlme libraries, this motivation no longer applies. Arguably, an MAR analysis is the preferred choice. Of course, the correctness of an MAR analysis is in its own right never completely verifiable. Purely resorting to MNAR analyses (Chapters 29 and 30) is not satisfactory either since important sensitivity issues (Chapter 31) then arise. See also Verbeke and Molenberghs (2000).

27.4 Bias in LOCF, CC, and Ignorable Likelihood Methods

It is often quoted that LOCF or CC, though problematic for parameter estimation, produce randomization-valid hypothesis testing, but this is questionable. First, in a CC analysis partially observed data are selected out, with probabilities that may depend on post-randomization outcomes, thereby undermining any randomization justification. Second, if the focus is on one particular time point, e.g., the last one scheduled, then LOCF plugs in data. Such imputations, apart from artificially inflating the information content, may deviate in complicated ways from the underlying data. In contrast, a likelihood-based MAR analysis uses all available data, with the need for neither deletion nor imputation, which suggests that a likelihood-based MAR analysis would usually be the preferred one for testing as well. Third, although the size of a randomization-based LOCF test may reach its nominal size under the null hypothesis of no difference in treatment profiles, there will be other regions of the alternative space where the power of the LOCF test procedure is equal to its size, which is completely unacceptable.

Using the simple but insightful setting of two repeated follow-up measures, the first of which is always observed while the second can be missing, we establish some properties of the LOCF and CC estimation procedures under different missing data mechanisms, against the background of an MAR process operating. In this way, we bring LOCF and CC within a general framework that makes clear their relationships with more formal modeling approaches, enabling us to make a coherent comparison among the different approaches. The use of a moderate amount of algebra leads to some interesting conclusions.

It is most convenient to consider continuous outcomes, although similar arguments hold for non-Gaussian outcomes as well. Let us assume each subject i is to be measured on two occasions $t_i = 0, 1$. Subjects are randomized to one of two treatment arms: $T_i = 0$ for the standard arm and $T_i = 1$ for the experimental arm. The probability of an observation being observed on the second occasion ($D_i = 2$) is p_0 and p_1 for treatment groups 0 and 1, respectively. We can write the means of the observations in the two dropout groups as follows:

$$\text{dropouts } D_i = 1 \;:\; \beta_0 + \beta_1 T_i + \beta_2 t_i + \beta_3 T_i t_i, \tag{27.1}$$

$$\text{completers } D_i = 2 \;:\; \gamma_0 + \gamma_1 T_i + \gamma_2 t_i + \gamma_3 T_i t_i. \tag{27.2}$$

The true underlying population treatment difference at time $t_i = 1$, as determined from (27.1)–(27.2), is equal to:

$$\begin{aligned}\Delta_{\text{true}} =\;& p_1(\gamma_0 + \gamma_1 + \gamma_2 + \gamma_3) + (1 - p_1)(\beta_0 + \beta_1 + \beta_2 + \beta_3) \\ & - [p_0(\gamma_0 + \gamma_2) + (1 - p_0)(\beta_0 + \beta_2)]. \end{aligned} \tag{27.3}$$

If we use LOCF, the expectation of the corresponding estimator equals:

$$\Delta_{\text{LOCF}} = p_1(\gamma_0 + \gamma_1 + \gamma_2 + \gamma_3) + (1-p_1)(\beta_0 + \beta_1)$$
$$- [p_0(\gamma_0 + \gamma_2) + (1-p_0)\beta_0]. \qquad (27.4)$$

Alternatively, if we use CC, the above expression changes to:

$$\Delta_{\text{CC}} = \gamma_1 + \gamma_3. \qquad (27.5)$$

Hence, in general, both procedures yield biased estimators.

We will now consider the special but important cases where the true missing data mechanisms are MCAR and MAR, respectively. Each of these will impose particular constraints on the β and γ parameters in Model (27.1)–(27.2). Under MCAR, the β parameters are equal to their γ counterparts and (27.3) simplifies to

$$\Delta_{\text{MCAR,true}} = \beta_1 + \beta_3 \equiv \gamma_1 + \gamma_3. \qquad (27.6)$$

Suppose we apply the LOCF procedure in this setting, the expectation of the resulting estimator then simplifies to:

$$\Delta_{\text{MCAR,LOCF}} = \beta_1 + (p_1 - p_0)\beta_2 + p_1 \beta_3. \qquad (27.7)$$

The bias is given by the difference between (27.6) and (27.7):

$$B_{\text{MCAR,LOCF}} = (p_1 - p_0)\beta_2 - (1-p_1)\beta_3. \qquad (27.8)$$

While of a simple form, we can learn several things from this expression by focusing on each of the terms in turn. First, suppose $\beta_3 = 0$ and $\beta_2 \neq 0$, implying that there is no differential treatment effect between the two measurement occasions, but there is an overall time trend. Then, the bias can go in either direction depending on the sign of $p_1 - p_0$ and the sign of β_2. Note that $p_1 = p_0$ only in the special case that the dropout rate is the same in both treatment arms. Whether or not this is the case has no impact on the status of the dropout mechanism (it is MCAR in either case, even though in the second case dropout is treatment-arm dependent), but is potentially very important for the bias implied by LOCF. Second, suppose $\beta_3 \neq 0$ and $\beta_2 = 0$. Again, the bias can go in either direction depending on the sign of β_3, i.e., depending on whether the treatment effect at the second occasion is larger or smaller than the treatment effect at the first occasion. In conclusion, even under the strong assumption of MCAR, we see that the bias in the LOCF estimator typically does not vanish and, even more importantly, the bias can be positive or negative and can even induce an apparent treatment effect when one does not exist.

In contrast, as can be seen from (27.5) and (27.6), the CC analysis is unbiased.

27.4 Bias in LOCF, CC, and Ignorable Likelihood

Let us now turn to the MAR case. In this setting, the constraint implied by the MAR structure of the dropout mechanism is that the conditional distribution of the second observation given the first is the same in both dropout groups (Molenberghs et al 1998). Based on this result, the expectation of the second observation in the standard arm of the dropout group is

$$E(Y_{i2}|D_i = 1, T_i = 0) = \gamma_0 + \gamma_2 + \sigma(\beta_0 - \gamma_0), \quad (27.9)$$

where $\sigma = \sigma_{21}\sigma_{11}^{-1}$, σ_{11} is the variance of the first observation in the fully observed group and σ_{12} is the corresponding covariance between the pair of observations. Similarly, in the experimental group we obtain

$$E(Y_{i2}|D_i = 1, T_i = 1) = \gamma_0 + \gamma_1 + \gamma_2 + \gamma_3 + \sigma(\beta_0 + \beta_1 - \gamma_0 - \gamma_1). \quad (27.10)$$

The true underlying population treatment difference (27.3) then becomes

$$\begin{aligned}\Delta_{\text{MAR,true}} &= \gamma_1 + \gamma_3 + \sigma[(1-p_1)(\beta_0 + \beta_1 - \gamma_0 - \gamma_1)\\ &\quad - (1-p_0)(\beta_0 - \gamma_0)].\end{aligned} \quad (27.11)$$

In this case, the bias in the LOCF estimator can be written as:

$$\begin{aligned}B_{\text{MAR,LOCF}} &= p_1(\gamma_0 + \gamma_1 + \gamma_2 + \gamma_3) + (1-p_1)(\beta_0 + \beta_1)\\ &\quad - p_0(\gamma_0 + \gamma_2) - (1-p_0)\beta_0 - \gamma_1 - \gamma_3\\ &\quad - \sigma[(1-p_1)(\beta_0 + \beta_1 - \gamma_0 - \gamma_1)\\ &\quad - (1-p_0)(\beta_0 - \gamma_0)].\end{aligned} \quad (27.12)$$

Again, although involving more complicated relationships, it is clear that the bias can go in either direction, thus contradicting the claim often put forward that the bias in LOCF leads to conservative conclusions. Further, it is far from clear what conditions need to be imposed in this setting for the corresponding estimator to be either unbiased or conservative.

The bias in the CC estimator case takes the form:

$$B_{\text{MAR,CC}} = -\sigma[(1-p_1)(\beta_0 + \beta_1 - \gamma_0 - \gamma_1) - (1-p_0)(\beta_0 - \gamma_0)]. \quad (27.13)$$

Even though this expression is simpler than in the LOCF case, it is still true that the bias can operate in either direction.

Thus, in all cases, LOCF typically produces bias of which the direction and magnitude depend on the true but unknown treatment effects. Hence, caution is needed when using this method. In contrast, an ignorable likelihood based analysis, as outlined in Section 27.3, provides a consistent estimator of the true treatment difference at the second occasion under both MCAR and MAR. Although this is an assumption, it is rather a mild one in contrast to the stringent conditions required to justify the LOCF method, even when the qualitative features of the bias are considered more important than the quantitative ones. Note that the LOCF method is not valid even under the strong MCAR condition, whereas the CC approach is valid under MCAR.

27.5 Weighted Generalized Estimating Equations

In the previous sections, in particular in the last one, it was shown that direct likelihood is a method of choice, due to the ease with which it can be implemented and the validity under MAR.

For categorical outcomes, as we have seen before, the GEE approach could be adopted. However, as Liang and Zeger (1986) pointed out, inferences with the GEE are valid only under the strong assumption that the data are missing completely at random (MCAR). To allow the data to be missing at random (MAR), Robins, Rotnitzky, and Zhao (1995) proposed a class of weighted estimating equations. These can be viewed as an extension of generalized estimating equations.

The idea of weighted generalized estimating equations (WGEE) is to weight each subject's measurements in the GEEs by the inverse probability that a subject drops out at that particular measurement occasion. Such a weight can be calculated as

$$\nu_{ij} \equiv P(D_i = j) = \prod_{k=2}^{j-1}[1 - P(R_{ik} = 0 | R_{i2} = \ldots = R_{i,k-1} = 1)] \times$$
$$P(R_{ij} = 0 | R_{i2} = \ldots = R_{i,j-1} = 1)^{I\{j \leq n_i\}} \quad (27.14)$$

if dropout occurs by time j or we reach the end of the measurement sequence, and

$$\nu_{ij} \equiv P(D_i = j) = \prod_{k=2}^{j}[1 - P(R_{ik} = 0 | R_{i2} = \ldots = R_{i,k-1} = 1)] \quad (27.15)$$

otherwise.

Recall that we partitioned $\boldsymbol{Y}_i$ into the unobserved components $\boldsymbol{Y}_i^m$ and the observed components $\boldsymbol{Y}_i^o$. Similarly, we can make the exact same partition of $\boldsymbol{\mu}_i$ into $\boldsymbol{\mu}_i^m$ and $\boldsymbol{\mu}_i^o$. In the weighted GEE approach, which is proposed to reduce possible bias of $\widehat{\boldsymbol{\beta}}$, the score equations to be solved are:

$$S(\boldsymbol{\beta}) = \sum_{i=1}^{N} W_i \frac{\partial \boldsymbol{\mu}_i}{\partial \boldsymbol{\beta}'} (A_i^{1/2} R_i A_i^{1/2})^{-1} (\boldsymbol{y}_i - \boldsymbol{\mu}_i) = \boldsymbol{0},$$

where W_i is a diagonal matrix with the elements of $\boldsymbol{\nu}_i$ along the diagonal, or

$$S(\boldsymbol{\beta}) = \sum_{i=1}^{N} \sum_{d=2}^{n_i+1} \frac{I(D_i = d)}{\nu_{id}} \frac{\partial \boldsymbol{\mu}_i(d)}{\partial \boldsymbol{\beta}'} (A_i^{1/2} R_i A_i^{1/2})^{-1}(d)(\boldsymbol{y}_i(d) - \boldsymbol{\mu}_i(d)) = \boldsymbol{0},$$

where $\boldsymbol{y}_i(d)$ and $\boldsymbol{\mu}_i(d)$ are the first $d-1$ elements of $\boldsymbol{y}_i$ and $\boldsymbol{\mu}_i$, respectively. We define

$$\frac{\partial \boldsymbol{\mu}_i}{\partial \boldsymbol{\beta}'}(d)$$

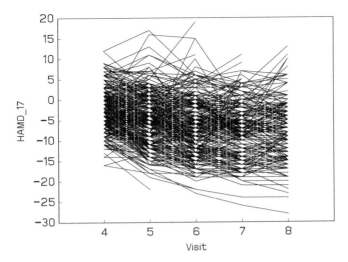

FIGURE 27.1. *Depression Trial. Individual profiles.*

and $(A_i^{1/2} R_i A_i^{1/2})^{-1}(d)$ analogously, in line with the definition of Robins, Rotnitzky and Zhao (1995).

Thus, not only likelihood methods but also appropriately adapted generalized estimating equations can be used with ease, under MAR. Both can be adapted to the MNAR setting as well (Chapters 29 and 30). Although it is beneficial to have both of these tools in one's toolkit, it is also important to realize that both 'schools' have strong supporters. An important discussion of these issues is given in Davidian, Tsiatis, and Leon (2005). Lipsitz *et al* (2001) studied bias in weighted estimating equations.

27.6 The Depression Trial

We will illustrate various methods discussed in this chapter by means of a clinical trial in depression, analyzed before by Molenberghs *et al* (2004), Jansen *et al* (2005), Dmitrienko *et al* (2005, Chapter 5), and Molenberghs *et al* (2005).

27.6.1 The Data

The depression trial data come from a clinical trial including 342 patients with post-baseline data. The Hamilton Depression Rating Scale ($HAMD_{17}$) is used to measure the depression status of the patients. For each patient, a baseline assessment is available.

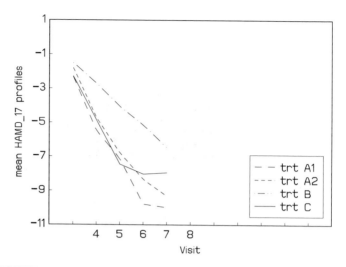

FIGURE 27.2. *Depression Trial. Mean profiles per treatment arm.*

For blinding purposes, therapies are coded as A1 for primary dose of experimental drug, A2 for secondary dose of experimental drug, and B and C for non-experimental drugs. Individual profiles and mean profiles of the changes from baseline in $HAMD_{17}$ scores per treatment arm are shown in Figures 27.1 and 27.2 respectively.

The contrast of primary interest is between A1 and C. Emphasis is on the difference between arms at the end of the study. A graphical representation of the dropout, per arm, is given in Figure 27.3. Part of the depression data set is given below. Therapies A1, A2, B, and C are denoted as treatment 1, 2, 3, and 4 respectively. Dots represent unobserved measurements.

We will focus on the analysis of the binary outcome, defined as 1 if the $HAMD_{17}$ score is larger than 7, and 0 otherwise. These analyses are in line with Jansen *et al* (2004), Dmitrienko *et al* (2005, Chapter 5), and Molenberghs *et al* (2005).

The primary null hypothesis will be tested using both GEE and WGEE, as well as GLMM. We include the fixed categorical effects of treatment, visit, and treatment-by-visit interaction, as well as the continuous, fixed covariates of baseline score and baseline score-by-visit interaction. A random intercept will be included when considering the random-effect models.

Analyses will be implemented using the SAS procedures GENMOD, GLIMMIX, and NLMIXED.

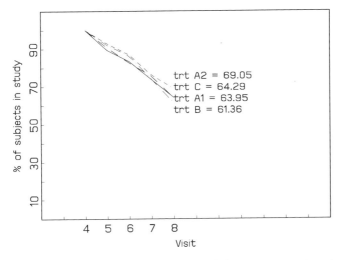

FIGURE 27.3. *Depression Trial. Evolution of dropout per treatment arm.*

27.6.2 Marginal Models

First, let us consider the GEE approach. Although we can consider both empirically corrected and model-based standard errors (Chapter 8), it is sensible to confine inferences to the empirically corrected ones. Several contrasts are of interest as well. The first one to test for treatment effect at the endpoint, the second one for the average treatment effect over the course of the study. Depending on the primary and secondary scientific questions, more of these can be considered. Both standard GEE (Section 8.2) as well as linearization-based GEE (Section 8.8) are considered. It will allow us to assess similarities and differences in this context, knowing how closely they agree from, for example, Chapter 8.

Of course, given the incomplete nature of the data, it is careful to consider weighted generalized estimating equations, unless one has strong belief that the MCAR assumption holds. This implies that weights have to be constructed, based on the probability to drop out at a given time, given the patient is still in the study, given his or her past measurements, and given covariates. We restrict attention to the previous outcome and treatment indicator. The resulting model is of a standard logistic regression or probit regression type, and can be easily fitted using standard logistic regression software, such as the SAS procedures GENMOD and LOGISTIC. The code is exemplified in Section 32.5. The result of fitting this logistic regression did not reveal strong evidence for a dependence on the previous outcome (estimate -0.097, s.e. 0.351), nor on the treatment allocation (estimate 0.065, s.e. 0.314).

TABLE 27.1. *Depression Trial. Results of marginal models: Parameter estimates (model-based standard errors; empirically corrected standard errors) for standard unweighted and weighted GEE (denoted GEE and WGEE, respectively) and the linearization based method (interaction terms are not shown).*

Effect	GEE	WGEE	Linearization
Intercept	-1.22 (0.77;0.79)	-0.56 (0.63;0.91)	-1.23 (0.75;0.79)
Treatment	-0.71 (0.38;0.38)	-0.91 (0.32;0.41)	-0.67 (0.37;0.38)
Visit 4	0.43 (1.05;1.22)	-0.15 (0.85;1.90)	0.45 (1.05;1.22)
Visit 5	-0.45 (0.91;1.23)	-0.23 (0.68;1.54)	-0.47 (0.92;1.23)
Visit 6	0.06 (0.86;1.03)	0.15 (0.69;1.13)	0.05 (0.86;1.03)
Visit 7	-0.25 (0.89;0.91)	-0.27 (0.78;0.89)	-0.25 (0.89;0.91)
Baseline	0.08 (0.04;0.04)	0.06 (0.03;0.05)	0.08 (0.04;0.04)

Results of fitting the standard GEE as well as weighted GEE, combined with the results of the linearization-based method, are presented in Table 27.1. Apart from treatment allocation, the effect of baseline value and indicators for time at visits 4, 5, 6, and 7 were included into the model. Further, the interactions between treatment and visit and between baseline and visit were included in the model.

Although GEE and its linearization based version produce very similar results, in line with earlier observations, there are differences with the weighted version, in parameter estimates as well as standard errors. The difference in standard errors (often, but not always, larger under WGEE) are explained by the fact that additional sources of uncertainty, due to missingness, are taken into account. The resulting inferences can be different. For example, the treatment effect parameter is non-significant with GEE ($p = 0.0633$ with standard GEE and $p = 0.1184$ with the linearized version) while a significant difference is found under the correct WGEE analysis ($p = 0.0268$). Also, the difference is marked for treatment effect at endpoint: $p = 0.0658$ with standard GEE and $p = 0.0631$ with the linearized version, while a significant difference is found under the correct WGEE analysis ($p = 0.0289$).

Thus, one may fail to detect such important effects as treatment differences when GEE is used rather than the, admittedly, somewhat more laborious WGEE.

27.6.3 Random-effects Models

Because the generalized linear mixed model is typically fitted using maximum likelihood, based on numerical integration or data approximations (Chapter 14), standard fitting algorithms can be used, without modification, provided the MAR assumption and the mild regularity conditions

TABLE 27.2. *Depression Trial. Results of random-effects model fitting. Parameter estimates (standard errors) for GLMM with adaptive Gaussian quadrature (Num. int.) and penalized-quasi likelihood methods (PQL) (interaction terms are not shown).*

Effect	PQL	Num. int.
Intercept	-1.70 (1.06)	-2.31 (1.34)
Treatment	-0.84 (0.55)	-1.20 (0.72)
Visit 4	0.66 (1.48)	0.64 (1.75)
Visit 5	-0.44 (1.29)	-0.78 (1.51)
Visit 6	0.17 (1.22)	0.19 (1.41)
Visit 7	-0.23 (1.25)	-0.27 (1.43)
Baseline	0.10 (0.06)	0.15 (0.07)
R.I. var.	2.53 (0.53)	5.71 (1.53)

for ignorability are fulfilled, as presented in Section 26.2.3. Dmitrienko et al (2005, Chapter 5) and Molenberghs et al (2005) have indicated that also here the choice between adaptive and non-adaptive quadrature, the number of quadrature points, and the choice between quasi-Newton and Newton-Raphson, has a noticeable impact on the results, where adaptive quadrature and Newton-Raphson iteration produce the most reliable results, with no difference in the parameter estimates and standard errors observed, whether 10, 20, or 50 quadrature points are used. These results are contrasted with PQL based estimates in Table 27.2.

Once again, there are considerable differences between both approaches, and the PQL estimates are rather close to the GEE estimates. This indicates that, though the method is in principle likelihood based, the poverty of the approximation jeopardizes its validity under MAR even more than when data are complete and, if at all possible, the numerical integration method ought to be the preferred one. Turning to the treatment effect, the treatment effect at endpoint is not significant in either of the analyses, but the difference in p-value is noticeable: $p = 0.0954$ for numerical integration and $p = 0.1286$ with PQL.

27.7 Age Related Macular Degeneration Trial

In Section 24.4 we considered a longitudinal analysis, jointly for the binary and continuous outcomes at 4, 12, 24, and 52 weeks, for the ARMD study introduced in Section 2.9. Results were reported in Table 24.7. All analyses done in Section 24.4 were based on 190 subjects with complete information at weeks 24 and 52. However, the total number of subjects equals 240, meaning that a substantial portion of the data is subject to missingness.

TABLE 27.3. *Age Related Macular Degeneration Trial. Overview of missingness patterns and the frequencies with which they occur. 'O' indicates observed and 'M' indicates missing.*

Measurement occasion					
4 wks	12 wks	24 wks	52 wks	Number	%
Completers					
O	O	O	O	188	78.33
Dropouts					
O	O	O	M	24	10.00
O	O	M	M	8	3.33
O	M	M	M	6	2.50
M	M	M	M	6	2.50
Non-monotone missingness					
O	O	M	O	4	1.67
O	M	M	O	1	0.42
M	O	O	O	2	0.83
M	O	M	M	1	0.42

Both intermittent missingness as well as dropout occurs. An overview is given in Table 27.3.

Thus, 78.33% of the profiles are complete, while 18.33% exhibit monotone missingness. Out of the latter group, 2.5% or 6 subjects have no follow-up measurements. The remaining 3.33%, representing 8 subjects, have intermittent missing values. Although the group of dropouts is of considerable magnitude, the ones with intermittent missingness is much smaller. Nevertheless, it is cautious to include all into the analyses. This is certainly possible for direct likelihood analyses and for standard GEE, but WGEE is more complicated in this respect. One solution is to monotonize the missingness patterns by means of multiple imputation (Section 28.2) and then conduct WGEE.

In the analysis of Section 24.4, 190 'completers' were used, even though Table 27.3 shows there are 188 completers only. However, the analyses in Section 24.4 were done on subjects with measurements at weeks 24 and 52. The table shows that these can come from either profile 'OOOO,' the completers, but also from 'MOOO,' thus amounting to $188 + 2 = 190$ subjects.

Analogous to the analysis presented in Section 27.6, and inspired by the model for the binary data reported in Table 24.4, we compare analyses performed on the completers only (CC), on the LOCF imputed data, as well as on the observed data. In all cases, standard GEE, and linearization-based GEE will be considered. For the observed, partially incomplete data,

27.7 Age Related Macular Degeneration Trial

GEE is supplemented with WGEE. Further, a random-intercepts GLMM is considered, based on both PQL and numerical integration. The GEE analyses are reported in Table 27.4 and the random-effects models in Table 27.6. In all cases, we use the logit link. For GEE, a working exchangeable correlation matrix is considered. The model has four intercepts and four treatment effects. The advantage of having separate treatment effects at each time is that particular attention can be given at the treatment effect assessment at the last planned measurement occasion, i.e., after one year. From Table 27.4 it is clear that there is very little difference between the standard GEE and linearization-based GEE results. This is undoubtedly the case for CC, LOCF, and unweighted GEE on the observed data. For these three cases, also the model-based and empirically corrected standard errors agree extremely well. This is due to the unstructured nature of the full time by treatment mean structure. However, we do observe differences in the WGEE analyses. Not only are the parameter estimates mildly different between the two GEE versions, there is a dramatic difference between the model-based and empirically corrected standard errors. This is entirely due to the weighting scheme. The weights were not calibrated to add up to the total sample size, which is reflected in the model-based standard errors. In the linearization case, part of the effect is captured as overdispersion. This can be seen from adding the parameters σ^2 and τ^2. In all other analyses, the sum is close to one, as it should be when there is no residual overdispersion, but in the last column these add up to 3.14. Nevertheless, the two sets of empirically corrected standard errors agree very closely, which is reassuring.

When comparing parameter estimates across CC, LOCF, and observed data analyses, it is clear that LOCF has the effect of artificially increasing the correlation between measurements. The effect is mild in this case. The parameter estimates of the observed-data GEE are close to the LOCF results for earlier time points and close to CC for later time points. This is to be expected, as at the start of the study the LOCF and observed populations are virtually the same, with the same holding between CC and observed populations near the end of the study. Note also that the treatment effect under LOCF, especially at 12 weeks and after 1 year, is biased downward in comparison to the GEE analyses. To properly use the information in the missingness process, WGEE can be used. To this end, a logistic regression for dropout, given covariates and previous outcomes, needs to be fitted. Parameter estimates and standard errors are given in Table 27.5. Intermittent missingness will be ignored. Covariates of importance are treatment assignment, the level of lesions at baseline (a four-point categorical variable, for which three dummies are needed), and time at which dropout occurs. For the latter covariates, there are three levels, since dropout can occur at times 2, 3, or 4. Hence, two dummy variables are included. Finally, the previous outcome does not have a significant impact, but will be kept in the model nevertheless. In spite of there being

TABLE 27.4. *Age Related Macular Degeneration Trial. Parameter estimates (model-based standard errors; empirically corrected standard errors) for the marginal models: standard and linearization-based GEE on the CC and LOCF population, and on the observed data. In the latter case, also WGEE is used.*

Effect	Par.	CC	LOCF	Observed data Unweighted	WGEE
			Standard GEE		
Int.4	β_{11}	-1.01(0.24;0.24)	-0.87(0.20;0.21)	-0.87(0.21;0.21)	-0.98(0.10;0.44)
Int.12	β_{21}	-0.89(0.24;0.24)	-0.97(0.21;0.21)	-1.01(0.21;0.21)	-1.78(0.15;0.38)
Int.24	β_{31}	-1.13(0.25;0.25)	-1.05(0.21;0.21)	-1.07(0.22;0.22)	-1.11(0.15;0.33)
Int.52	β_{41}	-1.64(0.29;0.29)	-1.51(0.24;0.24)	-1.71(0.29;0.29)	-1.72(0.25;0.39)
Tr.4	β_{12}	0.40(0.32;0.32)	0.22(0.28;0.28)	0.22(0.28;0.28)	0.80(0.15;0.67)
Tr.12	β_{22}	0.49(0.31;0.31)	0.55(0.28;0.28)	0.61(0.29;0.29)	1.87(0.19;0.61)
Tr.24	β_{32}	0.48(0.33;0.33)	0.42(0.29;0.29)	0.44(0.30;0.30)	0.73(0.20;0.52)
Tr.52	β_{42}	0.40(0.38;0.38)	0.34(0.32;0.32)	0.44(0.37;0.37)	0.74(0.31;0.52)
Corr.	ρ	0.39	0.44	0.39	0.33
			Linearization-based GEE		
Int.4	β_{11}	-1.01(0.24;0.24)	-0.87(0.21;0.21)	-0.87(0.21;0.21)	-0.98(0.18;0.44)
Int.12	β_{21}	-0.89(0.24;0.24)	-0.97(0.21;0.21)	-1.01(0.22;0.21)	-1.78(0.26;0.42)
Int.24	β_{31}	-1.13(0.25;0.25)	-1.05(0.21;0.21)	-1.07(0.23;0.22)	-1.19(0.25;0.38)
Int.52	β_{41}	-1.64(0.29;0.29)	-1.51(0.24;0.24)	-1.71(0.29;0.29)	-1.81(0.39;0.48)
Tr.4	β_{12}	0.40(0.32;0.32)	0.22(0.28;0.28)	0.22(0.29;0.28)	0.80(0.26;0.67)
Tr.12	β_{22}	0.49(0.31;0.31)	0.55(0.28;0.28)	0.61(0.28;0.29)	1.85(0.32;0.64)
Tr.24	β_{32}	0.48(0.33;0.33)	0.42(0.29;0.29)	0.44(0.30;0.30)	0.98(0.33;0.60)
Tr.52	β_{42}	0.40(0.38;0.38)	0.34(0.32;0.32)	0.44(0.37;0.37)	0.97(0.49;0.65)
	σ^2	0.62	0.57	0.62	1.29
	τ^2	0.39	0.44	0.39	1.85
Corr.	ρ	0.39	0.44	0.39	0.59

no strong evidence for MAR, the results between GEE and WGEE differ quite a bit. It is noteworthy that at 12 weeks, a treatment effect is observed with WGEE which goes unnoticed with the other marginal analyses. This finding is mildly confirmed by the random-intercept model, when the data as observed are used.

The results for the random-intercept models are given in Table 27.6. We observe the usual downward bias in the PQL *versus* numerical integration analysis, as well as the usual relationship between the marginal parameters of Table 27.4 and their random-effects counterparts. Note also that the random-intercepts variance is largest under LOCF, underscoring again that this method artificially increases the association between measurements on the same subject. In this case, unlike for the marginal models, LOCF and in fact also CC, slightly to considerably overestimates the treatment effect at certain times, in particular at 4 and 24 weeks.

TABLE 27.5. *Age Related Macular Degeneration Trial. Parameter estimates (standard errors) for a logistic regression model to describe dropout.*

Effect	Parameter	Estimate (s.e.)
Intercept	ψ_0	0.14 (0.49)
Previous outcome	ψ_1	0.04 (0.38)
Treatment	ψ_2	-0.86 (0.37)
Lesion level 1	ψ_{31}	-1.85 (0.49)
Lesion level 2	ψ_{32}	-1.91 (0.52)
Lesion level 3	ψ_{33}	-2.80 (0.72)
Time 2	ψ_{41}	-1.75 (0.49)
Time 3	ψ_{42}	-1.38 (0.44)

27.8 The Analgesic Trial

The binary satisfaction outcome in the analgesic trial (Section 2.2) was given extensive treatment in Chapter 17 and its ordinal counterpart was studied in Section 18.4. An important feature of the data is that a subgroup of patients does not complete the study but rather leaves prior to the scheduled end of the trial. Out of the 491 patients available for analysis, 223 are complete, and there are 55, 54, and 63 dropouts after the third, second, and first visit, respectively. Further, 96 patients have no follow up measurements. Among these, 63 have intermediate missing values as well. To further illustrate the impact of missingness on generalized estimating equations, we will conduct an analysis on the monotone sequences, with both ordinary and weighted generalized estimating equations, using the same marginal model (17.2) as fitted in Chapter 17.

A logistic regression is built for the dropout indicator, in terms of the previous outcome (for which the ordinal version is used by means of 4 dummies), pain control assessment at baseline, physical functioning at baseline, and genetic disorder measured at baseline. All of these are significant and parameter estimates are given in Table 27.7. This implies that there is evidence against MCAR in favor of MAR. This is a stronger result than observed in Section 27.6.2 for the depression trial.

In agreement with the procedure outlined in Section 27.5 and as illustrated on the depression trial, the predicted probabilities from this logistic regression are then used to calculate the weights, to be used in weighted GEE. Parameter estimates and standard errors for these are presented in Table 27.8. Clearly, though the evidence against MCAR is strong, the effect of the method chosen is noticeable but not terribly strong. We also note the impact on the standard errors. Weighted analyses are typically less precise, but more correct, than unweighted ones. Correction for the missingness mechanism has the effect of reducing the magnitude of the pa-

TABLE 27.6. *Age Related Macular Degeneration Trial. Parameter estimates (standard errors) for the random-intercept models: PQL and numerical-integration based fits on the CC and LOCF population, and on the observed data (direct-likelihood).*

Effect	Parameter	CC	LOCF	Direct lik.
		PQL		
Int.4	β_{11}	-1.19(0.31)	-1.05(0.28)	-1.00(0.26)
Int.12	β_{21}	-1.05(0.31)	-1.18(0.28)	-1.19(0.28)
Int.24	β_{31}	-1.35(0.32)	-1.30(0.28)	-1.26(0.29)
Int.52	β_{41}	-1.97(0.36)	-1.89(0.31)	-2.02(0.35)
Trt.4	β_{12}	0.45(0.42)	0.24(0.39)	0.22(0.37)
Trt.12	β_{22}	0.58(0.41)	0.68(0.38)	0.71(0.37)
Trt.24	β_{32}	0.55(0.42)	0.50(0.39)	0.49(0.39)
Trt.52	β_{42}	0.44(0.47)	0.39(0.42)	0.46(0.46)
R.I. s.d.	τ	1.42(0.14)	1.53(0.13)	1.40(0.13)
R.I. var.	τ^2	2.03(0.39)	2.34(0.39)	1.95(0.35)
		Numerical integration		
Int.4	β_{11}	-1.73(0.42)	-1.63(0.39)	-1.50(0.36)
Int.12	β_{21}	-1.53(0.41)	-1.80(0.39)	-1.73(0.37)
Int.24	β_{31}	-1.93(0.43)	-1.96(0.40)	-1.83(0.39)
Int.52	β_{41}	-2.74(0.48)	-2.76(0.44)	-2.85(0.47)
Trt.4	β_{12}	0.64(0.54)	0.38(0.52)	0.34(0.48)
Trt.12	β_{22}	0.81(0.53)	0.98(0.52)	1.00(0.49)
Trt.24	β_{32}	0.77(0.55)	0.74(0.52)	0.69(0.50)
Trt.52	β_{42}	0.60(0.59)	0.57(0.56)	0.64(0.58)
R.I. s.d.	τ	2.19(0.27)	2.47(0.27)	2.20(0.25)
R.I. var.	τ^2	4.80(1.17)	6.08(1.32)	4.83(1.11)

rameter estimates. In both cases, unstructured working assumptions were used. There is a noticeable effect on the working correlation matrix as well. With GEE, we obtain

$$R_{\text{UN, GEE}} = \begin{pmatrix} 1 & 0.173 & 0.246 & 0.201 \\ & 1 & 0.177 & 0.113 \\ & & 1 & 0.456 \\ & & & 1 \end{pmatrix},$$

TABLE 27.7. *Analgesic Trial. Parameter estimates (standard errors) for a logistic regression model to describe dropout.*

Effect	Parameter	Estimate (s.e.)
Intercept	ψ_0	-1.80 (0.49)
Previous GSA= 1	ψ_{11}	-1.02 (0.41)
Previous GSA= 2	ψ_{12}	-1.04 (0.38)
Previous GSA= 3	ψ_{13}	-1.34 (0.37)
Previous GSA= 4	ψ_{14}	-0.26 (0.38)
Basel. PCA	ψ_2	0.25 (0.10)
Phys. func.	ψ_3	0.009 (0.004)
Genetic disfunc.	ψ_4	0.59 (0.24)

TABLE 27.8. *Analgesic Trial. Parameter estimates (empirically corrected standard errors) for standard GEE and weighted GEE (WGEE) fitted to the monotone sequences.*

Effect	Parameter	GEE	WGEE
Intercept	β_1	2.95 (0.47)	2.17 (0.69)
Time	β_2	-0.84 (0.33)	-0.44 (0.44)
Time^2	β_3	0.18 (0.07)	0.12 (0.09)
Basel. PCA	β_4	-0.24 (0.10)	-0.16 (0.13)

whereas the WGEE version is

$$R_{\text{UN, WGEE}} = \begin{pmatrix} 1 & 0.215 & 0.253 & 0.167 \\ & 1 & 0.196 & 0.113 \\ & & 1 & 0.409 \\ & & & 1 \end{pmatrix}.$$

Of course, in line with general warnings issued in Section 8.2, care should be taken with interpreting the working correlation structure. In principle, it is a set of nuisance parameters, merely included to obtain reasonably efficient GEE estimates.

28
Multiple Imputation and the Expectation-Maximization Algorithm

28.1 Introduction

In Section 27.4, we have suggested direct likelihood as a preferred mode for analyzing incomplete (longitudinal) data, when the MAR assumption is deemed plausible. Two alternative methods are multiple imputation (MI) and the expectation-maximization (EM) algorithm. We will consider these in turn (Sections 28.2 and 28.3) and indicate the relative use of these methods next to direct likelihood in Section 28.4. The methods will be exemplified in Section 28.5 using the Age Related Macular Degeneration study, introduced in Section 2.9 and analyzed before in Sections 24.4 and 27.7.

28.2 Multiple Imputation

Multiple imputation (MI) was formally introduced by Rubin (1978). Rubin (1987) provides a comprehensive treatment. Several other sources, such as Rubin and Schenker (1986), Little and Rubin (1987), Tanner and Wong (1987), and Schafer's (1997) book give excellent and easy-to-read descriptions of the technique.

The key idea of the multiple imputation procedure is to replace each missing value with a set of M plausible values, i.e., values "drawn" from the distribution of one's data, that represent the uncertainty about the right value to impute. The imputed datasets are then analyzed by using standard procedures for complete data and combining the results from these analyses. Multiple imputation, at least in its basic form, requires the missingness mechanism to be MAR. However, the technique has been applied in MNAR settings as well (Thijs et al 2002). A number of variations to the theme have been developed. For example, Aerts et al (2002) developed a local multiple imputation method and Lipsitz, Zhao, and Molenberghs (1998) proposed a semi-parametric multiple imputation approach.

Multiple imputation involves three distinct phases or, using Rubin's (1987) terminology, tasks:

1. The missing values are filled in M times to generate M complete data sets.

2. The M complete data sets are analyzed by using standard procedures.

3. The results from the M analyses are combined into a single inference.

It is worth to note that the first and third tasks can be conducted by the SAS procedures MI and MIANALYZE, respectively. The second task is performed using one of the standard data analytic procedures.

28.2.1 Theoretical Justification

Suppose we have a sample of N, i.i.d. $n \times 1$ random vectors $\boldsymbol{Y}_i$. Our interest lies in estimating some parameter vector $\boldsymbol{\theta}$ of the distribution of $\boldsymbol{Y}_i$. Multiple imputation fills in the missing data $\boldsymbol{Y}^m$ using the observed data $\boldsymbol{Y}^o$, several times, and then the completed data are used to estimate $\boldsymbol{\theta}$.

If we knew the distribution of $\boldsymbol{Y}_i = (\boldsymbol{Y}_i^o, \boldsymbol{Y}_i^m)$, with parameter vector $\boldsymbol{\theta}$, then we would be able to impute $\boldsymbol{Y}_i^m$ by drawing a value of $\boldsymbol{Y}_i^m$ from the conditional distribution

$$f(\boldsymbol{y}_i^m | \boldsymbol{y}_i^o, \boldsymbol{\theta}).$$

The objective of the imputation process is to sample from this true predictive distribution. Because we do not know $\boldsymbol{\theta}$, we must estimate it from the data, say $\widehat{\boldsymbol{\theta}}$, and use

$$f(\boldsymbol{y}_i^m | \boldsymbol{y}_i^o, \widehat{\boldsymbol{\theta}})$$

to impute the missing data. Frequentists sometimes favor incorporating uncertainty in $\boldsymbol{\theta}$ in the multiple imputation scheme using bootstrap or other methods. However, in Bayesian terms, $\boldsymbol{\theta}$ is a random variable, in which the distribution is a function of the data, so we must account for its uncertainty. The Bayesian approach relies on integrating over $\widehat{\boldsymbol{\theta}}$, which provides a more natural and unifying framework for accounting for the uncertainty in $\boldsymbol{\theta}$. Thus, $\boldsymbol{\theta}$ is a random variable with mean equal to the estimated $\widehat{\boldsymbol{\theta}}$ from the data. Given this distribution, using multiple imputation, we first draw a random $\boldsymbol{\theta}^*$ from the distribution of $\boldsymbol{\theta}$, and then put this $\boldsymbol{\theta}^*$ in to draw a random $\boldsymbol{Y}_i^m$ from

$$f(\boldsymbol{y}_i^m | \boldsymbol{y}_i^o, \boldsymbol{\theta}^*).$$

The imputation algorithm is as follows:

1. Draw $\boldsymbol{\theta}^*$ from the distribution of $\boldsymbol{\theta}$.
2. Draw $\boldsymbol{Y}_i^{m*}$ from $f(\boldsymbol{y}_i^m|\boldsymbol{y}_i^o,\boldsymbol{\theta}^*)$.
3. To estimate a parameter of interest, $\boldsymbol{\beta}$ say, we then calculate the estimate of the parameter of interest, and its estimated variance, using the completed data, $(\boldsymbol{Y}^o, \boldsymbol{Y}^{m*})$:

$$\widehat{\boldsymbol{\beta}} = \widehat{\boldsymbol{\beta}}(\boldsymbol{Y}) = \widehat{\boldsymbol{\beta}}(\boldsymbol{Y}^o, \boldsymbol{Y}^{m*}),$$

and the *within* imputation variance is $\boldsymbol{U} = \widehat{\text{var}}(\widehat{\boldsymbol{\beta}})$.

4. Repeat steps 1, 2, and 3 a number of M times, producing $\widehat{\boldsymbol{\beta}}^m$ and $\boldsymbol{U}^m$, for $m = 1, ..., M$.

Steps 1 and 2 are referred to as the *Imputation Task*. Step 3 is the *Estimation Task*.

28.2.2 Pooling Information

Of course, one needs to combine the M inferences into a single one. In this section, we will discuss parameter and precision estimation and defer hypothesis testing to the next section.

When data would be complete, suppose that inference about the parameter $\boldsymbol{\beta}$ is made by

$$(\boldsymbol{\beta} - \widehat{\boldsymbol{\beta}}) \sim N(\boldsymbol{0}, \boldsymbol{U}).$$

The M within-imputation estimates for $\boldsymbol{\beta}$ are pooled to give the multiple imputation estimate

$$\widehat{\boldsymbol{\beta}}^* = \frac{\sum_{m=1}^M \widehat{\boldsymbol{\beta}}^m}{M}.$$

Further, one can make normal-based inferences for $\boldsymbol{\beta}$ based upon

$$(\boldsymbol{\beta} - \widehat{\boldsymbol{\beta}}^*) \sim N(\boldsymbol{0}, \boldsymbol{V}),$$

where

$$\boldsymbol{V} = \boldsymbol{W} + \left(\frac{M+1}{M}\right)\boldsymbol{B},$$

$$\boldsymbol{W} = \frac{\sum_{m=1}^M \boldsymbol{U}^m}{M}$$

is the average within imputation variance, and

$$\boldsymbol{B} = \frac{\sum_{m=1}^M (\widehat{\boldsymbol{\beta}}^m - \widehat{\boldsymbol{\beta}}^*)(\widehat{\boldsymbol{\beta}}^m - \widehat{\boldsymbol{\beta}}^*)'}{M-1}$$

is the *between* imputation variance (Rubin, 1987).

28.2.3 Hypothesis Testing

In case of multiple imputation, the asymptotic results and hence the χ^2 reference distributions do not only depend on the sample size N, but also on the number of imputations M. Therefore, Li, Raghunathan, and Rubin (1991) propose the use of an F reference distribution. To test the hypothesis $H_0 : \boldsymbol{\theta} = \boldsymbol{\theta}_0$, they advocate the following method to calculate p-values:

$$p = P(F_{k,w} > F),$$

where k is the length of the parameter vector $\boldsymbol{\theta}$, $F_{k,w}$ is an F random variable with k numerator and w denominator degrees of freedom, and

$$F = \frac{(\boldsymbol{\theta}^* - \boldsymbol{\theta}_0)' W^{-1} (\boldsymbol{\theta}^* - \boldsymbol{\theta}_0)}{k(1+r)},$$

$$w = 4 + (\tau - 4)\left[1 + \frac{(1 - 2\tau^{-1})}{r}\right]^2,$$

$$r = \frac{1}{k}\left(1 + \frac{1}{M}\right)\mathrm{tr}(BW^{-1}),$$

$$\tau = k(M-1).$$

Here, r is the average relative increase in variance due to nonresponse across the components of $\boldsymbol{\theta}$. The limiting behavior of this F variable is that if $M \to \infty$, then the reference distribution of F approaches an $F_{k,\infty} = \chi^2/k$ distribution.

Clearly, this procedure is not only applicable when the full vector $\boldsymbol{\theta}$, but also when one component, a subvector, or a set of linear contrasts, is the subject of hypothesis testing. In case of a subvector, or as a special case one component, we use the corresponding submatrices of B and W in the formulas. For a set of linear contrasts $L\boldsymbol{\beta}$, one should use the appropriately transformed covariance matrices: $\tilde{W} = LWL'$, $\tilde{B} = LBL'$, and $\tilde{V} = LVL'$.

28.2.4 Efficiency

Multiple imputation is attractive because it can be highly efficient even for small values of M. In many applications, merely 3–5 imputations are sufficient to obtain excellent results. Rubin (1987, p. 114) shows that the efficiency of an estimate based on M imputations is approximately

$$\left(1 + \frac{\gamma}{M}\right)^{-1},$$

where γ is the fraction of missing information for the quantity being estimated. The fraction γ quantifies how much more precise the estimate might

TABLE 28.1. *Relative efficiency (percentage) of multiple imputation estimation by number of imputations M and fraction of missing information γ.*

	\multicolumn{5}{c}{γ}				
m	0.1	0.3	0.5	0.7	0.9
2	95	87	80	74	69
3	97	91	86	81	77
5	98	94	91	88	85
10	99	97	95	93	92
20	100	99	98	97	96

have been if no data had been missing. The efficiencies achieved for various values of M and rates of missing information are shown in Table 28.1. This table shows that gains rapidly diminish after the first few imputations. In most situations there simply is little advantage to producing and analyzing more than a few imputed datasets.

28.2.5 Imputation Mechanisms

The method of choice to create the imputed datasets depends on the missing data pattern.

For monotone missing data patterns, either a parametric regression method that assumes multivariate normality or a nonparametric method that uses propensity scores is possible. For an arbitrary missing data pattern, a Markov chain Monte Carlo (MCMC) method (Schafer 1997) that assumes multivariate normality can be used. All of these have been implemented in the SAS procedure MI.

In the *regression method*, a regression model is fitted for each variable with missing values, with the previous variables as covariates. Based on the resulting model, a new regression model is then fitted and is used to impute the missing values for each variable (Rubin 1987). Because the dataset has a monotone missing data pattern, the process is repeated sequentially for variables with missing values.

The propensity score is the conditional probability of assignment to a particular treatment given a vector of observed covariates (Rosenbaum and Rubin 1983). In the *propensity score method*, a propensity score is generated for each variable with missing values to indicate the probability of observations being missing. The observations are then grouped based on these propensity scores, and an approximate Bayesian bootstrap imputation (Rubin 1987) is applied to each group. The propensity score method uses only the covariate information that is associated with whether the imputed variable values are missing. It does not use correlations among variables. It is effective for inferences about the distributions of individual imputed variables, but it is not appropriate for analyses involving relationship among variables.

Broadly, in statistical applications, MCMC is used to generate pseudo-random draws from multidimensional and otherwise intractable probability distributions via Markov chains. A Markov chain is a sequence of random variables in which the distribution of each element depends on the value of the previous one(s). In the *MCMC method*, one constructs a Markov chain long enough for the distribution of the elements to stabilize to a common distribution. This stationary distribution is the one of interest. By repeatedly simulating steps of the chain, draws from the distribution of interest are generated. In more detail, the MCMC method works as follows. Assume that the data arise from a multivariate normal distribution. In the first step, starting values need to be chosen. This can be done by computing a vector of means and a covariance matrix from the complete data. These are used to estimate the prior distribution, i.e., to estimate the parameters of the prior distributions for means and variances of the multivariate normal distribution with an informative prior. The next step is then the imputation step: values for missing data items are simulated by randomly selecting a value from the available distribution of values, i.e., the predictive distribution of missing values given the observed values. In the posterior step, the posterior distribution of the mean and covariance parameters is updated, by updating the parameters governing their distribution (e.g., the inverted Wishart distribution for the variance-covariance matrix and the normal distribution for the means). This is then followed by sampling from the posterior distribution of mean and covariance parameters, based on the updated parameters. The imputation and the posterior steps are then iterated until the distribution is stationary. This implies that the mean vector and covariance matrix are unchanged throughout the iterative process. Finally, we use the imputations from the final iteration to yield a data set that has no missing values.

28.3 The Expectation-Maximization Algorithm

This section deals with the expectation-maximization algorithm, popularly known as the EM algorithm. A specific version, for the context of mixture distributions, was presented in Section 23. It is an alternative to direct-likelihood in settings where the observed-data likelihood is complicated and/or difficult to access. Note that direct likelihood is within reach for many settings, including Gaussian and non-Gaussian longitudinal data, as proposed in Section 27.4. A perspective on when to use the various methods is given in Section 28.4.

The EM algorithm is a general-purpose iterative algorithm to find maximum likelihood estimates in parametric models for incomplete data. Within each iteration of the EM algorithm, there are two steps, called the expectation step, or E step, and the maximization step, or M step. The name EM algorithm was given by Dempster, Laird, and Rubin (1977), who provided a general and unified formulation of the EM algorithm, its basic properties, and many examples and applications of it. The books by Little and Rubin (1987), Schafer (1997), and McLachlan and Krishnan (1997) provide detailed descriptions and applications of the EM algorithm.

The fundamental idea behind the EM algorithm is to associate with the given incomplete-data problem, a complete-data problem for which maximum likelihood estimation is computationally more tractable. Starting from suitable initial parameter values, the E and M steps are repeated until convergence. Given a set of parameter estimates, such as the mean vector and covariance matrix for a multivariate normal setting, the E-step calculates the conditional expectation of the complete-data log-likelihood given the observed data and the parameter estimates. This step often reduces to calculating simple sufficient statistics. Given the complete-data log-likelihood, the M-step then finds the parameter estimates to maximize the complete-data log-likelihood from the E step.

An initial criticism was that the algorithm did not produce estimates of the covariance matrix of the maximum likelihood estimators. However, a number of developments have provided methods for such estimation (Louis 1982). Another issue is the slow convergence in certain cases. This has resulted in the development of modified versions of the algorithm as well as many simulation-based methods and other extensions of it (McLachlan and Krishnan 1997). As a matter of fact, precision estimation and speed of convergence are intimately linked, as both are based upon the matrix of second derivatives of the observed data likelihood, i.e., the Hessian matrix or, similarly, the information matrix.

The condition for the EM algorithm to be valid, in its basic form, is ignorability and hence MAR. The use of EM in the MNAR context is exemplified in Section 29.2.

28.3.1 The Algorithm

28.3.1.1 The Initial Step

Let $\boldsymbol{\theta}^{(0)}$ be an initial parameter vector, which can be found from, e.g., a complete case analysis, an available case analysis, or a simple method of imputation. Based on such a, possibly biased, estimate, the algorithm can then start.

28.3.1.2 The E Step

Given current values $\boldsymbol{\theta}^{(t)}$ for the parameters, the E step computes the objective function, which is in the case of the missing data problem equal to the expected value of the observed data loglikelihood, given the observed data and the current parameters

$$Q(\boldsymbol{\theta}|\boldsymbol{\theta}^{(t)}) = \int \ell(\boldsymbol{\theta}, \boldsymbol{Y}) f(\boldsymbol{Y}^m|\boldsymbol{Y}^o, \boldsymbol{\theta}^{(t)}) d\boldsymbol{Y}^m = E\left[\ell(\boldsymbol{\theta}|\boldsymbol{Y})|\boldsymbol{Y}^o, \boldsymbol{\theta}^{(t)}\right], (28.1)$$

i.e., substituting the expected value of $\boldsymbol{Y}^m$, given $\boldsymbol{Y}^o$ and $\boldsymbol{\theta}^{(t)}$. In some cases, this substitution can take place directly at the level of the data, but often it is sufficient to substitute only the function of $\boldsymbol{Y}^m$ appearing in the complete data log-likelihood. For exponential families, the E step reduces to the computation of complete data sufficient statistics.

28.3.1.3 The M Step

The M step determines $\boldsymbol{\theta}^{(t+1)}$, the parameter vector maximizing the log-likelihood of the imputed data (or the imputed log-likelihood). Formally, $\boldsymbol{\theta}^{(t+1)}$ satisfies

$$Q(\boldsymbol{\theta}^{(t+1)}|\boldsymbol{\theta}^{(t)}) \geq Q(\boldsymbol{\theta}|\boldsymbol{\theta}^{(t)}), \qquad \text{for all } \boldsymbol{\theta}.$$

One can show that the observed-data likelihood increases at every step. Because the log-likelihood is bounded from above, convergence is forced to apply.

The fact that the EM algorithm is guaranteed to converge to a, possibly local, maximum is a great advantage. However, a disadvantage is that this convergence is slow (linear or super-linear), and that precision estimates are not automatically provided.

28.3.2 Missing Information

In view of convergence monitoring, acceleration, and precision estimation, we will now turn attention to the principle of missing information. We use obvious notation for the observed and expected information matrices for the complete and observed data. Let

$$I(\boldsymbol{\theta}, Y^o) = \frac{\partial^2 \ln \ell(\boldsymbol{\theta})}{\partial \boldsymbol{\theta} \partial \boldsymbol{\theta}'}$$

be the matrix of the negative of the second-order partial derivatives of the (incomplete data) log-likelihood function with respect to the elements of $\boldsymbol{\theta}$, i.e., the observed information matrix for the observed data model. The expected information matrix for observed data model is termed $\mathcal{I}(\boldsymbol{\theta}, \boldsymbol{Y}^o)$. In analogy with the complete data $\boldsymbol{Y} = (\boldsymbol{Y}^o, \boldsymbol{Y}^m)$, we let $I_c(\boldsymbol{\theta}, \boldsymbol{Y})$ and $\mathcal{I}_c(\boldsymbol{\theta}, \boldsymbol{Y})$, be the observed and expected information matrices for the complete data model, respectively. Now, both likelihoods are connected via:

$$\ell(\boldsymbol{\theta}) = \ell_c(\boldsymbol{\theta}) - \ln \frac{f_c(y^0, y^m|\boldsymbol{\theta})}{f_c(y^0|\boldsymbol{\theta})} = \ell_c(\boldsymbol{\theta}) - \ln f(y^m|y^o, \boldsymbol{\theta}).$$

This equality carries over onto the information matrices:

$$I(\boldsymbol{\theta}, \boldsymbol{Y}^o) = I_c(\boldsymbol{\theta}, \boldsymbol{Y}) + \frac{\partial^2 \ln f(\boldsymbol{y}^m | \boldsymbol{y}^o, \boldsymbol{\theta})}{\partial \boldsymbol{\theta} \partial \boldsymbol{\theta}'}.$$

Taking expectation over $\boldsymbol{Y}|\boldsymbol{Y}^o = \boldsymbol{y}^o$ leads to

$$I(\boldsymbol{\theta}, \boldsymbol{y}^o) = \mathcal{I}_c(\boldsymbol{\theta}, \boldsymbol{y}^o) - \mathcal{I}_m(\boldsymbol{\theta}, \boldsymbol{y}^o),$$

where $\mathcal{I}_m(\boldsymbol{\theta}, \boldsymbol{y}^o)$ is the expected information matrix for $\boldsymbol{\theta}$ based on $\boldsymbol{Y}^m$ when conditioned on $\boldsymbol{Y}^o$. This information can be viewed as the 'missing information,' resulting from observing $\boldsymbol{Y}^o$ only and not also $\boldsymbol{Y}^m$. This leads to the *missing information principle*:

$$\mathcal{I}_c(\boldsymbol{\theta}, \boldsymbol{y}) = I(\boldsymbol{\theta}, \boldsymbol{y}) + \mathcal{I}_m(\boldsymbol{\theta}, \boldsymbol{y}),$$

which has the following interpretation: the (conditionally expected) complete information equals the observed information plus the missing information.

28.3.3 *Rate of Convergence*

The notion that the rate at which the EM algorithm converges depends upon the amount of missing information in the incomplete data compared to the hypothetical complete data, will be made explicit by deriving results regarding the rate of convergence in terms of information matrices (McLachlan and Krishnan 1997).

Under regularity conditions, the EM algorithm will converge linearly. By using a Taylor series expansion we can write

$$\boldsymbol{\theta}^{(t+1)} - \boldsymbol{\theta}^* \simeq J(\boldsymbol{\theta}^*)[\boldsymbol{\theta}^{(t)} - \boldsymbol{\theta}^*],$$

where $\boldsymbol{\theta}^*$ is the parameter vector value for which the likelihood attains its maximum. Thus, in a neighborhood of $\boldsymbol{\theta}^*$, the EM algorithm is essentially a linear iteration with rate matrix $J(\boldsymbol{\theta}^*)$, as $J(\boldsymbol{\theta}^*)$ is typically nonzero. For this reason, $J(\boldsymbol{\theta}^*)$ is often referred to as the matrix rate of convergence, or simply, the rate of convergence. For vector $\boldsymbol{\theta}^*$, a measure of the actual observed convergence rate is he global rate of convergence, which can be assessed by

$$r = \lim_{t \to \infty} \frac{||\boldsymbol{\theta}^{(t+1)} - \boldsymbol{\theta}^*||}{||\boldsymbol{\theta}^{(t)} - \boldsymbol{\theta}^*||},$$

where $|| \cdot ||$ is any norm on d-dimensional Euclidean space $\mathbb{R}^d$, and d is the number of missing values. In practice, during the process of convergence, r is typically assessed as

$$r = \lim_{t \to \infty} \frac{||\boldsymbol{\theta}^{(t+1)} - \boldsymbol{\theta}^{(t)}||}{||\boldsymbol{\theta}^{(t)} - \boldsymbol{\theta}^{(t-1)}||}.$$

Under regularity conditions, it can be shown that r is the largest eigenvalue of the $d \times d$ rate matrix $J(\boldsymbol{\theta}^*)$.

Now, $J(\boldsymbol{\theta}^*)$ can be expressed in terms of the observed and missing information:

$$J(\boldsymbol{\theta}^*) = I_d - \mathcal{I}_c(\boldsymbol{\theta}^*, \boldsymbol{Y}^o)^{-1} I(\boldsymbol{\theta}^*, \boldsymbol{Y}^o) = \mathcal{I}_c(\boldsymbol{\theta}^*, \boldsymbol{Y}^o)^{-1} \mathcal{I}_m(\boldsymbol{\theta}^*, \boldsymbol{Y}^o).$$

This means the rate of convergence of the EM algorithm is given by the largest eigenvalue of the information ratio matrix $\mathcal{I}_c(\boldsymbol{\theta}, \boldsymbol{Y}^o)^{-1} \mathcal{I}_m(\boldsymbol{\theta}, \boldsymbol{Y}^o)$, which measures the proportion of information about $\boldsymbol{\theta}$ that is missing by not observing $\boldsymbol{Y}^m$ in addition to $\boldsymbol{Y}^o$. The greater the proportion of missing information, the slower the rate of convergence. The fraction of information loss may vary across different components of $\boldsymbol{\theta}$, suggesting that certain components of $\boldsymbol{\theta}$ may approach $\boldsymbol{\theta}^*$ rapidly using the EM algorithm, while other components may require a large number of iterations. Further, exceptions to the convergence of the EM algorithm to a local maximum of the likelihood function occur if $J(\boldsymbol{\theta}^*)$ has eigenvalues exceeding unity.

28.3.4 EM Acceleration

Using the concept of rate matrix

$$\boldsymbol{\theta}^{(t+1)} - \boldsymbol{\theta}^* \simeq J(\boldsymbol{\theta}^*)[\boldsymbol{\theta}^{(t)} - \boldsymbol{\theta}^*],$$

we can solve this for $\boldsymbol{\theta}^*$, to yield

$$\widetilde{\boldsymbol{\theta}^*} = (I_d - J)^{-1}(\boldsymbol{\theta}^{(t+1)} - J\boldsymbol{\theta}^{(t)}).$$

The J matrix can be determined empirically, using a sequence of subsequent iterates. It also follows from the observed and complete (or, equivalently) missing information:

$$J = I_d - \mathcal{I}_c(\boldsymbol{\theta}^*, \boldsymbol{Y})^{-1} I(\boldsymbol{\theta}^*, \boldsymbol{Y}).$$

Here, $\widetilde{\boldsymbol{\theta}^*}$ can then be seen as an accelerated iterate.

28.3.5 Calculation of Precision Estimates

The observed information matrix is not directly accessible. Now, it has been shown by Louis (1982) that

$$\mathcal{I}_m(\boldsymbol{\theta}, \boldsymbol{Y}^o) = E[\boldsymbol{S}_c(\boldsymbol{\theta}, \boldsymbol{Y}) \boldsymbol{S}_c(\boldsymbol{\theta} \boldsymbol{Y})' | \boldsymbol{y}^o] - \boldsymbol{S}(\boldsymbol{\theta}, \boldsymbol{Y}^o) \boldsymbol{S}(\boldsymbol{\theta}, \boldsymbol{Y}^o)'.$$

This leads to an expression for the observed information matrix in terms of quantities that are available (McLachlan and Krishnan 1997):

$$I(\boldsymbol{\theta}, \boldsymbol{Y}^o) = \mathcal{I}_m(\boldsymbol{\theta}, \boldsymbol{Y}^o) - E[\boldsymbol{S}_c(\boldsymbol{\theta}, \boldsymbol{Y}) \boldsymbol{S}_c(\boldsymbol{\theta}, \boldsymbol{Y})' | \boldsymbol{y}^o] + \boldsymbol{S}(\boldsymbol{\theta}, \boldsymbol{Y}^o) \boldsymbol{S}(\boldsymbol{\theta}, \boldsymbol{Y}^o)'.$$

28.3 The Expectation-Maximization Algorithm

Complete data:	Y_{11}	Y_{12}	Y_2	Y_3	Y_4
Complete data model:	$\frac{1}{2}$	$\frac{1}{4}\theta$	$\frac{1}{4}(1-\theta)$	$\frac{1}{4}(1-\theta)$	$\frac{1}{4}\theta$

Observed data:	Y_1^o	Y_2^o	Y_3^o	Y_4^o
Observed data model:	$\frac{1}{2}+\frac{1}{4}\theta$	$\frac{1}{4}(1-\theta)$	$\frac{1}{4}(1-\theta)$	$\frac{1}{4}\theta$
Observed counts:	125	18	20	34

FIGURE 28.1. *Multinomial Example. Complete and observed data and model.*

From this equation, the observed information matrix can be estimated as

$$I(\widehat{\boldsymbol{\theta}}, \boldsymbol{Y}^o) = \mathcal{I}_m(\widehat{\boldsymbol{\theta}}, \boldsymbol{Y}^o) - E[\boldsymbol{S}_c(\widehat{\boldsymbol{\theta}}, \boldsymbol{Y})\boldsymbol{S}_c(\widehat{\boldsymbol{\theta}}, \boldsymbol{Y})'|\boldsymbol{y}^o],$$

where $\widehat{\boldsymbol{\theta}}$ is the maximum likelihood estimator.

28.3.6 A Simple Illustration

Let us exemplify the EM algorithm using a simple, artificial, yet illustrative multinomial setting, considered by Dempster, Laird, and Rubin (1977) in their original paper on the EM algorithm and also in Little and Rubin.

The data and the complete and incomplete data models are presented in Figure 28.1. The key feature, which turns this problem into an incomplete data problem, is the fact that the counts Y_{11} and Y_{12} are not separately observed, but their total Y_i^o is.

The data can be analyzed in at least three obvious ways: (1) by means of direct likelihood, using a non-iterative solution; (2) also by direct likelihood, but using an iterative solution; and (3) using the EM algorithm.

The log-likelihood for the (hypothetical) complete data is

$$\begin{aligned}
\ell_c(\theta) &= \sum_{j=1}^{5} \ln[\pi_j(\theta)] \\
&= Y_{11}(125;\theta)\ln\left(\frac{1}{2}\right) + Y_{12}(125;\theta)\ln\left(\frac{1}{4}\theta\right) + 18\ln\left(\frac{1}{4}(1-\theta)\right) \\
&\quad + 20\ln\left(\frac{1}{4}(1-\theta)\right) + 34\ln\left(\frac{1}{4}\theta\right),
\end{aligned} \quad (28.2)$$

and its counterpart for the observed data is

$$\ell(\theta) = \sum_{j=1}^{4} \ln[\pi_j^o(\theta)]$$

$$= 125 \ln\left(\frac{1}{2} + \frac{1}{4}\theta\right) + 18 \ln\left(\frac{1}{4}(1-\theta)\right)$$

$$+ 20 \ln\left(\frac{1}{4}(1-\theta)\right) + 34 \ln\left(\frac{1}{4}\theta\right). \tag{28.3}$$

A non-iterative solution starts from the first-order derivative $S(\theta)$ of the observed data log-likelihood (28.3):

$$4 \cdot S(\theta) = \frac{y_1}{2+\theta} - \frac{y_2}{1-\theta} - \frac{y_3}{1-\theta} + \frac{y_4}{\theta} = 0. \tag{28.4}$$

Rewriting (28.4) produces a quadratic equation:

$$-197 \cdot \theta^2 + 15 \cdot \theta + 68 = 0,$$

with two solutions $\theta_1 = 0.6268$ and $\theta_2 = -0.5507$, of which the proper solution obviously is: $\widehat{\theta} = 0.626821497871$. The unusually large number of decimal places is given to monitor the convergence of the iterative procedures in what follows.

Turning to an iterative solution of the observed data likelihood, let us first define the matrix that connects the observed to the complete data:

$$C = \begin{pmatrix} 1 & 1 & 0 & 0 & 0 \\ 0 & 0 & 1 & 0 & 0 \\ 0 & 0 & 0 & 1 & 0 \\ 0 & 0 & 0 & 0 & 1 \end{pmatrix}. \tag{28.5}$$

This matrix is called *coarsening matrix* by Molenberghs and Goetghebeur (1997). Using (28.5), $\pi^o(\theta) = C\pi(\theta)$. Writing

$$\pi(\theta) = \begin{pmatrix} 0.50 \\ 0 \\ 0.25 \\ 0.25 \\ 0 \end{pmatrix} + \begin{pmatrix} 0 \\ 0.25 \\ -0.25 \\ -0.25 \\ 0.25 \end{pmatrix} \theta = \boldsymbol{X}_0 + \boldsymbol{X}_1\theta,$$

the score function (28.4) can be written as

$$S(\theta) = \boldsymbol{X}_1' C'(C\text{cov}(\boldsymbol{Y})C')^-(\boldsymbol{Y}^o - nC\pi),$$

and the second derivative is

$$H(\theta) = n\boldsymbol{X}_1' C'(C\text{cov}(\boldsymbol{Y})C')^- C\boldsymbol{X}_1,$$

from which the updating algorithm follows:

$$\theta^{(t+1)} = \theta^{(t)} + \frac{S(\theta^{(t)})}{H(\theta^{(t)})}.$$

As always, at maximum, $W(\theta)$ can be used to estimate standard errors.

Before applying the direct-likelihood iterative solution, we first turn to the EM algorithm. Likelihood (28.2) for the complete data gives rise to the objective function:

$$\begin{aligned} Q(\theta|\theta^{(t)}) &= Y_{11}(125;\theta^{(t)}) \ln\left(\frac{1}{2}\right) + Y_{12}(125;\theta^{(t)}) \ln\left(\frac{1}{4}\theta\right) \\ &+ 18 \ln\left(\frac{1}{4}(1-\theta)\right) + 20 \ln\left(\frac{1}{4}(1-\theta)\right) \\ &+ 34 \ln\left(\frac{1}{4}\theta\right). \end{aligned} \quad (28.6)$$

The E step requires the calculation of $Y_{11}(125;\theta^{(t)})$ and $Y_{12}(125;\theta^{(t)})$:

$$Y_{11}(125;\theta^{(t)}) = 125 \cdot \frac{2}{2+\theta^{(t)}},$$

$$Y_{12}(125;\theta^{(t)}) = 125 \cdot \frac{\theta^{(t)}}{2+\theta^{(t)}}.$$

For the M step, observe first the complete-data objective function is

$$4 \cdot S_c(\theta) = \frac{Y_{12}}{\theta} - \frac{Y_2}{1-\theta} - \frac{Y_3}{1-\theta} + \frac{Y_4}{\theta} = 0,$$

which, upon rewriting, is seen to produce a linear equation:

$$Y_{12}^{(t)} + Z_4 = \theta[Y_{12}^{(t)} + Y_2 + Y_3 + Y_4],$$

leading to the solution

$$\theta^{(t+1)} = \frac{Y_{12}^{(t)} + Y_4}{Y_{12}^{(t)} + Y_2 + Y_3 + Y_4} = \frac{Y_{12}^{(t)} + 34}{Y_{12}^{(t)} + 18 + 20 + 34}.$$

The iteration history for both iterative methods is given in Table 28.2. The iteration history of the sufficient statistics $Y_{11}^{(t)}$ and $Y_{12}^{(t)}$ is given in Table 28.3.

Note that the convergence of the EM algorithm is quite a bit slower than the Newton-Raphson based convergence. In addition, note that convergence is faster if the convergence rate is smaller, as the rate described

TABLE 28.2. *Multinomial Example. Iteration history for direct-likelihood maximization using Newton-Raphson and for the EM algorithm.*

	Newton-Raphson		EM	
t	$\theta^{(t)}$	rate	$\theta^{(t)}$	rate
1	0.500000000000	0.0506	0.500000000000	0.1464
2	0.633248730964	0.0447	0.608247422680	0.1346
3	0.626534069270	0.0449	0.624321050369	0.1330
4	0.626834428416	0.0449	0.626488879080	0.1328
5	0.626820916320	0.0449	0.626777322347	0.1327
6	0.626821524027	0.0449	0.626815632110	0.1327
7	0.626821496695	0.0449	0.626820719019	0.1327
8	0.626821497924	0.0453	0.626821394456	0.1327

TABLE 28.3. *Multinomial Example. Iteration history of the sufficient statistics $Y_{11}^{(t)}$ and $Y_{12}^{(t)}$ with the EM algorithm.*

t	$Y_{11}^{(t)}$	$Y_{12}^{(t)}$
1	100.000	25.0000
2	95.8498	29.1502
3	95.2627	29.7373
4	95.1841	29.8159
5	95.1737	29.8263
6	95.1723	29.8277
7	95.1721	29.8279
8	95.1721	29.8279

the contraction of the difference between subsequent parameter values and the maximum.

The observed data log-likelihood and its complete-data counterpart for two subsequent iterations is given in Figure 28.2. When considering the log-likelihood values at maximum *of the complete-data log-likelihoods*, they seemingly decrease between subsequent cycles. However, they cannot be compared directly, as the function itself changes at every cycle. The complete-data log-likelihood is merely a device for optimization and cannot be used directly for likelihood ratio tests or precision estimation. As stated in Sections 28.3.4 and 28.3.5, asymptotic covariance matrices and thus standard errors do not follow immediately, but rather a bit of extra work is required.

Regarding precision estimation, it is easy enough to use direct likelihood methods, i.e., to use the information matrix deriving from the observed

28.3 The Expectation-Maximization Algorithm

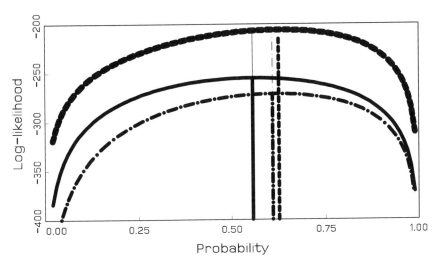

FIGURE 28.2. *Multinomial Example. Observed data log-likelihood (dashes) and two subsequent complete-data log-likelihoods (1: solid line; 2: dots and dashes).*

data likelihood:
$$I(\theta) = \frac{y_1}{(2+\theta)^2} + \frac{(y_2+y_3)}{(1-\theta)^2} + \frac{y_4}{\theta^2},$$

which evaluated in the maximum likelihood estimator $\hat{\theta} = 0.6268$, yields $(\hat{\theta}) = 377.516$. The asymptotic standard error is the inverse square root of this quantity or 0.051.

Now, the complete data score is
$$S_c(\theta, \boldsymbol{Y}) = \frac{Y_{12} + y_4}{\theta} - \frac{y_2 + y_3}{1 - \theta},$$

and the complete data information is
$$I_c(\theta, \boldsymbol{Y}) = \frac{Y_{12} + y_4}{\theta^2} + \frac{y_2 + y_3}{(1-\theta)^2},$$

with expectation
$$\mathcal{I}_c(\theta, \boldsymbol{y}^o) = \frac{E[Y_{12}|y_1] + y_4}{\theta^2} + \frac{y_2 + y_3}{(1-\theta)^2},$$

and
$$E(Y_{12}|y_1) = y_1 \cdot \frac{\frac{1}{4}\theta}{\frac{1}{2} + \frac{1}{4}\theta}.$$

The missing information is

$$\begin{aligned}
\mathcal{I}_m(\theta, \boldsymbol{y}^o) &= \mathrm{var}[S_c(\theta, \boldsymbol{Y})|\boldsymbol{y}^o] \\
&= \mathrm{var}\left[\left(\frac{Y_{12}+y_4}{\theta} - \frac{y_2+y_3}{1-\theta}\right)\Big| y\right] \\
&= \frac{1}{\theta^2}\mathrm{var}(Y_{12}|y) \\
&= \frac{1}{\theta^2}\cdot y_1 \cdot \frac{\frac{1}{4}\theta}{\frac{1}{2}+\frac{1}{4}\theta}\cdot\frac{\frac{1}{2}}{\frac{1}{2}+\frac{1}{4}\theta} = \frac{1}{\theta^2}\cdot y_1 \cdot \frac{\frac{1}{8}\theta}{(\frac{1}{2}+\frac{1}{4}\theta)^2}.
\end{aligned}$$

Substituting the observed data values and the MLE for θ yields $\mathcal{I}_c(\widehat{\theta}, \boldsymbol{y}^o) = 435.318$, $\mathcal{I}_m(\widehat{\theta}, \boldsymbol{y}^o) = 57.801$ and hence $I(\widehat{\theta}, \boldsymbol{y}^o) = 435.318 - 57.801 = 377.516$, in perfect agreement with the direct-likelihood derivation.

To conclude, note that the ratio

$$J(\widehat{\theta}) = \frac{\mathcal{I}_m(\widehat{\theta}, y)}{\mathcal{I}_c(\widehat{\theta}, y)} = \frac{57.801}{435.318} = 0.1328,$$

in agreement with the convergence rate observed earlier.

28.4 Which Method to Use?

An important question is when to use multiple imputation and the EM algorithm. Indeed, given the availability of flexible software tools allowing to conduct direct likelihood, such as the SAS procedures MIXED, NLMIXED, and GLIMMIX, it may appear there is little room for the alternative methods.

Nevertheless, we see at least four broad settings where MI can be of use. First, when there is a combination of missing covariates and missing outcomes, multiple imputation can be useful to deal with the missing covariates. A direct likelihood approach could then follow the imputation of covariates. Second and related, when incomplete outcomes are of a heterogeneous type, e.g., when a longitudinal process is measured jointly with a time-to-event outcome, MI can be very useful as well.

Third, when several mechanisms for missingness are postulated, and one would like to consider all of them, imputations could be drawn under all of these schemes and inferences could later be combined into a single one. This is a basic but important form of sensitivity analysis and was advocated in Rubin (1987).

Fourth, MI can be used as a tool to change non-monotone missingness into monotone missingness. Often, non-monotone missingness comes from a simpler mechanism on the one hand but tremendously complicates analysis on the other hand. Upon imputation in as far as to create monotone missingness, the monotonized datasets can then be analyzed with techniques for MAR *but also for MNAR* missingness. It is interesting to note that this particular application of MI is possible with the SAS procedure MI. Of course, there are ample situations where one would prefer to impute all missing values, and not just the intermittent ones. We merely want to point to the additional flexibility stemming from the ability to impute intermittent missing values.

Whereas MI is a method providing an alternative estimator to the one produced by direct likelihood, the EM algorithm typically produces exactly the same estimator. Thus, the difference between EM and direct likelihood is much smaller than between these and MI. Broadly, the algorithm is of use when the direct likelihood (observed data likelihood) is so complicated that it becomes intractable. In addition, it is often used as an auxiliary tool in a wider optimization task. For example, EM is used when generating multiple imputations within the SAS procedure MI. Finally, the stability of the algorithm is an attractive feature. Although it comes at the price of slow convergence, it can be useful to at least start maximization of a complex likelihood using EM and then switch to direct likelihood once the current value of the parameter is sufficiently close to the maximum. The elegance of EM lies in the ease with which it deals with unobserved variables, be it missing data, random effects, latent variables, component membership in mixture models, etc. (McLachlan and Krishnan 1997).

28.5 Age Related Macular Degeneration Study

In Section 27.7, the data were analyzed using GEE and generalized linear mixed models, on the complete cases, the LOCF imputed data, and using the observed data. In the latter case, also WGEE was considered. For the generalized estimating equations, both classical GEE and linearization-based GEE were considered. For GLMM, the models were fitted with PQL and based on numerical integration.

One complication with WGEE is that the calculation of the weights is difficult with non-monotone missingness. Standard GEE on the incomplete data is valid only when the missing data are MCAR. Precisely here, multiple imputation is an appealing alternative.

The binary indicators were created by dichotomizing the continuous visual acuity outcomes, as negative *versus* non-negative. The continuous outcomes were defined as the change from baseline in number of letters read. Therefore, multiple imputation could start from the continuous outcomes. Ten multiply-imputed datasets were created. The imputation model included, apart from the four continuous outcomes variables, also the four-

TABLE 28.4. *Age Related Macular Degeneration Trial. Parameter estimates (standard errors) for the standard GEE and numerical-integration based random-intercept models, after generating 10 multiple imputations.*

Effect	Par.	GEE	GLMM
Int.4	β_{11}	-0.84(0.20)	-1.46(0.36)
Int.12	β_{21}	-1.02(0.22)	-1.75(0.38)
Int.24	β_{31}	-1.07(0.23)	-1.83(0.38)
Int.52	β_{41}	-1.61(0.27)	-2.69(0.45)
Trt.4	β_{12}	0.21(0.28)	0.32(0.48)
Trt.12	β_{22}	0.60(0.29)	0.99(0.49)
Trt.24	β_{32}	0.43(0.30)	0.67(0.51)
Trt.52	β_{42}	0.37(0.35)	0.52(0.56)
R.I. s.d.	τ		2.20(0.26)
R.I. var.	τ^2		4.85(1.13)

point categorical variable 'lesions.' For simplicity, the latter was treated as continuous. Separate imputations were conducted for each of the two treatment groups. These choices imply that the imputed values depend on lesions and treatment assignment, and hence analysis models that include one or both of these effects are *proper* in the sense of Rubin (1987). This means, broadly speaking, that the model used for imputation should include all relationships that later will be considered in the analysis and inference tasks. The added advantage of including 'lesions' into the imputation model, is that even individuals for which none of the four follow-up measurements are available, are still imputed. The MCMC method was used, with EM starting values, and a single chain for all imputations.

Upon imputation, the same marginal GEE and random-intercept models as in Section 27.7 were fitted in the analysis task. Results from the inference task are reported in Table 28.4. Details on the practical implementation of the various tasks are described in Section 32.6. The parameter estimates and standard errors are very similar to their counterparts in Table 27.4 and 27.6. Of course, in the GEE case, there is no direct counterpart, since the WGEE method is different from GEE after multiple imputation, even though both are valid under MAR. However, in particular the similarity between the direct likelihood method (bottom right column of Table 27.6) is clear, with only a minor deviation in estimate for the treatment effect after 1 year.

Section 32.6 also contains a brief illustration of how to implement the EM algorithm, based on the continuous visual acuity outcomes.

28.6 Concluding Remarks

The direct-likelihood method (Chapter 27), the expectation-maximization algorithm, and multiple imputation constitute a set of three powerful tools to conduct likelihood inference when missing data are considered missing at random. In addition, the weighted generalized estimating equations (Section 27.5) methodology ensures also GEE can be applied under MAR. As we have seen in Section 28.4, each fulfills its proper role and thus incomplete longitudinal data, whether Gaussian or not, can be analyzed flexibly, without the need for deletion nor single imputation.

Of course, the MAR assumption, though flexible, can be questioned in a number of applications and therefore MNAR should not be ruled out. It is interesting to note that all methods, direct likelihood, EM, MI, and WGEE, can be extended to MNAR settings where then the missing data process itself will be modeled and its parameters estimated jointly with the measurement model parameters. We will provide several illustrations of this in Chapter 29 on selection models and in Chapter 30 dedicated to pattern-mixture models. Such extended frameworks will be useful in particular when conducting a sensitivity analysis, as discussed in Chapter 31.

29
Selection Models

29.1 Introduction

Chapters 27 and 28 have shown that, if MAR can be guaranteed to hold, a standard analysis would follow. This is certainly true for likelihood methods, while others, in particular GEE, can be adjusted for the MAR case (Section 27.5).

However, only rarely is such an assumption known to hold (Murray and Findlay 1988). Nevertheless, ignorable analyses may provide reasonably stable results, even when the assumption of MAR is violated, in the sense that such analyses constrain the behavior of the unseen data to be similar to that of the observed data (Mallinckrodt *et al* 2001ab). A discussion of this phenomenon in the survey context has been given in Rubin, Stern, and Vehovar (1995). These authors argue that, in rigidly controlled experiments (some surveys and many clinical trials), the assumption of MAR is often reasonable. Second, and very importantly for such studies as confirmatory trials, an MAR analysis can be specified *a priori* without additional work relative to a situation with complete data. Third, though MNAR models are more general and explicitly incorporate the dropout mechanism, the inferences they produce are typically highly dependent on untestable and often implicit assumptions regarding the distribution of the unobserved measurements given the observed measurements. The quality of the fit to the observed data need not reflect at all the appropriateness of the implied structure governing the unobserved data. This point is irrespective of the MNAR route taken, whether a parametric model of the type of

Diggle and Kenward (1994) or Molenberghs, Kenward, and Lesaffre (1997) is chosen, or a semiparametric approach such as in Robins, Rotnitzky, and Scharfstein (1998). Hence, in incomplete-data settings, a definitive MNAR analysis does not exist. To explore the impact of deviations from the MAR assumption on the conclusions, one should ideally conduct a sensitivity analysis (Chapter 31), within which MNAR models of the selection type as described in this chapter and pattern-mixture models (Chapter 30) can play a major role. See also Verbeke and Molenberghs (2000, Chapter 17–20), for a discussion in the context of continuous longitudinal data.

Diggle and Kenward (1994) describe a modeling procedure for continuous longitudinal data, also discussed in Diggle *et al* (2002, Chapter 11) and Verbeke and Molenberghs (2000, Chapter 17). Based on the multivariate Dale model (Section 7.7), Molenberghs, Kenward, and Lesaffre (1997) proposed a model for repeated ordinal outcomes with MNAR dropout. This model will be described in Section 29.2. The work on incomplete categorical data is vast. Baker and Laird (1988) develop the original work of Fay (1986) and give a thorough account of the modelling of contingency tables in which there is one response dimension and an additional dimension indicating whether the response is absent. Baker and Laird use loglinear models and the EM algorithm for the analysis. They pay particular attention to the circumstances in which no solution exists for the non-random dropout models. Such non-estimability is also a feature of the models we use below, but the more complicated setting makes a systematic account more difficult. Stasny (1986) and Conaway (1992, 1993) consider non-random missingness models for categorical longitudinal data. Baker (1995) allows for intermittent missingness in repeated categorical outcomes. Baker, Rosenberger, and DerSimonian (1992) present a method for incomplete bivariate binary outcomes with general patterns of missingness. The model was adapted for the use of covariates by Jansen *et al* (2003) and is presented in Section 29.3. In both cases, the method is illustrated using the fluvoxamine study, introduced in Section 2.4 and analyzed before in Sections 6.5, 7.2.4, and 7.11. These methods will be employed in Chapter 32 to develop sensitivity analysis tools.

29.2 An MNAR Dale Model

Molenberghs, Kenward, and Lesaffre (1997) proposed a model for longitudinal ordinal data with non-random dropout, i.e., the missingness mechanism was assumed to be MNAR, which combines the multivariate Dale model for longitudinal ordinal data with a logistic regression model for dropout. The resulting likelihood can be maximized relatively simply, using the fact that all stochastic outcomes are of a categorical type, using the EM algorithm. It means that the integration over the missing data, needed to maximize the likelihood of Diggle and Kenward (1994), is replaced by finite summation.

29.2.1 Likelihood Function

We will derive a general form for the likelihood for longitudinal categorical data with non-random dropout and introduce particular functional forms for the response, using the multivariate Dale model developed by Molenberghs and Lesaffre (1994), see also Section 7.7, and for the dropout process, using a simple logistic regression formulation.

We adopt the contingency table notation, outlined in Section 7.1. Assume we have $r = 1, \ldots, N$ design levels in the study, characterized by covariate information X_r. Let there be N_r subject at design level r. Let the outcome for subject i at level r be a␣c level ordinal categorical outcome is designed to be measured at occasions $j = 1, \ldots, n$, denoted by Y_{rij}. In principle, we could allow the number of measurement occasions to be different across subjects, but in an incomplete data setting, it is often sensible to assume that the number of measurements at the design stage is constant. Extension to the more general case is straightforward.

As in (7.1), the outcomes at level r are grouped into a contingency table $Z_r^{c*}(k_1 \ldots k_n)$. The cumulative version is $Z_r^c(k_1 \ldots k_n)$ as in (7.2). We have added the superscript c to refer to the (possibly hypothetical) complete data. Shorthand notation is $Z_r^{c*}(\boldsymbol{k})$ and $Z_r^c(\boldsymbol{k})$, and the corresponding cell probabilities are $\mu_r^{c*}(\boldsymbol{k})$ and $\mu_r^c(\boldsymbol{k})$. The corresponding vectors are $\boldsymbol{Z}^{c*}$, $\boldsymbol{Z}^c$, $\boldsymbol{\mu}^{c*}$, and $\boldsymbol{\mu}^c$, respectively.

Any model of the general family described in Section 7.3 can be used, with in particular the multivariate Dale model. The essence is a set of link functions:

$$\eta_r^c(\boldsymbol{\mu}_r^c) = X_r^c \boldsymbol{\beta}. \qquad (29.1)$$

Specific choices are discussed in Section 7.3, with in particular the multivariate probit model (Section 7.6) and the multivariate Dale model (Section 7.7). Also the Bahadur model (Section 7.2) can be employed.

We now also need to model the missingness or, in this particular case, the dropout process. Assume the random variable D can take values $2, \ldots, n+1$, the time at which a subject drops out, where $D = n+1$ indicates no dropout. The value $D = 1$ is not included since we assume at least one follow-up measurement is available. The hypothetical full data consist of complete data and the dropout indicator. The full data, $\boldsymbol{Z}_r^{c*}$, contain components $Z_{rdk_1\ldots k_n}^{c*}$ with joint probabilities:

$$\nu_{rdk_1\ldots k_n}^{c*} = \mu_{rk_1\ldots k_n}^{c*}(\boldsymbol{\beta})\, \phi_{rd|k_1\ldots k_n}(\boldsymbol{\psi}), \qquad (29.2)$$

where the $\boldsymbol{\psi}$ parameterizes the dropout probabilities $\phi_{rd|k_1\ldots k_n}$. We typically assume both parameters are distinct but this is, strictly speaking, not necessary.

Assume that the distribution of D may depend both on the past history of the process, denoted by $H_d = (k_1, \ldots, k_{d-1})$ for $D = d$, and the current outcome category k_d, but not on the process after that time. The advantage in modeling terms is that the set of unobserved outcomes, relevant to the modeling taks, is a singleton. Also, it is usually deemed plausible in time-ordered longitudinal data, that there is no additional information on the dropout process in the future measurements, given the history and the current, possibly unobserved, measurement.

Factorization (29.2) was made in terms of cell probabilities, superscripted with $*$. The factorization in terms of cumulative probabilities is identical and obtained upon dropping the superscript $*$.

Consequently,

$$\phi^{c*}_{rd|k_1\ldots k_n}(\boldsymbol{\psi})$$

$$= \phi^{c*}_{rd|k_1\ldots k_d}(\boldsymbol{\psi})$$

$$= \begin{cases} \prod_{t=2}^{d-1}[1 - p_{rt}(H_t, k_t; \boldsymbol{\psi})]\, p_{rd}(H_d, k_d; \boldsymbol{\psi}) & \text{if } D \leq n, \\ \prod_{t=2}^{T}[1 - p_{rt}(H_t, k_t; \boldsymbol{\psi})] & \text{if } D = n+1. \end{cases} \quad (29.3)$$

where

$$p_{rd}(H_d, k_d; \boldsymbol{\psi}) = P(D = d | D \geq d, H_d, k_d; W_r; \boldsymbol{\psi}).$$

Here, W_r is a set of covariates, used to model the dropout process. Expression (29.3) is similar to (27.14)–(27.15), used in the context of weighted generalized estimating equations. The difference is that here dropout is allowed to depend on the current, possibly unobserved, measurement.

Molenberghs, Kenward, and Lesaffre (1997) specified the model for the dropout probabilities by logit links, and assuming a linear relationship between the log-odds and the original response. However, the latter is not necessary. For example, non-linear relations and ones involving interactions between the response variables and the covariates could be used. Here, we expect that dropout does not depends on observations preceding k_{d-1}, and thus only depends on k_{d-1} and k_d, but an extension would be straightforward:

$$\operatorname{logit}[p_{rd}(H_d, k_d; \boldsymbol{\psi})] = \psi_0 + \psi_1 k_{d-1} + \psi_2 k_d.$$

This model can also be extended by allowing dependence on covariates W_r. The case $\psi_2 = 0$ corresponds to a MAR dropout process and the case $\psi_1 = \psi_2 = 0$ to a MCAR dropout process.

With dropout occurring, we will not observe $\boldsymbol{Z}^c_r$ but only $\boldsymbol{Z}_r$, a partially classified table, with corresponding probabilities ν_r. The components of ν_r are simple linear functions of the components ν^c_r. This is true for both the cell counts and the cumulative counts.

The multinomial log-likelihood is

$$\ell(\boldsymbol{\beta}, \boldsymbol{\psi}; \boldsymbol{Z}^*) = \ln\left(\frac{1}{\prod_1^N \boldsymbol{Z}_r^*!}\right) + \sum_{r=1}^{N}(\boldsymbol{Z}_r^*)' \ln(\boldsymbol{\nu}_r), \qquad (29.4)$$

with the components of ν_r summing to one. The kernel of the log-likelihood is the sum of two contributions. For the complete sequences we have,

$$\ell_1(\boldsymbol{\beta}, \boldsymbol{\psi}; \boldsymbol{Z}^*) = \sum_{r=1}^{N} \sum_{(k_1,\ldots,k_n)} Z^*_{r,n+1,k_1,\ldots,k_n}$$
$$\times \log\left\{\mu^*_{rk_1\ldots k_n}(\boldsymbol{\beta}) \prod_{t=2}^{n}[1 - p_{rt}(H_t, k_d; \boldsymbol{\psi})]\right\},$$

and similarly for the incomplete sequences (say $r = N_1 + 1, \ldots, N = N_1 + N_2$):

$$\ell_2(\boldsymbol{\beta}, \boldsymbol{\psi}; \boldsymbol{Z}^*)$$
$$= \sum_{r=1}^{N} \sum_{d=2}^{n} \sum_{(k_1,\ldots,k_{d-1})} Z^*_{rdk_1,\ldots,k_{d-1}}$$
$$\times \ln\left\{\prod_{t=2}^{d-1}[1 - p_{rt}(H_t, k_t; \boldsymbol{\psi})] \sum_{k_d=1}^{c} \mu^*_{rk_1\ldots k_d} p_{rd}(H_d, k_d; \boldsymbol{\psi})\right\}.$$

We note that, when the probability of dropout does not depend on k_d, i.e., when the dropout process is MAR, the second part of the likelihood partitions into two components, the first for the response process involving $\boldsymbol{\beta}$ only and the second for the dropout process involving $\boldsymbol{\psi}$ only. When the missingness mechanism is MNAR, the resulting likelihood is complex, but the processes of maximization for $\boldsymbol{\beta}$ and for $\boldsymbol{\psi}$ can be separated through the use of the EM algorithm (Dempster, Laird, and Rubin 1977), outlined in Section 28.3. Details are provided in the next section.

29.2.2 *Maximization Using the EM Algorithm*

We will now show how the likelihood derived in Section 29.2.1 can be maximized using the EM algorithm (Dempster, Laird, and Rubin, 1977; see also Section 28.3), where dropout and response components of the likelihood are maximized separately within each iteration of the algorithm.

Let $(\boldsymbol{\beta}^{(0)}, \boldsymbol{\psi}^{(0)})$ be initial parameters, which can be found from, e.g., a complete case analysis, an available case analysis, or a simple method of imputation. Given current values $(\boldsymbol{\beta}^{(t)}, \boldsymbol{\psi}^{(t)})$ for the parameters, the E step computes the objective function, which is in the case of the missing data problem equal to the expected value of the observed data log-likelihood, given the observed data and the current parameters:

$$Q\left[(\boldsymbol{\beta},\boldsymbol{\psi})|(\boldsymbol{\beta}^{(t)},\boldsymbol{\psi}^{(t)})\right] = E\left\{\ell\left[(\boldsymbol{\beta},\boldsymbol{\psi})|Z^{c*}_{r,d,k_1...k_n}\right] |Z^*_{rdk_1...k_{d-1}},(\boldsymbol{\beta}^{(t)},\boldsymbol{\psi}^{(t)})\right\}.$$

Due to the linearity of the complete data log-likelihood, it is natural to consider the expectations in terms of counts of contingency table Z_r^{c*}. Consider now the cell count for a particular joint outcome $(k_1, \ldots, k_n)$ with dropout time d, i.e., $Z^{c*}_{rdk_1...k_n}$. The corresponding observed count is $Z^*_{rdk_1...k_{d-1}}$. It can be shown that the conditional expectation for this cell count given the history can be written as

$$E(Z^{c*}_{rdk_1...k_d}|Z^*_{rdk_1...k_{d-1}},\boldsymbol{\beta},\boldsymbol{\psi})$$

$$= Z^*_{rdk_1...k_{d-1}} \frac{\mu^{c*}_{rk_1...k_d}(\boldsymbol{\beta})p_{rd}(H_d,k_d,\boldsymbol{\psi})}{\sum_{k_d}\mu^{c*}_{rk_1...k_{d-1}k_d}(\boldsymbol{\beta})p_{rd}(H_d,k_d,\boldsymbol{\psi})}. \quad (29.5)$$

Consequently, the maximization step of the EM cycle requires as input only the expectations $E(Z^{c*}_{rdk_1...k_d}|Z_{rdk_1...k_{d-1}},\boldsymbol{\beta},\boldsymbol{\psi})$ for $k_d = 1,\ldots c$. Given this the likelihood can be partitioned into separate components for the response variable and dropout measurements. Each can be maximized separately using conventional likelihood methods.

To summarize, the two steps of the EM algorithm are as follows.

1. *Expectation.* Predict $Z^{c*}_{rdk_1...k_d}$, $k_d = 1,\ldots,c$ for $d < n+1$, given current estimates of $\boldsymbol{\beta}$ and $\boldsymbol{\psi}$, $\left(\boldsymbol{\beta}^{(t)},\boldsymbol{\psi}^{(t)}\right)$:

$$E\left(Z^{c*}_{rdk_1...k_d}|Z^*_{rdk_1...k_{d-1}},\boldsymbol{\beta}^{(t)},\boldsymbol{\psi}^{(t)}\right)$$

$$= Z^*_{rdk_1...k_{d-1}} \cdot \frac{\mu^{c*}_{rk_1...k_d}\left(\boldsymbol{\beta}^{(t)}\right)p_{rd}\left(H_d,k_d,\boldsymbol{\psi}^{(t)}\right)}{\sum_{k_d}\mu^{c*}_{rk_1...k_{d-1}k_d}\left(\boldsymbol{\beta}^{(t)}\right)p_{rd}\left(H_d,k_d,\boldsymbol{\psi}^{(t)}\right)}.$$

2. *Maximization.* Maximize separately the kernels of the two components of the likelihood corresponding to the response variable and dropout measurements with respect to $\boldsymbol{\beta}$ and $\boldsymbol{\psi}$:

$$\ell^c(\boldsymbol{\beta},Z^{c*}) = \sum_{i=1}^{N}\sum_{d=2}^{n+1}\sum_{(k_1,\ldots,k_d)} Z^{c*}_{rdk_1...k_d}\ln\left(\mu^*_{rk_1...k_d}(\boldsymbol{\beta})\right),$$

$$\ell^c(\boldsymbol{\psi},Z^{c*}) = \sum_{i=1}^{N}\sum_{(k_1,\ldots,k_n)} Z^{c*}_{r,n+1,k_1...k_n}\ln\left(\prod_{t=2}^{n}\{1-p_{rt}(H_t,k_t;\boldsymbol{\psi})\}\right)$$

$$+ \sum_{i=1}^{N}\sum_{d=2}^{n}\sum_{(k_1,\ldots,k_d)} Z^{c*}_{rdk_1...k_d}$$

$$\times \ln\left(\prod_{t=2}^{d-1}[1-p_{rt}(H_t,k_t;\boldsymbol{\psi})]\,p_{rd}(H_d,k_d;\boldsymbol{\psi})\right).$$

The log-likelihood for the measurement model can be maximized using a Fisher scoring algorithm, as discussed in Sections 7.3 and 7.7.

For the dropout portion of the model, one proceeds as follows. By taking each time of measurement and conditioning on the number of units still present at that time, an overall likelihood can be assembled from independent components and, given k_d, this can be seen to be the likelihood of a conventional logistic regression. The maximum likelihood estimate of ψ can then be obtained simply using iteratively reweighted least squares (McCullagh and Nelder 1989, Section 4.4), or any other tool to maximize a logistic regression based likelihood.

Observe that not only the EM algorithm itself is iterative, but that each M step consists of a pair of iterative maximizations. A way to speed up the EM algorithm is to restrict the iterative schemes in the M step to only a few iterations. This yields a so-called generalized EM algorithm (GEM, Dempster, Laird, and Rubin 1977). Rather than fully maximizing the response log-likelihood and the dropout log-likelihood, one can reduce the number of iterations for either or both of the two maximizations, possibly to one.

Two of the main drawbacks of the EM algorithm are its typically very slow rate of convergence and its lack of direct provision of a measure of precision for the maximum likelihood estimates. Several proposals for overcoming these limitations have been made in the literature, and were discussed in some detail in Sections 28.3.3, 28.3.4, and 28.3.5. Molenberghs, Kenward, and Lesaffre (1997) accelerated convergence using a diagonal matrix analogous to the rate matrix introduced by Meng and Rubin (1991, Eq. 2.2.1). Approximations to the observed Fisher information were found through the technique termed EM-aided differentiation by Meilijson (1989). This technique is easy to implement as it requires a negligible amount of extra code. Standard errors and Wald statistics were computed directly from the observed information and score tests are also relatively simple to compute; calculation of the scores being straightforward. Alternatively, inferences can be based on likelihood ratios; the observed data likelihood is not difficult to evaluate in the current multinomial setting.

All computations were carried out in the statistical programming language GAUSS. As a convergence criterion the L_∞ norm of the relative *observed* data score vector was required to be smaller than 10^{-3}.

29.2.3 *Analysis of the Fluvoxamine Data*

The data were introduced in Section 2.4 and analyzed before in Sections 6.5, 7.2.4, and 7.11. Analyses of the data, assuming MAR, are described in

TABLE 29.1. *Fluvoxamine Trial. Summary of the ordinal therapeutic outcomes at three follow-up times. (For example, category 241 corresponds to a classification of 2 on the first visit, 4 on the second visit, and 1 on the third visit; a * in one of the positions indicates dropout.)*

Cat	#	Cat	#	Cat	#	Cat	#
				Completers			
111	10	211	32	311	12	411	1
112		212	1	312	1	412	
113		213		313		413	
114		214	1	314		414	
121	1	221	13	321	35	421	5
122		222	16	322	14	422	5
123	1	223	1	323	1	423	
124		224	3	324	1	424	1
131		231	1	331	6	431	13
132		232	2	332	5	432	13
133		233	2	333	3	433	5
134		234		334	1	434	
141		241	1	341	1	441	4
142		242		342	2	442	2
143		243	1	343		443	4
144		244		344		444	3
			Dropout after 2nd visit				
11*	3	21*	3	31*		41*	
12*		22*	7	32*	7	42*	2
13*		23*	3	33*	3	43*	5
14*		24*	2	34*	1	44*	8
			Dropout after 1st visit				
1**	4	2**	6	3**	9	4**	12

Molenberghs and Lesaffre (1994) and Kenward, Lesaffre, and Molenberghs (1994).

From the initially recruited subjects, 14 were not observed at all after the start, 31 and 44 patients, respectively, were observed on the first only and first and second occasions and 224 had complete observations. We omit from the current analyses two patients with non-monotone missing values, leaving 299 in the current analyses. We summarize the therapeutic and side effects results in two sets of contingency tables, Tables 29.1 and 29.2.

TABLE 29.2. *Fluvoxamine Trial. Summary of the ordinal side effects outcomes at three follow-up times. (For example, category 241 corresponds to a classification of 2 on the first visit, 4 on the second visit, and 1 on the third visit; a * in one of the positions indicates dropout.)*

Cat	#	Cat	#	Cat	#	Cat	#
\multicolumn{8}{c}{Completers}							

Cat	#	Cat	#	Cat	#	Cat	#
111	86	211	25	311	1	411	2
112	5	212	6	312		412	1
113	1	213		313		413	
114		214		314		414	
121	3	221	28	321	1	421	
122		222	39	322	5	422	1
123	7	223	4	323		423	
124		224		324		424	
131		231		331		431	
132		232	4	332	3	432	
133		233		333	2	433	
134		234		334		434	
141		241		341		441	
142		242		342		442	
143		243		343		443	
144		244		344		444	

Dropout after 2nd visit

Cat	#	Cat	#	Cat	#	Cat	#
11*	13	21*	3	31*	1	41*	
12*	4	22*	9	32*	1	42*	
13*		23*	3	33*	5	43*	
14*		24*	1	34*	2	44*	2

Dropout after 1st visit

Cat	#	Cat	#	Cat	#	Cat	#
1**	9	2**	6	3**	7	4**	9

For the data on therapeutic effect as well as on side effects we present four sets of parameter estimates. Each set is the result of fitting a marginal proportional odds model to the response and, for non-ignorable models, a logistic regression model to the dropout process. In the first set, the response model alone is fitted to the data from those subjects with complete records. Such an analysis will be consistent with an analysis of the full data set if the dropout process is completely random. The remaining three sets of estimates are obtained from fitting models with non-random, random,

TABLE 29.3. *Fluvoxamine Trial. Maximum likelihood estimates (standard errors) for side effects.*

Parameter	Completers	MCAR	MAR	MNAR
	Measurement model			
intercept 1	1.38(1.00)	-0.60(0.82)	-0.60(0.82)	-0.78(0.79)
intercept 2	4.42(1.04)	1.59(0.83)	1.59(0.83)	1.31(0.80)
intercept 3	6.32(1.14)	2.90(0.85)	2.90(0.85)	2.51(0.82)
age	-0.22(0.08)	-0.20(0.07)	-0.20(0.07)	-0.19(0.07)
sex	-0.35(0.25)	-0.03(0.22)	-0.03(0.22)	0.00(0.21)
duration (visit 1)	-0.05(0.08)	-0.13(0.05)	-0.13(0.05)	-0.12(0.05)
duration (visit 2)	-0.10(0.08)	-0.20(0.06)	-0.20(0.06)	-0.21(0.05)
duration (visit 3)	-0.13(0.08)	-0.19(0.07)	-0.19(0.07)	-0.23(0.06)
severity (visit 1)	0.00(0.16)	0.26(0.13)	0.26(0.13)	0.28(0.12)
severity (visit 2)	0.09(0.16)	0.33(0.13)	0.33(0.13)	0.34(0.13)
severity (visit 3)	0.17(0.16)	0.41(0.13)	0.41(0.13)	0.40(0.13)
Association				
visits 1 and 2	2.89(0.33)	3.12(0.30)	3.12(0.30)	3.26(0.29)
visits 1 and 3	2.06(0.32)	2.33(0.35)	2.33(0.35)	2.30(0.32)
visits 2 and 3	2.86(0.34)	3.16(0.37)	3.16(0.37)	3.18(0.36)
visits 1, 2, and 3	0.45(0.76)	0.48(0.79)	0.48(0.79)	0.61(0.71)
	Dropout model			
ψ_0		-1.90(0.13)	-3.68(0.34)	-4.26(0.48)
ψ_1				1.08(0.54)
ψ_2			0.94(0.15)	0.18(0.45)
-2 log-likelihood		1631.97	1591.98	1587.72

and completely random dropout, defined in terms of constraints on the ψ parameters.

We consider first the analysis of the side-effects data, Table 29.3. Covariates have been included in the response component of the model. The relationships with two covariates, sex and age, have been held constant across visits, the relationships with the other two covariates, duration and severity, have been allowed to differ among visits.

Conditional on acceptance of the validity of the overall model we can, by examining the statistical significance of the parameters in the dropout model, test for different types of dropout process. Three statistics, likelihood-ratio, Wald, and score can be computed for each null hypothesis, and we present each in Table 29.4 for comparisons of (1) MNAR *versus* MAR and

TABLE 29.4. *Fluvoxamine Trial. Side effects. Test statistics for dropout mechanism.*

	MNAR vs MAR		MAR vs MCAR	
Wald	4.02	$(p = 0.045)$	38.91	$(p < 0.001)$
LR	4.26	$(p = 0.039)$	39.99	$(p < 0.001)$
score	4.24	$(p = 0.040)$	45.91	$(p < 0.001)$

of (2) MAR *versus* MCAR. In line with Diggle and Kenward (1994) and Molenberghs, Kenward, and Lesaffre (1997), it is tempting to assume both statistics follow a null asymptotic χ_1^2 distribution. Jansen *et al* (2005) show that great care has to be taken with the test for MNAR against MAR (see Chapter 31).

All tests provide weak evidence for MNAR in the context of the assumed model. They also strongly support MAR over MCAR. But again, one has to be very cautious with such conclusions. Section 31.3 will study sensitivity of the MNAR model to the model assumptions made. Further detail on the precise nature of sensitivity can be found in Jansen *et al* (2005).

The estimated dropout model is, with simplified notation:

$$\text{logit}[P(\text{dropout})] = -4.26 + 1.08 Y_c + 0.18 Y_{pr}$$

for Y_{pr} and Y_c the previous and current observations, respectively. It is instructive to rewrite this in terms of the increment and sum of the successive measurements. Standard errors of the estimated parameters have been added in square brackets.

$$\text{logit}[P(\text{dropout})] = -4.26 + 0.63[0.08](Y_c + Y_{pr}) + 0.45[0.49](Y_c - Y_{pr}).$$

It can be seen that the estimated probability of dropout increases greatly with large side effects. The corresponding standard error is comparatively small. Although the coefficient of the increment does not appear negligible in terms of its absolute size, in the light of its standard error it cannot be said to be significantly different from zero. This reflects the lack of information in these data on the coefficient of the increment in the dropout model.

Although the evidence of dependence of the dropout process on previous observation is overwhelming, that for MNAR is borderline.

It is worth noting that there are substantial differences between the analyses of the completers only and full datasets with respect to the parameter estimates of the response model. In the presence of an MAR and MNAR process, the former analysis produces inconsistent estimators. Given the clear association of side-effect occurrence and the covariates age, duration, and severity, we investigated the relationship between these and dropout, but found only marginal evidence for a dependence on sex and severity.

TABLE 29.5. *Fluvoxamine Trial. Maximum likelihood estimates (standard errors) for therapeutic effect.*

Parameter	Completers	MCAR	MAR	MNAR
	Measurement model			
intercept 1	-2.36(0.17)	-2.32(0.15)	-2.32(0.15)	-2.33(0.14)
intercept 2	-0.53(0.13)	-0.53(0.12)	-0.53(0.11)	-0.52(0.10)
intercept 3	1.03(0.14)	0.90(0.11)	0.90(0.12)	0.90(0.09)
visit 2 - visit 1	1.38(0.12)	1.22(0.10)	1.22(0.10)	1.32(0.11)
visit 3 - visit 1	2.70(0.19)	2.58(0.18)	2.58(0.18)	2.83(0.19)
association				
visits 1 and 2	2.58(0.24)	2.57(0.22)	2.57(0.22)	2.46(0.20)
visits 1 and 3	0.85(0.23)	0.86(0.24)	0.86(0.24)	0.77(0.19)
visits 2 and 3	1.79(0.25)	1.79(0.25)	1.79(0.25)	1.59(0.20)
visits 1, 2 and 3	0.39(0.52)	0.27(0.52)	0.27(0.52)	0.22(0.23)
	Dropout model			
ψ_0		-1.88 (0.13)	-2.56(0.37)	-2.00(0.48)
ψ_1				-1.11(0.42)
ψ_2			0.26(0.13)	0.77(0.19)
-2 log-likelihood		2156.91	2152.87	2145.93

In Table 29.5, the results from the analyses of the therapeutic effect are presented. Here, apart from overall effects of time, no covariates are included because all showed negligible association with the response. Interestingly the comparison of the three dropout models (Table 29.6) produces somewhat different conclusions about the dropout mechanism, when compared to those of the side-effects analysis (Table 29.4).

Here, the three classes of tests again behave consistently. The evidence for MNAR is strong, but the same warnings about the sensitivity of the MNAR model to modeling assumptions apply here. The tests comparing the MAR and MCAR processes show only moderate evidence of a difference. The latter tests are not strictly valid however in the presence of MNAR missingness. It is interesting that a comparison of the MCAR and MAR models, which is much easier to accomplish than the comparison of MAR and MNAR, gives little suggestion that such a relationship might exist between dropout and response. This is partly a consequence of the nature of the dropout relationship in this example. With the side-effects the association between dropout and response was dominated by the average response. With the therapeutic observations however dependence of dropout probability is largely on the measurement increment, also a fea-

TABLE 29.6. *Fluvoxamine Trial. Therapeutic effect. Test statistics for dropout mechanism.*

	MNAR vs MAR		MAR vs MCAR	
Wald	6.98	($P = 0.008$)	3.98	($P = 0.046$)
LR	6.94	($P = 0.008$)	4.03	($P = 0.044$)
score	9.31	($P = 0.002$)	4.02	($P = 0.045$)

ture of the analyses in Diggle and Kenward (1994). From the fitted MNAR model we have:

$$\text{logit}\{P(\text{dropout})\} = -2.00 - 1.11 Y_c + 0.77 Y_{\text{pr}}$$
$$= -2.00 - 0.17[0.17](Y_c + Y_{\text{pr}}) - 0.94[0.28](Y_c - Y_{\text{pr}}).$$

A plausible interpretation would be that dropout decreases when there is a favorable change in therapeutic effect, and increases only comparatively slightly when there is little therapeutic effect. Larger differences can also be seen among the parameter estimates of the response component, between the MCAR and MAR models on one hand and the non-random dropout model on the other, than are apparent in the analysis of the side effects. The estimated differences between visits are greater in the MNAR model; in the MAR analysis no account is taken of the dependence of dropout on increment, so the sizes of the changes between visits is biased downwards. These differences are however of little practical importance given the sizes of the associated standard errors. Similarly, the statistical dependence between repeated measurements as measured by the log odds-ratios is smaller under the MNAR model, possibly because of the effect of selection under the MAR model.

29.3 A Model for Non-monotone Missingness

In Section 29.2, we presented a model for ordinal data but confined missingness to the dropout type. Here, general missingness will be studied, in the specific context of a bivariate binary outcome.

Baker, Rosenberger, and DerSimonian (1992) considered a log-linear type of model for two binary outcomes subject to incompleteness. A main advantage of this method is that it can easily deal with non-monotone missingness.

As in Section 29.2, let $r = 1, \ldots, N$ index distinct covariate levels. In this section, the index r will be suppressed from notation. Let $j, k = 1, 2$ correspond to the outcome categories of the first and second measurement, respectively and let $r_1, r_2 = 0, 1$ correspond to the missingness indicators

(1 for an observed and 0 for a missing measurement). Such a setup leads to a four-way classification. The complete data and observed data cell probabilities $\pi_{r_1 r_2, jk}$ for this setting are presented in Figure 29.1.

To accommodate (possibly continuous) covariates, as proposed by Jansen et al (2003), we will use a parameterization, different from and extending the original one, which belongs to the selection model family (Little 1994):

$$\pi_{r_1 r_2, jk} = p_{jk} q_{r_1 r_2 | jk}, \quad (29.6)$$

where p_{jk} parameterizes the measurement process and $q_{r_1 r_2 | jk}$ describes the missingness mechanism, conditional on the measurements. In particular, we will assume

$$p_{jk} = \frac{\exp(\boldsymbol{\theta}_{jk})}{\sum_{j,k=1}^{2} \exp(\boldsymbol{\theta}_{jk})}, \quad (29.7)$$

$$q_{r_1 r_2 | jk} = \frac{\exp[\beta_{jk}(1 - r_2) + \alpha_{jk}(1 - r_1) + \gamma(1 - r_1)(1 - r_2)]}{1 + \exp(\beta_{jk}) + \exp(\alpha_{jk}) + \exp(\beta_{jk} + \alpha_{jk} + \gamma)}, \quad (29.8)$$

for unknown parameters θ_{jk}, β_{jk}, α_{jk}, and γ. A priori, no ordering is imposed on the outcomes. The advantage is that genuine multivariate settings (e.g., several questions in a survey) can be handled as well. When deemed necessary, the implications of ordering can be imposed by considering specific models and leaving out others. For example, one may want to avoid missingness on future observations. In the current bivariate case, the index k would have to be removed from α in the above model. To identify the model, we set $\theta_{22} = \mathbf{0}$ and further $\boldsymbol{\theta}_{jk} = X_{jk} \boldsymbol{\eta}$. This allows the inclusion of covariate effects that, together with (29.7), is similar in spirit to the multigroup logistic model (Albert and Lesaffre 1986). Even though the parameters $\boldsymbol{\eta}$ are conditional in nature and therefore somewhat difficult to directly interpret in case planned sequences are of unequal length (but not in the case considered here), (29.7) allows easy calculation of the joint probabilities. Such computational advantages become increasingly important as the length of the response vector grows. If necessary, specific functions of interest, such as a marginal treatment effect, can be derived. They will typically take the form of non-linear functions. Arguably, a model of the type here can be most useful as a component of a sensitivity analysis, in conjunction with the use of different (e.g., marginal) models.

In many examples, the design matrices X_{jk} will be equal to each other. Stacking all parameters will lead to the following design:

$$\boldsymbol{\theta} = X \boldsymbol{\eta}. \quad (29.9)$$

Likewise, a design can be constructed for the non-response model parameters:

$$\boldsymbol{\delta} = W \boldsymbol{\psi}, \quad (29.10)$$

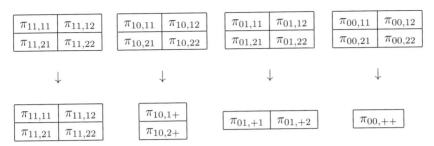

FIGURE 29.1. *Theoretical distribution over complete and observed cells of a bivariate binary outcome. Tables correspond to completely observed subjects and subjects with the second, the first, and both measurements missing, respectively.*

where the vector $\boldsymbol{\delta}$ stacks the β_{jk}, α_{jk} and γ and W is an appropriate design matrix. The vector $\boldsymbol{\psi}$ groups the parameters of interest. For example, if MCAR would be considered, the α and β parameters do not depend on neither j nor k and then $\boldsymbol{\psi}' = (\alpha, \beta, \gamma)$. Both designs (29.9) and (29.10) can be combined into one, using $\boldsymbol{\xi} = (\boldsymbol{\theta}', \boldsymbol{\delta}')'$,

$$T = \begin{pmatrix} X & 0 \\ 0 & W \end{pmatrix},$$

and

$$\boldsymbol{\phi} = (\boldsymbol{\eta}', \boldsymbol{\psi}')'. \tag{29.11}$$

The corresponding log-likelihood function can be written as:

$$\begin{aligned}
\ell &= \sum_{j,k=1}^{2} y_{11jk} \ln \pi_{11jk} + \sum_{j=1}^{2} y_{10j+} \ln(\pi_{10j1} + \pi_{10j2}) \\
&\quad + \sum_{k=1}^{2} y_{01+k} \ln(\pi_{011k} + \pi_{012k}) \\
&\quad + y_{00++} \ln(\pi_{0011} + \pi_{0012} + \pi_{0021} + \pi_{0022}) \\
&= \sum_{j,k=1}^{2} \sum_{s=1}^{y_{11jk}} \ln \pi_{11jk} + \sum_{j=1}^{2} \sum_{s=1}^{y_{10j+}} \ln \pi_{10j+} \\
&\quad + \sum_{k=1}^{2} \sum_{s=1}^{y_{01+k}} \ln \pi_{01+k} + \sum_{s=1}^{y_{00++}} \ln \pi_{00++}.
\end{aligned}$$

Computation of derivatives, needed for optimization and for the calculation of influence measures, is straightforward. A technical report can be obtained from the authors upon request.

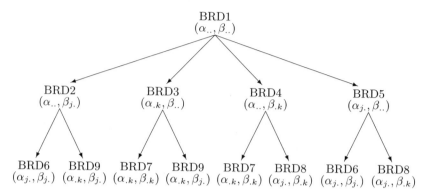

FIGURE 29.2. *Graphical representation of the BRD model nesting structure.*

To include covariates, the design level $r = 1, \ldots, N$ needs to be introduced again. In particular, with subject-specific covariates, it may be sensible to use $i = 1, \ldots, N$ to index individuals.

Baker, Rosenberger, and DerSimonian (1992, BRD) consider nine identifiable models, based on setting α_{jk} and β_{jk} constant in one or more indices. An overview, together with the nesting structure, is given in Figure 29.2.

Whereas these authors considered the nine models in terms of the original parameterization, they do carry over to parameterization (29.8). Interpretation is straightforward. For example, BRD1 is MCAR, in BRD4 missingness in the first variable is constant, while missingness in the second variable depends on its value. Two of the main advantages of this family are ease of computation in general, and the existence of a closed-form solution for several of its members (BRD2 to BRD9).

29.3.1 Analysis of the Fluvoxamine Data

In the analysis, all patients with known duration level are considered, leaving a total of 310 out of 315 subjects in the study. In the measurement model, the effect of duration is held constant over both visits. Regarding the missingness model, an effect of duration is assumed in both the α and the β parameters. Each of the 9 models is represented by a specific choice for the design. For example, for BRD1, and using the index i for individual, we obtain:

$$\phi = (\eta_1, \eta_2, \eta_3, \eta_4, \alpha, \alpha_{\text{dur}}, \beta, \beta_{\text{dur}}, \gamma)',$$

$$X_i = \begin{pmatrix} 1 & 0 & 0 & \text{duration}_i \\ 0 & 1 & 0 & \text{duration}_i \\ 0 & 0 & 1 & \text{duration}_i \end{pmatrix}$$

29.3 A Model for Non-monotone Missingness

TABLE 29.7. *Fluvoxamine Trial. Maximum likelihood estimates and standard errors of BRD models. All observations included. No covariates. Part I.*

Effect	BRD1	BRD2	BRD3	BRD4	BRD5
Measurement model					
Intercept$_{11}$	0.22(0.15)	0.20(0.15)	0.28(0.15)	0.03(0.17)	0.32(0.15)
Intercept$_{12}$	-1.72(0.30)	-1.74(0.30)	-1.72(0.30)	-1.61(0.30)	-1.62(0.30)
Intercept$_{21}$	-0.12(0.18)	-0.12(0.18)	-0.05(0.18)	-0.42(0.23)	-0.13(0.18)
Dropout model					
α	-4.72(0.71)	-4.72(0.71)		-4.72(0.71)	
$\alpha_{1.}$					-3.87(0.71)
$\alpha_{2.}$					$-\infty$
$\alpha_{.1}$			-4.27(0.71)		
$\alpha_{.2}$			$-\infty$		
β	-1.09(0.13)		-1.09(0.13)		-1.09(0.13)
$\beta_{1.}$		-1.37(0.22)			
$\beta_{2.}$		-0.91(0.17)			
$\beta_{.1}$				-1.57(0.38)	
$\beta_{.2}$				-0.55(0.29)	
γ	3.04(0.77)	3.04(0.77)	3.04(0.77)	3.04(0.77)	3.04(0.77)
- loglik	565.96	564.55	565.07	564.55	565.34

and

$$W_i = \begin{pmatrix} 1 & \text{duration}_i & 0 & 0 & 0 \\ 1 & \text{duration}_i & 0 & 0 & 0 \\ 1 & \text{duration}_i & 0 & 0 & 0 \\ 1 & \text{duration}_i & 0 & 0 & 0 \\ 0 & 0 & 1 & \text{duration}_i & 0 \\ 0 & 0 & 1 & \text{duration}_i & 0 \\ 0 & 0 & 1 & \text{duration}_i & 0 \\ 0 & 0 & 1 & \text{duration}_i & 0 \\ 0 & 0 & 0 & 0 & 1 \end{pmatrix}.$$

The matrix X_i includes a time dependent intercept and a time independent effect of duration. The W_i matrix indicates which of the nine BRD models is considered; changing the model also changes the vector ψ.

We will consider three sets of BRD models in some detail. Tables 29.7 and 29.8 presents models (parameter estimates, standard errors, negative log-likelihoods) without duration. In Tables 29.9 and 29.10, duration is added as a covariate to the measurement model but not yet to the missingness model, whereas in the final set (Tables 29.11 and 29.12) the effect of duration is included in both measurement and missingness parts of the

TABLE 29.8. *Fluvoxamine Trial. Maximum likelihood estimates and standard errors of BRD models. All observations included. No covariates. Part II.*

Effect	BRD6	BRD7	BRD8	BRD9
Measurement model				
Intercept$_{11}$	0.32(0.15)	0.14(0.16)	0.16(0.17)	0.27(0.15)
Intercept$_{12}$	-1.62(0.30)	-1.61(0.30)	-1.44(0.32)	-1.72(0.30)
Intercept$_{21}$	-0.13(0.18)	-0.31(0.21)	-0.39(0.22)	-0.04(0.17)
Dropout model				
α				
$\alpha_{1.}$	-3.93(0.71)		-3.93(0.71)	
$\alpha_{2.}$	$-\infty$		$-\infty$	
$\alpha_{.1}$		-4.29(0.71)		-4.29(0.71)
$\alpha_{.2}$		$-\infty$		$-\infty$
β				
$\beta_{1.}$	-1.37(0.22)			-1.37(0.22)
$\beta_{2.}$	-0.91(0.17)			-0.91(0.17)
$\beta_{.1}$		-1.57(0.38)	-1.56(0.37)	
$\beta_{.2}$		-0.56(0.29)	-0.56(0.29)	
γ	3.31(0.79)	3.51(0.84)	3.31(0.79)	3.11(0.77)
- loglik	563.97	563.70	563.97	563.70

model. Sampling zeroes in some of the cells forces some parameters to lie on the boundary of their corresponding parameter space which, due to the parameterization, is equal to ∞. This should not be seen as a disadvantage of our model, as boundary solutions are a well-known feature of MNAR models (Rubin 1996). The advantage of our parameterization is that either an interior or a boundary solution is obtained, and never an invalid solution.

From Tables 29.7 and 29.8, we learn that likelihood ratio tests fail to reject BRD1 in favor of a more complex model, implying the simplest mechanism, MCAR would be adequate. However, this conclusion changes when duration is included in the measurement model (Tables 29.9 and 29.10). The effect of duration is highly significant, whichever of the nine BRD models is chosen to conduct a likelihood ratio test. In addition, within Tables 29.9 and 29.10, not BRD1 but rather BRD4 provides the most adequate description. The likelihood ratio test statistic for comparing BRD1–4 equals 7.10, while those for BRD4–7 and BRD4–8 are 2.10 and 1.52, respectively. Thus, from this set of models, one observes that duration improves the fit and, moreover, one would be inclined to believe duration, included in the measurement model, has the effect of changing the nature of the missingness mechanism, by making it more complex, even though it is often

TABLE 29.9. *Fluvoxamine Trial. Maximum likelihood estimates and standard errors of BRD models. All observations included. Duration as covariate in the measurement model. Part I.*

Effect	BRD1	BRD2	BRD3	BRD4	BRD5
Measurement model					
Intercept$_{11}$	0.46(0.17)	0.45(0.17)	0.53(0.17)	0.23(0.20)	0.57(0.17)
Intercept$_{12}$	-1.46(0.31)	-1.48(0.31)	-1.46(0.31)	-1.26(0.32)	-1.37(0.31)
Intercept$_{21}$	0.10(0.20)	0.10(0.19)	0.17(0.20)	-0.25(0.23)	0.09(0.21)
Duration	-0.02(0.01)	-0.02(0.01)	-0.02(0.01)	-0.02(0.01)	-0.02(0.01)
Dropout model					
α	-4.71(0.71)	-4.71(0.71)		-4.71(0.71)	
$\alpha_{1.}$					-3.85(0.71)
$\alpha_{2.}$					$-\infty$
$\alpha_{.1}$			-4.24(0.71)		
$\alpha_{.2}$			$-\infty$		
β	-1.11(0.13)		-1.11(0.13)		-1.11(0.13)
$\beta_{1.}$		-1.44(0.23)			
$\beta_{2.}$		-0.90(0.17)			
$\beta_{.1}$				-1.86(0.45)	
$\beta_{.2}$				-0.43(0.25)	
γ	2.98(0.77)	2.98(0.77)	2.98(0.77)	2.98(0.77)	2.98(0.77)
- loglik	550.15	548.31	549.12	546.60	549.39

believed that including explanatory variables (either in the model for the outcomes or in the missingness model) may help to explain structure in the missingness mechanism. BRD4 states that missingness at the second occasion depends on the (possibly unobserved) value at that same occasion, a so-called type I model, in the typology of Baker (2000), in contrast to type II models, where missingness in a variable depends at least also on other, possibly incomplete, assessments. Obviously, such models are particularly vulnerable to assumptions made.

A key conclusion is that, up to this point, no covariate effects have been considered on the missingness parameters. An analysis including duration in the missingness part of the model should be entertained and examined carefully. When switching to Tables 29.11 and 29.12, the conclusions do change drastically. First, all evidence for non-MCAR missingness disappears as, based on likelihood ratio tests, BRD1 comes out as the most adequate description of all nine models. Second, comparing corresponding BRD models between Tables 29.9 and 29.10 on the one hand and Tables 29.11 and 29.12 (p-values in bottom line of Tables 29.11 and 29.12),

TABLE 29.10. *Fluvoxamine Trial. Maximum likelihood estimates and standard errors of BRD models. All observations included. Duration as covariate in the measurement model. Part II.*

Effect	BRD6	BRD7	BRD8	BRD9
Measurement model				
Intercept$_{11}$	0.57(0.17)	0.35(0.18)	0.36(0.19)	0.52(0.18)
Intercept$_{12}$	-1.37(0.31)	-1.26(0.32)	-1.06(0.33)	-1.46(0.31)
Intercept$_{21}$	0.09(0.20)	-0.13(0.21)	-0.21(0.22)	0.18(0.20)
Duration	-0.02(0.01)	-0.02(0.01)	-0.02(0.01)	-0.02(0.01)
Dropout model				
α				
$\alpha_{1\cdot}$	-3.92(0.71)		-3.94(0.71)	
$\alpha_{2\cdot}$	$-\infty$		$-\infty$	
$\alpha_{\cdot 1}$		-4.28(0.71)		-4.26(0.71)
$\alpha_{\cdot 2}$		$-\infty$		$-\infty$
β				
$\beta_{1\cdot}$	-1.44(0.23)			-1.44(0.23)
$\beta_{2\cdot}$	-0.90(0.17)			-0.90(0.17)
$\beta_{\cdot 1}$		-1.87(0.46)	-1.86(0.45)	
$\beta_{\cdot 2}$		-0.43(0.25)	-0.43(0.25)	
γ	3.31(0.79)	3.74(0.89)	3.39(0.79)	3.07(0.77)
- loglik	547.57	545.55	545.84	547.30

it is clear that the effect of duration on the missingness model cannot be neglected.

Important modeling and data analytic conclusions can be drawn from this. First, it clearly does not suffice to consider covariate effects on the measurement model, but one has to carefully contemplate such effects on the missingness model as well. Therefore, the models in Tables 29.11 and 29.12, should be regarded as the ones of primary interest. Second, it is found that a longer duration implies a less favorable side-effects outcome, as well as an increased change of missing visits. Obviously, duration acts as a confounding variable which, unless included in both parts of the model, may suggest a relationship between the measurement and missingness models and thus one may erroneously be led to believe that the missing data are MNAR. Third, it should be noted that the parameter estimates of duration are remarkably stable. This implies that, in case one is primarily interested in the effect of duration on the occurrence of side effects all 18 models containing this effect provide very similar evidence. Although this need not be the case in general, it is a comforting aspect of this particular data analysis.

29.3 A Model for Non-monotone Missingness

TABLE 29.11. *The Fluvoxamine Trial. Maximum likelihood estimates and standard errors of BRD models. All observations included. Duration as covariate in both measurement and missingness model. Part I.*

Effect	BRD1	BRD2	BRD3	BRD4	BRD5
Measurement model					
Intercept$_{11}$	0.46(0.18)	0.45(0.17)	0.53(0.18)	0.30(0.20)	0.57(0.17)
Intercept$_{12}$	-1.46(0.31)	-1.48(0.31)	-1.46(0.31)	-1.37(0.31)	-1.37(0.31)
Intercept$_{21}$	0.10(0.20)	0.10(0.20)	0.17(0.20)	-0.15(0.24)	0.09(0.20)
Duration	-0.02(0.01)	-0.02(0.01)	-0.02(0.01)	-0.02(0.01)	-0.02(0.01)
Dropout model					
$\alpha_{..}$	-4.57(0.72)	-4.57(0.72)		-4.57(0.72)	
$\alpha_{1.}$					-3.82(0.73)
$\alpha_{2.}$					$-\infty$
$\alpha_{.1}$			-4.20(0.72)		
$\alpha_{.2}$			$-\infty$		
α_{dur}	-0.02(0.02)	-0.02(0.02)	-0.01(0.02)	-0.02(0.02)	-0.01(0.02)
$\beta_{..}$	-1.40(0.16)		-1.40(0.16)		-1.40(0.16)
$\beta_{1.}$		-1.63(0.24)			
$\beta_{2.}$		-1.22(0.20)			
$\beta_{.1}$				-1.79(0.36)	
$\beta_{.2}$				-0.87(0.33)	
β_{dur}	0.02(0.01)	0.02(0.01)	0.02(0.01)	0.02(0.01)	0.02(0.01)
γ	3.10(0.78)	3.10(0.78)	3.10(0.77)	3.10(0.78)	3.09(0.78)
- loglik	543.78	542.74	542.86	542.63	543.14
$p^{\dagger}$	0.0017	0.0038	0.0019	0.0189	0.0019

† *p*-value for the comparison with the corresponding BRD model in Table 29.9, to test the null hypothesis of no effect of duration in the missingness model.

However, though we have reached plausible conclusions, one should still exercise caution, as non-random missingness models heavily rely on untestable assumptions (Verbeke and Molenberghs 2000). Therefore, it is important to search for observations that may drive these conclusions. This naturally leads to the concept of sensitivity analysis. In Sections 31.4 and 31.5, sensitivity analysis tools applicable to the BRD model, or its extension to covariates used here, will be introduced.

TABLE 29.12. *Fluvoxamine Trial. Maximum likelihood estimates and standard errors of BRD models. All observations included. Duration as covariate in both measurement and missingness model. Part II.*

Effect	BRD6	BRD7	BRD8	BRD9
Measurement model				
Intercept$_{11}$	0.57(0.17)	0.41(0.18)	0.43(0.19)	0.52(0.18)
Intercept$_{12}$	-1.37(0.31)	-1.37(0.31)	-1.22(0.33)	-1.46(0.31)
Intercept$_{21}$	0.09(0.21)	-0.04(0.22)	-0.13(0.23)	0.18(0.20)
Duration	-0.02(0.01)	-0.02(0.01)	-0.02(0.01)	-0.02(0.01)
Dropout model				
$\alpha_{..}$				
$\alpha_{1.}$	-3.87(0.73)		-3.88(0.73)	
$\alpha_{2.}$	$-\infty$		$-\infty$	
$\alpha_{.1}$		-4.23(0.73)		-4.22(0.72)
$\alpha_{.2}$		$-\infty$		$-\infty$
α_{dur}	-0.01(0.02)	-0.01(0.02)	-0.00(0.02)	-0.01(0.02)
$\beta_{..}$				
$\beta_{1.}$	-1.63(0.24)			-1.63(0.24)
$\beta_{2.}$	-1.22(0.20)			-1.22(0.20)
$\beta_{.1}$		-1.79(0.36)	-1.77(0.35)	
$\beta_{.2}$		-0.88(0.33)	-0.88(0.33)	
β_{dur}	0.02(0.01)	0.02(0.01)	0.02(0.01)	0.02(0.01)
γ	3.33(0.79)	3.50(0.84)	3.32(0.79)	3.16(0.78)
- loglik	542.14	541.77	542.05	541.86
$p^{\dagger}$	0.0044	0.0228	0.0226	0.0043

† p-value for the comparison with the corresponding BRD model in Table 29.10, to test the null hypothesis of no effect of duration in the missingness model.

29.4 Concluding Remarks

In Section 29.2, a modeling approach for incomplete ordinal outcomes with dropout was presented. The approach is very general and any measurement model can be used. In fact, it is easy enough to adapt the method to any type of outcome. Not only marginal models, also random-effects models can be used by way of measurement model. In Section 29.3, a model specifically for binary data, but then with general missingness patterns, has been presented. The one limitation of the model in Section 29.2 is its suitability to dropout only. Several extensions to general missingness have been studied in the literature. Troxel, Harrington, and Lipsitz (1998) presented methods for non-ignorable non-monotone missingness. Baker (1995) presented a modification of Diggle and Kenward (1994) to accommodate non-monotone missingness. Jansen and Molenberghs (2005) modify the model of Section 29.2 to account for non-monotone missingness by replacing the logistic regressions for dropout with a second multivariate Dale model to describe the vector of missingness indicators, given the outcomes.

Thus, a wide variety of selection models is available for incomplete longitudinal data, under MNAR and possibly also with non-monotone missingness. Nevertheless, care has to be taken with such models. As with all model fitting the conclusions drawn are conditional on the appropriateness of the assumed model. Especially here, there are aspects of the model that are in a fundamental sense not testable, namely the relationship between dropout and the missing observations. It is assumed in the modeling approach taken here that the relationships among the measurements from a subject are the same whether or not some of these measurements are unobserved due to dropout. It is this assumption, combined with the adoption of an explicit model linking outcome and dropout probability, that allows us to infer something about the MNAR nature of the dropout process. Given the dependence of the inferences on untestable assumptions, care is needed in the interpretation of the analysis.

The absence of evidence for non-random dropout may simply mean that a non-random dropout process is operating in a quite different manner, and in practice it is likely that many such processes are operating simultaneously.

Thus, the sensitivity of the posited model to modeling assumption needs to be addressed with great caution. Verbeke and Molenberghs (2000, Chapter 19 and 20) discussed ways to assess such sensitivities with continuous longitudinal data. We refer to Chapter 31 for a discussion of sensitivity analysis in the non-Gaussian setting.

30
Pattern-mixture Models

30.1 Introduction

Pattern-mixture models (PMM) were introduced in Section 26.2.1 as one of the three major frameworks within which missing data models can be developed, next to selection models (Chapter 29) and shared-parameter models.

Little (1993, 1994a, 1995) has been promoting the use of pattern-mixture models as a viable alternative to selection models. His work is based on, for example, Rubin (1977), where the idea was used in a sensitivity analysis within a fully Bayesian framework. Further references include Glynn, Laird, and Rubin (1993), Little and Rubin (1987), and Rubin (1987). In 1989, an entire issue of the *Journal of Educational Statistics* was devoted to this theme. A key reference is Hogan and Laird (1997). Several authors have contrasted selection models and pattern-mixture models. This is done either (1) to answer the same scientific question, such as marginal treatment effect or time evolution, based on these two rather different modeling strategies, or (2) to gain additional insight by supplementing the selection model results with those from a pattern-mixture approach. Examples include Verbeke, Lesaffre, and Spiessens (2001) or Michiels *et al* (2002) for continuous outcomes, and Molenberghs, Michiels, and Lipsitz (1999), or Michiels, Molenberghs, and Lipsitz (1999) for categorical outcomes. Further references include Cohen and Cohen (1983), Muthén, Kaplan, and Hollis (1987), Allison (1987), McArdle and Hamagani (1992), Little and Wang (1996), Hedeker and Gibbons (1997), Ekholm and Skinner (1998),

Molenberghs, Michiels, and Kenward (1998), Park and Lee (1999), and Thijs *et al* (2002).

An important issue is that pattern-mixture models are by construction under-identified, i.e., overspecified. Little (1993, 1994a) solves this problem through the use of identifying restrictions: inestimable parameters of the incomplete patterns are set equal to (functions of) the parameters describing the distribution of the completers. Identifying restrictions are not the only way to overcome under-identification and we will discuss alternative approaches in Section 30.2. Although some authors perceive this under-identification as a drawback, we believe it is an asset because it forces one to reflect on the assumptions made. This can serve as a starting point for sensitivity analysis, as outlined in Verbeke and Molenberghs (2000, Chapter 20).

A general framework for pattern-mixture modeling is sketched in Section 30.2 and the strategy based on identifying restrictions is developed in Section 30.3. A general modeling framework, within which both selection models and pattern-mixture models can be placed, is sketched in Sections 30.4 and 30.5. Finally, the fluvoxamine study, introduced in Section 2.4 and analyzed before in Sections 6.5, 7.2.4, 7.11, 29.2.3, and 29.3.1, is used to illustrate the proposed methods, in Section 30.6.

30.2 Pattern-mixture Modeling Approach

Fitting pattern-mixture models can be approached in several ways. It is important to decide whether pattern-mixture and selection modeling are to be contrasted with one another or rather the pattern-mixture modeling is the central focus. In the latter case, it is natural to conduct an analysis, and preferably a sensitivity analysis, *within* the pattern-mixture family. We will explicitly consider two strategies to deal with under-identification.

Strategy 1. Little (1993, 1994a) advocated the use of identifying restrictions and presented a number of examples. One of those, ACMV (available case missing values), is the natural counterpart of MAR in the PMM framework, as was established by Molenberghs *et al* (1998). Specific counterparts to MNAR selection models were studied by Kenward, Molenberghs, and Thijs (2003). More detail about this strategy is provided in Section 30.3.

Strategy 2. As opposed to identifying restrictions, model simplification can be done to identify the parameters. Thijs *et al* (2002) discussed several sub-strategies in detail, in the context of continuous longitudinal outcomes.

Although the second strategy is computationally simple, it is important to note that there is a price to pay. Indeed, simplified models, qualified as *assumption rich* by Sheiner, Beale, and Dunne (1997), also make untestable assumptions, just as in the selection model case. From a technical point of view, Strategy 2 only requires to either consider 'pattern' as an extra covariate in the model, or to conduct an analysis 'by pattern,' such that a separate analysis is obtained for each of the dropout patterns. In the identifying restrictions setting on the other hand (Strategy 1), the assumptions are clear from the start.

Pattern-mixture models do not always automatically provide estimates and standard errors of marginal quantities of interest, such as overall treatment effect or overall time trend. Hogan and Laird (1997) provided a way to derive selection model quantities from the pattern-mixture model. An example of such a marginalization is given by Thijs et al (2002). See also Verbeke and Molenberghs (2000, Chapter 20).

30.3 Identifying Restriction Strategies

In this section, we provide an introduction to the identifying restriction strategies, incorporating results of Molenberghs et al (1998) and Kenward, Molenberghs, and Thijs (2003). Ample detail can be found in Verbeke and Molenberghs (2000, Chapter 20). While these authors focus on continuous longitudinal outcomes, the general principles are entirely the same.

In line with Molenberghs et al (1998), we restrict attention to monotone patterns. In general, let us assume we have $t = 1, \ldots, n = T$ dropout patterns where the dropout indicator, introduced earlier, is $d = t+1$. The indices j for measurements occasions and t for dropout patterns assume the same values, but it is useful to dispose of both, to properly distinguish between the measurement and dropout processes.

For pattern t, the complete data density is given by

$$f_t(y_1, \ldots, y_T) = f_t(y_1, \ldots, y_t) f_t(y_{t+1}, \ldots, y_T | y_1, \ldots, y_t). \qquad (30.1)$$

The first factor is clearly identified from the observed data, while the second factor is not. It is assumed that the first factor is known or, more realistically, modeled using the observed data. Then, identifying restrictions are applied in order to identify the second component.

Although, in principle, completely arbitrary restrictions can be used by means of any valid density function over the appropriate support, strategies which relate back to the observed data deserve privileged interest. One can base identification on all patterns for which a given component, y_s say, is identified. A general expression for this is

$$f_t(y_s | y_1, \ldots y_{s-1}) = \sum_{j=s}^{T} \omega_{sj} f_j(y_s | y_1, \ldots y_{s-1}), \quad s = t+1, \ldots, T. \qquad (30.2)$$

We will use $\boldsymbol{\omega}_s$ as shorthand for the set of ω_{sj}'s used, the components of which are typically positive. Every $\boldsymbol{\omega}_s$ that sums to one provides a valid identification scheme.

Let us incorporate (30.2) into (30.1):

$$f_t(y_1,\ldots,y_T)$$
$$= f_t(y_1,\ldots,y_t) \prod_{s=0}^{T-t-1} \left[\sum_{j=T-s}^{T} \omega_{T-s,j} f_j(y_{T-s}|y_1,\ldots,y_{T-s-1}) \right]. \quad (30.3)$$

Let us consider three special but important cases, associated with these choices of $\boldsymbol{\omega}_s$ in (30.2). Little (1993) proposes CCMV (complete case missing values) which uses the following identification:

$$f_t(y_s|y_1,\ldots y_{s-1}) = f_T(y_s|y_1,\ldots y_{s-1}), \quad s = t+1,\ldots,T, \quad (30.4)$$

corresponding to $\omega_{sT} = 1$ and all others zero. In other words, information which is unavailable is always borrowed from the completers. Alternatively, the nearest identified pattern can be used:

$$f_t(y_s|y_1,\ldots y_{s-1}) = f_s(y_s|y_1,\ldots y_{s-1}), \quad s = t+1,\ldots,T, \quad (30.5)$$

corresponding to $\omega_{ss} = 1$ and all others zero. We will refer to these restrictions as *neighboring case missing values* or NCMV.

The third special case of (30.2) will be ACMV. ACMV is reserved for the counterpart of MAR in the PMM context. The corresponding $\boldsymbol{\omega}_s$ vectors can be shown (Molenberghs et al 1998) to have components:

$$\omega_{sj} = \frac{\alpha_j f_j(y_1,\ldots,y_{s-1})}{\sum_{\ell=s}^{T} \alpha_\ell f_\ell(y_1,\ldots,y_{s-1})}, \quad (30.6)$$

($j = s,\ldots,T$) where α_j is the fraction of observations in pattern j (Molenberghs et al 1998).

This MAR–ACMV link connects the selection and pattern-mixture families. It is further of interest to consider specific sub-families of the MNAR family. In the selection model context, one typically restricts attention to a class of mechanisms where dropout may depend on the current, possibly unobserved, measurement, but not on future measurements. The entire class of such models will be termed missing non-future dependent (MNFD). Although they are natural and easy to consider in a selection model context, there exist important examples of mechanisms that do not satisfy MNFD, such as shared-parameter models (Wu and Bailey 1989, Little 1995).

Kenward, Molenberghs, and Thijs (2003) have shown there is a counterpart to MNFD in the pattern-mixture context. The conditional probability of pattern t in the MNFD selection models obviously satisfies

$$f(r = t|y_1,\ldots,y_T) = f(r = t|y_1,\ldots,y_{t+1}). \quad (30.7)$$

Within the PMM framework, we define non-future dependent missing value restrictions (NFMV) as follows:

$$\forall t \geq 2, \forall j < t-1 \ :$$
$$f(y_t|y_1,\ldots,y_{t-1}, r = j) = f(y_t|y_1,\ldots,y_{t-1}, r \geq t-1). \quad (30.8)$$

```
SEM  :  MCAR   ⊂   MAR    ⊂   MNFD   ⊂   general MNAR
              ↕             ↕            ↕              ↕
PMM  :  MCAR   ⊂   ACMV   ⊂   NFMV   ⊂   general MNAR
                       ⊂    ≠
                         interior
```

FIGURE 30.1. *Relationship between nested families within the selection model (SEM) and pattern-mixture model (PMM) families. MCAR: missing completely at random; MAR: missing at random; MNAR: missing not at random; MNFD: missing non-future dependence; ACMV: available-case missing values; NFMV: non-future missing values; interior: restrictions based on a combination of the information available for other patterns. The '⊂' symbol here indicates 'is a special case of.' The '↕' symbol indicates correspondence between a class of SEM models and a class of PMM models.*

NFMV is not a single set of restrictions, but rather leaves one conditional distribution per incomplete pattern unidentified:

$$f(y_{t+1}|y_1,\ldots,y_t, r = t). \tag{30.9}$$

In other words, the distribution of the "current" unobserved measurement, given the previous ones, is unconstrained. Note that (30.8) excludes such mechanisms as CCMV and NCMV. Kenward, Molenberghs, and Thijs (2003) have shown that, for longitudinal data with dropouts, MNFD and NFMV are equivalent.

For pattern t, the complete data density is given by

$$\begin{aligned}f_t(y_1,\ldots,y_T) &= f_t(y_1,\ldots,y_t)f_t(y_{t+1}|y_1,\ldots,y_t)\\ &\times f_t(y_{t+2},\ldots,y_T|y_1,\ldots,y_{t+1}).\end{aligned} \tag{30.10}$$

It is assumed that the first factor is known or, more realistically, modeled using the observed data. Then, identifying restrictions are applied in order to identify the second and third components. First, from the data, estimate $f_t(y_1,\ldots,y_t)$. Second, the user has full freedom to choose

$$f_t(y_{t+1}|y_1,\ldots,y_t). \tag{30.11}$$

Substantive considerations can be used to identify this density. Alternatively, a family of densities can be considered by way of sensitivity analysis. Third, using (30.8), the densities $f_t(y_j|y_1,\ldots,y_{j-1})$, $(j \geq t+2)$ are identified. This identification involves not only the patterns for which y_j is observed, but also the pattern for which y_j is the current, the first unobserved measurement. An overview of the connection between selection and pattern-mixture models is given in Figure 30.1.

Two obvious mechanisms, within the MNFD family but outside MAR, are NFD1 (NFD standing for 'non-future dependent'), i.e., choose (30.11) according to CCMV, and NFD2, i.e., choose (30.11) according to NCMV. NFD1 and NFD2 are strictly different from CCMV and NCMV.

30.3.1 How to Use Restrictions?

We will briefly outline a general strategy. Several points which require further specification will be discussed in what follows. (1) Fit a model to the pattern-specific identifiable densities: $f_t(y_1, \ldots, y_t)$. This results in a parameter estimate, $\hat{\gamma}_t$. (2) Select an identification method of choice. (3) Using this identification method, determine the conditional distributions of the unobserved outcomes, given the observed ones:

$$f_t(y_{t+1}, \ldots, y_T | y_1, \ldots, y_t). \tag{30.12}$$

(4) Using standard multiple imputation methodology (Rubin 1987, Schafer 1997, Verbeke and Molenberghs 2000, Minini and Chavence 2004ab, Section 28.2 of this volume), draw multiple imputations for the unobserved components, given the observed outcomes and the correct pattern-specific density (30.12). (5) Analyze the multiply-imputed sets of data using the method of choice. This can be another pattern-mixture model, but also a selection model or any other desired model. (6) Inferences can be conducted in the standard multiple imputation way (Section 28.2 of this volume, Rubin 1987, Schafer 1997, Verbeke and Molenberghs 2000).

We have seen how general identifying restrictions (30.2), with CCMV, NCMV, and ACMV as special cases, lead to the conditional densities for the unobserved components, given the observed ones. This came down to deriving expressions for ω, such as in (30.6) for ACMV. In addition, we need to draw imputations from the conditional densities.

Let us proceed by studying the special case of three measurements. To this end, we consider an identification scheme and we start off by avoiding the specification of a parametric form for these densities. The following steps are required: (1) Estimate the parameters of the identifiable densities: from pattern 3, $f_3(y_1, y_2, y_3)$; from pattern 2, $f_2(y_1, y_2)$; and from pattern 1, $f_1(y_1)$. (2) To properly account for the uncertainty with which the parameters are estimated, we need to draw from them as is customarily done in multiple imputation. It will be assumed that in all densities from which we draw, this parameter vector is used. (3) **For pattern 2.** Given an observation in this pattern, with observed values (y_1, y_2), calculate the conditional density $f_3(y_3|y_1, y_2)$ and draw from it. (4) **For pattern 1.** We now have to distinguish three sub steps.

1. There is now only one ω involved: for pattern 1, in order to determine $f_1(y_2|y_1)$, as a combination of $f_2(y_2|y_1)$ and $f_3(y_2|y_1)$. Every ω in the unit interval is valid. Specific cases are: for NCMV, $\omega = 1$; for CCMV, $\omega = 0$; for ACMV, ω identifies a linear combination across patterns. Note that, given y_1, this is a constant, depending on α_2 and α_3. For

NFD1 and NFD2, the first unidentified conditional density can be chosen freely, thereafter a system of ω's has to be chosen as well.

To pick one of the two components f_2 or f_3, we need to generate a random uniform variate, U say, except in the boundary NCMV and CCMV cases.

2. If $U \leq \omega$, calculate $f_2(y_2|y_1)$ and draw from it. Otherwise, do the same based on $f_3(y_2|y_1)$.

3. Given the observed y_1 and given y_2 which has just been drawn, calculate the conditional density $f_3(y_3|y_1, y_2)$ and draw from it.

All steps but the first one have to be repeated M times, and further inferential steps proceed as in Section 28.2.

In case the observed densities are assumed to be normal, the corresponding conditional densities are particularly straightforward. However, in several cases, the conditional density is a mixture of normal densities. Then an additional and straightforward draw from the components of the mixture is necessary. Similar developments are possible with categorical data, ensuring that draws from the proper conditional multinomial distributions are made.

30.4 A Unifying Framework for Selection and Pattern-mixture Models

The developments in Section 30.3 can be followed whenever identifying restrictions are invoked, regardless of whether the outcomes are continuous or non-continuous. In this section, we present a different unification, in the sense that a versatile framework for modeling incomplete categorical data is presented. From this, selection models and pattern-mixture models will follow as a special case. These developments are based on work by Molenberghs and Goetghebeur (1997) and Michiels, Molenberghs, and Lipsitz (1999).

We will adopt the same notational conventions as in Section 29.2, based upon Section 7.1. In summary, there are $r = 1, \ldots, N$ design levels, grouping subjects $i = 1, \ldots, N_r$, which are measured at occasions $j = 1, \ldots, n$, producing outcomes Y_{rij} with corresponding design X_r. Restricting attention to dropout, D_{ri} is the dropout indicator. It is convenient to state that the categorical outcome Y_{rij} can take values $k_j = 1, \ldots, c_j$ and to let D_{ri}, which is categorical as well, range over $k_0 = 1, \ldots, c_0$. Typically $c_0 = n$, but it could be smaller if, for example, some dropout patterns do not occur by design.

All information about the responses on the units at the rth design level is contained in a cross-classification of the dropout indicator D_{ri} and the outcomes Y_{rij} into the $c_0 \times \ldots \times c_n$ dimensional contingency table with cell counts $Z^c_{rdk_1\ldots k_n}$, grouped into the vector $\boldsymbol{Z}^c_r$. The superscript c here and in what follows refers to 'complete' or 'full.' This notational convention is similar to Section 29.2. Since we will not distinguish between cell counts and cumulative counts, we assume that the above notation refers to cell counts, and we will not consider the version superscripted by a $*$.

The corresponding cell probability vector $\boldsymbol{\nu}^c_r$ has entries

$$\nu^c_{rdk_1\ldots k_n}. \qquad (30.13)$$

A selection model, such as the models described in Sections 29.2 and 29.3, is obtained by factorizing (30.13) as

$$\nu^c_{rdk_1\ldots k_n}(\boldsymbol{\theta}^S, \boldsymbol{\psi}^S) = \mu^{Sc}_{rk_1\ldots k_n}(\boldsymbol{\theta}^S)\, \phi^{Sc}_{rd|k_1\ldots k_n}(\boldsymbol{\psi}^S). \qquad (30.14)$$

A general pattern-mixture model is then based upon the factorization

$$\nu^c_{rdk_1\ldots k_n}(\boldsymbol{\theta}^P, \boldsymbol{\psi}^P) = \phi^{Pc}_{rd}(\boldsymbol{\psi}^P)\, \mu^{Pc}_{rk_1\ldots k_n|d}(\boldsymbol{\theta}^P). \qquad (30.15)$$

A certain amount of symmetry between the two frameworks is seen by assuming the data are collected following a multinomial sampling scheme and further assuming composite generalized linear models to hold:

- for the parameters of the selection model:

$$\eta^S_r(\boldsymbol{\mu}^{Sc}_r) = \boldsymbol{X}^S_{\eta r} \boldsymbol{\theta}^S, \qquad (30.16)$$

$$\xi^S_r(\boldsymbol{\phi}^{Sc}_r) = \boldsymbol{X}^S_{\xi r} \boldsymbol{\psi}^S, \qquad (30.17)$$

- and for the parameters of the pattern-mixture model:

$$\eta^P_r(\boldsymbol{\mu}^{Pc}_{r|d}) = \boldsymbol{X}^P_{\eta r} \boldsymbol{\theta}^P_d, \qquad d = 1, \ldots, n, \qquad (30.18)$$

$$\xi^P_r(\boldsymbol{\phi}^{Pc}_r) = \boldsymbol{X}^P_{\xi r} \boldsymbol{\psi}^P. \qquad (30.19)$$

Denote $\boldsymbol{\theta}^P = (\boldsymbol{\theta}^P_d)_{d=1,\ldots,n}$, $\boldsymbol{X}^S_r = (\boldsymbol{X}^S_{\eta r}, \boldsymbol{X}^S_{\xi r})$, $\boldsymbol{X}^P_r = (\boldsymbol{X}^P_{\eta r}, \boldsymbol{X}^P_{\xi r})$.

General choices for the vector link functions η^S_r, η^P_r are possible, inspired by the general framework laid out in Section 7.3.

The observed data are not $\boldsymbol{Z}^c_r$ but merely $\boldsymbol{Z}_r$, a partially classified table, arising by summing over the appropriate rows or columns in the corresponding complete table. We then have a linear relationship between observed and complete quantities: $\boldsymbol{Z}_r = C_r \boldsymbol{Z}^c_r$ and $\boldsymbol{\nu}_r = C_r \boldsymbol{\nu}^c_r$. We call the matrix C_i which consists of 0's and 1's the *coarsening matrix* in agreement with Heitjan and Rubin (1991) and Molenberghs and Goetghebeur (1997). See Section 28.3.6 for an example.

Illustration. As an illustration, assume complete data consist of a design matrix and a categorical outcome (with c levels) measured on two occasions for each subject, and further that each subject is seen at the first occasion, with only part of them measured at the second occasion. The observed multinomial data consist of a set of complete $c \times c$ tables $\mathbf{Z}_{r2}$ with counts Z_{r2jk} ($j, k = 1, \ldots, c$) and a supplemental margin $\mathbf{Z}_{r1}$ with counts Z_{r1j}, where $j = 1, \ldots, c$. The (hypothetical) full data amount to two $c \times c$ tables Z^c_{rdjk} with $d = 1, 2$ and $j, k = 1, \ldots, c$. Obviously, the relation between complete and observed counts is $Z_{r2jk} = Z^c_{r2jk}$ and $Z_{r1j} = \sum_{k=1}^c Z^c_{r1jk}$. Adopting the convention that the counts of all tables corresponding to design level r are represented as vectors in lexicographic ordering, and that $\mathbf{Z}_r = (\mathbf{Z}'_{r2}, \mathbf{Z}'_{r1})'$ with a similar expression for $\mathbf{Z}^c_r$, the coarsening matrix C_r is given by

$$C = C_r = \left(\begin{array}{c|c} C_{r0} & 0 \\ \hline 0 & C_{r1} \end{array} \right) = \left(\begin{array}{c|c} I_{c^2} & 0_{c^2, c^2} \\ \hline 0_{c, c^2} & I_c \otimes 1_{1,c} \end{array} \right), \qquad (30.20)$$

with I. the identity matrix, 0. a matrix of zeros, 1. a matrix of ones and $\otimes$ the Kronecker product.

The kernel of the multinomial (observed) log-likelihood is

$$\ell(\boldsymbol{\theta}, \boldsymbol{\psi}; \mathbf{Z}) = \sum_{r=1}^N \mathbf{Z}'_r \ln(\boldsymbol{\nu}_r),$$

subject to the constraints $\sum_k \nu_{rk} = 1$, where the summation index k cycles through all (multi-indexed) cells of $\boldsymbol{\nu}_r$.

We develop estimation of the parameters $\boldsymbol{\theta}$ and $\boldsymbol{\psi}$, which are either the selection model or the pattern-mixture model parameters. Following McCullagh and Nelder (1989), the score equations are given by

$$\frac{\partial \ell}{\partial \boldsymbol{\theta}} = \sum_{r=1}^N \left(\frac{\partial \boldsymbol{\nu}_r}{\partial \boldsymbol{\theta}} \right)' \mathbf{V}_r^- (\mathbf{Z}_r - n_r \boldsymbol{\nu}_r),$$

with $\mathbf{V}_r = \mathrm{diag}(\boldsymbol{\nu}_r) - \boldsymbol{\nu}_r \boldsymbol{\nu}'_r$. Further,

$$\left(\frac{\partial \boldsymbol{\nu}_r}{\partial \boldsymbol{\theta}} \right)' = \left(\frac{\partial \boldsymbol{\nu}^c_r}{\partial \boldsymbol{\theta}} \right)' \left(\frac{\partial \boldsymbol{\nu}_r}{\partial \boldsymbol{\nu}^c_r} \right)' = \left(\frac{\partial \boldsymbol{\nu}^c_r}{\partial \boldsymbol{\theta}} \right)' C'_r. \qquad (30.21)$$

30.5 Selection Models *versus* Pattern-mixture Models

A specific model choice is based on the form of (30.16) and (30.17), or (30.18) and (30.19), reflected in the matrix $\partial \boldsymbol{\nu}^c_r / \partial \boldsymbol{\theta}$ in (30.21). We will discuss selection models and pattern-mixture models in turn. The specific setting of a bivariate outcome will be considered, extension to the general case being straightforward.

30.5.1 Selection Models

Model (30.14), restricted to two outcomes, becomes

$$\nu^{Sc}_{rdjk}(\boldsymbol{\theta}^S, \boldsymbol{\psi}^S) = \mu^{Sc}_{rjk}(\boldsymbol{\theta}^S) \phi^{Sc}_{rd|jk}(\boldsymbol{\psi}^S).$$

Drop the superscript S throughout Section 30.5.1. For each r, the constraints on these probabilities are:

$$\sum_{d=1}^{2}\sum_{j=1}^{c}\sum_{k=1}^{c} \nu^c_{rdjk} = \sum_{j=1}^{c}\sum_{k=1}^{c} \mu^c_{rjk} = 1 \text{ and } \sum_{d=1}^{2} \phi^c_{rd|jk} = 1 \text{ for all } j,k.$$

In this section, we define $\phi_{rjk} = \phi^c_{r2|jk} = 1 - \phi^c_{r1|jk}$, the probability that a measurement is made at the second occasion, given that the complete data are $(Y_{ri1} = j, Y_{ri2} = k)$.

When the complete data $\boldsymbol{Z}^c_r$ would be available, the information required to estimate the measurement parameters $\boldsymbol{\theta}$ could be obtained from the collapsed table with entries $Z^c_{r1jk} + Z^c_{r2jk}$, while the parameters of $\boldsymbol{\psi}$ would follow from the pairs (Z^c_{r1jk}, Z^c_{r2jk}) for all (j,k). For the partially observed table however, we have to fit the observed data likelihood with cell probabilities ν_{r2jk} and

$$\nu_{r1j+} = \sum_{k=1}^{c} \nu^c_{r1jk} = \sum_{k=1}^{c} \mu^c_{rjk}(1 - \phi_{rjk}).$$

In general, the latter expression does not split into $\boldsymbol{\mu}$ and $\boldsymbol{\phi}$ parts.

To fully specify (30.16) and (30.17), we will choose link functions for the left hand sides of the form:

$$\boldsymbol{\eta}_r(\boldsymbol{\mu}^c_r) = D_\mu \ln(A_\mu \boldsymbol{\mu}^c_r), \qquad (30.22)$$

$$\boldsymbol{\xi}_r(\boldsymbol{\phi}^c_r) = D_\phi \ln(A_\phi \boldsymbol{\phi}^c_r), \qquad (30.23)$$

where A_μ and A_ϕ are matrices containing zeros and ones, used to construct sums of probabilities (e.g., probabilities of collapsed tables), and D_μ and D_ϕ are contrast matrices (with entries equal to 0, 1 or -1). This choice is in agreement with (7.17).

Observing that $\boldsymbol{\nu}^c_r = \boldsymbol{\nu}^c_r(\boldsymbol{\mu}^c_r, \boldsymbol{\phi}^c_r)$ and

$$\frac{\partial \boldsymbol{\nu}^c_r}{\partial(\boldsymbol{\mu}^c_r, \boldsymbol{\phi}^c_r)} = \left(\begin{array}{c|c} F_r & M_r \\ I - F_r & -M_r \end{array} \right),$$

with $F_r = \text{diag}(\boldsymbol{\phi}^c_r)$ and $M_r = \text{diag}(\boldsymbol{\mu}^c_r)$, and introducing the notation

$$T_{\eta r} = \left(\frac{\partial \boldsymbol{\eta}_r}{\partial \boldsymbol{\mu}^c_r}\right) = D_\mu (\text{diag}[A_\mu \boldsymbol{\mu}^c_r])^{-1} A_\mu,$$

$$T_{\xi r} = \left(\frac{\partial \boldsymbol{\xi}_r}{\partial \boldsymbol{\phi}^c_r}\right) = D_\phi (\text{diag}[A_\phi \boldsymbol{\phi}^c_r])^{-1} A_\phi,$$

the score equations become

$$\frac{\partial \ell}{\partial(\boldsymbol{\theta},\boldsymbol{\psi})} = \sum_{r=1}^{N} \left(\begin{array}{c|c} X_{\eta r} & 0 \\ \hline 0 & X_{\xi r} \end{array} \right)' \left(\begin{array}{c|c} T_{\eta r}^{-1} & 0 \\ \hline 0 & T_{\xi r}^{-1} \end{array} \right)'$$

$$\times \left(\begin{array}{c|c} F_r & M_r \\ \hline I - F_r & -M_r \end{array} \right)' C_r' V_r^- S_r, \qquad (30.24)$$

with $\boldsymbol{S}_r = \boldsymbol{Z}_r - N_r \boldsymbol{\nu}_r$. Solving these equations can be done using a Newton-Raphson algorithm, as discussed in the previous section. The inverse of the matrix of second derivatives, evaluated at the maximum of the likelihood function, provides an estimator of the precision.

30.5.2 Pattern-mixture Models

For pattern-mixture models, we factorize the complete data probabilities as products of marginal dropout parameters and measurement probabilities conditional on the dropout pattern: $\nu_{rdjk}^{Pc}(\boldsymbol{\theta}^P, \boldsymbol{\psi}^P) = \phi_{rd}^{Pc}(\boldsymbol{\psi}^P) \mu_{rjk|d}^{Pc}(\boldsymbol{\theta}^P)$. Because in this section it is clear that we work in the pattern-mixture model setting, the superscript P will be omitted. The constraints on these probabilities are, for each i:

$$\sum_{j=1}^{c} \sum_{k=1}^{c} \mu_{rjk|d}^{c} = 1 \text{ for all } d \quad \text{and} \quad \sum_{d=1}^{2} \phi_{rd}^{c} = 1.$$

To derive the score equation, we need to adapt the notation slightly. The measurement probabilities for pattern $d = 1, 2$ are collected into a vector $\boldsymbol{\mu}_{r|d}^{c}$ and the dropout parameters into $\boldsymbol{\phi}_r^c$. The design for the measurement part has 2 components $\boldsymbol{\eta}_{r|d} = X_{\eta r|d} \boldsymbol{\beta}$ $(d = 1, 2)$ and

$$T_{\eta r|d} = \left(\frac{\partial \boldsymbol{\eta}_{r|d}}{\partial \boldsymbol{\mu}_r^c} \right) = D_{\mu|d}(\text{diag}[A_{\mu|d}\boldsymbol{\mu}_{r|d}^c])^{-1} A_{\mu|d}.$$

This yields

$$\frac{\partial \ell}{\partial(\boldsymbol{\theta},\boldsymbol{\psi})} = \sum_{r=1}^{N} \left(\begin{array}{c|c|c} X_{\eta r|1} & 0 & 0 \\ X_{\eta r|2} & 0 & 0 \\ 0 & X_{\xi r} & \end{array} \right)' \left(\begin{array}{c|c|c} T_{\eta r|1}^{-1} & 0 & 0 \\ 0 & T_{\eta r|2}^{-1} & 0 \\ 0 & 0 & T_{\xi r}^{-1} \end{array} \right)'$$

$$\times \left(\begin{array}{c|c|c} F_r & 0 & \boldsymbol{\mu}_{r|1}^c \\ 0 & I - F_r & -\boldsymbol{\mu}_{r|2}^c \end{array} \right)' C_r' V_r^- S_r. \qquad (30.25)$$

To maximize the pattern-mixture likelihood, we need to discuss identifying restrictions, as discussed in Section 30.3.

30.5.3 Identifying Restrictions

A feature of the pattern-mixture approach is that the model is chronically overspecified. This is because the measurement probabilities are modeled separately in both patterns, but the incomplete pattern ($d = 1$) is only partially observed (Little 1993). In the case described above, the incomplete pattern would provide information about the first measurement, but not about the second one, nor about the association between both. Thus, only the probabilities $\mu_{rj|1}$ are identified, leaving the $\mu^c_{rk|1j}$ inestimable. We will describe a solution to this problem, by first considering a measurement model and secondly combining it with a particular form of identifying restrictions on the model parameters.

A possible modeling approach is to consider a bivariate model for the completers, e.g., a Dale model, and a univariate model for the incomplete observations, e.g., a logistic regression model. We will term this the *minimal approach*.

We can then translate the identifying restrictions of Section 30.3. In the case of the illustration in Section 30.4, $\mu^c_{rk|1j}$ are identified by equating them to appropriate functions of μ_{r2jk}. For two patterns only, CCMV, ACMV, and NCMV, all amount to: $\mu^c_{rk|1j} = \mu^c_{rk|2j} = \mu_{rk|2j}$.

To apply CCMV to the Dale model directly, we have to proceed in a different way. First, the minimal approach is followed. From the observed data $\widehat{\boldsymbol{\theta}}_0^P$ and $\widehat{\boldsymbol{\psi}}_0^P$ follow and hence the underlying probabilities $\widehat{\mu}_{rjk|2}$ and $\widehat{\mu}_{rj|1}$ can be estimated. Then, CCMV implies that $\widehat{\mu}_{rk|1j} \equiv \widehat{\mu}_{rk|2j}$ and hence the partial count $Z_{rj|1}$ can be used to impute $\widetilde{Z}_{rjk|1} = Z_{rj|1}\widehat{\mu}_{rk|2j}$. From these completed counts and $Z^c_{rjk|2}$, one can estimate the parameters of interest, i.e., a Dale model for both patterns, yielding $\widehat{\boldsymbol{\theta}^P}$ and $\widehat{\boldsymbol{\psi}^P} \equiv \widehat{\boldsymbol{\psi}_0^P}$. This approach implies that the odds ratio for both outcomes, after correction for the covariate effects on the marginal probabilities, is carried over from for the completers' table to the incompleters' table.

This two-step procedure is clearly not restricted to the Dale model. In the case of monotone dropout, extension to more than two measurement occasions is straightforward. Although parameter estimation is very elegant and computationally simple with the two-step procedure, precision estimation is less simple, since treating the filled-in table as if it represented real data fails to reflect random variability in the unobserved counts. Strategies to determine confidence intervals will be discussed in Section 30.5.4.

30.5.4 Precision Estimation with Pattern-mixture Models

We propose two methods to calculate 95% confidence intervals: profile likelihood (Clayton and Hills 1993, Welsh 1996) and multiple imputation (Section 28.2).

Let us discuss profile likelihood first. For each component θ_s^P of the measurement parameter vector $\boldsymbol{\theta}^P$, the profile likelihood is constructed by keeping θ_s^P fixed and maximizing the observed data log-likelihood

$$\ell(\boldsymbol{\theta}^P) = \sum_{r=1}^{N}\sum_{j=1}^{c}\left[\sum_{k=1}^{c} Z_{r2jk} \ln \nu_{r2jk}(\boldsymbol{\theta}^P, \boldsymbol{\psi}^P) + Z_{r1j}\ln \nu_{r1j}(\boldsymbol{\theta}^P, \boldsymbol{\psi}^P)\right],$$

with respect to the remaining parameters. In particular, lower and upper bounds θ_{sl}^P and θ_{su}^P of a 95% confidence interval for $\widehat{\theta_s^P}$ are found by solving $2[\ell(\widehat{\boldsymbol{\theta}}^P) - \ell(\widehat{\boldsymbol{\theta}}_{(s)}^P)] = \chi_1^2(0.05)$, where $\widehat{\boldsymbol{\theta}}_{(s)}^P$ is the constrained maximization over $\theta_s^P = \theta_{sl}^P$ or $\theta_s^P = \theta_{su}^P$ and $\chi_1^2(0.05)$ is the 95% quantile of the χ^2 distribution with a single degree of freedom. The advantage of profile likelihood is that it is able to reflect asymmetry in the log-likelihood function.

Alternatively, multiple imputation can be used to construct an asymptotic covariance matrix for $\widehat{\boldsymbol{\theta}}^P$, from which asymptotic 95% confidence intervals readily follows. Recall that, for each covariate level s, the observed data are $\boldsymbol{Z}_r$ and the complete data are $\boldsymbol{Z}_r^c$. If we knew the distribution of $\boldsymbol{Z}_r^c$, with parameter vector $\boldsymbol{\theta}$, then we could impute $\boldsymbol{Z}_r^c$ by drawing from the conditional distribution $f(\boldsymbol{Z}_r^c|\boldsymbol{Z}_r, \boldsymbol{\theta})$. Because $\boldsymbol{\theta}$ is unknown, we estimate it from the data, yielding $\widehat{\boldsymbol{\theta}}$, and use the distribution $f(\boldsymbol{Z}_r^c|\boldsymbol{Z}_r, \widehat{\boldsymbol{\theta}})$. Because $\widehat{\boldsymbol{\theta}}$ is a random variable, we obviously take its variability into account in drawing imputations. In the analysis task, the Dale model is used to estimate model parameters. The inference task is straightforward and in line with Section 28.2. Hypothesis testing can proceed using the methodology of Section 28.2.3, which can be applied when the number of imputations is small. Alternatively, if the number of imputations is large, then asymptotic approximations can be used.

These two methods do not need to give the same results for the variances. Apart from sampling variation, introduced through multiple imputation, and different reference distribution approximations, the main difference is that multiple imputation based confidence intervals are symmetric by construction, while profile likelihood confidence intervals are not.

30.6 Analysis of the Fluvoxamine Data

The fluvoxamine study was introduced in Section 2.4 and analyzed before in Sections 6.5, 7.2.4, 7.11, 29.2.3, and 29.3.1. We will use this study to illustrate the general selection and pattern-mixture modeling framework, in agreement with Michiels, Molenberghs, and Lipsitz (1999).

A dichotomized version of the side effects, at the first and at the last visit, will be considered, where category 1 (no side effect) is contrasted with the others for both outcomes (category 0). So, we model the probability of

TABLE 30.1. *Fluvoxamine Trial. Selection model parameter estimates and 95% confidence intervals (full model).*

Parameter	First measurement		Last measurement	
intercept	0.786	[-0.083;1.654]	1.432	[0.397;2.467]
age/30	-0.669	[-1.218;-0.119]	-0.676	[-1.318;-0.034]
sex	-0.318	[-0.811;0.175]	0.254	[-0.337;0.846]
antecedents	0.134	[-0.366;0.633]	-0.057	[-0.649;0.536]
Association				
log odds ratio	2.038	[1.335;2.740]		
Dropout model				
intercept	1.583	[0.571;2.595]		
previous	-0.556	[-1.119;0.007]		
age/30	-0.261	[-0.874;0.352]		
sex	0.608	[0.052;1.164]		
antecedents	-0.254	[-0.836;0.327]		

no side effects. 299 patients have at least one measurement, including 242 completers.

30.6.1 Selection Modeling

Table 30.1 represents parameter estimates and asymptotic confidence intervals for a selection model including *age, sex*, and *psychiatric antecedents*, both into the marginal measurement model as well as in the logistic model for dropout. Note that *age* is a continuous covariate, whereas the other two are dichotomous. To allow for MAR, the first response is also entered in the dropout model. The association is modeled in terms of a constant log odds ratio.

In the marginal model, *sex* and *antecedents* seem to have little effect, whereas *age* is borderline and its coefficients at both measurement occasions are very similar. Likewise, *age* and *antecedents* add little to the dropout model, and further *sex* and the outcome at the first occasion are borderline, albeit at different sides of the critical level. The association between both measurements, even with adjustment of the marginal regression for covariate effects, remains very high, with an odds ratio of $\exp(2.038) = 7.675$.

A backward selection procedure was performed on the measurement and dropout processes separately, based on the likelihood ratio test. Parameters were removed in the following order. For the measurement model: both *antecedents* effects and both *sex* effects were removed. Subsequently, the two *age* parameters were combined into a common *age* effect. For the dropout model, *age* and *antecedents* were removed. The result is shown in

30.6 Analysis of the Fluvoxamine Data

TABLE 30.2. *Fluvoxamine Trial. Selection model parameter estimates and 95% confidence intervals after model reduction.*

Parameter	First measurement		Last measurement	
intercept	0.661	[-0.043;1.365]	1.560	[0.823;2.297]
common age (/30)	-0.664	[-1.141;-0.188]		
Association				
log odds ratio	1.956	[1.270;2.642]		
Dropout model				
intercept	1.085	[0.547;1.624]		
previous	-0.584	[-1.140;-0.028]		
sex	0.568	[0.025;1.110]		

Table 30.2. From this model, it is seen that the probability of side effects is higher at the first measurement occasion than at the last one, and increases with *age*. In particular, for an increase of 1 year, the odds of side effects increase with a factor $\exp(0.664/30) = 1.022$, because *age* was divided by 30 for ease of display of the estimates. The probability of dropout is higher if side effects are observed at the first occasion, and is lower for males than for females. In particular, the dropout probabilities are 0.256 (0.161) for males with (without) previous side effects, and 0.377 (0.253) for females with (without) side effects. The association, as well as the other parameters, except for the intercept, are similar to the ones found in Table 30.1.

30.6.2 Pattern-mixture Modeling

For the pattern-mixture approach, the parameter estimates and confidence intervals for the variables *age*, *sex*, and *antecedents* can be found in Table 30.3. The model is parameterized as follows: intercepts and covariate effects are given for the complete observations, together with the differences between effects for incomplete and complete observations. The latter ones would be zero if the distribution among completers would equal the distribution among dropouts. This model is used for the first as well as for the last observation. A constant log odds ratio is assumed for the association between both measurements. The confidence intervals are calculated using profile likelihood, as well as using multiple imputation. For the multiple imputation technique, the results are given for 100 imputations. As a check, Michiels, Molenberghs, and Lipsitz (1999) have also calculated the confidence intervals for 1000 and 4000 imputations, leading to negligible differences. Both methods to calculate confidence intervals (results not shown here) gave approximately the same results. The same variables are used to fit the dropout model, and because the data needed to estimate this model

TABLE 30.3. *Fluvoxamine Trial. Pattern-mixture model. Profile likelihood (PL) and multiple imputation (MI) (full model).*

Parameter	Meth.	First measurement		Last measurement	
		\multicolumn{4}{c}{Complete observations}			
intercept	PL	1.296	[0.289;2.339]	1.664	[0.616;2.767]
	MI	1.296	[0.268;2.325]	1.663	[0.596;2.731]
age/30	PL	-0.849	[-1.519;-0.203]	-0.756	[-1.440;-0.091]
	MI	-0.849	[-1.500;-0.198]	-0.756	[-1.414;-0.097]
sex	PL	-0.593	[-1.189;-0.007]	0.127	[-0.497;0.739]
	MI	-0.593	[-1.182;-0.004]	0.127	[-0.483;0.737]
antecedents	PL	0.222	[-0.353;0.805]	-0.016	[-0.634;0.594]
	MI	0.222	[-0.357;0.800]	-0.016	[-0.621;0.589]
		\multicolumn{4}{c}{Incomplete minus complete observations}			
intercept	PL	-2.151	[-4.300;-0.084]	-0.913	[-4.376;3.204]
	MI	-2.156	[-4.224;-0.087]	-1.018	[-4.393;2.357]
age/30	PL	0.869	[-0.396;2.142]	0.366	[-1.845;2.435]
	MI	0.871	[-0.396;2.139]	0.395	[-1.503;2.292]
sex	PL	0.879	[-0.268;2.050]	0.382	[-1.413;2.236]
	MI	0.879	[-0.274;2.033]	0.347	[-1.477;2.171]
antecedents	PL	-0.234	[-1.428;0.986]	-0.107	[-2.271;1.802]
	MI	-0.234	[-1.439;0.970]	-0.012	[-1.858;1.834]
		\multicolumn{4}{c}{Association}			
log odds ratio	PL	2.038	[1.354;2.789]		
	MI	2.065	[1.346;2.784]		
		\multicolumn{4}{c}{Dropout model, CI based on asymptotic variance (AV)}			
intercept	AV	1.390	[0.450;2.370]		
age/30	AV	-0.349	[-0.953;0.255]		
sex	AV	0.559	[0.010;1.108]		
antecedents	AV	-0.232	[-0.809;0.345]		

are complete, we have calculated confidence intervals based on the asymptotic variance. Although multiple imputation is only performed to estimate the precision, we also display the corresponding parameter estimates as an extra indication for convergence of the algorithm.

Antecedents and *sex* have nearly no effect on the measurement model, but the *sex* parameter for the first measurement gives a borderline influence. *Age* has an effect on the measurement outcomes, but there is no difference between this effect for the complete and incomplete observations. The association between both measurements is very strong. The odds ratio

TABLE 30.4. *Fluvoxamine Trial. Pattern-mixture model. Profile likelihood (PL) and multiple imputation (MI) after model reduction.*

Parameter	Meth.	First measurement		Last measurement	
		Complete observations			
intercept	PL	0.762	[0.036;1.478]	1.590	[0.846;2.333]
	MI	0.747	[0.029;1.466]	1.576	[0.836;2.315
		Incomplete minus complete observations			
intercept	PL	-0.499	[-1.065;0.050]	-0.268	[-1.123;0.704]
	MI	-0.499	[-1.055;0.056]	-0.275	[-1.071;0.521]
		Common age effect (/30)			
	PL	-0.650	[-1.132;-0.162]		
	MI	-0.639	[-1.121;-0.158]		
		Association			
log odds ratio	PL	1.977	[1.291;2.682]		
	MI	1.943	[1.263;2.623]		
		Dropout model, CI based on asymptotic variance (AV)			
intercept	AV	0.766	[0.353;1.179]		
sex	AV	0.517	[-0.021;1.056]		

is $\exp(2.038) = 7.675$. *Age* and *antecedents* have no effect on the dropout model, but *sex* has.

We reduced our model using a backward selection procedure. For the measurement model, we dropped *antecedents*, the additional *age* effect for the incomplete observations, and all the *sex* effects. Finally, a joint *age* effect for both time points is assumed. In the dropout model, *antecedents* and *age* were removed. *Sex* was kept, although it is borderline. The final model can be found in Table 30.4.

From this model one can see that the probability of dropout is higher for males than for females: 0.253 and 0.168, respectively. The probability of having side effects is higher at the first occasion than at the last, and increases for those who did not show up at the last visit. This probability also increases with *age*. For an increase of 1 year, the odds of having side effects increases with 1.022. The association is similar to its value in the full model, found in Table 30.3.

Note that the pattern-mixture model assumed a common odds ratio among completers and dropouts. This implies that the conditional distribution of the missing second measure follows the same conditional distribution given the first variable as do the complete variable. This ACMV restriction, as discussed in Section 3.3, is equivalent to the MAR assumption in the selection model.

30.6.3 Comparison

Both reduced models include *age* as a predictor for side effects. For the selection model, this effect is the same at both measurement occasions. The same is true for the pattern-mixture model and although it could in principle differ for completers and dropouts, it is the same for both subgroups. As a result, the estimates of the *age* effects in both frameworks become comparable and their numerical values are indeed very close. By construction, the association parameters are also comparable; they are certainly of the same magnitude. Of course, the dropout models differ, since only in a selection model measurements can be included into the dropout part as covariates. The *sex* effect is similar in both models, but its effect is borderline.

It is important to note that the pattern-mixture model can yield valuable insight in its own right. Specifically, the probability of side effects, after adjusting for *age*, is higher in the dropout group than in the completers group, both at the first as well as at the last measurement occasion. For someone aged 30 say, the probabilities of side effects at the first measurement occasion for in the completers' group and the dropouts' groups are 0.4720 and 0.5956, respectively. At the last measurement occasion these probabilities are 0.2809 and 0.3380, respectively. These values can be obtained in a selection framework as well, but less straightforwardly so. Another advantage of the pattern-mixture model is that the model building can be done for the different dropout groups separately. For example, if *sex* would be a prognostic factor for side effects in the dropout group but not in the completers group, this is easily incorporated in the pattern-mixture analysis.

30.7 Concluding Remarks

Pattern-mixture models are tied to restrictions, whereas selection models apparently are not. This issue is easily discussed in the setting of the illustration of page 563. It is useful to start our discussion with the MAR case. For the selection model, such a mechanism entails $\phi^c_{rd|jk} = \phi^c_{rd|j}$. For a pattern-mixture model, it implies $\mu^c_{rk|1j} = \mu^c_{rk|2j}$. In other words, MAR naturally translates into assumptions about the dropout probabilities in a selection model, but into a restriction in the pattern-mixture section. Data to estimate $\phi^c_{rd|jk}$ (in particular $\phi^c_{rd|j}$) are available, but the data to estimate $\mu^c_{rk|1j}$ are not.

Both procedures rest on untestable assumptions. Although this is clearly true for the pattern-mixture models, it is less obvious for the selection models, since wide classes of models for $\phi^c_{rd|jk}$ are estimable. However, to correctly test for MAR, one would need to observe both measurements in both patterns, which is by definition impossible (Glynn, Laird, and Rubin 1986, and discussion).

30.7 Concluding Remarks

The same is true for non-random missingness mechanisms. For pattern-mixture models, MNAR mechanisms are reflected by different restrictions (e.g., protective restrictions: Brown 1990, Michiels and Molenberghs 1997). For selection models, MNAR is encompassed by models for $\phi^c_{rd|jk}$ that depend explicitly on k. In Molenberghs and Goetghebeur (1997), it is seen how two non-random selection models can be supported by the observed data almost equally, but yield radically different interpretations for the unobserved data, in the sense that different models distribute an observed count Z_{r1j} in entirely different ways over the full data cells Z^c_{r1jk}.

An advantage of pattern-mixture models in the context of non-random dropout, quoted by Little (1995), is that no explicit model for the dropout process is needed, as long as the restrictions imposed are acceptable. However, this claim is less fulfilling at second glance, as there is no symmetry between the ϕ parameters in the two families. In a selection model, $\phi^c_{rd|jk}$ contains all information about the dropout process, whereas the same information is spread out over ϕ_{rd} and $\mu^c_{rjk|d}$ in a pattern-mixture model. This is seen through the fact that MAR is emanated by the ϕ's in the first case but by the μ's in the latter. Furthermore, the interdependence between dropout and measurement processes is modeled in $\phi^c_{rd|jk}$ in the first case and in $\mu^c_{rjk|d}$ in the latter one. The pattern-mixture dropout probabilities ϕ_{rd} can be seen as the *covariate dependent* part of the dropout mechanism.

Arguably, a framework has to be chosen based on the questions of scientific interest. For instance, in case one is interested in the population as a whole, a selection model might be the natural choice. However, investigators who would like to explore differences among subgroups that are identified by their response patterns, should consider fitting pattern-mixture models. The latter situation could be of interest to differentiate therapies between subgroups. For instance, if males would suffer more from dropout than females, one may want to establish sex dependent treatment protocols. In addition, *both* models can be fitted in a sensitivity analysis.

It may even be possible, rather than to choose between selection models and pattern-mixture models, to combine aspects of both. Such a route was chosen by Molenberghs, Michiels, and Kenward (1998).

31
Sensitivity Analysis

31.1 Introduction

Even though the assumption of likelihood ignorability encompasses both MAR and the more stringent and often implausible MCAR mechanisms, it is difficult to exclude the option of a more general missingness mechanism. One solution is to fit an MNAR model as proposed by Diggle and Kenward (1994) or Molenberghs, Kenward, and Lesaffre (1997). However, as pointed out by several authors (discussion to Diggle and Kenward 1994, Verbeke and Molenberghs 2000, Chapter 18), one has to be extremely careful with interpreting evidence for or against MNAR using only the data under study. A detailed treatment of the issue is provided in Jansen *et al* (2005).

A sensible compromise between blindly shifting to MNAR models or ignoring them altogether is to make them a component of a sensitivity analysis. It is important to consider the effect on key parameters such as treatment effect. In many instances, a sensitivity analysis can strengthen one's confidence in the MAR model (Molenberghs *et al* 2001, Verbeke *et al* 2001).

Broadly speaking, we could define a sensitivity analysis as one in which several statistical models are considered simultaneously and/or where a statistical model is further scrutinized using specialized tools (such as diagnostic measures). This rather loose and very general definition encompasses a wide variety of useful approaches. The simplest procedure is to fit a selected number of (MNAR) models that are all deemed plausible or one in which a preferred (primary) analysis is supplemented with a number of variations. The extent to which conclusions (inferences) are stable across such ranges provides an indication about the belief one can put into them. Variations to a basic model can be constructed in different ways. The most obvious strategy is to consider various dependencies of the missing data process on the outcomes and/or covariates. Alternatively, the distributional assumptions of the model can be changed. Thus clearly, several routes to sensitivity analysis are possible and in fact the area is fully in expansion.

Sensitivity analysis can be conducted within the selection model family itself. A perspective is given in Section 31.2. Another promising tool, proposed by Verbeke *et al* (2001), and employed by Thijs, Molenberghs, and Verbeke (2000) and Molenberghs *et al* (2001), is based on local influence (Cook 1986). These authors considered the Diggle and Kenward (1994) model, which is based on a selection model, integrating a linear mixed model for continuous outcomes with logistic regression for dropout.

These ideas have been developed for categorical data as well. Van Steen *et al* (2001) developed a local influence based sensitivity analysis for the MNAR Dale model of Section 29.2. It is presented in Section 31.3. Section 31.4 discusses related ideas for the general Baker, Rosenberger, and DerSimonian (1992) model, introduced in Section 29.3. It is based upon work by Jansen *et al* (2003). Hens *et al* (2005) developed kernel weighted influence measures.

Although classical inferential procedures account for the imprecision resulting from the stochastic component of the model and for finite sampling, less attention is devoted to the uncertainty arising from (unplanned) incompleteness in the data, even though the majority of studies in humans suffer from incomplete follow-up. Molenberghs *et al* (2001) acknowledge both the status of imprecision, due to (finite) random sampling, as well as ignorance, due to incompleteness. Both can be combined into uncertainty (Kenward, Goetghebeur, and Molenberghs 2001). An overview is given in Section 31.5.

Another option is to consider pattern-mixture models as a complement to selection models (Thijs *et al* 2002, Michiels *et al* 2002). The analysis conducted in Section 30.6, along the lines outlined in Sections 30.4 and 30.5, can be viewed as a sensitivity analysis of this type. A perspective is given in Section 31.6.

31.2 Sensitivity Analysis for Selection Models

When data are incomplete, the analysis of the actually observed data is subject to further untestable modeling assumptions. The methodologically simplest case is discussed in Section 27.3, where it is assumed that the missing data are MCAR. However, the MCAR assumption is a strong one and made too often in practice.

When more flexible assumptions, such as MAR or even MNAR, are considered, several choices have to be made. For example, one has to choose between selection and pattern-mixture models, or an alternative framework such as shared-parameter models (Section 26.2.1).

Particularly within the selection modeling framework, there has been an increasing literature on MNAR. At the same time, concern has been growing precisely about the fact that models often rest on strong assumptions and relatively little evidence from the data themselves.

In response to these concerns, there is growing awareness of the need for methods that investigate the sensitivity of the results with respect to the model assumptions. See, for example, Nordheim (1984), Little (1994b), Rubin (1994), Laird (1994), Fitzmaurice, Molenberghs, and Lipsitz (1995), Molenberghs *et al* (1999), Kenward (1998), and Kenward and Molenberghs (1999). Many of these are to be considered useful but *ad hoc* approaches. Whereas such informal sensitivity analyses are an indispensable step in the analysis of incomplete longitudinal data, it is desirable to conduct more formal sensitivity analyses.

At any rate, fitting an MNAR model should be subject to careful scrutiny. The modeler needs to pay attention, not only to the assumed distributional form of the model (Little 1994b, Kenward 1998), but also to the impact one or a few influential subjects may have on the dropout and/or measurement model parameters. Because fitting an MNAR model is feasible by virtue of strong assumptions, such models are likely to pick up a wide variety of influences in the parameters describing the nonrandom part of the dropout mechanism. Hence, a good level of caution is in place. This issue has been studied in detail by Jansen *et al* (2005). These authors not only study the behavior of local influence methods in the presence of a variety of deviations from the posited model, not only in terms of the dropout mechanism, they also study the behavior of the likelihood ratio test statistic, used to test MNAR *versus* MAR. Their conclusion is that such a test is surrounded with both philosophical issues, as well as technical problems. There are philosophical issues because two models, similar or even identical in terms of their fit to the observed data, may produce widely varying predictions of the unobserved data. When unrecognized, this is a problem, as such models cannot be distinguished in terms of statistical arguments only. When the scientific question is, at least in part, in terms of the fit to the unobserved outcomes, it is very difficult to distinguish between such models solely in statistical terms. The technical issues occur because the likelihood ratio test statistic for MNAR *versus* MAR, of the type used in the Diggle and Kenward (1994) and MNAR Dale (Section 29.2) models, exhibits non-standard behavior. This should not come as a surprise, as most of the information on the MNAR parameter(s) comes from distributional assumptions, and not from genuine information in the data. Therefore, classical asymptotics should not be taken for granted. This problem is studied by Jansen *et al* (2005); see also Scharfstein, Rotnitzky, and Robins (1999). By using a semi-parametric framework, it becomes clear that, under MNAR, semi-parametric assumptions, i.e., moment-based assumptions, are not sufficient to identify model parameters.

31.3 A Local Influence Approach for Ordinal Data with Dropout

Incomplete longitudinal ordinal data can be modeled using a simple logistic regression formulation for the dropout process and using a multivariate Dale model for the response (Molenberghs and Lesaffre 1994, 1999, Molenberghs, Kenward, and Lesaffre, 1997), as described in Section 29.2. To explore the sensitivity of this selection model for repeated ordinal outcomes, Van Steen et al (2001), considered a local influence approach.

31.3.1 General Principles

Cook (1986) suggests that more confidence can be put in a model that is relatively stable under small modifications. The best known perturbation schemes are based on case-deletion (Cook and Weisberg 1982) in which the effect is studied of completely removing cases from the analysis. A quite different paradigm is the local influence approach where one investigates how the results of an analysis are changed under small perturbations of the model. In the framework of the linear mixed model Beckman, Nachtsheim, and Cook (1987) used local influence to assess the effect of perturbing the error variances, the random-effects variances and the response vector. In the same context, Lesaffre and Verbeke (1998) have shown that the local influence approach is also useful for the detection of influential subjects in a longitudinal data analysis. Verbeke et al (2001) and Verbeke and Molenberghs (2000, Chapter 19) use the same idea to explore the sensitivity of a selection model for repeated continuous outcomes. The principal idea is to explore how small perturbations around MAR, in the direction of MNAR, can have a large impact. These authors have shown that various types of influential subjects can cause a model to apparently be of the MNAR type. This implies that caution should be used before concluding that the model really is MNAR, as many types of influential subjects, different from an MNAR mechanism, can force such a conclusion. This view was confirmed by Jansen et al (2005).

Consider the following perturbed dropout model:

$$\text{logit}[p_{id}(H_d, k_d; \boldsymbol{\psi})] = H_d \boldsymbol{\psi} + \omega_i k_d. \qquad (31.1)$$

which are the components of the ϕ's in (29.3). We choose to use the individual-level index i, rather than the design-level index r, as the perturbations ω_i are defined at the individual level.

31.3 A Local Influence Approach for Ordinal Data with Dropout

When $\omega_i = 0$ for all i, MAR is obtained. Due to ignorability, no influence on the measurement model parameters is then possible. When small perturbations in a specific ω_i lead to relatively large differences in the model parameters, then this suggests that these subjects may have a large impact on the final analysis. Note that the ω_i are not to be seen as fixed or random subject-specific parameters, but rather as (infinitesimal) perturbations, to which differential geometry will be applied, rather than ordinary parameter estimation.

We first give a general introduction of the local influence methodology as introduced by Cook (1986). In Section 31.3.2, it will be applied to the fluvoxamine study.

We denote the log-likelihood function corresponding to the model including perturbed dropout model (31.1) by

$$\ell(\boldsymbol{\gamma}|\boldsymbol{\omega}) = \sum_{i=1}^{N} \ell_i(\boldsymbol{\gamma}|\omega_i),$$

in which $\ell_i(\boldsymbol{\gamma}|\omega_i)$ is the contribution of the ith individual to the log-likelihood, and where $\boldsymbol{\gamma} = (\boldsymbol{\theta}, \boldsymbol{\psi})$ is the s-dimensional vector, grouping the parameters of the measurement model and the dropout model, not including the $N \times 1$ vector $\boldsymbol{\omega} = (\omega_1, \omega_2, \ldots, \omega_N)'$ of weights defining the perturbation of the MAR model. It is assumed that $\boldsymbol{\omega}$ belongs to an open subset Ω of $\mathbb{R}^N$. For $\boldsymbol{\omega}$ equal to $\boldsymbol{\omega_0} = (0, 0, \ldots, 0)'$, $\ell(\boldsymbol{\gamma}|\boldsymbol{\omega_0})$ is the log-likelihood function that corresponds to a MAR dropout model.

Let $\widehat{\boldsymbol{\gamma}}$ be the maximum likelihood estimator for $\boldsymbol{\gamma}$, obtained by maximizing $\ell(\boldsymbol{\gamma}|\boldsymbol{\omega_0})$, and let $\widehat{\boldsymbol{\gamma}}_\omega$ denote the maximum likelihood estimator for $\boldsymbol{\gamma}$ under $\ell(\boldsymbol{\gamma}|\boldsymbol{\omega})$. The local influence approach now compares $\widehat{\boldsymbol{\gamma}}_\omega$ with $\widehat{\boldsymbol{\gamma}}$. Similar estimates indicate that the parameter estimates are robust with respect to perturbations of the MAR model in the direction of MNAR. Very different estimates suggest that the estimation procedure is highly sensitive to such perturbations, which suggests that the choice between a random and a non-random dropout model highly affects the results of the analysis. Cook (1986) proposed to measure the distance between $\widehat{\boldsymbol{\gamma}}_\omega$ and $\widehat{\boldsymbol{\gamma}}$ by the so-called likelihood displacement, defined by $LD(\boldsymbol{\omega}) = 2[\ell(\widehat{\boldsymbol{\gamma}}|\boldsymbol{\omega_0}) - \ell(\widehat{\boldsymbol{\gamma}}_\omega|\boldsymbol{\omega_0})]$. This takes into account the variability of $\widehat{\boldsymbol{\gamma}}$. Indeed, $LD(\boldsymbol{\omega})$ will be large if $\ell(\boldsymbol{\gamma}|\boldsymbol{\omega_0})$ is strongly curved at $\widehat{\boldsymbol{\gamma}}$, which means that $\boldsymbol{\gamma}$ is estimated with high precision, and small otherwise. Therefore, a graph of $LD(\boldsymbol{\omega})$ versus $\boldsymbol{\omega}$ contains essential information on the influence of perturbations. It is useful to view this graph as the geometric surface formed by the values of the $N + 1$ dimensional vector $\boldsymbol{\xi}(\boldsymbol{\omega}) = [\boldsymbol{\omega}', LD(\boldsymbol{\omega})]'$ as $\boldsymbol{\omega}$ varies throughout Ω. Because this so-called influence graph can only be depicted when $N = 2$, Cook (1986) proposed to consider local influence, i.e., at the normal curvatures $C_{\boldsymbol{h}}$ of $\boldsymbol{\xi}(\boldsymbol{\omega})$ in $\boldsymbol{\omega_0}$, in the direction of some N dimensional vector

h of unit length. Let $\mathbf{\Delta}_i$ be the s dimensional vector defined by

$$\mathbf{\Delta}_i = \left.\frac{\partial^2 \ell_i(\boldsymbol{\gamma}|\omega_i)}{\partial \omega_i \partial \boldsymbol{\gamma}}\right|_{\boldsymbol{\gamma}=\widehat{\boldsymbol{\gamma}}, \omega_i=0}$$

and define $\boldsymbol{\Delta}$ as the $(s \times N)$ matrix with $\boldsymbol{\Delta}_i$ as its ith column. Further, let $\ddot{L}$ denote the $(s \times s)$ matrix of second-order derivatives of $\ell(\boldsymbol{\gamma}|\boldsymbol{\omega}_0)$ with respect to $\boldsymbol{\gamma}$, also evaluated at $\boldsymbol{\gamma} = \widehat{\boldsymbol{\gamma}}$. Cook (1986) has then shown that C_h can be easily calculated by $C_h = 2|h' \boldsymbol{\Delta}' \ddot{L}^{-1} \boldsymbol{\Delta} h|$.

Obviously, C_h can be calculated for any direction h. One evident choice is the vector h_i containing one in the ith position and zero elsewhere, corresponding to the perturbation of the ith weight only. This reflects the influence of allowing the ith subject to drop out non-randomly, whereas the others can only drop out at random. The corresponding local influence measure, denoted by C_i, then becomes $C_i = 2|\boldsymbol{\Delta}_i' \ddot{L}^{-1} \boldsymbol{\Delta}_i|$. Another important direction is the direction $h_{\max}$ of maximal normal curvature $C_{\max}$. It shows how to perturb the MAR model to obtain the largest local changes in the likelihood displacement. It is readily seen that $C_{\max}$ is the largest eigenvalue of $-2\,\boldsymbol{\Delta}'\,\ddot{L}^{-1}\,\boldsymbol{\Delta}$, and that $h_{\max}$ is the corresponding eigenvector.

When a subset $\boldsymbol{\gamma}_1$ of $\boldsymbol{\gamma} = (\boldsymbol{\gamma}_1', \boldsymbol{\gamma}_2')'$ is of special interest, a similar approach can be used, replacing the log-likelihood by the profile log-likelihood for $\boldsymbol{\gamma}_1$, and the methods discussed above for the full parameter vector directly carry over. Details can be found in Lesaffre and Verbeke (1998), Verbeke et al (2001), and Verbeke and Molenberghs (2000, Chapters 11 and 19).

It will be clear from the previous derivations that calculation of local influence measures merely reduces to evaluation of $\boldsymbol{\Delta}$ and $\ddot{L}$. In the linear mixed model case, Verbeke et al (2001) and Verbeke and Molenberghs (2000) have proposed closed form expressions, with some emphasis on the case of compound symmetry. For the multivariate Dale model, as will be the case for many other non-normal models, this is algebraically very involved and may not yield the same type of insightful expressions. However, when a program is available to fit the full non-random model (3.11), a particularly convenient computational scheme can be used. Indeed, in this case there are usually tools available to obtain a Hessian matrix evaluated in a point of interest (e.g., through EM-aided differentiation, see also page 537). Note that in our situation, it suffices to compute the second derivatives of the likelihood, for each observation separately, after which the subvector $\boldsymbol{\Delta}_i$ pertaining to the $(\boldsymbol{\gamma}, \omega)$-block can be selected.

In practice, the parameter $\boldsymbol{\theta}$ in the measurement model is often of primary interest. Because $\ddot{L}$ is block-diagonal with blocks $\ddot{L}(\boldsymbol{\theta})$ and $\ddot{L}(\boldsymbol{\psi})$, we have that for any unit vector h, C_h equals $C_h(\boldsymbol{\theta}) + C_h(\boldsymbol{\psi})$, with

$$C_h(\boldsymbol{\theta}) = -2h' \left[\left.\frac{\partial^2 \ell_{i\omega}}{\partial \boldsymbol{\theta} \partial \omega_i}\right|_{\omega_i=0}\right]' \ddot{L}^{-1}(\boldsymbol{\theta}) \left[\left.\frac{\partial^2 \ell_{i\omega}}{\partial \boldsymbol{\theta} \partial \omega_i}\right|_{\omega_i=0}\right] h$$

$$C_{\boldsymbol{h}}(\boldsymbol{\psi}) = -2\boldsymbol{h}'\left[\frac{\partial^2 \ell_{i\omega}}{\partial\boldsymbol{\psi}\partial\omega_i}\bigg|_{\omega_i=0}\right]' \ddot{L}^{-1}(\boldsymbol{\psi})\left[\frac{\partial^2 \ell_{i\omega}}{\partial\boldsymbol{\psi}\partial\omega_i}\bigg|_{\omega_i=0}\right]\boldsymbol{h},$$

evaluated at $\boldsymbol{\gamma} = \widehat{\boldsymbol{\gamma}}$.

31.3.2 Analysis of the Fluvoxamine Data

Van Steen et al (2001) applied the local influence ideas of Section 31.3 to the fluvoxamine study introduced in Section 2.4 and analyzed at various instances.

To investigate the sensitivity of inferences reported in Section 29.2.3 with respect to modeling assumptions for the dropout process, the overall C_i, influences $C_i(\boldsymbol{\theta})$ and $C_i(\boldsymbol{\psi})$ for the measurement parameters and dropout parameters, as well as $\boldsymbol{h}_{\max}$ of maximal curvature are displayed in Figure 31.1. Note that the largest C_i are observed for patients #34 and #252 (both having side effects surpassing the therapeutic effect at visit 1 and visit 2), followed by patients #182, #64, #122, #28, #108, #287, #232, #112, and #245, all of whom yield the worst score on side effects at visit 1 and drop out at visit 2. We pay special attention to patient #239, showing side effects interfering significantly with functionality at visit 1, after which dropout occurs.

In addition, Figure 31.1 shows some evidence of the fact that influence on measurement model parameters can theoretically only arise from those measurement occasions at which dropout occurs, a fact already observed by Verbeke et al (2001). Nevertheless, it should be noted that influence on the measurement model parameters can also arise from complete observations. Indeed, when small perturbations in a specific ω_i lead to relatively large differences in the model parameters, the subject's impact on dropout parameters indirectly influences all functions that include these dropout parameters. An example of such a function is the conditional mean of an unobserved measurement, given the observed measurements and given the fact that the patient belongs to a certain dropout pattern. As a consequence, the corresponding measurement model parameters will *indirectly* be affected as well (Verbeke et al 2001).

Influential completers occur in the index plots of C_i, $C_i(\boldsymbol{\psi})$, and of the components of the direction $\boldsymbol{h}_{\max}$ of maximal curvature, but are absent in the index plot for $C_i(\boldsymbol{\theta})$. Focusing on $C_i(\boldsymbol{\theta})$, Figure 31.1 reveals the highest peaks for patients #239 and #128. It appears that the influence of allowing subject #239 to drop out non-randomly, is best visible on the measurement model parameters. Patient #128 has an incomplete sequence, with a relatively mild score for side effects (side effects not interfering with functionality). Hence, the relatively large value for $C_i(\boldsymbol{\theta})$ is somewhat unusual, especially because other index plots do not show evidence of any influential effect, not even globally. One could ask the question whether other, unmeasured factors could have caused this phenomenon.

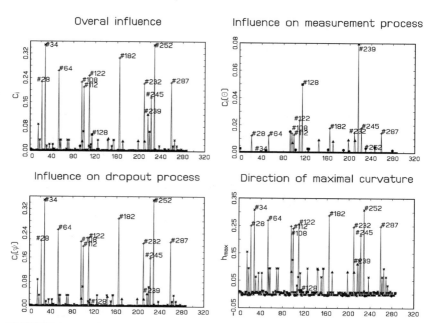

FIGURE 31.1. *Fluvoxamine Trial. Index plots of C_i, $C_i(\boldsymbol{\theta})$, $C_i(\boldsymbol{\psi})$, and of the components of the direction $\boldsymbol{h}_{\max}$ of maximal curvature. The x-axis merely contains sequential indicators. Relevant patient IDs have been added to the plot. Completers (patients with observed responses at visit 1 and visit 2) are indicated with a solid star. A solid circle, a solid square, a solid triangle, or a solid plus is used for subjects whose score on side effects at visit 1 respectively ranges from (1) to (4). Patients with a non-monotone dropout pattern are discarded.*

Before addressing this question, we turn attention to $C_i(\boldsymbol{\psi})$ and $\boldsymbol{h}_{\max}$. To avoid confusion, observe that the scale is different from the one of $C_i(\boldsymbol{\theta})$. The most influential patients appear to be the same as for the overall C_i (#34, #252 and #182, #64, #122, #28, #108, #287, #232, #112, #245). The same patients are also shown in the index plot for $\boldsymbol{h}_{\max}$.

Observe that in all plots, 'layers' of influential cases may be distinguished. The higher the layers, the more they seem to be associated with particular response levels. For instance, in Figure 31.1, patients #34 and #252 give rise to components of $\boldsymbol{h}_{\max}$ that are larger than 0.3. Patients #182, #64, #122, #28, #108, #287, #232, #112 and #245 (corresponding to the influential patients in the previous paragraph) refer to $\boldsymbol{h}_{\max}$ components that are all smaller than 0.3 but larger than 0.2. The layer formation is not clear though, and recalling the particular behavior of patient #128, one is led to believe that another distorting factor is involved, blurring the picture. Therefore, we investigate the effect of covariates on the ability to interpret influence plots.

31.3 A Local Influence Approach for Ordinal Data with Dropout

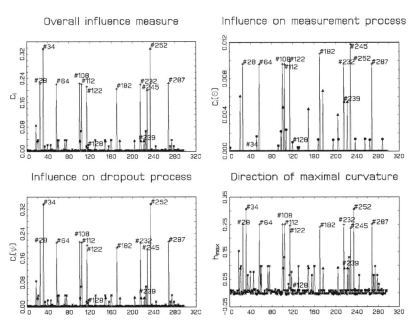

FIGURE 31.2. *Fluvoxamine Trial. Index plots of C_i, $C_i(\boldsymbol{\theta})$, $C_i(\boldsymbol{\psi})$, and of the components of the direction $\mathbf{h}_{\max}$ of maximal curvature, where 'age' is considered as the sole covariate in the Dale model. The x-axis contains sequential indicators. Completers are indicated with a solid star. A solid circle, a solid square, a solid triangle, or a solid plus is used for subjects whose score at visit 1 on side effects respectively ranges from (1) to (4).*

To this end, we consider two additional models. The first one includes 'sex' as the only covariate in the measurement model, the second one uses 'age' as the only covariate. These models perform worse than the model including both 'age' and 'sex,' augmented with 'duration' and 'severity,' but they are merely intended for illustrative purposes. The resulting influence plots are enlightening. Figure 31.2 shows the index plots when 'age' is included as only covariate, Figure 31.3 displays the corresponding pictures in case 'sex' is the only source of covariate information. In both cases, much smaller values are obtained for $C_i(\boldsymbol{\theta})$. The high peaks for patients #239 and #128 have disappeared. Patients #122, #245, and #182 also show up in Figure 31.2 with the highest peaks for $C_i(\boldsymbol{\theta})$, although hard to distinguish from the peaks for patients #287, #232, #28, #108, #64, and #112. The variability observed in $C_i(\boldsymbol{\theta})$ values also appears in Figure 31.3. However, in this case, it seems to be caused by the fact that patients #108, #182, #287, and #232 have $C_i(\boldsymbol{\theta})$ equal to about 0.0116 compared to approximately 0.0097 for patients #28, #245, #64, #122, and #112. This layer effect may be explained by the binary character of 'sex' as opposed to 'age,' the latter of which entered the model as a continuous variable. Also note that patients #108, #182, #287, and #232 are all male, whereas patients #28, #245, #64, #122, and #112 are all female. All these patients drop out at visit 2 and showed side effects surpassing therapeutic effect at visit 1. In Figures 31.2 and 31.3, the same patient group (i.e., patients #34, #252, #287, #108, #28, #112, #64, #232, #122, #182, and #245) is distinguished as globally influential, with highest C_i values for #34 and #252. The layering effect is again the most explicit when 'sex' is considered as only covariate (Figure 31.3). Influential patients for $C_i(\psi)$ and $h_{\max}$ appear to be the same as before, where 'sex' and 'age' were both considered in the pool of covariates, with the exception of subject #239 whose corresponding component in $h_{\max}$ is now less than 0.1000. The distribution over potential values becomes more discrete when 'age' is considered to be the only covariate in the multivariate Dale model. Changing 'age' for 'sex' causes the distribution to be even more discrete and therefore the layer effect more explicit.

In an attempt to improve insight into the driving forces present in the set of data, which may explain possible deviations from a random dropout process, we exclude patients #34 and #252 from the data set and apply the same measurement model as in the beginning of Section 5 (thus including the covariates 'age,' 'sex,' 'duration,' and 'severity'). Provided MAR is the correct alternative hypothesis and provided the parametric form for the MAR process is correct (again, no covariates were included), there seems to be even less evidence for MAR; the likelihood ratio test statistic comparing MCAR with MAR equals $G^2 = 0.94$, based on 1 degree of freedom ($p = 0.333$). Note that now borderline evidence for MNAR is observed, since a comparison between the non-random and random dropout model generates a likelihood ratio test statistic of $G^2 = 3.74$ with 1 degree of freedom ($p = 0.053$). Hence, the suggested local influence approach bridges the gap between the random and the non-random model: some of the mechanisms that cannot be explained by the random model and are captured by the non-random model, the latter resting on untestable assumptions, can be attributed to the observations for patients #34 and #252.

Repeating the previous analysis on a reduced data set, where patient #239 is excluded instead of patients #34 and #252, we find no evidence for MAR against MCAR ($G^2 = 0.01$, $p = 0.913$). After investigating the likelihood ratio test statistic for comparing the non-random with the random dropout model ($G^2 = 2.13$, $p = 0.145$), we may conclude that the MCAR assumption is fairly plausible. It is not surprising that conclusions remain similar. Indeed, although patient #239 appeared to be most influential patient with respect to the measurement model parameters, it should be noted that (i) the value for $C_i(\boldsymbol{\theta})$ is "only" 0.079 (further investigation is required to define some critical value above which $C_i(\boldsymbol{\theta})$ can be said to be

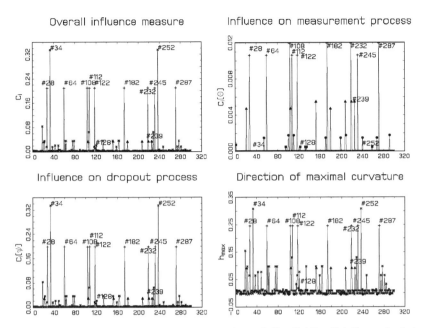

FIGURE 31.3. *Fluvoxamine Trial. Index plots of C_i, $C_i(\boldsymbol{\theta})$, $C_i(\boldsymbol{\psi})$, and of the components of the direction $\boldsymbol{h}_{\max}$ of maximal curvature, where 'sex' is considered as only covariate in the Dale model. The x-axis contains sequential indicators. Completers are indicated with a solid star. A solid circle, a solid square, a solid triangle, or a solid plus is used for non-completers whose score at visit 1 on side effects respectively ranges from (1) to (4).*

statistically significantly large) and that (ii) patient #239 did not appear to be influential overall.

31.4 A Local Influence Approach for Incomplete Binary Data

31.4.1 General Principles

For multivariate and longitudinal binary data, subject to non-monotone missingness, one can focus on the model proposed by Baker, Rosenberger, and DerSimonian (1992). They considered a log-linear type of model for two possibly binary outcomes, subject to non-monotone missingness. Jansen *et al* (2003) reformulated the model such that its membership of the selection model family is unambiguously clear. Next, they extended the original model to accommodate for, possibly continuous, covariates, turning the model into a regression tool for several categorical outcomes. Further, a parameterization was proposed that avoids the risk of invalid solutions. In other words, all combinations of the natural parameters produce probabilities between 0 and 1. The model is introduced in Section 29.3.

As a consequence of these extensions, the closed-form solutions of Baker, Rosenberger, and DerSimonian (1992) no longer apply. Of course, given the focus on continuous covariates, the derivation of closed-form solutions should not be of primary concern. Finally, Jansen et al (2003) coupled a local influence approach with the model strategy, to assess which observations have a strong impact on the comparison of two nested models within the BRD family.

Jansen et al (2005) consider perturbations of a given BRD model in the direction of a model with one more parameter in which the original model is nested, implying that perturbations lie along the edges of Figure 29.2: for each of the nested pairs in Figure 29.2, the simpler of the two models equates two parameters from the more complex one. For example, BRD4 includes $\beta_{.k}$, $(k = 1, 2)$, whereas in BRD1 only $\beta_{..}$ is included. For the influence analysis, ω_i is then included as a contrast between two such parameters; for the perturbation of BRD1 in the direction of BRD4, one considers $\beta_{..}$ and $\beta_{..} + \omega_i$. Such an ω_i is not a subject-specific parameter, but rather an infinitesimal perturbation. The vector of all ω_i's defines the direction in which such a perturbation is considered. Clearly, other perturbation schemes are possible as well, or one could consider a different route of sensitivity analysis altogether. Ideally, several could be considered within an integrated sensitivity analysis. Note that our influence analysis focuses on the missingness model, rather than on the measurement model parameters. This may be seen as slightly odd, because often, scientific interest focuses on the measurement model parameters. However, it has been documented (discussion to Diggle and Kenward 1994, Kenward 1998, Verbeke et al 2001) that the missingness model parameters are often the most sensitive ones to take up all kinds of misspecification and influential features. These may then, in turn, impact conclusions coming from the measurement model parameters (e.g., time evolution) or combinations from both (e.g., covariate effects for certain groups of responders).

31.4.2 Analysis of the Fluvoxamine Data

We will now apply the local influence ideas, outlined in the previous section, to the BRD models in order to contradict or strengthen the conclusions of Section 29.3.1. Whereas all comparisons along the edges of Figure 29.2 are possible, we propose to primarily focus on the comparison of BRD1 with BRD4 (Figure 31.4), as the first one was the most adequate model when no duration effect is included and when duration is included in both parts of the model, whereas the second one was the model of choice when duration

31.4 A Local Influence Approach for Incomplete Binary Data   587

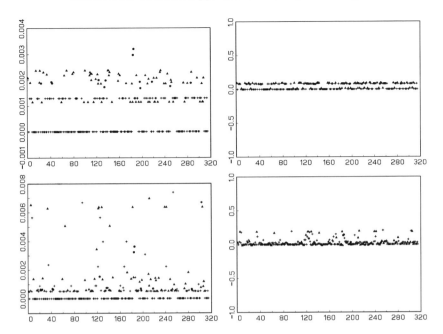

FIGURE 31.4. *Fluvoxamine Trial. Index plots of C_i (left panels) and of the components of the direction $h_{\max}$ of maximal curvature (right panels) for comparison BRD1–4, without (top panels) or with (bottom panels) duration as a covariate in the missingness models.*

is included in the measurement model only. In addition, we will consider the comparisons BRD4–7 (Figure 31.5) and BRD4–8 (plot not shown), the supermodels of BRD4. The symbols used in these figures are the following: +: both observations are available, (1,1) type; black triangle: only the first observation is available, (1,0) type; black square: only the second observation is available, (0,1) type; •: both measurements are missing, (0,0) type.

The overall C_i are considered, as well as the components of the direction of maximal curvature $h_{\max}$. The top right panel in Figure 31.4 shows essentially no structure, whereas in the top left there are two important observations. First, a clear layering effect is present, consistent with the analysis in Section 31.3.2. Again, this is not surprising, as there are quite a number of discrete features to the model: the responses and the missingness patterns. On the other hand, the continuous covariate duration is included in the measurement model. In this case, mainly the missingness patterns are noticeable, although the top layer shows a good deal of variability. These layers are reminiscent of a pattern-mixture structure (Little 1995) even though the model is of a selection nature.

Two views can be taken. Either, focus can be on two observations, #184 and #185, that stand out. These subjects have no measurements at all for

TABLE 31.1. *Fluvoxamine Trial. Negative log-likelihood values for three additional sets of analysis. I: #184 and #185 removed, no covariates; II: #184 and #185 removed, duration as covariate in the measurement model; III: all observations in the (0,0) group removed, duration as covariate in the measurement model.*

Set	BRD1	BRD2	BRD3	BRD4	BRD5
I	559.59	558.18	558.70	558.18	558.97
II	543.65	541.87	542.16	540.35	542.43
III	496.19	494.33	495.26	492.53	495.53
Set	BRD6	BRD7	BRD8	BRD9	
I	557.59	557.32	557.59	557.32	
II	540.61	538.53	538.81	540.34	
III	493.71	491.67	491.95	493.43	

side effects. Alternatively, the entire pattern without follow up measurements can be given further consideration. We will return to this issue later in this section. This phenomenon is in contrast to the analyses made by Verbeke *et al* (2001) and Molenberghs *et al* (2001) who found that the influential observations are invariably completers. In this case, the situation is different since the "empty" observations are explicitly modeled in the BRD models. Therefore, assumptions about the perturbations in the direction of such observations have an impact on the values such an individual *would have had* had the measurements been made; hence a strong sensitivity. This is an illustration of the fact that studying influence by means of perturbations in the missingness model may lead to important conclusions regarding the measurement model parameters. Indeed, the measurement model conclusions depend, not only on the observations actually made, but also on the expectation of the missing measurements. In an MNAR model, such expectations depend on the missingness model as well, since they are made *conditional on an observation being missing*. A high level of sensitivity means that the expectations of the missing outcomes and the resulting measurement model parameters strongly depend on the missingness model (Verbeke *et al* 2001). As stated earlier, the only continuous characteristics of the observations are the levels for duration. These are 38 and 41, respectively, the largest values within the group without observations and the 91st and 92nd percentile values within the entire sample. Thus, the conclusions are driven by a very high value of duration.

Let us now turn to the bottom panels of Figure 31.4. The right hand panel still shows little or no structure. On the left hand side, the layering has been blurred due to the occurrence of duration as a continuous feature into the missingness model. The fact that no sets of observations stand

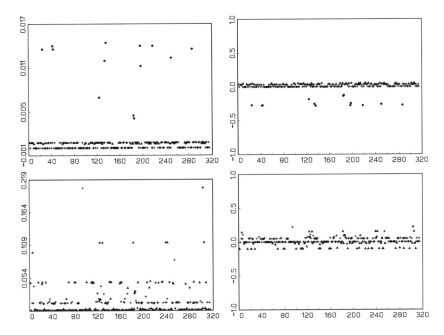

FIGURE 31.5. *Fluvoxamine Trial. Index plots of C_i (left panels) and of the components of the direction $h_{\max}$ of maximal curvature (right panels) for comparison BRD4–7, without (top panels) or with (bottom panels) duration as a covariate in the missingness models.*

out as such, confirms the impression that a good fit has been obtained by including duration in both parts of the model.

Let us now turn to Figure 31.5. A qualitative difference with Figure 31.4 (top left panels) is that now the entire group with no follow-up measurements shows more influential than all other subjects. In this case, $h_{\max}$ displays the same group of subjects with no follow-up. However, all of this disappears when one turns to the bottom panels, again underscoring the importance of duration in the missingness model.

The consequence of these findings is that, as soon as duration is included in the missingness model, a reasonable amount of confidence can be put into the conclusions so obtained. Nevertheless, based on the comparison BRD1–4, it seems wise to further study the effect of subjects #184 and #185, as well as from the group without follow up measurements. To this effect, three additional analyses are considered (Table 31.1): two sets pertain to removal of subjects #184 and #185: without (I) and with (II) duration as a covariate in the measurement model. Note that we do not consider removal in case duration is included in the missingness model because, in this case, these two subjects did not show up as locally influential. Finally, removing all subjects without follow-up measurements and using duration as covariate in the measurement model is reported as family III.

In analysis I, BRD1 is still the preferred model; in II, evidence still points towards BRD4, although slightly less extreme than before: likelihood ratio test statistics for BRD1–4, BRD4–7, and BRD4–8 are 6.60, 3.64, and 3.08, respectively, compared to 7.10, 2.10, and 1.52 obtained initially. However, while the two subjects deleted in I and II cannot explain the apparent non-random missingness, the same conclusions are reached when all subject in pattern (0,0) are deleted (analysis III), as then a few likelihood ratios are above the significance threshold (7.17, attained for BRD3–7 and for BRD5–8; and 7.32 for BRD1–4). Thus, removing these subjects does not change the conclusions about the non-random nature of the data. This is useful supplemental information. Indeed, it is confirmed that the largest impact on the conclusion regarding the nature of the missingness mechanism, is coming from the inclusion of the covariate duration, and neither from isolated individuals, nor from a specific missingness pattern (those without measurements). A nice side effect of this conclusion is that the selected analysis encompasses all subjects and therefore avoids the need of subject deletion, which, if at all possible, should be avoided in statistical analysis.

These analyses can be seen as a useful component of a sensitivity analysis. Given the intrinsic problems with incomplete data models, one can never be completely sure the nature of the missingness mechanism is as posited in the model of choice and therefore several sensitivity assessments simultaneously and/or substantive knowledge have to be considered. When a number of possible causes for the observed non-randomness are found, one might ideally add substantive arguments as to their relative plausibility.

Subjects in an influence graph are displayed without a particular order. Several alternatives are possible, each with pros and cons. For example, one could order the subjects by covariate level, but this method cannot be considered when there are several covariates. Alternatively, the subjects could be ordered by C_i or h_i level, but then different orderings would exist on different plots.

31.5 Interval of Ignorance

Classical inferential procedures induce conclusions from a set of data to a population of interest, accounting for the imprecision resulting from the stochastic component of the model. This is usually done by means of precision or interval estimates. Less attention is devoted to the uncertainty arising from (unplanned) incompleteness in the data. Through the choice of an identifiable model for MNAR missingness, one narrows the possible data generating mechanisms to the point where inference only suffers from imprecision. Some proposals have been made for assessing the sensitivity of these model assumptions; many are based on fitting several plausible but competing models.

Molenberghs, Kenward, and Goetghebeur (2001) and Kenward, Goetghebeur, and Molenberghs (2001) showed an approach that identifies and incorporates both sources of uncertainty in inference: imprecision due to finite sampling, and ignorance due to incompleteness. A simple sensitivity analysis considers a finite set of plausible models. This idea can be taken one step further, by considering more degrees of freedom than the data support. This produces sets of estimates, termed *region of ignorance*, and sets of confidence region, combined into so-called *regions of uncertainty*.

We focus on the model proposed by Baker, Rosenberger, and DerSimonian (1992) and used before in Sections 29.3 and 31.4. Two of the main advantages of this family are ease of computation in general, and the existence of a closed-form solution for several of its members, at least in the initial formulation. Molenberghs, Kenward, and Goetghebeur (2001) used this family of models in a reanalysis of the Slovenian plebiscite data of Rubin, Stern, and Vehovar (1995).

31.5.1 General Principle

It is useful to distinguish between two types of statistical uncertainty. The first, statistical imprecision, is due to finite sampling. The second source of uncertainty, due to incompleteness, will be called statistical ignorance. Statistical imprecision is classically quantified by means of estimators (standard error and variance, confidence regions, etc.) and properties of estimators (consistency, asymptotic distribution, efficiency, etc.). To quantify statistical ignorance, it is useful to distinguish between complete and observed data.

For the BRD model, the 16 complete-data degrees of freedom and the 9 observed-data degrees of freedom are represented in Table 29.1. A sample from this table produces empirical proportions representing the π's with error. This imprecision disappears as the sample size tends to ∞. What remains is ignorance regarding the redistribution of all except the first four πs over the missing outcome value. This leaves ignorance regarding any probability in which at least one of the first or second indices is equal to 0 and hence regarding any derived parameter of scientific interest. For such a parameter, θ say, a region of possible values that is consistent with Table 29.1 is called a *region of ignorance*. Analogously, an observed incomplete table leaves ignorance regarding the would-be observed complete table, which in turn leaves imprecision regarding the true complete probabilities. The region of estimators for θ consistent with the observed data provides an estimated region of ignorance. The $100(1-\alpha)\%$ *region of uncertainty* is a larger region in the spirit of a confidence region, designed to capture the combined effects of imprecision and ignorance. Various ways of constructing regions of ignorance and regions of uncertainty are conceivable.

In standard statistical practice, ignorance is hidden in the consideration of a single identified model, such as models BRD1–BRD9. Among those,

BRD6–BRD9 are said to saturate the degrees of freedom. To be precise, they saturate the *observed data* degrees of freedom. A model that would saturate the *complete data* degrees of freedom, would need 15 rather than 8 parameters. From a (classical) observed data perspective, such a model would be overspecified, as would be any model with 9 or more parameters. Note that it is possible to construct an overspecified model with degrees of freedom less than those in an identifiable saturated model at the observed level.

We construct three such overspecified models. Write the missingness part of the model as (29.8). We will consider two models (Models 10 and 11) with a single sensitivity parameter, while Model 12 will include two sensitivity parameters. Model 10 is defined as (α_k, β_{jk}) with

$$\beta_{jk} = \beta_0 + \beta_j + \beta_k, \tag{31.2}$$

an additive decomposition for missingness on the independence question.

Similarly, Model 11, (α_{jk}, β_j), uses

$$\alpha_{jk} = \alpha_0 + \alpha_j + \alpha_k, \tag{31.3}$$

an additive decomposition of the missingness parameter on the attendance question.

Finally, we define Model 12, $(\alpha_{jk}, \beta_{jk})$, as a combination of both (31.2) and (31.3).

We will now outline the general principle behind considering such overspecified models and then focus on the sensitivity parameter approach.

We start from the classical approach of fitting a single identifiable model M_0 to incomplete data (e.g., a particular BRD model). Maximum likelihood estimation produces a parameter estimate $\widehat{\pi}$ along with measures of imprecision (estimated standard errors). From $\widehat{\pi}$ four predicted contingency tables can be derived as in Table 29.1.

The fitted complete tables collapse back to fitted values for the incomplete Table 29.1. Contrasting the latter with the observed data shows the goodness-of-fit of model M_0. If there is substantial lack of fit, the original model M_0 needs to be reconsidered. Lack of fit has strong bearings on imprecision and, as we want to focus on ignorance, we will assume the fit is acceptable. In what follows, models with poor fit (or boundary solutions) will be dropped.

One can now range through *all possible* complete tables, which collapse back to the M_0 predicted incomplete table. One could call such tables 'M_0 compatible' and we denote the set by $\mathcal{S}(M_0)$. The general principle is that to each table in $\mathcal{S}(M_0)$ an extended model M^* will be fitted. This implies that each table produces an estimated parameter vector and a confidence region. The union of those are termed *region of ignorance* and *region of uncertainty*, respectively. For scalar parameters the terms interval of ignorance (II) and interval of uncertainty (IU) will be used.

Apart from explicitly constructing the (real-valued) set of complete tables, one can proceed in an alternative way. This is done by fitting the model M^* directly to the observed data. This implies that the general principle translates to fitting an overspecified model to the observed data, which will produce a *range* of parameters maximizing the observed data likelihood. This range is then the region of ignorance. If this route is followed, there are technically several ways to find the region. One method is described next.

31.5.2 Sensitivity Parameter Approach

The overspecification can be removed by considering a minimal set of parameters $\boldsymbol{\eta}$, conditional upon which the others, $\boldsymbol{\mu}$, are identified. We term $\boldsymbol{\eta}$ the sensitivity parameter and $\boldsymbol{\mu}$ the estimable parameter. Such a technique has been proposed for specific examples by Nordheim (1984) and Vach and Blettner (1995). Foster and Smith (1998) expand on this idea and by referring to Baker and Laird (1988) and to Rubin, Stern, and Vehovar (1995), they suggest imposing a prior distribution on a range. Each value of $\boldsymbol{\eta}$ will produce an estimate $\hat{\boldsymbol{\mu}}(\boldsymbol{\eta})$. The union of these yields the region of ignorance. It is important to realize that in general there will not be a unique choice for $\boldsymbol{\eta}$ and hence for $\boldsymbol{\mu}$. Changing the partitioning will produce the same region for $\boldsymbol{\theta} = (\boldsymbol{\eta}', \boldsymbol{\mu}')'$. Models 10 and 11 have a single sensitivity parameter. We chose $\eta = \beta_k$ and $\eta = \alpha_k$ from (31.2) and (31.3), respectively. In Model 12, both these parameters $\boldsymbol{\eta} = (\beta_k, \alpha_k)'$ are treated as sensitivity parameters. In practice, an easy computation scheme is to consider a grid in the sensitivity parameter space, at each value of which the estimable parameter is maximized.

A natural estimate of the region of uncertainty is the union of confidence regions for each $\hat{\boldsymbol{\mu}}(\boldsymbol{\eta})$. Note that one has to ensure that $\boldsymbol{\eta}$ is within the allowable range. Because the choice of sensitivity parameter is non-unique and a proper choice can greatly simplify the treatment. Another issue is whether the parameters of direct scientific interest can overlap with the sensitivity set or not (White and Goetghebeur 1998). For example, if the scientific question is a sensitivity analysis for treatment effect, then one should consider the implications of including the treatment effect parameters in the sensitivity set. There will be no direct estimate of imprecision available for the sensitivity parameter. Clearly, the particular choice of sensitivity parameter will not affect the estimate of the region of ignorance. However, the region of uncertainty is built from confidence regions that are conditional on a particular value of the sensitivity parameter and hence will typically vary with the choice made.

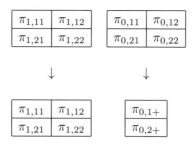

FIGURE 31.6. *Monotone Patterns. Theoretical distribution over complete and observed cells. (Monotone patterns).*

31.5.3 Models for Monotone Patterns and a Bernoulli Experiment

To further illustrate the II ideas, let us focus on the relatively simple setting of two binary outcomes, of which the first one is always observed but the second one is missing for some subjects. This setting is depicted in Figure 31.6. Decompose the cell probabilities as

$$\pi_{r,ij} = p_{ij} q_{r|ij}, \qquad (31.4)$$

where p_{ij} parameterizes the measurement process and $q_{r|ij}$ describes the non-response (or dropout) mechanism. In what follows, we will leave p_{ij} unconstrained and consider various forms for $q_{r|ij}$, as listed in Table 31.2. In this setting, there are 7 complete-data degrees of freedom, d.f.(comp)= 7 and 5 observed-data degrees of freedom, d.f.(obs)= 5.

Model M_{sat} (Model 5) has 3 measurement parameters and 4 dropout parameters and saturates d.f.(comp). However, there are only 5 observed degrees of freedom, rendering this model overspecified when fitted to the observed data.

Three models are identified. Conventional restrictions result from assuming an MCAR or MAR model (Models 1 and 2, respectively). Another identified model lets dropout depend on the potentially unobserved second measurement, but not on the first one (Michiels and Molenberghs 1997). Brown (1990) who proposed this estimator for normally distributed endpoints, used the term *protective* estimator because it can be fitted without explicitly addressing the missingness model. We refer to it in Table 31.2 as MNAR 0. Models 2 and 3 both saturate d.f.(obs), and hence cannot be distinguished from each other purely on statistical grounds, in terms of the observed data. In Model 4, dropout is allowed to depend on both measurements but not on their interaction. As a consequence, it overspecifies d.f.(obs) and underspecifies d.f.(comp).

Before turning to setting (31.6), let us illustrate the ideas outlined in Section 31.5.1 by means of the simple setting of a Bernoulli experiment with N trials, where r denotes the number of observed successes, $n - r$

TABLE 31.2. *Monotone Patterns. Dropout models corresponding to the setting of Figure 31.6.*

	Dropout models			
Model	$q_{r|ij}$	Par.	Obs. d.f.	Comp. d.f.
1. MCAR	q_r	4	Non-sat.	Non-sat.
2. MAR	$q_{r|i}$	5	Sat.	Non-sat.
3. MNAR 0	$q_{r|j}$	5	Sat.	Non-sat.
4. MNAR I	$\text{logit}(q_{r|ij}) = \alpha + \beta_i + \gamma_j$	6	Oversp.	Non-sat.
5. M_{sat}	$\text{logit}(q_{r|ij}) = \alpha + \beta_i + \gamma_j + \delta_{ij}$	7	Oversp.	Sat.

the number of observed failures, and $N - n$ the number of unclassified subjects. Independent of the parameterization chosen, the observed data log-likelihood can be represented in the form

$$\ell = r \ln \alpha + (n - r) \ln \beta + (N - n) \ln(1 - \alpha - \beta), \quad (31.5)$$

with α the probability of an observed success and β the probability of an observed failure. It is sometimes useful to denote $\gamma = 1 - \alpha - \beta$. We consider two models, of which the parameterization is given in Table 31.3. The first one is identified, the second one is overparameterized. Here, p is the probability of a success (whether observed or not), q_1 (q_2) is the probability of being observed given a success (failure), and λ is the odds for being observed for failures versus successes. For Model I, the latter is assumed to be unity. Denote the corresponding log-likelihoods by ℓ_I and ℓ_{II} respectively. In both cases,

$$\widehat{\alpha} = \frac{r}{N}, \quad \widehat{\beta} = \frac{n-r}{N}.$$

Maximum likelihood estimates for p and q follow immediately under Model I, either by observing that the moments (α, β) map 1–1 onto the pair (p, q) or by directly solving ℓ_I. The solutions are given in Table 31.3. The asymptotic variance-covariance matrix for p and q is block-diagonal with well-known elements $p(1-p)/n$ and $q(1-q)/N$. Observe that we now obtain only one solution, a strong argument in favor of the current model.

A similar standard derivation is not possible for Model II, as the triplet (p, q_1, q_2) or, equivalently, the triplet (p, q, λ), is redundant. This follows directly from Catchpole and Morgan (1997) and Catchpole, Morgan, and Freeman (1998) whose theory shows that Model II is rank-deficient and Model I is of full rank. Because Model I is a submodel of Model II and saturates the observed data, so must every solution to ℓ_{II}, implying the relationships:

$$pq_1 = \frac{r}{N}, \quad (1-p)q_2 = \frac{n-r}{N}. \quad (31.6)$$

TABLE 31.3. *Bernoulli Experiment. Two transformations of the observed-data likelihood.*

Model I (MAR)	Model II (MNAR,M_{sat})
Parameterization:	
$\alpha = pq$	$\alpha = pq_1$
$\beta = (1-p)q$	$\beta = (1-p)q_2$
$\gamma = 1-q$	$\gamma = 1 - pq_1 - (1-p)q_2$
	$q_1 = q$
	$q_2 = q\lambda$
Solution:	
$\widehat{p} = \frac{\widehat{\alpha}}{\widehat{\alpha}+\widehat{\beta}} = \frac{r}{n}$	$pq_1 = \frac{r}{N}$
$\widehat{q} = \widehat{\alpha} + \widehat{\beta} = \frac{n}{N}$	$(1-p)q_2 = \frac{n-r}{N}$
	$\dfrac{r}{q_1} + \dfrac{n-r}{q_2} = N$
	$p \in \left[\dfrac{r}{N}, \dfrac{N-n+r}{N}\right]$

Constraints (31.6) imply

$$\widehat{p} = \frac{r}{Nq_1} = 1 - \frac{n-r}{Nq_2}$$

and hence

$$\frac{r}{q_1} + \frac{n-r}{q_2} = N. \tag{31.7}$$

The requirement that $q_1, q_2 \leq 1$ in (31.6) implies a range for p:

$$p \in \left[\frac{r}{N}, \frac{N-n+r}{N}\right]. \tag{31.8}$$

Such overspecification of the likelihood can be managed in a more general way using the method outlined in Section 31.5.2. It is not always the case that the range for η will be an entire line or real space and hence specific measures may be needed to ensure that η is within its allowable range. As the choice of sensitivity parameter is non-unique, a proper choice can greatly simplify the treatment. It will be seen in what follows that the choice of λ as in Table 31.3 is an efficient one from a computational point of view. In contrast, the choice $\theta = q_2 - q_1$ would lead to cumbersome computations and will not be pursued. Of course, what is understood by a proper choice will depend on the context.

TABLE 31.4. *Bernoulli Experiment. Limiting cases for the sensitivity parameter analysis.*

Estimator	λ	$\lambda = \frac{n-r}{N-r}$	$\lambda = 1$	$\lambda = \frac{N-(n-r)}{r}$
p_λ	$\frac{\lambda r}{n-r(1-\lambda)}$	$\frac{r}{N}$	$\frac{r}{n}$	$\frac{N-n+r}{N}$
q_λ	$\frac{n-r(1-\lambda)}{N\lambda}$	1	$\frac{n}{N}$	$\frac{r}{N-(n-r)}$
$q_\lambda \lambda$	$\frac{n-r(1-\lambda)}{N}$	$\frac{n-r}{N-r}$	$\frac{n}{N}$	1
$\frac{p_\lambda}{1-p_\lambda}$	$\lambda \frac{r}{n-r}$	$\frac{r}{N-r}$	$\frac{r}{n-r}$	$\frac{N-(n-r)}{n-r}$

For example, the sensitivity parameter can be chosen from the nuisance parameters, rather than from the parameters of direct scientific interest. Whether the latter parameters can overlap with the sensitivity set or not is itself an issue (White and Goetghebeur 1998). For example, if the scientific question is a sensitivity analysis for treatment effect, then one should consider the implications of including the treatment effect parameters in the sensitivity set. There will be no direct estimate of imprecision available for the sensitivity parameter. Alternatively, if, given a certain choice of sensitivity parameter, the resulting profile likelihood has a simple form (analogous to the Box-Cox transformation, where conditioning on the transformation parameter produces essentially a normal likelihood), then such a parameter is an obvious candidate.

Given our choice of sensitivity parameter λ, simple algebra yields estimates for p and q (subscripted by λ to indicate dependence on the sensitivity parameter):

$$p_\lambda = \frac{\widehat{\alpha}\lambda}{\widehat{\beta}+\widehat{\alpha}\lambda} = \frac{\lambda r}{n-r(1-\lambda)}, \qquad (31.9)$$

$$q_\lambda = \frac{\widehat{\beta}+\widehat{\alpha}\lambda}{\lambda} = \frac{n-r(1-\lambda)}{N\lambda}. \qquad (31.10)$$

Using the delta method, an asymptotic variance-covariance matrix of p_λ and q_λ is seen to be built from:

$$\widehat{\mathrm{Var}}(p_\lambda) = \frac{p_\lambda(1-p_\lambda)}{N\lambda q_\lambda}$$
$$\times \left\{1 + \frac{1-\lambda}{\lambda}(1-p_\lambda)[1-p_\lambda q_\lambda(1-\lambda)]\right\}, \qquad (31.11)$$

$$\widehat{\mathrm{Cov}}(p_\lambda, q_\lambda) = -\frac{1}{N}p_\lambda(1-p_\lambda)\frac{1-\lambda}{\lambda}q_\lambda, \qquad (31.12)$$

598   31. Sensitivity Analysis

TABLE 31.5. *Fluvoxamine Trial. The first subtable represents the complete observations. Subjects with only the first outcome, only the last outcome, or no outcome at all reported are presented in subtables 2, 3, and 4, respectively.*

Side effects:

		time 2				
time 1		yes	no	26	2 0	14
yes		89	13	49		
no		57	65			

Therapeutic effect:

		time 2				
time 1		no	yes	7	0 2	14
no		11	1	68		
yes		124	88			

$$\widehat{\text{Var}(q_\lambda)} = \frac{q_\lambda(1-q_\lambda)}{N}\left\{1 + \frac{1-p_\lambda}{1-q_\lambda}\frac{1-\lambda}{\lambda}\right\}.$$

Note that the parameter estimates are asymptotically correlated, except when $\lambda = 1$, i.e., under the MAR assumption, or under boundary values ($p_\lambda = 0, 1; q_\lambda = 0$). This is in line with the ignorable nature of the MAR model (Rubin 1976). We need to determine the set of allowable values for λ by requiring $0 \leq p_\lambda, q_\lambda, \lambda q_\lambda \leq 1$. These six inequalities reduce to

$$\lambda \in \left[\frac{n-r}{N-r}, \frac{N-(n-r)}{r}\right].$$

Table 31.4 presents estimates for limiting cases. The interval of ignorance for the success probability is thus seen to be as in (31.8). It is interesting to observe that the success odds estimator is linear in the sensitivity parameter; the resulting interval of ignorance equals

$$\text{odds}(p) \in \left[\frac{r}{N-r}, \frac{N-n+r}{n-r}\right].$$

For the success probability, the variance of p_λ is given by (31.11). For the success odds, we obtain:

$$\widehat{\text{Var}(\text{odds}(p_\lambda))} = \frac{1}{N\lambda q_\lambda}\frac{p_\lambda}{1-p_\lambda}\left\{1 + \frac{1-\lambda}{\lambda}(1-p_\lambda)[1 - p_\lambda q_\lambda(1-\lambda)]\right\}$$

31.5 Interval of Ignorance   599

TABLE 31.6. *Fluvoxamine Trial. Identifiable models, fitted to monotone patterns.*

	(1,1)		(1,0)		-2 logl
Side effects	83.7	12.2	28.0	4.1	495.8
Model 1 (MCAR)	59.9	68.3	20.0	22.9	
Side effects	89.0	13.0	22.7	3.3	494.4
Model 2 (MAR)	57.0	65.0	22.9	26.1	
Side effects	89.0	13.0	18.6	7.4	494.4
Model 3 (MNAR 0)	57.0	65.0	11.9	37.1	
Therapeutic effect	13.0	1.2	4.4	0.4	386.5
Model 1 (MCAR)	122.7	87.1	41.1	29.2	
Therapeutic effect	11.0	1.0	6.4	0.6	385.8
Model 2 (MAR)	124.0	88.0	39.8	28.2	
Therapeutic effect	11.0	1.0	7.1	-0.1	385.8
Model 3 (MNAR 0, Unconstr.)	124.0	88.0	80.5	-12.5	
Therapeutic effect	11.6	1.0	6.4	0.0	385.8
Model 3 (MNAR 0, Constr.)	123.4	88.0	68.5	0.0	

and for the success logit:

$$\widehat{\text{Var}}(\text{logit}(p_\lambda)) = \frac{1}{N\lambda q_\lambda} \frac{1}{p_\lambda(1-p_\lambda)} \left\{ 1 + \frac{1-\lambda}{\lambda}(1-p_\lambda)[1 - p_\lambda q_\lambda(1-\lambda)] \right\}.$$

For each λ, a confidence interval C_λ can be constructed for every point within the allowable range of λ. The union of the C_λ is the *interval of uncertainty*, for either p, its odds, or its logit.

31.5.4   Analysis of the Fluvoxamine Data

We focus on the setting of Table 29.1. A version for the fluvoxamine study, based on the first and last follow-up measurements, is given in Table 31.5. There are two patients with a non-monotone pattern of follow-up, whereas 14 subjects have no follow-up data at all. This enables us to treat these data both from the monotone non-response or dropout perspective, as well as from the more complicated but more general non-monotone point of view. We will first the identifiable models and then switch to sensitivity analysis.

31.5.4.1   Identified Models

We first consider the monotone patterns and the corresponding models of Table 31.2. Table 31.6 shows the predicted complete tables for Models 1, 2, and 3. The effect of ignorance is clearly seen by comparing the MAR and

TABLE 31.7. *Fluvoxamine Trial. Marginal probabilities and (log) odds ratio for monotone patterns of side-effects data. Models 1–3: point estimate and 95% confidence interval; Models 4–5: interval of ignorance (II) and interval of uncertainty (IU); these models are defined in Section 31.5.3.*

Parameter		Model 1/2	Model 3	Model 4	Model 5
First Marg.	II	0.43	0.43	0.43	0.43
	IU	[0.37;0.48]	[0.37;0.48]	[0.37;0.48]	[0.37;0.48]
Second Marg.	II	0.64	0.59	[0.49;0.74]	[0.49;0.74]
	IU	[0.58;0.70]	[0.53;0.65]	[0.43;0.79]	[0.43;0.79]
Log O.R.	II	2.06	2.06	[1.52;2.08]	[0.41;2.84]
	IU	[1.37;2.74]	[1.39;2.72]	[1.03;2.76]	[0.0013;2.84]
O.R.	II	7.81	7.81	[4.57;7.98]	[1.50;17.04]
	IU	[3.95;15.44]	[4.00;15.24]	[2.79;15.74]	[1.0013;32.89]

protective models: they provide a substantially different prediction for the partially observed table, while producing the same deviance. In addition, the protective model produces a boundary solution, or even an invalid solution if predicted proportions are not constrained to lie within the unit interval, for therapeutic effect.

We now interpret these results in terms of possible quantities of interest, for instance the first and second marginal probability of side effects and the odds ratio, capturing the association between both measurements (Table 31.7). Models 4 and 5 will be discussed in the sensitivity analysis. Models 1 and 2 are both ignorable and hence all measurement model quantities are independent of the choice between MAR and MCAR.

The quantities in Tables 31.6 and 31.7 differ in one important way. The former quantities are calculated conditional on the dropout pattern; the latter follow directly from the marginal measurement probabilities p_{ij}, which are common to all three models while the dropout probabilities $q_{r|ij}$ depend on the model. As a consequence, while MAR and MCAR are equivalent for the quantities in Table 31.7, this does not carry over to the predicted cell counts in Table 31.6. Further, the stability of the estimates in Table 31.7 (at least for Models 1–3) is in marked contrast to the variation among the predicted cell counts in Table 31.6. These considerations suggest that stability may be restricted to *certain* functions of parameters in *certain* sets of data.

We now introduce the non-monotone patterns into the analysis and fit the nine identifiable BRD models of Table 29.2. The fitted counts of the models with an interior solution are given in Table 31.8 and the marginal quantities of interest are displayed in Table 31.9. Note that a subgroup of

TABLE 31.8. *Fluvoxamine Trial. Complete data counts for models fitted to side effects data.*

	(1,1)		(1,0)		(0,1)		(0,0)		(+,+)	
BRD1	84.00	12.12	28.13	4.06	0.74	0.11	5.26	0.76	118.13	17.05
	60.21	67.67	20.16	22.66	0.53	0.60	3.77	4.23	84.67	95.16
BRD2	89.42	12.89	22.73	3.27	0.80	0.12	4.24	0.61	117.19	16.89
	57.27	64.42	23.06	25.94	0.51	0.58	4.30	4.82	85.14	95.76
BRD3	83.67	12.22	28.02	4.09	1.17	0.00	8.16	0.00	121.01	16.31
	59.85	68.25	20.04	22.85	0.83	0.00	5.84	0.00	86.57	91.11
BRD4	89.42	12.89	18.58	7.42	0.80	0.12	3.47	1.39	112.27	21.82
	57.27	64.42	11.90	37.10	0.51	0.58	2.22	6.93	71.90	109.03
BRD7	89.00	13.00	18.58	7.42	1.22	0.00	8.53	0.00	117.33	20.42
	57.00	65.00	11.90	37.10	0.78	0.00	5.47	0.00	75.15	102.10
BRD9	89.00	13.00	22.69	3.31	1.22	0.00	6.97	0.00	119.87	16.31
	57.00	65.00	22.89	26.11	0.78	0.00	7.03	0.00	87.71	91.11

models produces invalid solutions without appropriate constraints, such as automatically imposed by form (29.8) for the dropout model.

In spite of the fact that we are now looking at a larger class of models, the results are comparable with those obtained for the monotone patterns. Table 31.9 reveals that Models BRD1–9 show little variation in the marginal probabilities and in the measure of association. Considered as an informal sensitivity analysis, this could be seen as evidence for the robustness of these measures. We will revisit this conclusion following a more formal sensitivity analysis and deduce that it is strongly misleading.

31.5.4.2 Intervals of Ignorance

Turning to the overspecified models, let us consider the monotone patterns first. In addition to the three identifiable models from Table 31.2, we now fit overspecified Models 4 and 5 to the same data. Results for these additional models are also given in Table 31.7.

For Model 4, there is one sensitivity parameter, which we choose to be γ (measuring the extent of non-randomness). When $\gamma = 0$ the MAR Model 2 is recovered. The value of γ which corresponds to $q_{r|ij} = q_{r|j}$ in Table 31.2 yields the protective Model 3. Because there is only one sensitivity parameter, a graphical representation (Figure 31.7) is straightforward. Because among the monotone cases the first measurement is always obtained, there is no ignorance about the first marginal probability and hence the interval of ignorance for this quantity is still a point. This is not true for the other two quantities.

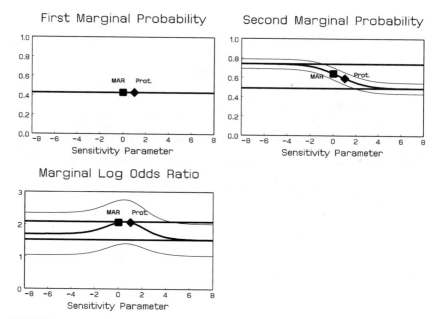

FIGURE 31.7. *Fluvoxamine Trial. Graphical representation of intervals of ignorance and intervals of uncertainty for monotone patterns of psychiatric study (side effects). The bold curve graphs the point estimates conditional on the sensitivity parameter. The bold horizontal lines project the interval of ignorance on the vertical axes. The extremes of the thin lines correspond to the interval of uncertainty. The MAR and protective point estimates have been added to the figure.*

Commonly, fitting a pair of identifiable models (e.g., Models 2 and 3) is regarded as a sensitivity analysis. This example shows how misleading this can be. Both models differ by about 0.05 in the second marginal probability, but the II of Model 4 shows the range is about 0.25! Similarly, Models 2 and 3 yield virtually the same result for the odds ratio, but the II of Model 4 shows that this proximity is fortuitous.

The impact of fitting an overspecified but, at the complete-data level, non-saturated model is seen by contrasting Model 4 with the fully saturated Model 5. The sensitivity parameter for Model 4 is γ_1 in Table 31.2. For Model 5, the two sensitivity parameters are γ_1 and δ_{11} (all other γ and δ parameters need to be set to zero for classical identifiability purposes). As expected, both models coincide for the first marginal probability. It turns out that their respective intervals of ignorance and uncertainty for the second marginal probability exhibit considerable overlap. In contrast, the length of the II for the log odds ratio is now about 5 times longer. The Model 5 lower limit of the IU is very close to zero, whereas its Model 4 counterpart shows clear evidence for a strong positive association between both outcomes.

TABLE 31.9. *Fluvoxamine Trial. Model fit for side effects (par: number of model parameters; G^2: likelihood ratio test statistic for model fit, corresponding p-value, estimates and 95% confidence limits for marginal probabilities and marginal (log) odds ratio.) For Model 10 (31.2), intervals of ignorance and uncertainty are presented instead.*

				Marg. prob.	
Model	par	G^2	p-value	First	Second
BRD1	6	4.5	0.104	0.43[0.37;0.49]	0.64[0.58;0.71]
BRD2	7	1.7	0.192	0.43[0.37;0.48]	0.64[0.58;0.70]
BRD3	7	2.8	0.097	0.44[0.38;0.49]	0.66[0.60;0.72]
BRD4	7	1.7	0.192	0.43[0.37;0.48]	0.58[0.49;0.68]
BRD7	8	0.0	-	0.44[0.38;0.49]	0.61[0.53;0.69]
BRD9	8	0.0	-	0.43[0.38;0.49]	0.66[0.60;0.72]
Model 10:II	9	0.0	-	[0.425;0.429]	[0.47;0.75]
Model 10:IU	9	0.0	-	[0.37;0.49]	[0.41;0.80]

	Odds ratio	
	Orig. scale	Log scale
BRD1	7.80[3.94;15.42]	2.06[1.37;2.74]
BRD2	7.81[3.95;15.44]	2.06[1.37;2.74]
BRD3	7.81[3.95;15.44]	2.06[1.37;2.74]
BRD4	7.81[3.95;15.44]	2.06[1.37;2.74]
BRD7	7.81[3.95;15.44]	2.06[1.37;2.74]
BRD9	7.63[3.86;15.10]	2.03[1.35;2.71]
Model 10:II	[4.40;7.96]	[1.48;2.07]
Model 10:IU	[2.69;15.69]	[0.99;2.75]

By construction, the data do not provide evidence for choosing between Models 4 and 5. Both are overspecified at the observed data level and both encompass Models 2 and 3. Model 5 is saturated at the observed data level as well and therefore the limits derived from it are not model-based. The reduced width of the intervals produced under Model 4 are entirely due to the unverifiable model assumption that the dropout probability depends on both outcomes through their main effects only and *not* on the interaction between both outcomes. If this assumption is deemed implausible, it can easily be avoided by including an extra degree of freedom. However, in more complicated settings, such as when covariates are included or with continuous responses, assumptions are unavoidable in the interest of model parsimony. Now including the non-monotone patterns, any model within the BRD family with more than 8 parameters is non-identifiable. To simplify the sensitivity analysis, let us consider a slightly different but equivalent parameterization

$$\pi_{r_1 r_1, ij} = p_{ij} \frac{\exp[\beta^*_{ij}(1-r_2) + \alpha^*_{ij}(1-r_1) + \gamma^*(1-r_1)(1-r_2)]}{1 + \exp(\beta^*_{ij}) + \exp(\alpha^*_{ij}) + \exp(\beta^*_{ij} + \alpha^*_{ij} + \gamma^*)}, \quad (31.13)$$

which contains the marginal success probabilities p_{ij} and forces the missingness probabilities to obey their range restrictions.

Although Models BRD1–9 have shown stability in the estimates of the marginal parameters of interest, it has been revealed in the monotone context, that such a conclusion could be deceptive. To study this further, we consider an overspecified model, analogous to Model 4 in Table 31.2. The choice can be motivated by observing that both BRD7 and BRD9 yield an interior solution and differ only in the β-model. Therefore, Model 10, defined by (31.2), will be fitted. Because one parameter is redundant, we propose using β_j as the sensitivity parameter. Although the II, obtained in this way, is acceptable, the IU shows aberrant behavior (plot not shown), toward larger values of the sensitivity parameter, leading to very wide IUs. This problem is entirely due to the zero count in pattern (0,1) (see Table 31.5), as can be seen by adding 0.5 to this zero count. The results are presented in Figure 31.8. The resulting II and IU are presented in Table 31.9, and they are very similar to the results for Model 4, as displayed in Table 31.7. Due to the non-monotone patterns, there is a (very small) ignorance in the first marginal probability as well. Once again, it is seen that fitting identifiable models only may be misleading because, for example, the log odds ratio shows much more variability than seen among Models BRD1–9.

31.6 Sensitivity Analysis and Pattern-mixture Models

Pattern-mixture models (Chapter 30) can be of use in the context of sensitivity analysis. Given there are several, quite distinct, strategies to formulate such models (Section 30.2), one can consider one strategy as a sensitivity analysis for another one. For example, the sensitivity of simple, identified models can be checked using identifying restrictions (Section 30.3). Also, a set of identifying restrictions can be considered, rather than a single one, by way of sensitivity analysis. Thijs et al (2002) and Molenberghs et al (2004) discuss strategies for fitting pattern-mixture models.

Obviously, one can formulate selection models for one's primary analysis, and then fit pattern-mixture models to assess sensitivity. This was done in Sections 30.4 and 30.5. Michiels et al (2002) followed this route.

Molenberghs, Michiels, and Kenward (1998) formulated models that combine aspects of both selection models and pattern-mixture models, and used pseudo-likelihood ideas to fit such models.

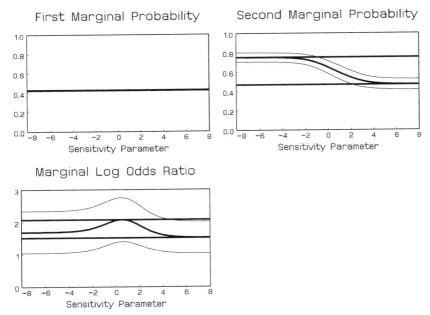

FIGURE 31.8. *Fluvoxamine Trial. Graphical representation of intervals of ignorance and intervals of uncertainty for monotone patterns (side effects). A value of 0.5 is added to the zero count in pattern (1,0). The bold curve graphs the point estimates conditional on the sensitivity parameter. The bold horizontal lines project the interval of ignorance on the vertical axes. The extremes of the thin lines correspond to the interval of uncertainty.*

31.7 Concluding Remarks

When fitting models to incomplete (longitudinal) data, especially of the MNAR type but also of the MAR and MCAR types, it is important to assess the sensitivity of the conclusions to unverifiable model assumptions. Generally, a sensitivity analysis can be conducted within different frameworks, and there are times where the setting will determine which framework is the more appropriate one (for example Bayesian or frequentist), in conjunction with technical and computational considerations. Draper (1995) has considered ways of dealing with model uncertainty in the very natural Bayesian framework. We have focused on local influence methods, the interval of ignorance, and the use of pattern-mixture models. Although these methods are useful, it ought to be clear they are by no means the only routes to sensitivity analysis. This field, in the context of incomplete data, is still in full development and more work will undoubtedly emerge in times to come.

32
Incomplete Data and SAS

32.1 Introduction

In this chapter, SAS implementations for several methods discussed in missing data Part VI will be discussed. In Section 32.2, complete case analysis is presented. Section 32.3 discusses how to conduct last observation carried forward (LOCF). The fact that these two simple methods, criticized in Section 27.3, are included does not imply an endorsement of the methodology. MAR-based methods are discussed in Section 32.4, devoted to likelihood methods, and in Section 32.5, where weighted generalized estimating equations are discussed. Multiple imputation is considered in Section 32.6, and the EM algorithm is the subject of Section 32.7. Finally, we conclude with some brief comments on the more advanced methods. Several macros have been developed and will be discussed in what follows. They are available from the authors.

32.2 Complete Case Analysis

The only step required to perform a complete case analysis is deletion of subjects for which not all designed measurements have been obtained. When the data are organized 'horizontally,' i.e., one record per subject, this is particularly easy. With 'vertically' organized data, slightly more data manipulation is needed and the following SAS macro, prepared by C. Beunckens, can be used:

```
%macro cc(data=,id=,time=,response=,out=);
%if %bquote(&data)= %then %let data=&syslast;
proc freq data=&data noprint;
tables &id /out=freqsub;
tables &time / out=freqtime;
run;
proc iml;
use freqsub;
read all var {&id,count};
nsub = nrow(&id);
use freqtime;
read all var {&time,count};
ntime = nrow(&time);
use &data;
read all var {&id,&time,&response};
n =  nrow(&response);
complete = j(n,1,1);
ind = 1;
do while (ind <= nsub);
  j = 1;
  do while (j <= ntime);
    if (&response[(ind-1)*ntime+j]=.) then
      complete[(ind-1)*ntime+1:(ind-1)*ntime+ntime]=0;
    j = j+1;
end;
  ind = ind+1;
end;
create help var {&id &time &response complete};
append;
quit;
data &out;
merge &data help;
if complete=0 then delete;
drop complete;
run;
%mend;
```

The CC macro requires four arguments. The 'data=' argument is the dataset to be analyzed. If not specified, the most recent dataset is used. The name of the variable in the dataset that contains the identification variable is specified by 'id=,' and 'time=' specifies the variable indicating the time ordering within a subject. The outcome variable is passed on by means of the 'response=' argument and the name of the output dataset, created with the macro, is defined through 'out=.'

For example, for the age related macular degeneration trial, running the next statement produces the complete case CC dataset:

```
%cc(data=armd111,id=subject,time=time,
 response=bindif,out=armdcc);
```

Upon performing this data pre-processing, a complete case analysis follows of any type requested by the user, including but not limited to longitudinal analysis. Of course, a totally different question is whether such an analysis is to be recommended, as discussed in Section 27.3.

The macro requires records, corresponding to missing values, to be present in the dataset. Otherwise, it is assumed that a measurement occasion not included is missing by design.

32.3 Last Observation Carried Forward

Similar steps as needed for a complete case analysis need to be performed when LOCF is the goal. For a vertically organized dataset, the following macro can be used to appropriately process the data:

```
%macro locf(data=,id=,time=,response=,out=);
%if %bquote(&data)= %then %let data=&syslast;
proc freq data=&data noprint;
tables &id /out=freqsub;
tables &time / out=freqtime;
run;
proc iml;
use freqsub;
read all var {&id,count};
nsub = nrow(&id);
use freqtime;
read all var {&time,count};
ntime = nrow(&time);
use &data;
read all var {&id,&time,&response};
n = nrow(&response);
locf = &response;
ind = 1;
print nsub;
print ntime;
do while (ind <= nsub);
   j=2;
   do while (j <= ntime);
     if (locf[(ind-1)*ntime+j]=.)
       then locf[(ind-1)*ntime+j]=locf[(ind-1)*ntime+j-1];
```

```
      j= j+1;
    end;
    ind = ind+1;
  end;
  create help var {&id &time &response locf};
  append;
quit;
data &out;
merge &data help;
run;
%mend;
```

The arguments are exactly the same and have the same meaning as in the CC macro of Section 32.2.

Running the next statement produces the dataset we need for the LOCF analysis.

```
%locf(data=armd111,id=subject,time=time,
  response=bindif,out=armdlocf);
```

It is instructive to consider a portion of the LOCF dataset:

Obs	subject	treat	time	bindif	LOCF
1	1	2	1	1	1
2	1	2	2	1	1
3	1	2	3	.	1
4	1	2	4	.	1
5	2	2	1	0	0
6	2	2	2	1	1
7	2	2	3	1	1
8	2	2	4	1	1
17	5	2	1	.	.
18	5	2	2	.	.
19	5	2	3	.	.
20	5	2	4	.	.
121	31	2	1	0	0
122	31	2	2	.	0
123	31	2	3	.	0
124	31	2	4	.	0
197	50	1	1	1	1
198	50	1	2	1	1
199	50	1	3	.	1

200	50	1	4	1	1
389	98	1	1	.	.
390	98	1	2	0	0
391	98	1	3	0	0
392	98	1	4	1	1

Subjects with complete records are obviously left untouched. Both values after dropout and intermittent values are substituted with the most recently observed value, except at the beginning of the sequence, when no prior information is available. This means, in particular, that someone without any follow up will be left blank.

32.4 Direct Likelihood

In contrast to CC and LOCF, no extra data processing is necessary when a direct likelihood analysis is envisaged, provided the software tool used for analysis is able to handle measurement sequences of unequal length. This is the case for virtually all longitudinal data analysis tools, including the SAS procedures MIXED, NLMIXED, and GLIMMIX.

One precaution is in place. When residual correlation structures are used for which the order of the measurements within a sequence is important, such as unstructured and AR(1), but not simple nor compound symmetry, and intermittent missingness occurs, care as to be taken to ensure the *design* order within the sequence, and not the *apparent* order, is passed on. In the SAS procedure MIXED, a statement such as

```
repeated / subject=subject type=un;
```

is fine when every subject has, say, four designed measurements. However, when for a particular subject the second measurement is missing, there is a risk that the remaining measurements are considered the first, second, and third, rather than the first, third, and fourth. Thus, it is careful to replace the above statement by:

```
repeated time / subject=subject type=un;
```

For the GENMOD procedure, the option 'withinsubject=time' to the REPEATED statement can be used. Note that this produces GEE and not direct likelihood. For the GLIMMIX procedure, there is no such feature.

In all cases, especially when GLIMMIX is used, the proper order is passed on when a record is included, even for the missing measurements, of course with a missing value instead of an actual measurement then.

When the NLMIXED procedure is used, only random effects can be included, and in such a case all relevant information is contained in the actual effects that define the random effects structure. For example, the order is immaterial for a random intercepts model, and for a random slope in time, all information needed about time is passed on, for example, by the RANDOM statement:

```
RANDOM intercept time / subject=subject type=un;
```

The following program could be used for fitting a generalized linear mixed-effects model to the age related macular degeneration data, regardless of whether data are complete or incomplete:

```
data help;
set m.armdwgee;
time1=0;
time2=0;
time3=0;
time4=0;
if time=1 then time1=1;
if time=2 then time2=1;
if time=3 then time3=1;
if time=4 then time4=1;
run;

proc nlmixed data=help qpoints=20 maxiter=100 technique=newrap;
eta = beta11*time1+beta12*time2+beta13*time3+beta14*time4 + b
    +(beta21*time1+beta22*time2+beta23*time3+beta24*time4)
       *(2-treat);
p = exp(eta)/(1+exp(eta));
model bindif ~ binary(p);
random b ~ normal(0,tau*tau) subject=subject;
estimate 'tau^2' tau*tau;
run;
```

Note that the dataset contains the suffix 'wgee' because it also contains the weights for weighted generalized estimating equations, to be discussed in Section 32.5.

Thus generally, with only a mild amount of precaution, a direct likelihood analysis is not any more complex than the corresponding analysis on a set of data free of missingness. The same holds for GEE by means of, for example, the GENMOD procedure. Of course, as discussed in Section 27.5, GEE is not valid unless the missing data mechanism is MCAR. Under MAR, weighted GEE is advisable and this will be discussed in the next section.

32.5 Weighted Estimating Equations (WGEE)

Let us illustrate WGEE by means of the analysis of the age related macular degeneration trial, discussed in Section 27.7.

A program for the standard GEE analysis would be:

```
proc genmod data=armdwgee;
class time treat subject;
model bindif = time treat*time
     / noint dist=binomial;
repeated subject=subject
         / withinsubject=time type=exch modelse;
run;
```

Alternatively, a linearization-based version can be fitted using:

```
proc glimmix data=armdwgee empirical;
nloptions maxiter=50 technique=newrap;
class time treat subject;
model bindif = time treat*time
     / noint solution dist=binary;
random _residual_ / subject=subject type=cs;
run;
```

Let us now discuss which steps have to be taken to conduct a weighted GEE analysis.

To compute the weights, we first have to fit the dropout model, using for example logistic regression. The outcome 'dropout' is binary and indicates whether or not dropout occurs at a given time from the start of the measurement sequence until the time of dropout or the end of the sequence. Covariates in the model are the outcomes at previous occasions ('prev'), supplemented with genuine covariate information. The DROPOUT macro is used to construct the variables 'dropout' and 'prev.'

```
%macro dropout(data=,id=,time=,response=,out=);
%if %bquote(&data)= %then %let data=&syslast;
proc freq data=&data noprint;
tables &id /out=freqid;
tables &time / out=freqtime;
run;
proc iml;
reset noprint;
use freqid;
read all var {&id};
nsub = nrow(&id);
use freqtime;
read all var {&time};
```

```
ntime = nrow(&time);
time = &time;
use &data;
read all var {&id &time &response};
n = nrow(&response);
dropout = j(n,1,0);
ind = 1;
do while (ind <= nsub);
  j=1;
  if (&response[(ind-1)*ntime+j]=.)
    then print "First Measurement is Missing";
  if (&response[(ind-1)*ntime+j]^=.) then
    do;
      j = ntime;
      do until (j=1);
        if (&response[(ind-1)*ntime+j]=.) then
          do;
            dropout[(ind-1)*ntime+j]=1;
j = j-1;
  end;
          else j = 1;
      end;
end;
  ind = ind+1;
end;
prev = j(n,1,1);
prev[2:n] = &response[1:n-1];
i=1;
do while (i<=n);
  if &time[i]=time[1] then prev[i]=.;
  i = i+1;
end;
create help var {&id &time &response dropout prev};
append;
quit;
data &out;
merge &data help;
run;
%mend;
```

Likewise, once a logistic regression has been fitted, these need to be translated into weights, preparing for the WGEE analysis. These weights are defined at the individual measurement level. They are equal to the product of the probabilities of not dropping out up to the measurement occasion. The last factor is either the probability of dropping out at that

32.5 Weighted Estimating Equations (WGEE)

time or continuing the study. This task can be performed with the following macro. The arguments are the same as in the DROPOUT macro, except that now also the predicted values from the logistic regression have to be passed on through the 'pred=' argument, and dropout indicator is passed on through the 'dropout=' argument.

```
%macro dropwgt(data=,id=,time=,pred=,dropout=,out=);
%if %bquote(&data)= %then %let data=&syslast;
proc freq data=&data noprint;
tables &id /out=freqid;
tables &time / out=freqtime;
run;
proc iml;
reset noprint;
use freqid;
read all var {&id};
nsub = nrow(&id);
use freqtime;
read all var {&time};
ntime = nrow(&time);
time = &time;
use &data;
read all var {&id &time &pred &dropout};
n = nrow(&pred);
wi = j(n,1,1);
ind = 1;
do while (ind <= nsub);
   wihlp = 1;
   stay = 1;
   /* first measurement */
   if (&dropout[(ind-1)*ntime+2]=1)
     then do;
         wihlp = pred[(ind-1)*ntime+2];
      stay = 0;
      end;
   else if (&dropout[(ind-1)*ntime+2]=0)
     then wihlp = 1-pred[(ind-1)*ntime+2];
   /* second to penultimate measurement */
   j=2;
   do while ((j <= ntime-1) & stay);
      if (&dropout[(ind-1)*ntime+j+1]=1)
         then do;
            wihlp = wihlp*pred[(ind-1)*ntime+j+1];
      stay = 0;
      end;
```

```
      else if (&dropout[(ind-1)*ntime+j+1]=0)
        then wihlp = wihlp*(1-pred[(ind-1)*ntime+j+1]);
          j = j+1;
      end;
      j = 1;
      do while (j <= ntime);
        wi[(ind-1)*ntime+j]=wihlp;
        j = j+1;
      end;
      ind = ind+1;
    end;
    create help var {&id &time &pred &dropout wi};
    append;
    quit;
    data &out;
    merge &data help;
    data &out;
    set &out;
    wi=1/wi;
    run;
    %mend;
```

Using both macros, the following code can be used to prepare for a WGEE analysis:

```
%dropout(data=armd111,id=subject,time=time,
 response=bindif,out=armdhlp);

proc genmod data=armdhlp descending;
class trt prev lesion time;
model dropout = prev trt lesion time
     / pred dist=binomial;
ods output obstats=pred;
run;

data pred;
set pred;
keep observation pred;
run;

data armdhlp;
merge pred armdhlp;
run;

%dropwgt(data=armdhlp,id=subject,time=time,
 pred=pred,dropout=dropout,out=armdwgee);
```

First, the dropout indicator and previous outcome variable are defined using the DROPOUT macro, whereafter an ordinary logistic regression is performed. Predicted values are first saved and then merged with the original data. Finally, the predicted values are translated into proper weights using the DROPWGT macro.

Let us take a look at a portion of the final dataset:

subject	time	bindif	DROPOUT	PREV	Pred	WI
1	1	1	0	.	.	58.4309
1	2	1	0	1	0.0120543	58.4309
1	3	.	1	1	0.017323	58.4309
1	4	.	1	.	.	58.4309
2	1	0	0	.	.	1.2741
2	2	1	0	0	0.031629	1.2741
2	3	1	0	1	0.0434131	1.2741
2	4	1	0	1	0.1526847	1.2741
5	1	.	0	.	.	.
5	2	.	0	.	.	.
5	3	.	0	.	.	.
5	4	.	0	.	.	.
31	1	0	0	.	.	5.7965
31	2	.	1	0	0.1725191	5.7965
31	3	.	1	.	.	5.7965
31	4	.	1	.	.	5.7965
50	1	1	0	.	.	.
50	2	1	0	1	0.0130651	.
50	3	.	0	1	0.0187673	.
50	4	1	0	.	.	.
98	1	.	0	.	.	.
98	2	0	0	.	.	.
98	3	0	0	0	0.0194998	.
98	4	1	0	0	0.0731861	.

Note that some individuals have a very high weight. This is the case when dropout occurs, in spite of a very low dropout probability. Further, non-monotone sequences are not taken into account in this analysis. Also, alternative weighting schemes that allow weights to differ by measurement, rather than by subject, are possible as well.

After this preparatory endeavor, we merely need to include the weights by means of the WEIGHT (or, equivalently, SCWGT) statement within the

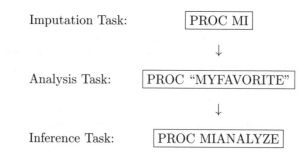

FIGURE 32.1. *The three multiple imputation tasks using SAS.*

GENMOD procedure. This statement identifies a variable in the input data set to be used as the exponential family dispersion parameter weight for each observation. The exponential family dispersion parameter is divided by the WEIGHT variable value for each observation. Whereas the inclusion of the REPEATED statement turns a univariate exponential family model into GEE, the addition of WEIGHT further switches to WGEE. In other words, we merely need to add:

```
weight wi;
```

Note that the use of the WEIGHT statement is equally possible in the GLIMMIX procedure, so that also a weighted version of the linearization based GEE method is feasible.

32.6 Multiple Imputation

Multiple imputation has been introduced in Section 28.2 and exemplified using the age related macular degeneration trial in Section 28.5.

The three tasks of multiple imputation, i.e., the imputation, analysis, and inference tasks, can be conducted within SAS. Two key procedures are the MI and MIANALYZE procedures. A schematic representation of the three tasks is given in Figure 32.1. We will discuss each of the tasks in turn. A specific use of the MI procedure is to change non-monotone missingness into monotone missingness. We will devote some attention to this specific job as well.

32.6.1 *The MI Procedure for the Imputation Task*

PROC MI is used to generate the imputations. It creates M imputed datasets from an input dataset, physically stored in a single data set with indicator variable _IMPUTATION_ to separate the imputed copies.

There is a variety of imputation mechanisms available (Section 28.2.5), distinguishing between non-monotone and monotone sequences, and between continuous and categorical variables.

The following program can be used:

```
proc mi data=armd13 seed=486048 out=armd13a
        simple nimpute=10 round=0.1;
var lesion diff4 diff12 diff24 diff52;
by treat;
run;
```

Let us describe some options available in the PROC MI statement. The option 'simple' displays simple descriptive statistics and pairwise correlations based on available cases in the input dataset. The number of imputations is specified by the option 'nimpute=,' with a default of five. The option 'round=' controls the number of decimal places in the imputed values, with no rounding by default. For example, 'round=0.1' requests a single decimal place. If more than one number is specified, one should use a VAR statement, and the specified numbers must correspond to the number of variables in the VAR statement. The 'seed=' option is used to specify a positive integer, which is used by PROC MI to start the pseudo-random number generator. The default is a value generated from the time of day from the computer's clock. Thus, though not needed, it is useful when an analysis needs to be checked afterwards or when a seed is specified by an external source such as, for example, a regulatory authority.

The imputation task is carried out separately for each level of the variables specified in the BY statement. For example, when there are several treatment arms, imputation can be done for each arm separately, thus not imposing any relationship between the outcome variables and such an important covariate as treatment assignment.

In PROC MI, one can choose between one of the three imputation mechanisms we discussed in Section 28.2.5. When missingness is confined to dropout, the MONOTONE statement can, but does not have to, be used. The parametric regression method 'method=reg' as well as the nonparametric propensity score method ('method=propensity') are available. For general patterns of missingness, the MCMC statement can be used, which is the default as well.

In all cases, especially with MCMC, a number of options is available to flexibly control the imputation task. For example, 'ngroups=' specifies the number of groups based on propensity scores when the propensity scores method is used. For the MCMC method, one can give the initial mean and covariance estimates to start the MCMC process by the 'initial=' option. The 'pmm' option in the MCMC statement uses the predictive mean matching method to impute an observed value that is closest to the predicted value in the MCMC method. The 'regpmm' option in the MONOTONE statement uses the predictive mean matching method to impute an observed value that is closest to the predicted value for data sets with monotone missingness. One can specify more than one method in the MONOTONE statement, and for each imputed variable, the covariates can be specified separately.

Whereas such methods as 'propensity' and 'regression' are used for incomplete continuous outcomes, incomplete categorical outcomes can be imputed by including them into the CLASS statement, in addition to their inclusion in the VAR statement. In such a case, the MONOTONE option should be used, and one can make use of logistic regression and discriminant analysis imputation by means of the options 'logistic' and 'discrim,' respectively.

With the (default) 'initial=EM' option, the procedure uses the means and standard deviations from available cases as the initial estimates for the EM algorithm. The final estimates after applying the EM algorithm are then used to start the MCMC process. One can also specify 'initial=*input SAS-data-set*' to use a SAS dataset with the initial estimates of the mean and covariance matrix for each imputation. Further, the 'niter=' option specifies the number of iterations between imputations in a single chain, the default being 100.

Let us illustrate the MI procedure by means of the analysis conducted on the age related macular degeneration trial in Section 28.5. At this point, the dataset is in a 'multivariate' format, i.e., each subject has got a single record, with different measurement occasions stored in different columns (variables). We started from the continuous outcomes 'diff4,' 'diff12,' 'diff24,' and 'diff52,' i.e., the difference from baseline in number of letters read, which was then dichotomized as negative *versus* non-negative. It is then sensible to multiply impute the continuous outcome first, and then dichotomize. The four outcomes were supplemented with 'lesion,' a count, which for the purpose of this analysis is treated as continuous. The imputation is conducted for each of the two treatment arms separately. This implies the lesion and treatment outcomes are taken into account. A consequence of this approach is that subjects for whom all four follow-up measurements are missing are still imputed, by virtue of the lesion covariate information. One has to ensure the data are sorted by treatment group, since otherwise the BY statement in the MI procedure will cause problems.

Ten imputations are requested by the 'nimpute=' option and the imputed values are rounded to one decimal place by including 'round=0.1.' The 'seed=' option is needed only to reproduce the analysis. Without the 'seed=' option, the random generator is started based on the computer's clock.

No imputation method has been specified, implying the user is satisfied with the defaults, as presented in the 'Model Information' panel:

```
Model Information
```

32.6 Multiple Imputation

```
Data Set                         ARMD13
Method                           MCMC
Multiple Imputation Chain        Single Chain
Initial Estimates for MCMC       EM Posterior Mode
Start                            Starting Value
Prior                            Jeffreys
Number of Imputations            10
Number of Burn-in Iterations     200
Number of Iterations             100
Seed for random number generator 486048
```

Multiple imputations are generated using Monte Carlo Markov Chain sampling, with a 'single chain' for all of the 10 imputations, as opposed to a different chain for each one of the iterations. Initial estimates for the MCMC algorithm are obtained using the EM algorithm, applied to the five-variate normal distribution assumed for the five outcomes ('lesion' and the four follow-up measurements). Initial values for the EM algorithm are generated using a complete case analysis.

Some of the descriptive statistics for treatment arm 1 are as follows. An overview is given of the missing data patterns:

Missing Data Patterns

Group	lesion	diff4	diff12	diff24	diff52	Freq	Percent
1	X	X	X	X	X	102	85.71
2	X	X	X	X	.	9	7.56
3	X	X	X	.	X	2	1.68
4	X	X	X	.	.	3	2.52
5	X	X	.	.	.	1	0.84
6	X	.	X	X	X	1	0.84
7	X	.	.	.	.	1	0.84

and the corresponding table for the second treatment arm is

Missing Data Patterns

Group	lesion	diff4	diff12	diff24	diff52	Freq	Percent
1	X	X	X	X	X	86	71.07
2	X	X	X	X	.	15	12.40
3	X	X	X	.	X	2	1.65
4	X	X	X	.	.	5	4.13
5	X	X	.	.	X	1	0.83
6	X	X	.	.	.	5	4.13
7	X	.	X	X	X	1	0.83
8	X	.	X	.	.	1	0.83

9	X	.	.	.	.	4	3.31
10	0	0	0	0	0	1	0.83

Next, group means per pattern are given (displayed for treatment arm 1):

Missing Data Patterns

```
------------------------------Group Means------------------
Group     lesion       diff4        diff12       diff24      diff52

  1      1.901961    -0.921569    -2.313725   -5.598039  -10.960784
  2      1.666667    -1.222222     2.111111   -7.666667        .
  3      1.500000   -12.500000   -19.000000         .    -18.500000
  4      2.000000    -4.000000    -4.000000         .          .
  5      4.000000   -10.000000         .             .          .
  6      1.000000         .        1.000000    1.000000  -19.000000
  7      1.000000         .            .             .          .
```

Then, unadjusted univariate statistics are given, based on the averages over the available information for each of the outcomes:

Univariate Statistics

						-Missing Values-	
Variable	N	Mean	Std Dev	Min	Max	Count	Percent
lesion	119	1.8823	0.9313	1.0	4.0	0	0.00
diff4	117	-1.2991	7.7183	-33.0	30.0	2	1.68
diff12	117	-2.2735	11.7345	-38.0	31.0	2	1.68
diff24	112	-5.7053	13.8281	-54.0	26.0	7	5.88
diff52	105	-11.1809	16.4292	-59.0	23.0	14	11.76

The posterior modes, obtained after applying the EM algorithm, together with the corresponding covariance parameters, are presented. These are used to draw imputations from:

EM (Posterior Mode) Estimates

TYPE	_NAME_	lesion	diff4	diff12	diff24	diff52
MEAN		1.8823	-1.2696	-2.3352	-5.9795	-11.3339
COV	lesion	0.8188	-0.9175	-1.1290	-0.8096	-0.7889
COV	diff4	-0.9175	56.0723	49.0903	45.1982	44.6498
COV	diff12	-1.1290	49.0903	130.0959	91.9756	100.8011
COV	diff24	-0.8096	45.1982	91.9756	188.6427	174.7665
COV	diff52	-0.7889	44.6498	100.8011	174.7665	264.5092

More detail on the specific use of the MI procedure to apply the EM algorithm is given in Section 32.6.

For each of the incomplete outcomes, which in our case excludes the 'lesion' variable, information on the between, within and total variances is given, as well as on the fraction of missing information:

Multiple Imputation Variance Information

Variable	Between	Within	Total	DF
diff4	0.004699	0.504802	0.509971	114.72
diff12	0.026864	1.161408	1.190959	112.3
diff24	0.159445	1.745878	1.921267	96.074
diff52	0.085476	2.405584	2.499607	109.76

Variable	Relative Increase in Variance	Fraction Missing Information	Relative Efficiency
diff4	0.010240	0.010159	0.998985
diff12	0.025444	0.024946	0.997512
diff24	0.100459	0.092967	0.990789
diff52	0.039085	0.037918	0.996223

Note that the amount of missing information is larger at 24 weeks than at 52 weeks, in spite of the reverse holding for the number of missing subjects at these occasions. The above information can then be used to test standard hypotheses about the imputed outcomes. This is useful when the scientific questions are stated in terms of the individual outcomes, as then the other two tasks (analysis and inference) are no further needed. However, one usually would be interested in fitting a (longitudinal) model to the imputed datasets and hence both tasks would be needed.

At this point, the data are still in a horizontal or multivariate mode. Thus, we first define the binary outcomes out of the multiply imputed continuous ones, and then store the data in longitudinal or vertical mode, as was done on page 455:

```
data armd13a;
set armd13a;
bindif4=0; if diff4 <= 0   then bindif4=1;
bindif12=0;if diff12 <= 0  then bindif12=1;
bindif24=0;if diff24 <= 0  then bindif24=1;
bindif52=0;if diff52 <= 0  then bindif52=1;
if diff4=. then bindif4=.;
if diff12=. then bindif12=.;
if diff24=. then bindif24=.;
```

```
if diff52=. then bindif52=.;
run;

data armd13b;
set armd13a;
array x (4) bindif4 bindif12 bindif24 bindif52;
array y (4) diff4 diff12 diff24 diff52;
do j=1 to 4;
   bindif=x(j);
   diff=y(j);
   time=j;
   output;
end;
run;
```

Taking a look at the first subject, in horizontal format for conciseness, we obtain (variable names have been shortened):

```
_Imp._  diff4  diff12  diff24  diff52  bin4  bin12  bin24  bin52

  1      -4     -14      3.2     3.1    1      1      0      0
  2      -4     -14    -31.6   -43.9    1      1      1      1
  3      -4     -14    -11.4   -18.4    1      1      1      1
  4      -4     -14    -30.4   -39.3    1      1      1      1
  5      -4     -14     -5.5   -24.9    1      1      1      1
  6      -4     -14      3.0   -15.9    1      1      0      1
  7      -4     -14    -22.3   -45.2    1      1      1      1
  8      -4     -14     -2.8   -33.6    1      1      1      1
  9      -4     -14    -27.1   -48.1    1      1      1      1
 10      -4     -14    -23.7   -46.9    1      1      1      1
```

Thus, the measurements at weeks 24 and 52 have been imputed 10 times. Of course, due to the coarsening occuring when dichotomizing a continuous outcome, the binary indicators show relatively little variability.

We are now ready to conduct the analysis task.

32.6.2 The Analysis Task

The imputed data sets are analyzed using a standard procedure, labeled 'MYFAVORITE' in Figure 32.1. It is important to ensure that the BY statement is used to force an analysis for each of the imputed sets of data separately, in the following way:

```
by _imputation_;
```

Parameter estimates and their estimated covariance matrices need to be stored in appropriate output datasets, so they can be passed on to the MI-

ANALYZE procedure in the inference task (Section 32.6.3). Although the MIANALYZE procedure is conceived very generally, it still is a bit of challenge because the estimates and their estimated covariances are called differently by different SAS procedures, and the output datasets corresponding to them may be organized somewhat differently as well. The procedure is able to handle CLASS effects as well, even though a number of columns in the corresponding output datasets are then needed to multi-index the effect.

In spite of this CLASS feature of the MIANALYZE procedure, we have chosen to create appropriate dummies for categorical effects and interactions, by way of defensive programming. It also facilitates direct mapping between GEE and GLMM parameters, using the GENMOD and NLMIXED procedures, respectively.

To prepare for the analysis, dummies are created and then the data are sorted by imputation number.

```
data armd13c;
set armd13b;
time1=0;
time2=0;
time3=0;
time4=0;
trttime1=0;
trttime2=0;
trttime3=0;
trttime4=0;
if time=1 then time1=1;
if time=2 then time2=1;
if time=3 then time3=1;
if time=4 then time4=1;
if (time=1 & treat=1) then trttime1=1;
if (time=2 & treat=1) then trttime2=1;
if (time=3 & treat=1) then trttime3=1;
if (time=4 & treat=1) then trttime4=1;
run;

proc sort data=armd13c;
by _imputation_ subject time;
run;
```

The latter is needed because the MI procedure performed imputation by treatment group, hence the imputations run from 1 through 10 within each treatment group, and hence the overall ordering by imputation needs to be restored first.

The GENMOD procedure can then be called for a GEE analysis, analogous to the one presented at the start of Section 32.5:

```
proc genmod data=armd13c;
class time subject;
by _imputation_;
model bindif = time1 time2 time3 time4
               trttime1 trttime2 trttime3 trttime4
       / noint dist=binomial covb;
repeated subject=subject
         / withinsubject=time type=exch modelse;
ods output ParameterEstimates=gmparms
           parminfo=gmpinfo CovB=gmcovb;
run;
```

Apart from an otherwise irrelevant change to user-defined dummy coding of the covariates in the model, the BY statement has been added, as well as the ODS statement, to store the parameter estimates and the covariance parameters. For the latter, the 'parminfo=' option is used next to the 'covb=' option, to ensure the proper names of the covariate effects are mapped to abbreviations of type 'Prm1,' etc. Note that the 'covb=' output option works only because the 'covb' option was included into the MODEL statement. The parameter estimates are generated by default. The direct output of the GENMOD procedure will be a GEE analysis for each of the ten imputed datasets. As such, they are of no direct scientific interest. Formal inference ought to be conducted only using the results from the inference task (Section 32.6.3).

Because the 'noint' option was included into the effect 'Prm1' formally exists but it is unavailable as a parameter estimate. It is therefore prudent to delete it from the parameter information:

```
data gmpinfo;
set gmpinfo;
if parameter='Prm1' then delete;
run;
```

It is one of many small data handling operations that might have to take place between the analysis and inference tasks. When problems occur, it is wise to print the output datasets needed and make the necessary adjustments.

A portion of the parameter-estimates set of data reads:

Obs	_Imputation_	Parameter	DF	Estimate
1	1	Intercept	0	0.0000
2	1	time1	1	-0.8473
3	1	time2	1	-1.0546
4	1	time3	1	-1.0986
5	1	time4	1	-1.6094
6	1	trttime1	1	0.2042

32.6 Multiple Imputation

```
 7        1        trttime2    1     0.6281
 8        1        trttime3    1     0.4555
 9        1        trttime4    1     0.2850
10        1        Scale       0     1.0000
...
12        2        time1       1    -0.8079
...
22        3        time1       1    -0.8079
...
32        4        time1       1    -0.8873
...
42        5        time1       1    -0.8473
...
52        6        time1       1    -0.8473
...
62        7        time1       1    -0.8079
...
72        8        time1       1    -0.8473
...
82        9        time1       1    -0.8873
...
92       10        time1       1    -0.8473
```

The full set of parameters for the first dataset is displayed, as well as the effect at 4 weeks ('time1') for each of the remaining nine datasets.

It is instructive to consider a portion of the variance-covariance dataset:

```
     I
     m
     p
     u
     t    R
     a    o
     t    w
     i    N
   0 o    a        P         P         P          P
   b n    m        r         r         r          r
   s _    e        m         m         m          m
                   2         3         4          5   ...

   1 1  Prm2  0.0396825      0         0          0   ...
   2 1  Prm3       0      0.043494     0          0   ...
   3 1  Prm4       0         0    0.0444444       0   ...
   4 1  Prm5       0         0         0       0.06   ...
   ...
   9 2  Prm2  0.0390752      0         0          0   ...
  10 2  Prm3       0      0.043494     0          0   ...
```

```
11  2  Prm4              0            0  0.0444444             0 ...
12  2  Prm5              0            0           0    0.0625326 ...
...
```

Not only this portion, but every one of the 10 variance-covariance matrices, is fully diagonal, in line with the fact that we have a full treatment by time interaction model, on rectangular sets of data. However, this need not be the case for the final variance-covariance matrix, as we will see from the inference task.

The parameter mapping dataset looks as follows:

```
Obs     _Imputation_    Parameter    Effect

 1           1            Prm2       time1
 2           1            Prm3       time2
 3           1            Prm4       time3
 4           1            Prm5       time4
 5           1            Prm6       trttime1
 6           1            Prm7       trttime2
 7           1            Prm8       trttime3
 8           1            Prm9       trttime4
...
```

Of course, once the imputation task is finished, in principle any (longitudinal) analysis can be done. For example, the GLMM from Section 32.4 can be conducted on the multiply imputed datasets:

```
proc nlmixed data=armd13c qpoints=20 maxiter=100
     technique=newrap cov ecov;
by _imputation_;
eta = beta11*time1+beta12*time2+beta13*time3+beta14*time4
      +b
     +beta21*trttime1+beta22*trttime2
     +beta23*trttime3+beta24*trttime4;
p = exp(eta)/(1+exp(eta));
model bindif ~ binary(p);
random b ~ normal(0,tau*tau) subject=subject;
estimate 'tau2' tau*tau;
ods output ParameterEstimates=nlparms
           CovMatParmEst=nlcovb
           AdditionalEstimates=nlparmsa
           CovMatAddEst=nlcovba;
run;
```

Apart from the BY statement, four output datasets are generated using the ODS statement. For the standard model parameters, we only need the 'parameterestimates=' and 'covmatparmest=' options. If, in addition, multiple imputation inference is requested about the additional estimates, then they can be saved as well using the 'additionalestimates=' and 'covmataddest=' options. However, it may be wiser to calculate the additional estimates directly from the results of the inference task, i.e., to conduct multiple imputation inference and then calculate additional estimates, rather than the other way around. For both covariance matrices to be generated, the options 'cov' and 'ecov,' respectively, need to be included into the PROC NLMIXED statement.

For both models, we can now conduct multiple imputation inference, as explained in Section 32.6.3.

32.6.3 The Inference Task

Finally, PROC MIANALYZE combines the M inferences into a single one, by making use of the theory laid out in Section 28.2.2. Parameter and standard errors are passed on through a combination of the 'data=,' 'parms=,' 'covb=,' and/or 'xpxi=' options to the PROC MIANALYZE statement. Using 'data=' datasets of types COV, CORR, or EST can be passed on, as well as a dataset containing parameter estimates and standard errors. When one wants to pass on parameter estimates and variance-covariance matrices instead, it is better to use 'parms=' and 'covb=' or 'parms=' and 'xpxi=.' When the 'covb=' matrices contain generic names ('Prm1,'...), the mapping between generic and actual parameter names is passed on using 'parminfo=.'

A number of fine tuning options is available as well in the PROC MIANALYZE statement. For example, the within-imputation, between-imputation and total covariance matrices are printed upon including the 'wcov', 'bcov', and 'tcov' options, respectively.

The parameters or effects for which multiple imputation inference is needed are passed on by means of the MODELEFFECTS statement (previously VAR statement). Categorical effects are handled as well, upon including them in the CLASS statement. As stated earlier, it could be cautious to create appropriate dummies and avoid the use of the CLASS statement, as sometimes the mapping between parameter estimates and the corresponding precision parameters is not straightforward. In principle, the MIANALYZE procedure works after applying any standard analysis, using a SAS procedure, in the analysis task, from SAS Version 9.1 onwards.

The TEST statement allows testing for hypotheses about linear combinations of the parameters. The statement is based on Rubin (1987), and uses a t-distribution which is the univariate version of the work by Li, Raghunathan, and Rubin (1991), described in Section 28.2.3.

Applying the procedure to the GEE analysis on the ARMD data, presented in Section 32.6.2, can be done using the following code:

```
proc mianalyze parms=gmparms covb=gmcovb
```

```
                parminfo=gmpinfo wcov bcov tcov;
modeleffects time1 time2 time3 time4
              trttime1 trttime2 trttime3 trttime4;
run;
```

Compared to the MI procedure, the MIANALYZE procedure is rather simple, in line with the simplicity and elegance of the pooling method of Section 28.2.2. For each of the parameters, their between, within, and total variance is presented:

Multiple Imputation Variance Information

Parameter	Between	Variance Within	Total	DF
time1	0.000856	0.039631	0.040573	16698
time2	0.003629	0.042843	0.046835	1238.9
time3	0.007760	0.043903	0.052440	339.63
time4	0.013950	0.060207	0.075551	218.18
trttime1	0.002235	0.076721	0.079179	9337.3
trttime2	0.003376	0.077934	0.081648	4350.7
trttime3	0.009839	0.081079	0.091902	648.95
trttime4	0.015836	0.108550	0.125969	470.66

based upon which the fraction of missing information can be calculated:

Multiple Imputation Variance Information

Parameter	Relative Increase in Variance	Fraction Missing Information	Relative Efficiency
time1	0.023768	0.023333	0.997672
time2	0.093173	0.086705	0.991404
time3	0.194438	0.167673	0.983509
time4	0.254868	0.210309	0.979402
trttime1	0.032041	0.031254	0.996884
trttime2	0.047649	0.045921	0.995429
trttime3	0.133485	0.120471	0.988096
trttime4	0.160474	0.141922	0.986006

This is similar in spirit to some of the output of the MI procedure (Section 32.6.1), but here the interest lies in parameters, whereas the MI procedure focuses on the imputed outcome variables. The information is useful to see how missingness decreases precision with which the various parameters are estimated.

32.6 Multiple Imputation

The key portion of the output is the parameter estimates, their standard errors, and related information:

```
            Multiple Imputation Parameter Estimates

Parameter    Estimate    Std Error   95% Confidence Limits      DF

time1       -0.843486    0.201427   -1.23831    -0.44867     16698
time2       -1.020910    0.216413   -1.44549    -0.59633      1238.9
time3       -1.069445    0.228997   -1.51988    -0.61901       339.63
time4       -1.607580    0.274866   -2.14931    -1.06585       218.18
trttime1     0.211407    0.281388   -0.34017     0.76299      9337.3
trttime2     0.604904    0.285740    0.04471     1.16510      4350.7
trttime3     0.429925    0.303153   -0.16535     1.02521       648.95
trttime4     0.366539    0.354921   -0.33089     1.06396       470.66
```

Some additional information is the range for the parameter estimates, assembled from the 10 imputations, and results from testing the null hypothesis of a zero true parameter value:

```
            Multiple Imputation Parameter Estimates
                                              t for H0:
Parameter    Minimum     Maximum    Theta0    Par=Theta0    Pr > |t|

time1       -0.887303   -0.807923     0         -4.19        <.0001
time2       -1.143564   -0.927987     0         -4.72        <.0001
time3       -1.236763   -0.927987     0         -4.67        <.0001
time4       -1.871802   -1.439215     0         -5.85        <.0001
trttime1     0.127354    0.281167     0          0.75        0.4525
trttime2     0.501468    0.717045     0          2.12        0.0343
trttime3     0.284850    0.593626     0          1.42        0.1566
trttime4     0.213264    0.645850     0          1.03        0.3023
```

The values for 'Theta0' can be specified by the user in the PROC MIANALYZE statement. In this case, for the final four parameters, the tests corresponds to the null hypothesis of no treatment effect at each of the four times.

It is instructive to pay attention to the within-imputation, between-imputation, and total covariance matrices. Although the within-imputation covariance matrix, being the average of the 10 matrices passed on through the 'covb=' option, is diagonal, the between-imputation matrix is not, as is seen from the following small fraction:

```
     Between-Imputation Covariance Matrix

                  time1              time2 ...
```

time1	0.0008563099	0.0004082521 ...
time2	0.0004082521	0.0036288964 ...
...		

Conducting multiple imputation inference for the NLMIXED analysis, presented in Section 32.6.2, is done by means of:

```
proc mianalyze parms=nlparms covb=nlcovb
              wcov bcov tcov;
modeleffects beta11 beta12 beta13 beta14
              beta21 beta22 beta23 beta24;
run;
```

with the following results for the model parameters:

Multiple Imputation Parameter Estimates

Parameter	Estimate	Std Error	95% Confidence Limits		DF
beta11	1.455346	0.356901	0.75556	2.15513	3139.1
beta12	1.749244	0.376606	1.01021	2.48827	999.52
beta13	1.826672	0.383498	1.07377	2.57957	726.52
beta14	2.686402	0.445717	1.80943	3.56338	313.46
beta21	-0.315416	0.480927	-1.25816	0.62733	8002.1
beta22	-0.988679	0.488167	-1.94574	-0.03162	4324.6
beta23	-0.673317	0.507420	-1.66922	0.32258	876.41
beta24	-0.515931	0.563860	-1.62394	0.59208	468.56
tau	2.203316	0.256697	1.69895	2.70768	488.15

and

Multiple Imputation Parameter Estimates

Parameter	Minimum	Maximum	Theta0	t for H0: Par=Theta0	Pr > |t|
beta11	1.338106	1.582843	0	4.08	<.0001
beta12	1.529515	1.882212	0	4.64	<.0001
beta13	1.653527	2.028812	0	4.76	<.0001
beta14	2.481554	3.074676	0	6.03	<.0001
beta21	-0.445510	-0.192473	0	-0.66	0.5119
beta22	-1.126595	-0.769312	0	-2.03	0.0429
beta23	-0.907306	-0.449662	0	-1.33	0.1849
beta24	-0.954038	-0.276338	0	-0.91	0.3607
tau	2.081615	2.332432	0	8.58	<.0001

32.6.4 The MI Procedure to Create Monotone Missingness

When missingness is non-monotone, one might think of several mechanisms operating simultaneously: e.g., a simple (MCAR or MAR) mechanism for the intermediate missing values and a more complex (MNAR) mechanism for the missing data past the moment of dropout. However, analyzing such data is complicated because many model strategies, especially those under the assumption of MNAR, but also WGEE, have been developed for dropout only or at least work in a considerably simpler way under monotone missingness. Therefore, a solution might be to generate multiple imputations that render the datasets monotone missing, by including into MI:

```
mcmc impute = monotone;
```

and then apply a method of choice to the so-completed multiple sets of data. Note that this is different from the monotone method in the MI procedure. The latter in fact does the opposite: it fully completes already monotone sets of data.

The other value for the 'impute=' option is 'impute=full,' which is also the default. This method implies that all missing values are imputed, whether monotone or non-monotone.

32.7 The EM Algorithm

A version of the EM algorithm, for multivariate normal data, can be conducted using the MI procedure in SAS. With the MCMC imputation method (for general non-monotone settings), the MCMC chain is started using EM-based starting values. It is possible to suppress the actual MCMC-based multiple imputation, thus restricting action of PROC MI to the EM algorithm.

The 'nimpute=' option in the MI procedure should be set equal to zero to skip multiple imputation. Then, only tables with model information, missing data patterns, descriptive statistics (in case the 'simple' option is given) and the results from the EM algorithm (EM statement) are displayed.

We have to specify the EM statement, so that the EM algorithm is used to compute the maximum likelihood estimate (MLE) of the data with missing values, assuming a multivariate normal distribution for the data. Clearly, this feature is as such not needed to estimate parameters of a multivariate normal based on incomplete data, since direct likelihood is well within reach using, for example, the MIXED procedure. However, it illustrates nicely the features of the EM algorithm.

The following options are available with the EM statement. The option 'converge=' option specifies the convergence criterion, with a value between 0 and 1. The iterations are considered to have converged when the maximum change in the parameter estimates between iteration steps is less than the value specified. The change is a relative change if the parameter is greater than 0.01 in absolute value; otherwise it is an absolute change. By default, 'converge' is set to 10^{-4}. The iteration history in the EM algorithm is printed if the option 'itprint' is given. The maximum number of iterations used in the EM algorithm is specified with the 'maxiter=' option. The default is 'maxiter=200.'

Initial values for the EM algorithm are computed using the method specified by means of the 'initial=' option. The default is the AC (available case) method, but also CC (complete cases) are possible. The correlations are set equal to zero when starting the procedure with AC.

The 'out=' option specifies an output dataset, equal to the input dataset with all incomplete values among the variables analyzed replaced by their final expectation under the EM algorithm. The option 'outem=' creates an output SAS data set containing the MLE of the parameter vector (μ, Σ), computed with the EM algorithm. Finally, 'outiter=' creates an output SAS data set containing parameters for each iteration. The dataset includes a variable named '_iteration_' to identify the iteration number.

Applying the method to the four continuous outcomes in the ARMD trial can be done using the following program:

```
proc mi data=armd14 seed=675938 simple nimpute=0;
em itprint;
var diff4 diff12 diff24 diff52;
by treat;
run;
```

When the complete data estimates have to be used as initial values, the option 'initial=cc' has to be added to the EM statement.

The initial estimates, obtained from the available cases, and in agreement with the 'simple' statistics on page 622, are

Initial Parameter Estimates for EM

TYPE	_NAME_	diff4	diff12	diff24	diff52
MEAN		-1.299145	-2.273504	-5.705357	-11.180952
COV	diff4	59.573534	0	0	0
COV	diff12	0	137.700413	0	0
COV	diff24	0	0	191.218710	0
COV	diff52	0	0	0	269.918864

The first line is for μ, the following four lines are for Σ. The evolution of the log-likelihood and each of the four parameters is displayed in the following panel:

EM (MLE) Iteration History

	-2 Log L	diff4	diff12	diff24	diff52
0	2677.623690	-1.299145	-2.273504	-5.705357	-11.180952
1	2499.142589	-1.299145	-2.273504	-5.705357	-11.180952
2	2490.124996	-1.288106	-2.337030	-5.920341	-11.287948
3	2489.821035	-1.284122	-2.338551	-5.968896	-11.326957
4	2489.809193	-1.282958	-2.338624	-5.981039	-11.336978
5	2489.808488	-1.282661	-2.338637	-5.984320	-11.339102
6	2489.808431	-1.282579	-2.338640	-5.985249	-11.339499
7	2489.808426	-1.282555	-2.338641	-5.985521	-11.339563
8	2489.808426	-1.282547	-2.338641	-5.985603	-11.339571
9	2489.808426	-1.282544	-2.338641	-5.985628	-11.339571

Then, a panel with the MLE estimates is given:

EM (MLE) Parameter Estimates

TYPE	_NAME_	diff4	diff12	diff24	diff52
MEAN		-1.282544	-2.338641	-5.985628	-11.339571
COV	diff4	58.922448	51.511233	47.562350	47.117941
COV	diff12	51.511233	136.639243	96.740432	106.108044
COV	diff24	47.562350	96.740432	198.718732	184.115237
COV	diff52	47.117941	106.108044	184.115237	279.107171

as well as with the posterior modes. The latter was given already on page 622.

When the 'initial=cc' option is included, the following starting values are used:

Initial Parameter Estimates for EM

TYPE	_NAME_	diff4	diff12	diff24	diff52
MEAN		-0.921569	-2.313725	-5.598039	-10.960784
COV	diff4	47.756164	35.628810	38.542419	38.838478
COV	diff12	35.628810	122.791691	84.968938	97.408464
COV	diff24	38.542419	84.968938	188.361580	176.993982
COV	diff52	38.838478	97.408464	176.993982	275.820229

In this case, the EM algorithm converges in about half the iterations needed for the AC starting values. Although the AC values may be closer to the true values for some, the use of the covariances here, unlike in the AC case, has the effect of considerably fastening convergence.

32.8 MNAR Models and Sensitivity Analysis Tools

The earlier sections in this chapter have shown that the simple methods, as well as methodology valid under MAR, are quite feasible using standard software, such as the SAS system. Models for MNAR and sensitivity analysis tools require more programming by the user, perhaps with the exception of simple pattern-mixture models (Section 30.2). Such tools have been developed by C. Beunckens and colleagues for continuous outcomes, as reported in Dmitrienko *et al* (2005, Chapter 5) and Molenberghs *et al* (2005). These include software to fit the model of Diggle and Kenward (1994), as well as implementation of the associated local influence methodology. We will gradually place such tools on our Web site as they become available.

References

Adams, R.J., Wilson, M., and Wang, W. (1997) The multidimensional random coefficients multinomial logit model, *Applied Psychological Measurement*, **21**, 1–23.

Aerts, M. and Claeskens, G. (1999) Bootstrapping pseudolikelihood models for clustered binary data. *Annals of the Institute of Statistical Mathematics*, **51**, 515–530.

Aerts, M., Claeskens, G., Hens, N., and Molenberghs, G. (2002) Local multiple imputation. *Biometrika*, **89**, 375–388.

Afifi, A. and Elashoff, R. (1966) Missing observations in multivariate statistics I: Review of the literature. *Journal of the American Statistical Association*, **61**, 595–604.

Agresti, A. (1990) *Categorical Data Analysis*. New York: John Wiley & Sons.

Agresti, A. (2002) *Categorical Data Analysis* (2nd ed.). New York: John Wiley & Sons.

Aitkin, M. and Rubin, D.B. (1985) Estimation and hypothesis testing in finite mixture models. *Journal of the Royal Statistical Society, Series B*, **47**, 67–75.

Akaike, H. (1974) A new look at the statistical model identification. *IEEE Transactions on Automatic Control*, **19**, 716–723.

Albert, A. and Lesaffre, E. (1986) Multiple group logistic discrimination. *Computers and Mathematics with Applications.* **12**, 209–224.

Allison, P.D. (1987) Estimation of linear models with incomplete data. *Sociology Methodology*, 71–103.

Altham, P.M.E. (1978) Two generalizations of the binomial distribution. *Applied Statistics*, **27**, 162-167.

Anderson, D.A. and Aitkin, M. (1985) Variance component models with binary response: interviewer variability. *Journal of the Royal Statistical Society, Series B*, **47**, 203–210.

Anderson, J.A. and Pemberton, J.D. (1985) The grouped continuous model for multivariate ordered categorical variables and covariate adjustment. *Biometrics*, **41**, 875–885.

Anscombe, F. J. (1981) *Computing in Statistical Science through APL.* New York: Springer-Verlag.

Arnold, B.C., Castillo, E. and Sarabia, J.M. (1992) *Conditionally Specified Distributions, Lecture Notes in Statistics* **73**, New York: Springer Verlag.

Arnold, B.C. and Strauss, D. (1991) Pseudolikelihood estimation: some examples. *Sankhya: the Indian Journal of Statistics - Series B*, **53**, 233–243.

Ashford, J.R. and Sowden, R.R. (1970) Multivariate probit analysis. *Biometrics*, **26**, 535–546.

Autian, J. (1973) Toxicity and health threats of phthalate esters: Review of the literature. *Environmental Health Perspectives*, **4**, 3–26.

Bahadur, R.R. (1961) A representation of the joint distribution of responses to n dichotomous items. In: *Studies in Item Analysis and Prediction,*, H. Solomon (Ed.). Stanford Mathematical Studies in the Social Sciences VI. Stanford, CA: Stanford University Press.

Baker, S.G. (1995) Marginal regression for repeated binary data with outcome subject to non-ignorable non-response. *Biometrics*, **51**, 1042–1052.

Baker, S.G. (1995) Analyzing a randomized cancer prevention trial with a missing binary outcome, an auxiliary variable, and all-or-none compliance. *Journal of the American Statistical Association*, **95**, 43–50.

Baker, S.G. and Laird, N.M. (1988) Regression analysis for categorical variables with outcome subject to non-ignorable non-response. *Journal of the American Statistical Association*, **83**, 62–69.

Baker, S.G., Rosenberger, W.F., and DerSimonian, R. (1992) Closed-form estimates for missing counts in two-way contingency tables. *Statistics in Medicine*, **11**, 643–657.

Barndorff-Nielsen, O.E. (1978) *Information and Exponential Families in Statistical Theory*. Chichester: John Wiley & Sons.

Barbosa, M.F. and Goldstein, H. (2000) Discrete response multilevel models for repeated measures: an application to voting intentions data. *Quality and Quantity*, **34**, 323–330.

Becker, M.P. (1989) On the bivariate normal distribution and association models for ordinal categorical data. *Statistics and Probability Letters*, **8**, 435–440.

Becker, M.P. and Balagtas, C.C. (1993). A log-nonlinear model for binary cross-over data. *Biometrics*, **49**, 997–1009.

Beckman, R.J., Nachtsheim, C.J., and Cook, R.D. (1987) Diagnostics for mixed-model analysis of variance. *Technometrics*, **29**, 413–426.

Besag, J., Green, P.J., Higdon, D., and Mengersen, K. (1995) Bayesian computation and stochastic systems, *Statistical Science*, **10**, 3–66.

Bishop, Y.M.M., Fienberg, S.E., and Holland, P.W. (1975) *Discrete Multivariate Analysis: Theory and Practice*. Cambridge: MIT Press.

Boeckmann, A.J., Sheiner, L.B., and Beal, S.L. (1992) *NONMEM User's Guide, Part V, Introductory Guide*. University of California, San Francisco.

Böhning D. (1999) *Computer-assisted Analysis of Mixtures and Applications: Meta-analysis, Disease Mapping, and Others*. London: Chapman & Hall.

Böhning, D. and Lindsay, B.G. (1988) Monotonicity of quadratic approximation algorithms. *The Annals of the Institute of Statistical Mathematics*, **40**, 641–663.

Box, G.E.P. and Tiao, G.C. (1992) *Bayesian Inference in Statistical Analysis*. Wiley Classics Library edition. New York: John Wiley & Sons.

Brant, L.J., Sheng, S.L., Morrell, C.H., Verbeke, G.N., Carter, H.B., and Lesaffre, E. (2003) Screening for prostate cancer using random-effects models, *Journal of the Royal Statistical Society, Series A*, **166**, 51–62.

Brenowitz, E.A., Margoliash, D., and Nordeen, K.W. (1997) An introduction to birdsong and the avian song system. *Journal of Neurobiology*, **33**, 495–500.

Breslow, N.E. and Clayton, D.G. (1993) Approximate inference in generalized linear mixed models. *Journal of the American Statistical Association*, **88**, 9–25.

Breslow, N.E. and Day, N.E. (1989) *Statistical methods in cancer research. Volume 1 : The analysis of case-control studies*, International Agency for Research on Cancer, Scientific Publications 32.

Breslow, N.E. and Lin, X. (1995) Bias correction in generalized linear mixed models with a single component of dispersion. *Biometrika*, **82**, 81–91.

Brown, C.H. (1990) Protecting against nonrandomly missing data in longitudinal studies. *Biometrics*, **46**, 143–155.

Brown, N.A. and Fabro, S. (1981) Quantitation of rat embryonic development in vitro: a morphological scoring system. *Teratology*, **24**, 65–78.

Brown, L.D. (1986) *Fundamentals of Statistical Exponential Families.* California: Institute of Mathematical Statistics.

Browne, W.J. and Draper, D. (2003) A comparison of bayesian and likelihood-based methods for fitting multilevel models, *Submitted*, **000**, 000–000.

Bryk, A.S. and Raudenbush, S.W. (1992) *Hierarchical Linear Models: Applications and Data Analysis Methods.* Newbury Park: Sage Publications.

Buck, S.F. (1960) A method of estimation of missing values in multivariate data suitable for use with an electronic computer. *Journal of the Royal Statistical Society, Series B*, **22**, 302–306.

Burnham, K.P. and Anderson, D.R. (1998) *Model Selection and Inference: A Practical Information-Theoretic Approach*, New York: Springer-Verlag.

Burton, S.W. (1991) A review of fluvoxamine and its uses in depression. *International Clinical Psychopharmacology, 6 (Suppl. 3)*, 1–17.

Burzykowski, T., Molenberghs, G., and Buyse, M. (2005) *The Evaluation of Surrogate Endpoints.* New York: Springer-Verlag.

Burzykowski, T., Molenberghs, G., Buyse, M., Geys, H., and Renard, D. (2001) Validation of surrogate endpoints in multiple randomized clinical trials with failure time end points, *Applied Statistics*, **50**, 405–422.

Butler, S.M. and Louis, T.A. (1992) Random effects models with nonparametric priors. *Statistics in Medicine*, **11**, 1981–2000.

Buyse, M. and Molenberghs, G. (1998) The validation of surrogate endpoints in randomized experiments. *Biometrics*, **54**, 1014–1029.

Buyse, M., Molenberghs, G., Burzykowski, T., Renard, D., and Geys, H. (2000) The validation of surrogate endpoints in meta-analyses of randomized experiments, *Biostatistics*, **1**, 49–67.

Carey, V.C., Zeger, S.L., and Diggle, P.J. (1993) Modelling multivariate binary data with alternating logistic regressions. *Biometrika*, **80**, 517–526.

Carlin, B.P. and Louis, T.A. (1996) *Bayes and Empirical Bayes Methods for Data Analysis*. London: Chapman & Hall.

Catalano, P.J. (1997) Bivariate modelling of clustered continuous and ordered categorical outcomes. *Statistics in Medicine*, **16**, 883–900.

Catalano, P.J. and Ryan, L.M. (1992) Bivariate latent variable models for clustered discrete and continuous outcomes. *Journal of the American Statistical Association*, **87**, 651–658.

Catchpole, E.A. and Morgan, B.J.T. (1997) Detecting parameter redundancy. *Biometrika*, **84**, 187–196.

Catchpole, E.A., Morgan, B.J.T., and Freeman, S.N. (1998) Estimation in parameter-redundant models. *Biometrika*, **85**, 462–468.

Chakraborty, H., Helms, R.W., Sen, P.K., and Cohen, M.S. (2003) Estimating correlation by using a general linear mixed model: Evaluation of the relationship between the concentration of HIV-1 RNA in blood and semen, *Statistics in Medicine*, **22**, 1457–1464.

Clayton, D. and Hills, M. (1993) *Statistical Methods in Epidemiology*. Oxford: Oxford University Press.

Cleveland, W.S. and Grosse, E. (1991) Computational methods for local regression. *Statistics and Computing*, **1**, 47–62.

Cohen, J. and Cohen, P. (1983) *Applied multiple regression/correlation analysis for the behavioral sciences* (2nd ed.). Hillsdale, NJ: Erlbaum.

Conaway, M. (1989) Analysis of repeated categorical measurements with conditional likelihood methods. *Journal of the American Statistical Association*, **84**, 53–62.

Conaway, M.R. (1992) The analysis of repeated categorical measurements subject to nonignorable nonresponse. *Journal of the American Statistical Association*, **87**, 817–824.

Conaway, M.R. (1993) Non-ignorable non-response models for time-ordered categorical variables. *Applied Statistics*, **42**, 105–115.

Conniffe, D. (2001) Score tests when a nuisance parameter is unidentified under the null hypothesis. *Journal of Statistical Planning and Inference*, **97**, 67–83.

Cook, R.D. (1986) Assessment of local influence. *Journal of the Royal Statistical Society, Series B*, **48**, 133–169.

Cook, R.D. and Weisberg, S. (1982) *Residuals and Influence in Regression*. London: Chapman & Hall.

Cox, D.R. (1972) The analysis of multivariate binary data. *Applied Statistics*, **21**, 113–120.

Cox, N.R. (1974) Estimation of the correlation between a continuous and a discrete variable. *Biometrics*, **30**, 171–178.

Cox, D.R. and Reid, N. (1987) On the stability of maximum-likelihood estimators of orthogonal parameters. *Canadian Journal of Statistics*, **49**, 1–39.

Cox, D.R. and Wermuth, N. (1992) Response models for mixed binary and quantitative variables. *Biometrika*, **79**, 441–461.

Cox, D.R. and Wermuth, N. (1994) A note on the quadratic exponential binary distribution. *Biometrika*, **81**, 403–408.

Cox, D.R. and Wermuth, N. (1994) *Multivariate Dependencies: Models, Analysis and Interpretation*. London: Chapman & Hall.

Cressie, N.A.C. (1991) *Statistics for Spatial Data*. New York: John Wiley & Sons.

Crowder, M. (1995) On the use of a working correlation matrix in using generalized linear models for repeated measurements. *Biometrika*, **82**, 407–410.

Csiszar, I. (1975) I-divergence geometry of probability distributions and minimisation problems. *Annals of Probability*, 3, 146–158.

Cytel Software Corporation (2000) *EGRET for Windows, User Manual*.

Dale, J.R. (1984) Local versus global association for bivariate ordered responses. *Biometrika*, **71**, 507–514.

Dale, J.R. (1986) Global cross-ratio models for bivariate, discrete, ordered responses. *Biometrics*, **42**, 721–727.

Davidian, M. and Giltinan, D.M. (1995) *Nonlinear Models for Repeated Measurement Data*. London: Chapman & Hall.

Davidian, M., Tsiatis, A.A., and Leon, S. (2005) Semiparametric estimation of treatment effect in a pretest-posttest study with missing data. *Statistical Science*, **00**, 000–000.

Davies, R.B. (2002) Hypothesis testing when a nuisance parameter is present only under the alternative: linear model case. *Biometrika*, **89**, 484–489.

De Boeck, P. and Wilson, M. (editors) (2004) *Explanatory item response models: A generalized linear and nonlinear approach*, New-York: Springer, statistics for social science and public policy edition.

De Backer, M., De Keyser, P., De Vroey, C., and Lesaffre, E. (1996) A 12-week treatment for dermatophyte toe onychomycosis: terbinafine 250mg/day vs. itraconazole 200mg/day–a double-blind comparative trial. *British Journal of Dermatology*, **134**, 16–17.

Declerck, L., Aerts, M., and Molenberghs, G. (1998) Behaviour of the likelihood ratio test statistic under a Bahadur model for exchangeable binary data. *Journal of Statistical Computations and Simulations*, **61**, 15–38.

DeGruttola, V., Lange, N., and Dafni, U. (1991) Modeling the progression of HIV infection. *Journal of the American Statistical Association*, **86**, 569–577.

DeGruttola, V. and Tu, X.M. (1994) Modelling progression of CD4 lymphocyte count and its relationship to survival time. *Biometrics*, **50**, 1003–1014.

Dempster, A.P., Laird, N.M., and Rubin, D. B. (1977) Maximum likelihood from incomplete data via the EM algorithm (with discussion). *Journal of the Royal Statistical Society, Series B*, **39**, 1–38.

Dempster, A.P. and Rubin, D.B. (1983) Overview. In: *Incomplete Data in Sample Surveys, Vol. II: Theory and Annotated Bibliography*, W.G. Madow, I. Olkin, and D.B. Rubin (Eds.). New York: Academic Press, pp. 3–10.

Dennis, J.E. and Schnabel, R.B. (1983) *Numerical methods for unconstrained optimization and nonlinear equations*. Englewood Cliffs: Prentice-Hall.

Diggle, P.J. (1983) *Statistical Analysis of Spatial Point Patterns*. Mathematics in Biology. London: Academic Press.

Diggle, P.J., Heagerty, P.J., Liang, K.-Y., and Zeger, S.L. (2002) *Analysis of Longitudinal Data (2nd ed.)*. Oxford Science Publications. Oxford: Clarendon Press.

Diggle, P.J. and Kenward, M.G. (1994) Informative drop-out in longitudinal data analysis (with discussion). *Applied Statistics*, **43**, 49–93.

Diggle, P.J., Liang, K.-Y., and Zeger, S.L. (1994) *Analysis of Longitudinal Data*. Oxford Science Publications. Oxford: Clarendon Press.

Dmitrienko, A., Offen, W.W., Faries, D., Christy Chuang-Stein, J.L., and Molenberghs, G. (2005). *Analysis of Clinical Trial Data Using the SAS System*. Cary, NC: Sas Publishing.

Draper, D. (1995) Assessment and propagation of model uncertainty (with discussion). *Journal of the Royal Statistical Society, Series B*, **57**, 45–97.

Drum M. and McCullagh P. (1993). Comment to Fitzmaurice, G. M., Laird, N. M., and Rotnitzky A. Regression models for discrete longitudinal responses. *Statistical Science*, **8** 300–301.

Ekholm, A., McDonald, J.W., and Smith, P.W.F. (2000) Association models for a multivariate binary response. *Biometrics*, **56**, 712–718.

Ekholm, A. and Skinner, C. (1998) The muscatine children's obesity data reanalysed using pattern mixture models. *Applied Statistics*, **47**, 251–263.

Ekholm, A., Smith, P.W.F., and McDonald, J.W. (1995) Marginal regression analysis of a multivariate binary response. *Biometrika*, **82**, 847–854.

Faes, C., Aerts, M., Geys, H., Molenberghs, G., Declerck, L. (2004) Bayesian testing for trend in a power model for clustered binary data. *Environmental and Ecological Statistics*, **11**, 305–322.

Fahrmeir, L. and Tutz, G. (1994) *Multivariate Statistical Modelling Based on Generalized Linear Models*. Heidelberg: Springer-Verlag.

Fahrmeir, L. and Tutz, G. (2001) *Multivariate statistical modelling based on Generalized Linear Models (2nd ed.)*. Springer Series in Statistics, Springer-Verlag, New York.

Faught, E., Wilder, B.J., Ramsay, R.E., Reife, R.A., Kramer, L.D., Pledger, G.W., and Karim, R.M. (1996) Topiramate placebo-controlled dose-ranging trial in refractory partial epilepsy using 200-, 400-, and 600-mg daily dosages, *Neurology*, **46**, 1684–1690.

Fay, R.E. (1986) Causal models for patterns of nonresponse. *Journal of the American Statistical Association*, **81**, 354–365.

Feller, W. (1968) *An Introduction to Probability Theory and Its Applications* (3rd ed). New York: John Wiley.

Fieuws, S., Spiessens, B., and Draney, K. (2004) Mixture models, in P. De Boeck and M. Wilson, editors, *Explanatory item response models: A generalized linear and nonlinear approach*, Statistics for Social Science and Public Policy, chapter 11, 317–340, Springer-Verlag, New York.

Fieuws, S. and Verbeke, G. (2004) Joint modelling of multivariate longitudinal profiles: Pitfalls of the random-effects approach, *Statistics in Medicine*, **23**, 3093–3104.

Fieuws, S. and Verbeke, G. (2005a) Pairwise fitting of generalized linear mixed models for multidimensional repeated discrete responses, *Submitted for publication*.

Fieuws, S. and Verbeke, G. (2005b) Pairwise fitting of mixed models for the joint modelling of multivariate longitudinal profiles, *Submitted for publication*.

Fieuws, S., Verbeke, G., and Brant, L.J. (2005) Classification of longitudinal profiles using nonlinear mixed-effects models, *Submitted for publication*.

Fitzmaurice, G.M. and Laird, N.M. (1993) A Likelihood-based method for analysing longitudinal binary responses. *Biometrika*, **80**, 141–151.

Fitzmaurice, G.M. and Laird, N.M. (1995) Regression models for a bivariate discrete and continuous outcome with clustering. *Journal of the American Statistical Association*, **90**, 845–852.

Fitzmaurice, G.M., Laird, N.M., and Rotnitzky, A. (1993) Regression models for discrete longitudinal responses. *Statistical Science*, **8**, 284–309.

Fitzmaurice, G.M., Laird, N.M., and Tosteson, T.D. (1996) Polynomial exponential models for clustered binary outcomes. *Technical report*.

Fitzmaurice, G.M., Laird, N.M., and Ware, J.H. (2004) *Applied Longitudinal Analysis*. New York: John Wiley & Sons.

Fitzmaurice, G.M. and Lipsitz, S.R. (1995) A model for binary time series data with serial oods ratio patterns. *Applied Statistics*, **44**, 51–61.

Fitzmaurice, G.M., Molenberghs, G., and Lipsitz, S.R. (1995) Regression models for longitudinal binary responses with informative dropouts. *Journal of the Royal Statistical Society, Series B*, **57**, 691–704.

Folk, V.G. and Green, B.F. (1989) Adaptive estimation when the unidimensionality assumption of irt is violated, *Applied Psychological Measurement*, **13**, 373–389.

Foster, J.J. and Smith, P.W.F. (1998) Model-based inference for categorical survey data subject to non-ignorable non-response. *Journal of the Royal Statistical Society, Series B*, **60**, 57–70.

Foulley, J.-L. and Gianola, D. (1996) Statistical analysis of ordered categorical data via a structural heteroskedastic threshold model. *Genetics Selection Evolution*, **28**, 249–273.

Fréchet, M. (1951) Sur les tableaux de corrélation dont les marges sont données. Annals Université Lyon, Section A, Series 3, **14**, 53–77.

Friedman, J.H., Bentley, J.L., and Finkel, R.A. (1977) An algorithm for finding best matches in logarithmic expected time. *ACM Transactions on Mathematical Software*, **3**, 209–226.

Gamerman, D. (1997) Efficient sampling from the posterior distribution in generalized linear mixed models, *Statistics and Computing*, **7**, 57–68.

Gelman, A., Carlin, J.B., Stern, H.S., and Rubin, D.B. (1995) *Bayesian Data Analysis*, Texts in Statistical Science. London: Chapman & Hall.

Gelman, A. and Speed, T.P. (1993) Characterizing a joint probability distribution by conditionals. *Journal of the Royal Statistical Society - Series B*, **55**, 185–188.

Geyer, C.J. and Thompson, E.A. (1992) Constrained Monte Carlo maximum likelihood for dependent data (with discussion). *Journal of the Royal Statistical Society, Series B*, **69**, 657–699.

Geys, H., Molenberghs, G., and Lipsitz, S.R. (1998) A note on the comparison of pseudo-likelihood and generalized estimating equations for marginal odds ratio models. *Journal of Statistical Computation and Simulation*, **62**, 45–72.

Geys, H., Molenberghs, G., and Ryan, L.M. (1997) Pseudo-likelihood inference for clustered binary data. *Communications in Statistics: Theory and Methods*, **26**, 2743–2767.

Geys, H., Molenberghs, G., and Ryan, L. (1999) Pseudolikelihood modeling of multivariate outcomes in developmental toxicology. *Journal of the American Statistical Association*, **94**, 734–745.

Geys, H., Regan, M.M., Catalano, P.J., and Molenberghs, G. (2001) Two latent variable risk assessment approaches for mixed continuous and discrete outcomes from developmental toxicity data. *Journal of Agricultural, Biological and Environmental Statistics*, **6**, 340–355.

Ghosh, J.K. and Sen, P.K. (1985) On the asymptotic performance of the log likelihood ratio statistic for the mixture model and related results. In: *Proceedings of the Berekely Conference in Honor or Jerzy Neyman and Jack Kiefer*, Vol. 2, L.M. Le Cam and R.A. Olshen (Eds.). Monterey: Wadsworth, Inc., pp. 789–806.

Glonek, G.F.V. and McCullagh, P. (1995) Multivariate logistic models. *Journal of the Royal Statistical Society, Series B*, **81**, 477–482.

Glynn, R.J., Laird, N.M., and Rubin, D.B. (1986) Selection modelling versus mixture modelling with non-ignorable nonresponse. In: *Drawing Inferences from Self Selected Samples*, H. Wainer (Ed.). New York: Springer-Verlag, pp. 115–142.

Glynn, R.J., Laird, N.M. and Rubin, D.B. (1993) Multiple Imputation in Mixture Models for Nonignorable Nonresponse With Follow-ups. *Journal of the American Statistical Association*, **88**, 984–993.

Goldstein, H. (1991) Nonlinear multilevel models with an application to discrete response data, *Biometrika*, **78**, 45–51.

Goldstein, H. (1995) *Multilevel Statistical Models*. Kendall's Libary of Statistics 3. London: Arnold.

Goldstein, H., Healy, M.J.R., and Rasbash, J. (1994) Multilevel time series models with applications to repeated measures data. *Statistics in Medicine*, **13**, 1643–1655.

Goldstein, H. and Rasbash, J. (1996) Improved approximations for multilevel models with binary responses. *Journal of the Royal Statistical Society, Series A*, **159**, 505–513.

Goldstein, H., Rasbash, J., Plewis, I., Draper, D., Browne, W., Yang, M. et al (1998). *A User's Guide to MLwiN*. London: Institute of Education.

Goodman, L.A. (1969) How to ransack social mobility tables and other kinds of cross-classification tables. *American Journal of Sociology*, **75**, 1–39.

Goodman, L.A. (1979) Simple models for the analysis of association in cross-classifications having ordered categories. *Journal of the American Statistical Association*, **74**, 537–552.

Goodman, L.A. (1981a) Association models and canonical correlation in the analysis of cross-classifications having ordered categories. *Journal of the American Statistical Association*, **76**, 320–334.

Goodman, L.A. (1981b) Association models and the bivariate normal for contingency tables with ordered categories. *Biometrika*, **68** (1981b), 347–355.

Goodman, L.A. (1985) The 1983 Henry L. Rietz memorial lecture. The analysis of cross-classified data having ordered and/or unordered categories: association models, correlation models, and asymmetry models for contingency tables with or without missing entries. *Annals of Statistics*, **13**, 10–69.

Grizzle, J.E., Starmer, C.F., and Koch, G.G. (1969) Analysis of categorical data by linear models. *Biometrics*, 25, 189–195.

Gueorguieva, R. (2001) A multivariate generalized linear mixed model for joint modelling of clustered outcomes in the exponential family, *Statistical Modelling*, **1**(3) 177–193.

Haber, F. (1924) Zur Geschichte des Gaskrieges (On the history of gas warfare). In: *Funf Vortrage aus den Jahren 1920-1923 (Five Lectures from the Years 1920-1923)*, Berlin: Springer-Verlag, pp. 76–92.

Hall, D.B. and Præstgaard, J.T. (2001) Order-restricted score tests for homogeneity in generalised linear and nonlinear mixed models. *Biometrika* **88**, 739–751.

Hannan, J.F. and Tate, R.F. (1965) Estimation of the parameters for a multivariate normal distribution when one variable is dichotomized. *Biometrika*, **52**, 664–668.

Hartley, H.O. and Hocking, R. (1971) The analysis of incomplete data. *Biometrics*, **27**, 7783–808.

Harville, D.A. (1974) Bayesian inference for variance components using only error contrasts. *Biometrika*, **61**, 383–385.

Heagerty, P.J. and Lele, S.R. (1998) A composite likelihood approach to binary spatial data. *Journal of the American Statistical Association*, **93**, 1099–1111.

Heagerty, P.J. and Zeger, S.L. (1996) Marginal regression models for clustered ordinal measurements. *Journal of the American Statistical Association*, **91**, 1024–1036.

Heagerty, P.J. and Zeger, S.L. (2000) Marginalized multilevel models and likelihood inference, *Statistical Science*, **15**(1) 1–26.

Heckman, J.J. (1976) The common structure of statistical models of truncation, sample selection and limited dependent variables and a simple estimator for such models. *Annals of Economic and Social Measurement*, **5**, 475–492.

Hedeker, D. and Gibbons, R.D. (1993) *MIXOR: a Computer Program for Mixed Effects Ordinal Probit and Logistic Regression.* Chicago: University of Illinois.

Hedeker, D. and Gibbons, R.D. (1994) A random-effects ordinal regression model for multilevel analysis. *Biometrics*, **50**, 933–944.

Hedeker, D. and Gibbons, R.D. (1996) MIXOR: A computer program for mixed-effects ordinal regression analysis. *Computer Methods and Programs in Biomedicine*, **49**, 157–176.

Hedeker, D. and Gibbons, R.D. (1997) Application of random-effects pattern-mixture models for missing data in longitudinal studies. *Psychological Methods*, **2**, 64–78.

Heitjan, D.F. and Rubin, D.B. (1991) Ignorability and coarse data. *The Annals of Statistics*, **19**, 2244–2253.

Henderson, C.R. (1984) *Applications of Linear Models in Animal Breeding.* Guelph, Canada: University of Guelph Press.

Hens, N., Aerts, M., Molenberghs, G., Thijs, H., and Verbeke, G. (2005) Kernel weighted influence measures. *Computational Statistics and Data Analysis*, **48**, 467–487.

Heyting, A., Tolboom, J.T.B.M., and Essers, J.G.A. (1992) Statistical handling of drop-outs in longitudinal clinical trials. *Statistics in Medicine*, **11**, 2043–2061.

Hobert, J.P. and Casella, G. (1996) The effect of improper priors on gibbs sampling in hierarchical linear mixed models, *Journal of the American Statistical Association*, **91**, 1461–1473.

Hogan, J.W. and Laird, N.M. (1997) Mixture models for the joint distribution of repeated measures and event times. *Statistics in Medicine*, **16**, 239–258.

Holland, P.W. (1986) A Comment on Remarks by Rubin and Hartigan. In H. Wainer (Ed.), *Drawing Inferences from Self-Selected Samples* (pp. 149–151). New York: Springer.

Holmes, L.B. (1988) Human teratogens: delineating the phenotypic effects, the period of greatest sensitivity, and the dose-response relationship and mechanisms of action. In: *Transplacental Effects on Fetal Health.* New York: Alan R. Liss, Inc., pp. 171–191.

Jaffrézic, F., Robert-Granié, C., and Foulley, J.-L. (1999) A quasi-score approach to the analysis of ordered categorical data via a mixed heteroskedastic threshold model. *Genetics Selection Evolution*, **31**, 301–318.

Jansen, I. and Molenberghs, G. (2005) A flexible marginal modeling strategy for non-monotone missing data. *Submitted for publication*.

Jansen, I., Molenberghs, G., Aerts, M., Thijs, H., and Van Steen, K. (2003) A Local influence approach applied to binary data from a psychiatric study. *Biometrics*, **59**, 410–419.

Jansen, I., Hens, N., Molenberghs, G., Aerts, M., Verbeke, G., and Kenward, M.G. (2005) The nature of sensitivity in missing not at random models. *Computational Statistics and Data Analysis*, **00**, 000–000.

Johnson, R.A. and Wichern, D.W. (1992) *Applied Multivariate Statistical Analysis* (3rd ed.). Englewood Cliffs, NJ: Prentice-Hall.

Jones, B. and Kenward, M.G. (1989) *The Analysis of Cross-Over Studies*. London: Chapman & Hall.

Kauermann, G. (1993) Notes on multivariate logistic models for contingency tables. *Technical Report: Forschungsberichte der Fachbereich Informatik*. Technical University Berlin.

Kay, S.R., Opler, L.A., and Lindenmayer, J.-P. (1988) Reliability and validity of the Positive and Negative Syndrome Scale for schizophrenia. *Psychiatric Research*, **23**, 99–110.

Kenward, M.G. (1998) Selection models for repeated measurements with nonrandom dropout: an illustration of sensitivity. *Statistics in Medicine*, **17**, 2723–2732.

Kenward, M.G, Goetghebeur, E.J.T., and Molenberghs, G. (2001) Sensitivity analysis of incomplete categorical data. *Statistical Modelling*, **1**, 31–48.

Kenward, M.G. and Jones, B. (1991) The analysis of categorical data from cross-over trials using a latent variable model. *Statistics in Medicine*, **10**, 1607–1619.

Kenward, M.G., Lesaffre, E., and Molenberghs, G. (1994) An application of maximum likelihood and generalized estimating equations to the analysis of ordinal data from a longitudinal study with cases missing at random. *Biometrics*, **50**, 945–953.

Kenward, M.G. and Molenberghs, G. (1998) Likelihood based frequentist inference when data are missing at random. *Statistical Science*, **12**, 236–247.

Kenward, M.G. and Molenberghs, G. (1999) Parametric models for incomplete continuous and categorical longitudinal studies data. *Statistical Methods in Medical Research*, **8**, 51–83.

Kenward, M.G., Molenberghs, G. and Lesaffre, E. (1994) An application of maximum likelihood and estimating equations to the analysis of ordinal data from a longitudinal study with cases missing at random. *Biometrics*, **50**, 945–953.

Kenward, M.G., Molenberghs, G., and Thijs, H. (2003) Pattern-mixture models with proper time dependence. *Biometrika*, **90**, 53–71.

Kesteloot, H., Geboers, J., and Joossens, J.V. (1989) On the within-population relationship between nutrition and serum lipids, the birnh study. *European Heart Journal*, **10**, 196–202.

Khoury, M.J., Adams, M.M., Rhodes, P., and Erickson, J.D. (1987) Monitoring multiple malformations in the detection of epidemics of birth defects. *Teratology*, **36**, 345–354.

Kiefer, J. and Wolfowitz, J. (1956) Consistency of the maximum likelihood estimator in the presence of infinitely many incidental parameters, *The Annals of Mathematical Statistics*, **27**, 887–906.

Kimmel, G.L., Cuff, J.M., Kimmel, C.A., Heredia, D.J., Tudor, N., and Silverman, P.M. (1993) Embryonic development in vitro following short-duration exposure to heat. *Teratology*, **47**, 243–251.

Kimmel, G.L., Williams, P.L., Kimmel, C.A., Claggett, T.W., and Tudor, N. (1994) The effects of temperature and duration of exposure on in vitro development and response-surface modelling of their interaction. *Teratology*, **49**, 366–367.

Kleinman, J. (1973) Proportions with extraneous variance: single and independent samples, *Journal of the American Statistical Association*, **68**, 46–54.

Kreft, I. and de Leeuw, J. (1998) *Introducing Multilevel Modeling*. London: Sage Publications.

Krzanowski, W.J. (1988) *Principles of Multivariate Analysis*. Oxford: Clarendon Press.

Kuk, A.Y.C. (1995) Asymptotically unbiased estimation in generalised linear models with random effects, *Journal of the Royal Statistical Society, Series B*, **57**, 395–407.

Kupper, L.L. and Haseman, J.K. (1978) The use of a correlated binomial model for the analysis of certain toxicology experiments., *Biometrics*, **34**, 69–76.

Kwan, K.C., Breault, G.O., Umbenhauer, E.R., McMahon, F.G., and Duggan, D.E. (1976) Kinetics of indomethacin absorption, eliminaton, and enterohepatic circulation in man. *Journal of Pharmacokinetics and Biopharmaceutics*, **4**, 255–280.

Laenen, A., Vangeneugden, T., Geys, H., and Molenberghs, G. (2004) Generalized reliability estimation using repeated measurements. *Submitted for publication.*

Laird, N.M. (1978) Nonparametric maximum likelihood estimation of a mixing distribution. *Journal of the American Statistical Association*, **73**, 805–811.

Laird, N.M. (1994) Discussion to Diggle, P.J. and Kenward, M.G.: Informative dropout in longitudinal data analysis. *Applied Statistics*, **43**, 84.

Laird, N.M. and Ware, J.H. (1982) Random effects models for longitudinal data. *Biometrics*, **38**, 963–974.

Lang, J.B. and Agresti, A. (1994) Simultaneously modeling joint and marginal distributions of multivariate categorical responses. *Journal of the American Statistical Association*, **89**, 625–632.

Lange, K. (1999) *Numerical analysis for statisticians.* New York: Springer-Verlag.

Lapp, K., Molenberghs, G., and Lesaffre, E. (1998) Local and global cross ratios to model the association between ordinal variables. *Computational Statistics and Data Analysis*, **28**, 387–411.

Lavori, P.W., Dawson, R., and Shera, D. (1995) A multiple imputation strategy for clinical trials with truncation of patient data. *Statistics in Medicine*, **14**, 1913–1925.

Le Cessie, S. and Van Houwelingen, J.C. (1994) Logistic regression for correlated binary data. *Applied Statistics*, **43**, 95–108.

Lee, Y. and Nelder, J.A. (1996) Hierarchical generalized linear models (with discussion). *Journal of the Royal Statistical Society, Series B*, **58**, 619–678.

Lee, Y. and Nelder, J.A. (2001) Hierarchical generalized linear models: a synthesis of generalized linear models, random-effect models and structured dispersions. *Biometrika*, **88**, 987–1006.

Lee, Y., and Nelder, J.A. (2003) Extended-REML estimators. *Journal of Applied Statistics*, **30**, 845–856.

Lefkopoulou, M. and Ryan, L. (1993) Global tests for multiple binary outcomes. *Biometrics*, **49**, 975–988.

Lesaffre, E. and Molenberghs, G. (1991) Multivariate Probit Analysis: A Neglected Procedure in Medical Statistics. *Statistics in Medicine*, **10**, 1391–1403.

Lesaffre, E. and Verbeke, G. (1998) Local influence in linear mixed models. *Biometrics*, **54**, 570–582.

Lesaffre, E., Verbeke, G., and Molenberghs, G. (1994) A sensitivity analysis of two multivariate response models. *Computational Statistics and Data Analysis*, **17**, 363–391.

Li, K.H., Raghunathan, T.E., and Rubin, D.B. (1991) Large-sample significance levels from multiply imputed data using moment-based statistics and an F reference distributions. *Journal of the American Statistical Association*, **86**, 1065–1073.

Liang, K.Y. and and Self, S. (1996) On the asymptotic behavior of the pseudolikelihood ratio test statistic. *Journal of the Royal Statistical Society, Series B*, **58**, 785–796.

Liang, K.-Y. and Zeger, S.L. (1986) Longitudinal data analysis using generalized linear models. *Biometrika*, **73**, 13–22.

Liang, K.–Y., Zeger, S.L., and Qaqish, B. (1992) Multivariate regression analyses for categorical data. *Journal of the Royal Statistical Society, Series B*, **54**, 3–40.

Lin, X. and Breslow, N.E. (1996) Bias correction in generalized linear mixed models with multiple components of dispersion, *Journal of the American Statistical Association*, **91**, 1007–1016.

Lindley, D.V. and Smith, A.F.M. (1972) Bayes estimates for the linear model. *Journal of the Royal Statistical Society, Series B*, **34**, 1–41.

Lindsay, B.G. (1983a) Efficiency of the conditional score in a mixture setting, *The Annals of Statistics*, **11**, 486–497.

Lindsay, B.G. (1983b) The geometry of mixture likelihoods, part I : A general theory, *The Annals of Statistics*, **11**, 86–94.

Lindsay, B.G. (1983c) The geometry of mixture likelihoods, part II : The exponential family, *The Annals of Statistics*, **11**, 783–792.

Lindsay, B.G. (1988) Composite likelihood methods. *Contemporary Mathematics*, **80**, 221–239.

Lindsay, B.G., Clogg, C.C., and Grego, J. (1991) Semiparametric estimation in the Rasch model and related exponential response models, including a simple latent class model for item analysis, *Journal of the American Statistical Association*, **86**, 96–107.

Lipsitz, S.R., Laird, N.M., and Harrington, D.P. (1991) Generalized estimating equations for correlated binary data: using the odds ratio as a measure of association. *Biometrika*, **78**, 153–160.

Lipsitz, S., Parzen, M., Molenberghs, G., and Ibrahim, J. (2001) Testing for bias in weighted estimating equations, *Biostatistics*, **2**, 295–308.

Lipsitz, S.R., Zhao, L.P., and Molenberghs, G. (1998) A semi-parametric method of multiple imputation. *Journal of the Royal Statistical Society, Series B*, **60**, 127–144.

Litière S., Alonso, A., Molenberghs, G., and Geys, H. (2005) Impact of misspecified random-effects distribution on maximum likelihood estimation in generalized linear mixed models. *Submitted for publication.*

Little, R.J.A. (1993) Pattern-mixture models for multivariate incomplete data. *Journal of the American Statistical Association*, **88**, 125–134.

Little, R.J.A. (1994a) A class of pattern-mixture models for normal incomplete data. *Biometrika*, **81**, 471–483.

Little, R.J.A. (1994b) Discussion to Diggle, P.J. and Kenward, M.G.: Informative dropout in longitudinal data analysis. *Applied Statistics*, **43**, 78.

Little, R.J.A. (1995) Modeling the drop-out mechanism in repeated measures studies. *Journal of the American Statistical Association*, **90**, 1112–1121.

Little, R.J.A. and Rubin, D.B. (1987) *Statistical Analysis with Missing Data*. New York: John Wiley & Sons.

Little, R.J.A. and Rubin, D.B. (2002) *Statistical Analysis with Missing Data* (2nd ed.). New York: John Wiley & Sons.

Little, R.J.A. and Schluchter, M.D. (1985) Maximum likelihood estimation for mixed continuous and categorical data with missing values. *Biometrika*, **72**, 497–512.

Little, R.J.A. and Wang, Y. (1996) Pattern-mixture models for multivariate incomplete data with covariates. *Biometrics*, **52**, 98–111.

Longford, N.T. (1993) *Random Coefficient Models*. Oxford: Oxford University Press.

Louis, T.A. (1982) Finding the observed information matrix when using the EM algorithm. *Journal of the Royal Statistical Society, Series B*, **44**, 226-233.

MacCallum, R., Kim, C., Malarkey, W., and Kiecolt-Glaser, J. (1997) Studying multivariate change using multilevel models and latent curve models, *Multivariate Behavioral Research*, **32**, 215–253.

Magder, L.S. and Zeger, S.L. (1996) A smooth nonparametric estimated of a mixing distribution using mixtures of Gaussians. *Journal of the American Statistical Association*, **91**, 1141–1152.

Mallinckrodt, C.H., Clark, W.S., and Stacy R.D. (2001a) Type I error rates from mixed-effects model repeated measures versus fixed effects analysis of variance with missing values imputed via last observation carried forward. *Drug Information Journal*, **35**, 4, 1215–1225.

Mallinckrodt, C.H., Clark, W.S., and Stacy R.D. (2001b) Accounting for dropout bias using mixed-effects models. *Journal of Biopharmaceutical Statistics*, **11**, (1 & 2), 9–21.

Mallinckrodt, C.H., Carroll, R.J., Debrota, D.J., Dube, S., Molenberghs, G., Potter, W.Z., Sanger, T.D., and Tollefson, G.D. (2003) Assessing and interpreting treatment effects in longitudinal clinical trials with subject dropout. *Biological Psychiatry*, **53**, 754–760.

Mallinckrodt, C.H., Scott Clark, W., Carroll, R.J., and Molenberghs, G. (2003) Assessing response profiles from incomplete longitudinal clinical trial data with subject dropout under regulatory conditions. *Journal of Biopharmaceutical Statistics*, **13**, 179–190.

Mardia, K.V. (1970). *Families of Bivariate Distributions*. London: Griffin.

McArdle, J.J. and Hamagami, F. (1992) Modeling incomplete longitudinal and cross-sectional data using latent growth structural models. *Experimental Aging Research*, **18**, 145–166.

McCullagh, P. (1987) *Tensor Methods in Statistics*. London: Chapman & Hall.

McCullagh, P. and Nelder, J.A. (1989) *Generalized Linear Models*. London: Chapman & Hall.

McCulloch, C.E. (1994) Maximum likelihood variance components estimation for binary data. *Journal of the American Statistical Association*, **89**, 330–335.

McCulloch, C.E. (1997) Maximum likelihood algorithms for generalized linear mixed models. *Journal of the American Statistical Association*, **92**, 162–170.

McLachlan, G.J. and Basford, K.E. (1988) *Mixture models. Inference and Applications to Clustering.* New York: Marcel Dekker.

McLachlan, G.J. and Krishnan, T. (1997) *The EM Algorithm and Extensions.* New York: John Wiley & Sons.

McLachlan, G.J. and Peel, D. (2000) *Finite mixture models.* New York: John Wiley & Sons.

Meilijson, I. (1989) A fast improvement to the EM algorithm on its own terms. *Journal of the Royal Statistical Society, Series B,* **51**, 127–138.

Meng, X.-L. and Rubin, D.B. (1991) Using EM to obtain asymptotic variance covariance matrices: the SEM algorithm. *Journal of the American Statistical Association,* **86**, 899–909.

Michiels, B. and Molenberghs, G. (1997) Protective Estimation of Longitudinal Categorical Data with Nonrandom Dropout. *Communications in Statistics,* **26**, 65–94.

Michiels, B., Molenberghs, G., Bijnens, L., and Vangeneugden, T. (2002) Selection models and pattern-mixture models to analyze longitudinal quality of life data subject to dropout. *Statistics in Medicine,* **21**, 1023–1041.

Michiels, B., Molenberghs, G., and Lipsitz, S.R. (1999). Selection models and pattern-mixture models for incomplete categorical data with covariates. *Biometrics,* **55**, 978–983.

Minini, P. and Chavance, M. (2004a) Observations longitudinales incomplètes : de la modélisation des observations disponibles à l'analyse de sensibilité. *Journal de la Société française de Statistique,* **145**, 000–000.

Minini, P. and Chavance, M. (2004b) Sensitivity analysis of longitudinal binary data with non-monotone missing values. *Biostatistics,* **5**, 531–544.

Molenberghs, G., Beunckens, C., Jansen, I., Thijs. H., Van Steen, K., Verbeke, G., and Kenward, M.G. (2005) The Analysis of Incomplete Data, In: *Pharmaceutical Statistics With SAS.* Chuang-Stein, C. and D'Agostino, R. (Eds). Cary, NC: SAS Publishing.

Molenberghs, G. and Danielson, L. (1999) Simple methods for the analysis of multivariate and longitudinal categorical data. In: *Proceedings of the 7th International Conference on Probability Theory and Mathematical Statistics and Vilnius Conference (1998),* B. Grigelionis et al (Eds.), TEV, Vilnius/VSP, Utrecht, pp. 499–514.

Molenberghs, G., Geys, H., and Buyse, M. (2001) Evaluation of surrogate endpoints in randomized experiments with mixed discrete and continuous outcomes. *Statistics in Medicine*, **20**, 3023–3038.

Molenberghs, G. and Goetghebeur, E. (1997) Simple fitting algorithms for incomplete categorical data. *Journal of the Royal Statistical Society, Series B*, **59**, 401–414.

Molenberghs, G., Goetghebeur, E.J.T., Lipsitz, S.R., Kenward, M.G. (1999) Non-random missingness in categorical data: strengths and limitations. *The American Statistician*, **53**, 110–118.

Molenberghs, G., Kenward, M.G., and Goetghebeur, E. (2001) Sensitivity analysis for incomplete contingency tables: the Slovenian plebiscite case. *Applied Statistics*, **50**, 15–29.

Molenberghs, G., Kenward, M. G., and Lesaffre, E. (1997) The analysis of longitudinal ordinal data with non-random dropout. *Biometrika*, **84**, 33–44.

Molenberghs, G. and Lesaffre, E. (1994) Marginal modelling of correlated ordinal data using a multivariate Plackett distribution. *Journal of the American Statistical Association*, **89**, 633–644.

Molenberghs, G. and Lesaffre, E. (1999) Marginal modelling of multivariate categorical data. *Statistics in Medicine*, **18**, 2237–2255.

Molenberghs, G., Michiels, B., and Kenward, M.G. (1998) Pseudo-likelihood for combined selection and pattern-mixture models for missing data problems. *Biometrical Journal*, **40**, 557–572.

Molenberghs, G., Michiels, B., Kenward, M.G., and Diggle, P.J. (1998) Missing data mechanisms and pattern-mixture models. *Statistica Neerlandica*, **52**, 153–161.

Molenberghs, G., Michiels, B., and Lipsitz, S.R. (1999) A pattern-mixture odds ratio model for incomplete categorical data. *Communications in Statistics: Theory and Methods*, **28**, 2843–2869.

Molenberghs, G. and Ritter, L. (1996) Likelihood and quasi-likelihood based methods for analysing multivariate categorical data, with the association between outcomes of interest. *Biometrics*, **52**, 1121–1133.

Molenberghs, G. and Ryan, L.M. (1999) Likelihood inference for clustered multivariate binary data. *Environmetrics*, **10**, 279–300.

Molenberghs, G., Thijs, H., Michiels, B., Verbeke, G., and Kenward, M.G. (2004) Pattern-mixture models. *Journal de la Société française de Statistique*, **145**, 49–77.

Molenberghs, G., Verbeke, G., Thijs, H., Lesaffre, E., and Kenward, M.G. (2001) Mastitis in dairy cattle: influence analysis to assess sensitivity of the dropout process. *Computational Statistics and Data Analysis*, **37**, 93–113.

Morimune, K. (1979) Comparison of normal and logistic models in the bivariate dichotomous analysis. *Econometrica*, **47**, 957–975.

Murray, G.D. and Findlay, J.G. (1988) Correcting for the bias caused by drop-outs in hypertension trials. *Statististics in Medicine*, **7**, 941-946.

Muthén, B., Kaplan, D., and Hollis, M. (1987) On structural equation modeling with data that are not missing completely at random. *Psychometrika*, **52**, 431–462.

Muthén, B. and Shedden, K. (1999) Finite mixture modeling with mixture outcomes using the EM-algorithm, *Biometrics*, **55**, 463–469.

Nelder, J.A. and Mead, R. (1965) A simplex method for function minimisation. *The Computer Journal*, **7**, 303–313.

Nelder, J.A. and Wedderburn, R.W.M. (1972) Generalized linear models. *Journal of the Royal Statistical Society, Series B*, **135**, 370–384.

Neuhaus, J.M. (1992) Statistical methods for longitudinal and clustered designs with binary responses. *Statistical Methods in Medical Research*, **1**, 249-273.

Neuhaus, J.M., Hauck, W.W., and Kalbfleisch, J.D. (1992) The effects of mixture distribution specification when fitting mixed-effects logistic models, *Biometrika*, **79**, 755–762.

Neuhaus, J.M., Kalbfleisch, J.D., and Hauck, W.W. (1991) A comparison of cluster-specific and population-averaged approaches for analyzing correlated binary data. *International Statistical Review*, **59**, 25–35.

Neyman, J. and Scott, E.L. (1948) Consistent estimates based on partially consistent observations, *Econometrica*, **16**, 1–32.

NIOSH (1983) U.S. Department of Health and Human Services, Public Health Service, Center for Disease Control, National Institute for Occupational Safety and Health (1983). *Current Intelligence Bulletin 39: Glycol Ethers 2-Methoxyethanol and 2-Ethoxyethanol.*

Nocedal, J. and Wright, S.J. (1999) *Numerical optimization.* New York: Springer-Verlag.

Nordheim, E.V. (1984) Inference from nonrandomly missing categorical data: an example from a genetic study on Turner's syndrome. *Journal of the American Statistical Association*, **79**, 772–780.

Ochi, Y. and Prentice, R.L. (1984) Likelihood inference in a correlated probit regression model. *Biometrika*, **71**, 531–543.

Olkin, I. and Tate, R.F. (1961) Multivariate correlation models with mixed discrete and continuous variables. *Annals of Mathematical Statistics*, **32**, 448–465 (with correction in **36**, 343–344).

Palmgren, J. (1989) *Regression models for bivariate responses*. Technical Report 101, Department of Biostatistics, Seattle, Washington.

Pearson, K. (1900) Mathematical contribution to the theory of evolution. vii. On the correlation of characters not quantitatively measurable. *Phil. Transactions Royal Society London A*, **195**, 1–47.

Park, T. and Lee, S.-L. (1999) Simple pattern-mixture models for longitudinal data with missing observations: analysis of urinary incontinence data. *Statistics in Medicine*, **18**, 2933–2941.

Pfeiffer, R.M., Hildesheim, A., Gail, M.H., Pee, D., Chen, C., Goldstein, A. M., and Diehl, S.R. (2003) Robustness of inference on measured covariates to misspecification of genetic random effects in family studies, *Genetic Epidemiology*, **24**, 14–23.

Pharmacological Therapy for Macular Degeneration Study Group (1997) Interferon α-IIA is ineffective for patients with choroidal neovascularization secondary to age-related macular degeneration. Results of a prospective randomized placebo-controlled clinical trial. *Archives of Ophthalmology*, **115**, 865–872.

Pinheiro, J.C. and Bates, D.M. (1995). Approximations to the log-likelihood function in the nonlinear mixed-effects model. *Journal of Computational and Graphical Statistics*, **4**, 12–35.

Pinheiro, J.C. and Bates, D.M. (2000) *Mixed effects models in S and S-Plus*. Springer-Verlag, New-York.

Plackett, R.L. (1965) A class of bivariate distributions. *Journal of the American Statistical Association*, **60**, 516–522.

Prentice, R.L. (1988) Correlated binary regression with covariates specific to each binary observation. *Biometrics*, **44**, 1033–1048.

Prentice, R.L. and Zhao, L.P. (1991) Estimating equations for parameters in means and covariances of multivariate discrete and continuous responses. *Biometrics*, **47**, 825–839.

Press, W.H., Teukolsky, S.A., Vetterling, W.T., and Flannery, B.P. (1992) *Numerical recipes in FORTRAN*, Cambridge University Press (second ed.).

Price, C.J., Kimmel, C.A., George, J.D., and Marr, M.C. (1987) The developmental toxicity of diethylene glycol dimethyl ether in mice. *Fundamental and Applied Toxicology*, **8**, 115–126.

Price, C. J., Kimmel, C. A., Tyl, R. W., and Marr, M. C. (1985) The developmental toxicity of ethylene glycol in mice. *Toxicology and Applied Pharmacology*, **81**, 113–127.

Rabe-Hesketh, S., Pickles, A., and Skrondal, A. (2001) Gllamm manual, Technical report, Department of Biostatistics and Computing, Institute of Psychiatry, King's College, University of London [Report # 2001/01].

Rao, C.R. (1973) *Linear Statistical Inference and Its Applications* (2nd ed.). New York: John Wiley & Sons.

Rao, J.N.K. and Scott, A.J. (1987) On simple adjustments to chi-square tests with sample survey data. *Annals of Statistics*, **15**, 385–397.

Raudenbush, S.W., Bryk, A.S., Cheong, Y.F., Fai, Y., and Congdon, R. (2001) *HLM5: Hierarchical linear and nonlinear modeling*, Lincolnwood, IL: Scientific Software International.

Raudenbush, S.W., Yang, M.L., and Yosef, M. (2000) Maximum likelihood for generalized linear models with nested random effects via high-order, multivariate laplace approximations, *Journal of Computational and Graphical Statistics*, **9**, 141–157.

Regan, M.M. and Catalano, P.J. (1999a) Likelihood models for clustered binary and continuous outcomes: Application to developmental toxicology. *Biometrics*, **55**, 760–768.

Regan, M.M. and Catalano, P.J. (1999b) Bivariate dose-response modeling and risk estimation in developmental toxicology. *Journal of Agricultural, Biological and Environmental Statistics*, **4**, 217–237.

Regan, M.M. and Catalano, P.J. (2000) Regression models for mixed discrete and continuous outcomes with clustering. *Risk Analysis*, **20**, 363–376.

Regan, M.M. and Catalano, P.J. (2002) Combined Continuous and Discrete Outcomes. In: *Topics in Modelling of Clustered Data*, Aerts, M., Geys, H., Molenberghs, G., and Ryan, L. (eds.), London: Chapman & Hall.

Renard, D., Geys, H., Molenberghs, G., Burzykowski, T., and Buyse, M. (2002) Validation of surrogate endpoints in multiple randomized clinical trials with discrete outcomes. *Biometrical Journal*, **44**, 921–935.

Renard, D., Molenberghs, G., and Geys, H. (2004) A pairwise likelihood approach to estimation in multilevel probit models. *Computational Statistics and Data Analysis*, **44**, 649–667.

Ripley, B.D. (1981) *Spatial Statistics*. New York: John Wiley & Sons.

Ripley, B.D. (1987) *Stochastic Simulation*. New York: John Wiley.

Roberts, D.T. (1992) Prevalence of dermatophyte onychomycosis in the United Kingdom : Results of an omnibus survey, *British Journal of Dermatology*, **126 Suppl. 39**, 23–27.

Roberts, J., Rao, J.N.K., and Kumar, S. (1987) Logistic regression analysis of sample survey data. *Biometrika*, **74**, 1–12.

Robins, J.M., Rotnitzky, A., and Scharfstein, D.O. (1998) Semiparametric regression for repeated outcomes with non-ignorable non-response. *Journal of the American Statistical Association*, **93**, 1321–1339.

Robins, J.M., Rotnitzky, A., and Zhao, L.P. (1995) Analysis of semiparametric regression models for repeated outcomes in the presence of missing data. *Journal of the American Statistical Association*, **90**, 106–121.

Rodríguez, G. and Goldman, N. (1995) An assessment of estimation procedures for multilevel models with binary responses. *Journal of the Royal Statistical Society, Series A*, **158**, 73–89.

Rosenbaum, P.R. and Rubin, D.B. (1983) The central role of the propensity score method in observational studies for causal effects. *Biometrika*, **70**, 41–55.

Rosner, B. (1984) Multivariate methods in ophtalmology with applications to other paired-data situations. *Biometrics*, **40**, 1025–1035.

Rotnitzky, A. and Jewell, N.P. (1990) Hypothesis testing of regression parameters in semiparametric generalized linear models for cluster correlated data. *Biometrika*, **77**, 485–497.

Rowe, V.K. (1963) Glycols. In: F.A. Patty (Ed.) *Industrial Hygiene and Toxicology*, New York: Wiley–Interscience, New York, Vol. 99, pp. 1497–1536.

Royston, P. and Altman, D.G. (1994) Regression using fractional polynomials of continuous covariates: parsimonious parametric modelling. *Applied Statistics*, **43**, 429–468.

Rubin, D.B. (1976) Inference and missing data. *Biometrika*, **63**, 581–592.

Rubin, D.B. (1977) Formalizing Subjective Notions About the Effect of Nonrespondents in Sample Surveys. *Journal of the American Statistical Association*, **72**, 538–543.

Rubin, D.B. (1978) Multiple imputations in sample surveys – a phenomenological Bayesian approach to nonresponse. In: *Imputation and Editing of Faulty or Missing Survey Data*. Washington, DC: U.S. Department of Commerce, pp. 1–23.

Rubin, D.B. (1987) *Multiple Imputation for Nonresponse in Surveys*. New York: John Wiley & Sons.

Rubin, D.B. (1994) Discussion to Diggle, P.J. and Kenward, M.G.: Informative dropout in longitudinal data analysis. *Applied Statistics*, **43**, 80–82.

Rubin, D.B. (1996) Multiple imputation after 18+ years. *Journal of the American Statistical Association*, **91**, 473–489.

Rubin, D.B. and Schenker, N. (1986) Multiple imputation for interval estimation from simple random samples with ignorable nonresponse. *Journal of the American Statistical Association*, **81**, 366–374.

Rubin, D.B., Stern H.S., and Vehovar V. (1995) Handling "don't know" survey responses: the case of the Slovenian plebiscite. *Journal of the American Statistical Association*, **90**, 822–828.

Ruppert, D., Wand, M.P., and Carroll, R.J. (2003) *Semiparametric Regression*. Cambridge: Cambridge Univeristy Press.

Sammel, M.D., Ryan, L.M., and Legler, J.M. (1997) Latent variable models for mixed discrete and continuous outcomes. *Journal of the Royal Statistical Society, Series B*, **59**, 667–678.

SAS Institute Inc. (1991) *SAS System for Linear Models* (3rd ed.). Cary, NC: SAS Institute Inc.

SAS Institute Inc. (1995) SAS/IML Software: Changes and Enhancements Through Release 6.11. SAS Institute Inc., Cary, NC.

SAS Institute Inc. (2004) *The GLIMMIX Procedure (Experimental)*. Cary, NC: SAS Institute Inc.

Satterthwaite, F.E. (1941) Synthesis of variance. *Psychometrika*, **6**, 309–316.

Schafer J.L. (1997) *Analysis of Incomplete Multivariate Data*. London: Chapman & Hall.

Scharfstein, D.O., Rotnitzky, A., and Robins, J.M. (1999) Adjusting for non-ignorable drop-out using semiparametric nonresponde models (with discussion). *Journal of the American Statistical Association*, **94**, 1096–1146.

Schwarz, G. (1978) Estimating the dimension of a model. *The Annals of Statistics*, **6**, 461–464.

Searle, S.R., Casella, G., and McCulloch, C.E. (1992) *Variance Components*. New York: John Wiley & Sons.

Seber, G.A.F. (1984) *Multivariate Observations*. New York: John Wiley & Sons.

Seber, G.A.F. and Wild, C.J. (2003) *Nonlinear Regression*. New York: John Wiley.

Self, S.G. and Liang, K.Y. (1987) Asymptotic properties of maximum likelihood estimators and likelihood ratio tests under nonstandard conditions. *Journal of the American Statistical Association*, **82**, 605–610.

Serroyen, J., Molenberghs, G., Verhoye, M., Van Meir, V., and Van der Linden, A. (2005) Dynamic manganese enhanced (DME) MRI signal intensity processing based on non-linear mixed modeling to study changes in neuronal activity. *Journal of Agricultural, Biological, and Environmental Statistics*, **10**, 000–000.

Severini, T.A. (2004) A modified likelihood ratio statistics for some non-regular models. *Biometrika*, **91**, 603–612.

Shah, A., Laird, N., and Schoenfeld, D. (1997) A random-effects model for multiple characteristics with possibly missing data, *Journal of the American Statistical Association*, **92**, 775–779.

Sheiner, L.B., Beal, S.L., and Dunne, A. (1997) Analysis of nonrandomly censored ordered categorical longitudinal data from analgesic trials. *Journal of the American Statistical Association*, **92**, 1235–1244.

Shervish, M. (1984) Multivariate normal probabilities with error bound. *Applied Statistics*, 33, 81–94.

Shih, W.J. and Quan, H. (1997) Testing for treatment differences with dropouts in clinical trials—a composite approach. *Statistics in Medicine*, **16**, 1225–1239.

Shiota, K., Chou, M.J., and Nishimura, H. (1980) Embryotoxic effects of di-2-ethylhexyl phthalate (DEHP) and di-n-butyl phthalate (DBP) in mice. *Environmental Research*, **22**, 245–253.

Siddiqui, O. and Ali, M.W. (1998) A comparison of the random-effects pattern-mixture model with last-observation-carried-forward (LOCF) analysis in longitudinal clinical trials with dropouts. *Journal of Biopharmaceutical Statistics*, **8**, 545–563.

Silvapulle, M.J. and Silvapulle, P. (1995) A score test against one-sided alternatives, *Journal of the American Statistical Association*, **90**, 342–349.

Skellam, J.G. (1948) A probability distribution derived from the binomial distribution by regarding the probability of success as variable between the sets of trials, *Journal of the Royal Statistical Society, Series B*, **10**, 257–261.

Skrondal, A. and Rabe-Hesketh, S. (2004) *Generalized latent variable modeling*. London: Chapman & Hall/CRC.

Smith, A.F.M. (1973) A general Bayesian linear model. *Journal of the Royal Statistical Society, Series B*, **35**, 67–75.

Stasny, E.A. (1986) Estimating gross flows using panel data with nonresponse: an example from the Canadian Labour Force Survey. *Journal of the American Statistical Association*, **81**, 42–47.

Stiratelli, R., Laird, N., and Ware, J. (1984) Random effects models for serial observations with dichotomous response. *Biometrics*, **40**, 961–972.

Stram, D.O. and Lee, J.W. (1994) Variance components testing in the longitudinal mixed effects model. *Biometrics*, **50**, 1171–1177.

Stram, D.A. and Lee, J.W. (1995) Correction to: Variance components testing in the longitudinal mixed effects model. *Biometrics*, **51**, 1196.

Strenio, J.F., Weisberg, H.J., and Bryk, A.S. (1983) Empirical Bayes estimation of individual growth-curve parameters and their relationship to covariates. *Biometrics*, **39**, 71–86.

Sutradhar, B.C. and Das, K. (1999) On the efficiency of regression estimators in generalized linear models for longitudinal data. *Biometrika*, **86**, 459–465.

Tanner, M.A. (1991) *Tools for Statistical Inference: Observed Data and Data Augmentation Methods*. Berlin: Springer-Verlag.

Tanner, M.A. and Wong, W.H. (1987) The calculation of posterior distributions by data augmentation. *Journal of the American Statistical Association*, **82**, 528–550.

Tate, R.F. (1954) Correlation between a discrete and a continuous variable. *Annals of Mathematical Statistics*, **25**, 603–607.

Tate, R.F. (1955) The theory of correlation between two continuous variables when one is dichotomized. *Biometrika*, **42**, 205–216.

Ten Have, T.R., Landis, R., and Weaver, S.L. (1995) Association models for periodontal disease progression: a comparison of methods for clustered binary data. *Statistics in Medicine*, **14**, 413–429.

Thélot, C. (1985) Lois logistiques à deux dimensions. *Annales de l'Insée*, **58**, 123–149.

Thiébaut, R., Jacqmin-Gadda, H., Chêne, G., and Commenges, D. (2002a) Bivariate longitudinal study of CD4+ cell count and HIV RNA taking into account informative drop-out and left censoring of HIV RNA values, in M. Stasinopoulos and G. Touloumi, editors, *Proceedings of the 17th International Workshop on Statistical Modelling*, 521–524, Odense, Denmark.

Thiébaut, R., Jacqmin-Gadda, H., Chêne, G., Leport, C., and Commenges, D. (2002b) Mixed effects models with bivariate and univariate association parameters for longitudinal bivariate binary response data, *Computer Methods and Programs in Biomedicine*, **69**, 249–256.

Thijs, H., Molenberghs, G., Michiels, B., Verbeke, G., and Curran, D. (2002) Strategies to fit pattern-mixture models. *Biostatistics*, **3**, 245–265.

Thijs, H., Molenberghs, G., and Verbeke, G. (2000) The milk protein trial: influence analysis of the dropout process. *Biometrical Journal*, **42**, 617–646.

Thum, Y.M. (1997) Hierarchical linear models for multivariate outcomes, *Journal of Educational and Behavioral Statistics*, **22**(1) 77–108.

Tierny, L. and Kadane, J.B. (1986) Accurate approximations for posterior moments and marginal densities, *Journal of the American Statistical Association*, **81**, 82–86.

Titterington, D.M., Smith, A.F.M., and Makov, U.E. (1985) *Statistical Analysis of Finite Mixture Distributions*. New York: John Wiley & Sons.

Tomasko, L., Helms, R.W., and Snapinn, S.M. (1999) A discriminant analysis extension to mixed models. *Statistics in Medicine*, **18**, 1249–1260.

Troxel, A.B., Harrington, D.P., and Lipsitz, S.R. (1998) Analysis of longitudinal data with non-ignorable non-monotone missing values. *Applied Statistics*, **47**, 425–438.

Tuerlinckx, F., Rijmen, F., Molenberghs, G., Verbeke, G., Briggs, D., Noortgate, W. Van den, Meulders, M., and Boeck, P. De (2004) Estimation and software, in P. De Boeck and M. Wilson, editors, *Explanatory item response models*, Statistics for Social Science and Public Policy, chapter 12, 343–373, Springer-Verlag, New York.

Tyl, R.W., Price, C.J., Marr, M.C., and Kimmel, C.A. (1988) Developmental toxicity evaluation of dietary di(2-ethylhexyl)phthalate in Fischer 344 rats and CD-1 mice. *Fundamental and Applied Toxicology*, **10**, 395–412.

Vach, W. and Blettner, M. (1995) Logistic regresion with incompletely observed categorical covariates–investigating the sensitivity against violation of the missing at random assumption. *Statistics in Medicine*, **12**, 1315–1330.

Van der Linden, A., Verhoye, A., Van Meir, V., Tindemans, I., Eens, M., Absil, P., and Balthazart, J. (2002) In vivo manganese-enhanced magnetic resonance imaging reveals connections and functional properties of the songbird vocal control system. *Neuroscience*, **112**, 467–474.

Van Meir, V., Verhoye, M., Absil, P., Eens, M., Balthazart, J., and Van der Linden, A. (2004) Differential effects of testosterone on neuronal populations and their connections in a sensorimotor brain nucleus controlling song production in songbirds: a manganese enhanced-magnetic resonance imaging study. *Neuroimage*, **21**, 914–923.

Vansteelandt, K. (2000) *Formal models for contextualized personality psychology*, PhD thesis, Catholic University of Leuven, Faculty of Psychology.

Van Steen, K., Molenberghs, G., Verbeke, G., and Thijs, H. (2001) A local influence approach to sensitivity analysis of incomplete longitudinal ordinal data. *Statistical Modelling: A International Journal*, **1**, 125–142.

Verbeke, G. (1995) *The linear mixed model. A critical investigation in the context of longitudinal data analysis*. Ph.D. thesis, Catholic University of Leuven, Faculty of Science, Department of Mathematics.

Verbeke, G. and Lesaffre, E. (1996) A linear mixed-effects model with heterogeneity in the random-effects population. *Journal of the American Statistical Association*, **91**, 217–221.

Verbeke, G. and Lesaffre, E. (1997) The effect of misspecifying the random effects distribution in linear mixed models for longitudinal data. *Computational Statistics and Data Analysis*, **23**, 541–556.

Verbeke, G., Lesaffre, E., and Spiessens, B. (2001) The practical use of different strategies to handle dropout in longitudinal studies. *Drug Information Journal*, **35**, 419–434.

Verbeke, G. and Molenberghs, G. (1997) *Linear Mixed Models in Practice: A SAS-Oriented Approach*. Lecture Notes in Statistics 126. New York: Springer-Verlag.

Verbeke, G. and Molenberghs, G. (2000) *Linear Mixed Models for Longitudinal Data*. New York: Springer-Verlag.

Verbeke, G. and Molenberghs, G. (2003) The use of score tests for inference on variance components, *Biometrics*, **59**, 254–262.

Verbeke, G., Molenberghs, G., Thijs, H., Lesaffre, E., and Kenward, M.G. (2001) Sensitivity analysis for non-random dropout: a local influence approach. *Biometrics*, **57**, 7–14.

Verbeke, G., Spiessens, B., and Lesaffre, E. (2001) Conditional linear mixed models, *The American Statistician*, **55**, 25–34.

Verbyla, A.P., Cullis, B.R., Kenward, M.G., and Welham, S.J. (1999) The analysis of designed experiments and longitudinal data by using smoothing splines. *Applied Statistics* **48**, 269–311.

Verloove, S.P. and Verwey, R.Y. (1988) *Project on preterm and small-for-gestational age infants in the Netherlands, 1983 (Thesis, University of Leiden)*. University Microfilms International, Ann Arbor, Michigan, USA, no. 8807276.

Vonesh, E.F., Wang, H., and Majumdar, D. (2001) Generalized least squares, Taylor series linearization, and Fisher's scoring in multivariate nonlinear regression. *Journal of the American Statistical Association*, **96**, 282–291.

Vonesh, E.F., Wang, H., Nie, L., and Majumdar, D. (2002) Conditional second-order generalized estimating equations for generalized linear and nonlinear mixed-effects models. *Journal of the American Statistical Association*, **97**, 271–283.

Wang, Y.J. (1987) The probability integrals of bivariate normal distributions: a contingency table approach. *Biometrika*, **74**, 185–190.

Waternaux, C., Laird, N.M., and Ware, J.H. (1989) Methods for analysis of longitudinal data: bloodlead concentrations and cognitive development. *Journal of the American Statistical Association*, **84**, 33–41.

Wedderburn, R.W.M. (1974) Quasi-likelihood functions, generalized linear models, and the Gauss-Newton method. *Biometrika*, **61**, 439–447.

Welsh, A.H. (1996) *Aspects of Statistical Inference*. New York: Wiley.

White, I.R. and Goetghebeur, E.J.T. (1998) Clinical trials comparing two treatment arm policies: which aspects of the treatment policies make a difference? *Statistics in Medicine*, **17**, 319–340.

Williams, P.L., Molenberghs, G., and Lipsitz, S.R. (1996) Analysis of multiple ordinal outcomes in developmental toxicity studies. *Journal of Agricultural, Biological, and Environmental Statistics*, **1**, 250–274.

Williamson, J.M., Lipsitz, S.R., and Kim, K.M. (1997) GEECAT and GEEGOR: Computer programs for the analysis of correlated categorical response data. *Technical Report*.

Windholz, M. (1983) *The Merck Index: An Encyclopedia of Chemicals, Drugs, and Biologicals* (M. Windholz, Ed.), 10th ed., Merck and Co., Rahway, NJ.

Wolfinger, R.D. (1998) Towards practical application of generalized linear mixed models, in B. Marx and H. Friedl, editors, *Proceedings of the 13th International Workshop on Statistical Modeling*, 388–395, New Orleans, Louisiana, USA.

Wolfinger, R. and O'Connell, M. (1993) Generalized linear mixed models: a pseudo-likelihood approach. *Journal of Statistical Computation and Simulation*, **48**, 233–243.

Wu, M.C. and Bailey, K.R. (1988) Analysing changes in the presence of informative right censoring caused by death and withdrawal. *Statistics in Medicine*, **7**, 337–346.

Wu, M.C. and Bailey, K.R. (1989) Estimation and comparison of changes in the presence of informative right censoring: conditional linear model. *Biometrics*, **45**, 939–955.

Wu, M.C. and Carroll, R.J. (1988) Estimation and comparison of changes in the presence of informative right censoring by modeling the censoring process. *Biometrics*, **44**, 175–188.

Yule, G.U. and Kendall, M.G. (1950) *An Introduction to the Theory of Statistics* (14 ed.). London: Griffin.

Zeger, S.L. and Karim, M.R. (1991) Generalised linear models with random effects: a Gibbs sampling approach. *Journal of the American Statistical Association*, **86**, 79–102.

Zeger, S.L. and Liang, K.-Y. (1986) Longitudinal data analysis for discrete and continuous outcomes. *Biometrics*, **42**, 121–130.

Zhao, L.P. and Prentice, R.L. (1990) Correlated binary regression using a quadratic exponential model. *Biometrika*, 77, 642–648.

Zhao, L.P., Prentice, R.L., and Self, S.G. (1992) Multivariate mean parameter estimation by using a partly exponential model. *Journal of the Royal Statistical Society B*, **54**, 805–811.

Index

age related macular degeneration trial, *see* ARMD trial
Akaike information criterion, 134
ALR, *see* alternating logistic regressions
alternating logistic regressions, 49, 152, 153, 165–167, 173, 310, 318, 319
    SAS, 205–206, 212–215
analgesic trial, 8, 309–323, 332–333, 383, 388–392, 507–509
ARE, *see* asymptotic relative efficiency
ARMD trial, 24–25, 448–455, 503–506
asymptotic normality, 189, 192, 396
asymptotic relative efficiency, 247
autocorrelation, *see* serial correlation
autoregressive model, 236, 239

background risk, 91

Bahadur model, *see* marginal model
balanced data, 483
balanced design, 483
baseline category, 327
Bayesian inference, 512, 555
beta-binomial model, 260–261
bi-exponential model, 352, 353, 361, 373
BIRNH study, 103–112, 119–121, 329
bootstrap, 195
    Bayesian, 515
    parametric, 195
boundary problem, 41, 379
boundary solution, 413, 548
British occupational study, 56, 62
bucket size, *see* smoothing splines

Caithness data, 56, 62–64
case-control study
    matching, 47, 51
cell probability, 141

CGI, *see* clinical global imression
clinical global imression, 401, 412
clustered data, 88–92, 132, 244
coarsening, 522
coefficient of determination, 398, 401
compartment model, 352, 361, 369, 375
complete case analysis, *see* missing data
complete data, *see* missing data
composite link function, 197
conditional independence, 258, 266, 443–445, 463
conditional logistic regression, 47, 51, 52
conditional model, 47, 49–50, 55–82, 225–254, 393, 437
    exponential family model, 227–233
    transition model, 47, 226, 236–242
consistency, 189, 192, 396
contingency table, 55–84, 92, 125, 135, 533
continuation-ratio model, 327, 329
convergence, 248, 453, 459, 462
Cramèr-Rao inequality, 192
cross ratio, 114, 129
    conditional, 143
    global, 59, 70, 75, 79, 114, 115
    infinite, 66
    local, 58, 60–62
cross-over trial, 84, 100–101, 127–131
    carry-over effect, 128–130
    period effect, 128
    treatment effect, 128, 129
cumulative count, 56, 85
cumulative probability, 126, 141

Dale model, *see* marginal model
data augmentation, 481
delta method, 93, 441, 597
dependence ratio, 95
depression trial, 499–503
design matrix, 85, 90, 97, 331, 444, 484, 544, 546
developmental toxicity study, 174, 251
    Haber's law, 176
    low dose extrapolation, 180
    segment II study, 174
direct likelihood method, *see* missing data
dose-response model, 92, 232, 249, 251, 253, 350, 377, 379
dropout, *see* missing data

efficiency, 396, 514
EGRET software, 296
EM algorithm, 481, 516–527, 532, 535, 580
    acceleration, 518, 520, 537
    convergence, 537
    E step, 425, 517–518, 523, 536
    heterogeneity model, 423–427
    initial step, 517
    M step, 426, 517–518, 523, 536, 537
    missing information, 526
    Monte Carlo EM, 394
    precision estimation, 517, 518, 520–521, 537
    rate matrix, 520
    rate of convergence, 519–520
    SAS, 633–635
empirical Bayes estimation (EB), *see* random effects
epilepsy data, 14, 337–345
    generalized estimating equations, 337–340

generalized linear mixed
    model, 340–345
  Poisson regression, 32–33
equicorrelation, 88
exchangeability, 88, 98, 195–198,
    226, 229, 231, 244, 505
expectation-maximization
    algorithm, see EM
    algorithm
exponential family, 27–28, 125,
    152, 226, 228, 243, 327,
    438, 443
  canonical parameter, 27,
    122, 124, 226
  multivariate, 123
  natural parameter, 27–30
  quadratic, 123, 168
  scale parameter, 27

Fisher information, 317
Fisher scoring, 61, 119, 125, 138,
    164, 197, 199, 201, 228,
    537
Fisher's z-transform, 89, 93, 97,
    112, 121
fluvoxamine trial, 12–14, 56,
    64–68, 74, 92–93,
    134–135, 234, 328–329,
    537–543, 567–572,
    581–590, 599–604
Fréchet inequality, 143
fractional polynomial, 249–254,
    348, 369, 373–374, 380,
    407
frequentist inference, 482, 485,
    512
full data, see missing data

GAUSS software, 441
Gaussian quadrature, 273–276,
    315, 393, 395, 403, 453,
    465
  adaptive, 275–280, 315, 503
  non-adaptive, 274–275,
    277–280, 315, 503

  order of approximation, 274,
    278–280
GEE, see generalized estimating
    equations
GEE2, see generalized
    estimating equations
general location model, 437
generalized estimating equations,
    49, 83, 90, 123,
    151–187, 189, 192,
    195–202, 225, 227,
    309–314, 316, 330, 332,
    438, 447, 465, 488, 507
  empirically corrected
    variance, 156, 159, 310,
    318, 334
  GEE2, 164–165, 200
  hybrid marginal-conditional
    model, 168–169
  linearization based method,
    169–170, 215–219, 310,
    320, 334, 450, 501, 527
  model-based variance, 156,
    310
  naive variance estimator,
    156
  Prentice, 162–164, 310
  robust variance, 156, 198,
    200
  sandwich estimator, 156
  SAS, 204–212, 215–219
  weighted, 498–500, 504, 527
    SAS, 613–618
  working assumption, 155,
    157, 204, 330
    auto-regressive, 157, 310,
      338
    autoregressive, 167
    banded, 167
    exchangeable, 157, 167,
      172, 204, 310, 338
    independence, 157, 172,
      204, 310, 334
    unstructured, 157, 160,
      204, 310, 318, 338, 508

674 Index

generalized linear mixed model, 262–263, 265–280, 393, 403, 406, 412, 439, 462, 500
  approximation of data, 269–273, 410
  approximation of integral, 273–276
  approximation of integrand, 268–269
  Bayesian inference, 266
  empirical Bayes estimation, *see* random effects
  inference, 276–277
  Laplace transformation, 268–269, 276–278, 341
  likelihood, 267
  marginalization, 300–301, 342–345
  maximum likelihood, 266–267
  MQL, *see* marginal quasi-likelihood
  parameter interpretation, 297–306
  Poisson model, 340–342
  PQL, *see* penalized quasi-likelihood
  SAS, 281–296
  software, 296
  versus marginal model, 297–306
generalized linear model, 28, 154, 169, 193, 198, 202, 236, 562
  linear regression, 29
  logistic regression, 29, 31, 56, 102, 105, 114, 135, 154, 157, 228, 237, 241, 245, 310, 326, 327, 332, 437, 440, 507, 537, 553, 566, 578
  maximum likelihood estimation, 30–31
  Poisson regression, 29–30, 32–33, 337–340
  probit regression, 29
GENMOD procedure, 152, 203–212, 238, 240, 318, 326, 331, 332, 334, 338, 440, 500, 501
  BY statement, 626
  CONTRAST statement, 319
  MODEL statement, 241
    'covb' option, 626
    'dist=' option, 205
    'link=' option, 321
    'noint' option, 626
  ODS statement, 626
    'covb=' option, 626
    'parminfo=' option, 626
  output, 206–215
  PROC GENMOD statement
    'descending option, 205
  program, 205–206
  REPEATED statement, 205–206, 313, 319, 334, 618
    'covb' option, 205
    'link=' option, 334
    'logor=' option, 205, 212
    'modelse' option, 205
    'subject=' option, 205
    'type=' option, 205, 212, 334
    'withinsubject=' option, 205, 611
  SCWGT statement, 617
  WEIGHT statement, 617
GLIMMIX macro, 169, 170, 215–219, 287–289, 320
  'empirical=' option, 216
  'error=' option, 215
  'hold=' option, 288
  'link=' option, 215
  'logor=' option, 215
  'printall' option, 216
  'procopt=' option, 215, 288

'rcorr' option, 216
'rcorr=' option, 320
'stmts=' option, 215, 288
'type=' option, 215
output, 216–217, 289
PARMS statement, 288
program, 215–216, 288
REPEATED statement, 216, 218
GLIMMIX procedure, 169, 170, 215–219, 282–287, 315, 320, 332, 340, 410, 416, 427, 451, 455, 460, 462, 465, 494, 500, 526
   CLASS statement, 283
   MODEL statement, 218, 283, 389
      'dist=' option, 284, 456, 457
      'link=' option, 284, 321, 456–458
      'noint' option, 458
   NLOPTIONS statement, 335, 416, 459
      'absftol=' option, 417
      'absgtol=' option, 417
      'technique=' option, 416
   output, 218–219, 284–287, 390–392
   PROC GLIMMIX statement, 283
      'empirical' option, 218
      'method=' option, 218, 283, 320
   program, 218, 283–284, 384–392
   R-side effects, 334
   RANDOM statement, 284, 389, 416
      '_residual_' option, 218
      'subject=' option, 284
      'type=' option, 218, 284, 416, 459
   WEIGHT statement, 618

GLM, see generalized linear model
GLMM, see generalized linear mixed model
global odds ratio, 96
Goodman model, 55, 57–59, 63, 68, 79, 80, 117, 329
goodness-of-fit, 65
   deviance, 75

Haber's law, see developmental toxicity study
heatshock study, 174–177
Hessian matrix, 189, 580
heterogeneity model, 421–423, 430
   classification, 427–428
   EM algorithm, 423–427
   empirical Bayes estimation, 427–428
   estimation, 423–427
   identifiability, 424
   inference, 423–427
   number of components, 422, 423
   posterior probability, 426
heteroscedasticity, 353
hierarchical generalized linear model, 263, 394, 417
HLM software, 296
homogeneity model, 421, 432
homoscedasticity, 353
hybrid marginal-conditional model, 122–127, 168–169, 174–187, 226

identifiability, 58, 379, 398, 599
identifying restrictions, see pattern-mixture model
ignorable missing data, see missing data
IML procedure, 409
imputation, 492–494
   conditional, 494

last observation carried
    forward, 489, 493,
    495–497, 505, 506
  SAS, 609–611
multiple, 482, 490, 492, 504,
    511–516, 526–527, 560,
    567, 569
  analysis task, 624–629
  hypothesis testing, 514
  MCMC method, 516, 528
  propensity score method,
    515
  regression method, 515
  SAS, 618–633
  semi-parametric, 512
single, 492
unconditional, 493
incomplete data, see missing
    data
indomethacin study, 351–355,
    361–363, 385–386
influence analysis, 545
influenza study, 99–102
information matrix, 90, 125
intraclass correlation, 322
iterative proportional fitting, 49,
    117, 125, 140, 141, 166,
    168
iteratively reweighted least
    squares, 169, 537

joint model
  bivariate model, 186, 469,
    472
  continuous and discrete,
    437–465
  dimensionality problem, 471
  generalized linear mixed
    model, 442–445,
    447–448, 454, 465,
    469–471
  high dimensional, 467–477
  inference, 471–473
  linear mixed model, 469–471
  model fitting, 471–473

  multivariate model, 469
  non-linear mixed model,
    469–471
  pairwise fitting, 471–472
  pairwise likelihood, 472
  Plackett-Dale model, 438,
    439, 441–442, 445,
    447–448, 453, 465
  probit-normal model,
    438–441, 446–447, 452,
    453, 465
  pseudo-likelihood, 472–473
  SAS, 455–464
  semiparametric model, 438
  shared-parameter model,
    470
  univariate model, 468

kappa coefficient, 221, 237
Kronecker delta, 139

Lagrange multiplier, 49
Laplace transformation, see
    generalized linear
    mixed model
last observation carried forward
    (LOCF), see
    imputation
latent variable, 79, 107, 110, 118,
    395, 398, 405, 406, 410,
    417, 445, 446, 449
likelihood function, 267, 327,
    335, 395, 487, 533, 545,
    563
  factorization, 487
  full data, 487
  observed data, 564
  perturbed, 579
likelihood ratio, 160, 192–195,
    200, 540, 548, 584, 590
linear mixed model, 36–39, 158,
    260, 345, 405, 452
  hierarchical model, 38, 299
  inference, 39–41
  marginal model, 38, 299

maximum likelihood, 40
parameter interpretation, 299
restricted maximum likelihood, 40, 272
linear predictor, 57, 61, 118, 124, 170, 237, 314, 317
linearization based method, *see* generalized estimating equations
link function, 57, 73, 94, 98, 118, 124, 127, 140, 170, 562
   complementary log-log, 57, 94, 334
   composite, 89
   cumulative, 334
   identity, 457
   logit, 57, 89, 94, 118, 124, 125, 130, 170, 321, 334, 404, 440, 443, 448, 450, 457
      adjacent-category, 57
      baseline-category, 57, 127
      cumulative, 57, 59, 334
   probit, 57, 94, 118, 321, 334, 394, 414, 440, 448, 450, 457
local dependence function, 79
log-linear model, 49, 58, 79, 143, 226, 543
LOGISTIC procedure, 238, 240, 329, 440, 501
logistic regression, *see* generalized linear model

macro, *see* SAS macro
marginal correlation coefficient, 87, 95
marginal model, 47–50, 55–149, 195, 225, 233–234, 309, 318, 325, 329–331, 568
   Bahadur model, 48, 61, 83, 86–93, 97, 131, 134, 142, 151, 157, 165, 169, 171, 189, 200, 230, 233, 261, 533
   Dale model, 56, 59–61, 83, 93–102, 113–135, 166, 189, 226, 325, 329, 450, 534, 566, 580
   generalized linear model, 443, 448, 452, 462
   parameter interpretation, 297–306
   probit model, 93–113, 132, 189, 325, 329, 394
   SAS, 203–221
   software, 221
   versus random-effects model, 297–306, 342–345
marginal quasi-likelihood, 270–273, 277–278, 315, 316, 320, 333, 334, 393, 403, 410, 418, 465
   maximum likelihood, 272, 277–278
   restricted maximum likelihood, 272, 277–278
   versus penalized quasi-likelihood, 277–278, 301–306, 340–342
Markov chain Monte Carlo, 243, 515
Markov model, 236
maximum likelihood, 61, 74, 83–149, 151, 177, 181, 189, 228, 234, 244, 246, 250, 395, 399, 526, 592, 595
measurement process, *see* missing data
meta-analysis, 401–403, 412–414, 447
MI procedure, 515, 527, 618–624, 633
   BY statement, 619, 620
   CLASS statement, 620

EM algorithm, 633–635
EM statement, 633
'converge=' option, 633
'initial=' option, 634
'itprint' option, 634
'maxiter=' option, 634
'out=' option, 634
'outem=' option, 634
'outiter=' option, 634
MCMC statement, 619
'impute=' option, 633
'initial=' option, 619, 620
'niter=' option, 620
'pmm' option, 619
MONOTONE statement, 619
'discrim' option, 620
'logistic' option, 620
'method=' option, 619
'ngroups=' option, 619
'regpmm' option, 619
PROC MI statement
'nimpute=' option, 619, 620, 633
'round=' option, 619, 620
'seed=' option, 619, 620
'simple' option, 619
VAR statement, 619, 620
MIANALYZE procedure, 625, 629–633
CLASS statement, 629
MODELEFFECTS statement, 629
PROC MIANALYZE statement
'bcov' option, 629
'covb=' option, 629, 631
'data=' option, 629
'parminfo=' option, 629
'parms=' option, 629
'tcov' option, 629
'wcov' option, 629
'xpxi=' option, 629
TEST statement, 629

missing at random (MAR), see missing data
missing completely at random (MCAR), see missing data
missing data, 135, 482–488
complete case analysis, 489, 492, 495–497, 505, 506
SAS, 607–609
complete data, 483
covariates, 526
direct likelihood, 521, 527, 611–612
GLIMMIX procedure, 611
MIXED procedure, 611
NLMIXED procedure, 611
dropout, 481, 483
full data, 483, 490
generalized estimating equations, 345, 531
identifiable parameter, 485
ignorability, 482, 487–488, 490, 491, 494–497, 531, 575
Bayesian inference, 487
frequentist inference, 487
imputation, see imputation
last observation carried forward (LOCF), see imputation
measurement process, 483
mechanism, 484
MAR, 482, 486, 489, 494, 496, 497, 503, 507, 512, 528, 531, 537, 542, 556, 571, 575, 584, 598
MCAR, 309, 482, 485–486, 489, 491, 496, 501, 507, 527, 542, 545, 549, 584
MNAR, 482, 486–487, 494, 512, 531, 535, 541, 542, 550, 553, 573, 575, 577, 584

missing data indicators, 483
missing data process, 483
observed data, 483, 490
overspecified model, 592
pattern, 483
   attrition, 483
   dropout, 491, 504, 533, 561, 566, 573
   intermittent missingness, 481, 505, 527
   monotone, 483, 504, 515, 526
   non-monotone, 483, 543–552
pattern-mixture model, 481, 484, 486, 532, 555–573, 587, 604
   ACMV, 556, 558, 560, 566
   CCMV, 558, 560, 566
   identifying restrictions, 556–561, 565–566, 604
   MNFD, 558
   NCMV, 558, 560, 566
   NFMV, 559
   precision, 566–567
SAS, 607–636
selection model, 481, 484, 485, 531–553, 555, 561, 568–569, 577
sensitivity analysis, 482, 494, 532, 555, 575–605
   ignorance, 590–604
   imprecision, 576, 590–604
   influence, 576
   influence graph, 583, 587
   interval of ignorance, 590–604
   local influence, 577–590
   uncertainty, 576, 590–604
separability condition, 487
shared-parameter model, 484
missing data indicators, *see* missing data

missing data mechanism, *see* missing data
missing data pattern, *see* missing data
missing data process, *see* missing data
missing not at random (MNAR), *see* missing data
MIXED procedure, 451, 494, 526
MIXOR software, 296, 315, 317, 321–322
MIXREG software, 296
mixture distribution
   number of components, 422, 423
   random effects, 380, 420, 421
MLwiN software, 315, 323, 401
   multilevel model, 393, 404, 405, 417
moment-based estimate, 157
Monte Carlo integration, 243
MQL, *see* marginal quasi-likelihood
multigroup logistic model, 70, 127, 327
multilevel model, *see* MLwiN
multiple imputation, *see* imputation
multiple outcomes, *see* joint model
multivariate Dale model, 117, 121
multivariate probit model, 96
multivariate regression, 36
multivariate repeated measures, *see* joint model

National Toxicology Program data, *see* NTP data
Newton-Raphson, 61, 90, 138, 197, 201, 228, 315, 442, 503, 523, 565
NLIN procedure, 351

NLMIXED procedure, 238,
    290–296, 315, 317, 329,
    332, 333, 335, 340, 362,
    427, 451, 460, 465, 494,
    500, 526
  BY statement, 628
  ESTIMATE statement, 388
  MODEL statement, 291,
    385
    general likelihood, 291
  ODS statement, 628
    'additionalestimates='
      option, 629
    'covmataddest=' option,
      629
    'covmatparmest=' option,
      628
    'parameterestimates='
      option, 628
  output, 293–296
  PARMS statement, 291, 385
  PREDICT statement, 385
  PROC NLMIXED
    statement, 290
    'alpha=' option, 295
    'cov' option, 629
    'ecov' option, 629
    'noad' option, 290, 321
    'qpoints=' option, 290,
      321
  program, 290–293
  RANDOM statement, 291,
    385, 612
    'out=' option, 293
    'subject=' option, 293
nominal data, 57, 78, 326, 335
non-ignorable missing data, see
    missing data
non-linear mixed model,
    357–392, 485
non-linear model, 347–392
  longitudinal, 355–378
    continuous, 357–376
    discrete, 376–378
    SAS, 384–392
  smoothing splines,
    379–383
  univariate, 349–355
nonparametric maximum
    likelihood (NPML),
    259, 380
notation, 84, 561
  contingency table notation,
    85, 93, 147
  regression notation, 84
NTP data, 17–23, 90–92,
    170–173, 200–202,
    234–236, 246–254, 315,
    316
  conditional model, 304–306
  DEHP, 18–22, 200, 219–221,
    304–306, 378
  DYME, 22–23, 200, 378
  EG, 18, 249–254, 378
  generalized linear mixed
    model, 277–278,
    304–306
  marginal model, 219–221,
    304–306
  non-linear mixed model,
    377–378, 388
numerical integration, see
    Gaussian quadrature

observed data, see missing data
odds ratio, 125, 165–167, 186,
    201, 253, 311–313, 318,
    319, 449, 568, 569
  conditional, 123, 141, 168
  exchangeable, 312
  global, 59, 114, 115, 127,
    138, 142, 329, 442
  local, 58, 78, 127, 141
  marginal, 48, 123, 124, 168,
    243
  three-way, 78
  unstructured, 312
offset, 32, 167
orange tree data, 358–359,
    384–385

ordinal data, 56, 57, 59, 67, 81, 85, 106, 110, 127, 141, 325–335, 438, 532
ordinal regression, 315
overdispersion, 88, 155, 230, 236, 323, 443, 459, 505
overdispersion parameter, 154, 155, 157, 169, 170

pairwise likelihood, *see* pseudo-likelihood
parameter space constraints, 48, 86, 89, 90, 92, 134, 151, 230, 232, 233
pattern-mixture model, *see* missing data
penalized quasi-likelihood, 270–273, 277–278, 315, 317, 333, 334, 393, 401, 403, 406, 410, 414, 417, 448, 453, 465, 503, 506, 527
   maximum likelihood, 272, 277–278
   restricted maximum likelihood, 272, 277–278
   versus marginal quasi-likelihood, 277–278, 301–306, 340–342
pharmacodynamics, 360–368
pharmacokinetics, 351, 360–369, 375
Plackett distribution, 49, 66, 80, 93, 114, 116, 118, 125, 142–148, 166, 196, 226, 438
Poisson regression, *see* generalized linear model
polychoric correlation, 104, 110, 112
POPS data, 14–16, 131–134
Positive and negative symptoms scale, 401, 412

PQL, *see* penalized quasi-likelihood
primary dysmenorrhoea study, 127–131
probit regression, *see* generalized linear model
probit-normal model, 262, 394–410
profile likelihood, 566, 597
proportional odds, 98, 118, 326, 328–332, 539
pseudo-likelihood, 49, 50, 189–202, 225, 227, 235, 243–254, 393–418, 447, 465
   definition, 190
   empirically corrected variance, 247
   joint model, 472–473
   model based variance, 247
   pairwise likelihood, 394, 408, 472
   robust variance, 192, 198, 200, 396, 409, 473
   weighted, 404
psycho-cognitive functioning study, 473–477

quasi-likelihood, 52, 151, 169, 200

R software, 221
   nlme, 494
radial base function, *see* smoothing splines
random effects, 38
   conjugate distribution, 263
   empirical Bayes estimation, 41–43, 268, 359, 419, 427–428
   heterogeneity model, 421–423, 430
   homogeneity model, 421, 432
   mixing distribution, 259

mixture of normals, 420, 421
normality assumption, 37, 43, 260, 419–435
posterior distribution, 42, 268
shrinkage, 42
random-effects model, 47, 50–51, 314–317, 320, 331, 393, 452
  parameter interpretation, 297–306
  versus marginal model, 297–306, 342–345
Rasch model, 128
RC model, *see* row-column model, 58–59
restricted maximum likelihood (REML), *see* linear mixed model
row-column model, 56, 57, 60, 61, 78

sampling zero, 187
SAS macro
  CC, 607–608
  DROPOUT, 240, 613–614
  DROPWGT, 615–616
  GLIMMIX, *see* GLIMMIX macro
  LOCF, 609–610
  PLRINT_CORR, 415
schizophrenia study, 401–403, 412–414
score equation, 136, 140, 169, 189, 197, 200, 498, 563, 565
score function, 90, 522
score test, 106, 110, 160, 193–194, 540
selection model, *see* missing data
sensitivity analysis, *see* missing data
separability condition, *see* missing data

serial correlation, 236, 403, 405–418, 442, 465
  AR(1), 410
  exponential decay, 407, 410, 413
  Gaussian decay, 407, 410
shared-parameter model, *see* joint model
smoothing parameter, *see* smoothing splines
smoothing splines, 380–383
  bucket size, 383, 389
  radial base function, 382
  SAS, 388–392
  smoothing parameter, 382
  spline coefficient, 382
  spline knot, 382
  thin-plate splines, 382
songbird data, 368–376, 387–388
spline coefficient, *see* smoothing splines
spline knot, *see* smoothing splines
splines, *see* smoothing splines
SPlus software, 221
  nlme, 494
sports injuries trial, 23–24, 181–187
SPSS software, 221
Stata software, 221, 296
  gllamm procedure, 296
structural zero, 186
subject-specific model, 47, 50–51, 257–263
  conditional approach, 258–259
  fixed-effects approach, 47, 258
  random-effects approach, 47, 259–260
SUDAAN software, 221
surrogate endpoint, 394, 405, 439
surrogate marker, 397–404, 412, 439, 448

temporal assocation, 98
tetrachoric correlation, 104, 107
theophylline data, 363–367, 386–387
thin-plate splines, *see* smoothing splines
toenail data, 8–12, 238–240
    alternating logistic regressions, 212–215
    generalized estimating equations, 204–212, 215–219, 297–298, 301–304
    generalized linear mixed model, 278–298, 301–304
    logistic regression, 31
    marginal models, 203–219
transition model, *see* conditional model

two-stage analysis, 355, 362, 366

underdispersion, 230
upward compatibility, 233

verbal aggression data, 428–434

Wald test, 186, 193, 248, 276, 312, 313, 319, 540
weighted estimating equations, *see* generalized estimating equations
working assumption, *see* generalized estimating equations

zero cell, 66
    sampling zero, 187
    structural zero, 186

Springer Series in Statistics *(continued from p. ii)*

Huet/Bouvier/Poursat/Jolivet: Statistical Tools for Nonlinear Regression: A Practical Guide with S-PLUS and R Examples, 2nd edition.
Ibrahim/Chen/Sinha: Bayesian Survival Analysis.
Jolliffe: Principal Component Analysis, 2nd edition.
Knottnerus: Sample Survey Theory: Some Pythagorean Perspectives.
Kolen/Brennan: Test Equating: Methods and Practices.
Kotz/Johnson (Eds.): Breakthroughs in Statistics Volume I.
Kotz/Johnson (Eds.): Breakthroughs in Statistics Volume II.
Kotz/Johnson (Eds.): Breakthroughs in Statistics Volume III.
Küchler/Sørensen: Exponential Families of Stochastic Processes.
Kutoyants: Statistical Influence for Ergodic Diffusion Processes.
Lahiri: Resampling Methods for Dependent Data.
Le Cam: Asymptotic Methods in Statistical Decision Theory.
Le Cam/Yang: Asymptotics in Statistics: Some Basic Concepts, 2nd edition.
Liu: Monte Carlo Strategies in Scientific Computing.
Longford: Models for Uncertainty in Educational Testing.
Manski: Partial Identification of Probability Distributions.
Mielke/Berry: Permutation Methods: A Distance Function Approach.
Molenberghs/Verbeke: Models for Discrete Longitudinal Data.
Pan/Fang: Growth Curve Models and Statistical Diagnostics.
Parzen/Tanabe/Kitagawa: Selected Papers of Hirotugu Akaike.
Politis/Romano/Wolf: Subsampling.
Ramsay/Silverman: Applied Functional Data Analysis: Methods and Case Studies.
Ramsay/Silverman: Functional Data Analysis, 2nd edition.
Rao/Toutenburg: Linear Models: Least Squares and Alternatives.
Reinsel: Elements of Multivariate Time Series Analysis, 2nd edition.
Rosenbaum: Observational Studies, 2nd edition.
Rosenblatt: Gaussian and Non-Gaussian Linear Time Series and Random Fields.
Särndal/Swensson/Wretman: Model Assisted Survey Sampling.
Santner/Williams/Notz: The Design and Analysis of Computer Experiments.
Schervish: Theory of Statistics.
Shao/Tu: The Jackknife and Bootstrap.
Simonoff: Smoothing Methods in Statistics.
Singpurwalla and Wilson: Statistical Methods in Software Engineering: Reliability and Risk.
Small: The Statistical Theory of Shape.
Sprott: Statistical Inference in Science.
Stein: Interpolation of Spatial Data: Some Theory for Kriging.
Taniguchi/Kakizawa: Asymptotic Theory of Statistical Inference for Time Series.
Tanner: Tools for Statistical Inference: Methods for the Exploration of Posterior Distributions and Likelihood Functions, 3rd edition.
van der Laan: Unified Methods for Censored Longitudinal Data and Causality.
van der Vaart/Wellner: Weak Convergence and Empirical Processes: With Applications to Statistics.
Verbeke/Molenberghs: Linear Mixed Models for Longitudinal Data.
Weerahandi: Exact Statistical Methods for Data Analysis.
West/Harrison: Bayesian Forecasting and Dynamic Models, 2nd edition.

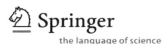 **Springer**
the language of science

springeronline.com

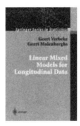

Linear Mixed Models for Longitudinal Data
G. Verbeke and G. Molenberghs

This book provides a comprehensive treatment of linear mixed models for continuous longitudinal data. Next to model formulation, this edition puts major emphasis on exploratory data analysis for all aspects of the model, such as the marginal model, subject-specific profiles, and residual covariance structure. Further, model diagnostics and missing data receive extensive treatment. Sensitivity analysis for incomplete data is given a prominent place. Several variations to the conventional linear mixed model are discussed (a heterogeity model, conditional linear mid models). This book will be of interest to applied statisticians and biomedical researchers in industry, public health organizations, contract research organizations, and academia. The book is explanatory rather than mathematically rigorous. Most analyses were done with the MIXED procedure of the SAS software package, and many of its features are clearly elucidated.

1997. 568 p. (Springer Series in Statistics) Hardcover ISBN 0-387-95027-3

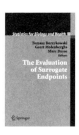

The Evaluation of Surrogate Endpoints
T. Burzykowski, G. Molenberghs, and M. Buyse

Surrogate endpoints are useful when they can be measured earlier, more conveniently, or more frequently than the "true" endpoints of primary interest. Regulatory agencies around the globe are introducing provisions and policies relating to the use of surrogate endpoints in registration studies. But how can one establish the adequacy of a surrogate? What kind of evidence is needed, and what statistical methods portray that evidence most appropriately? This book offers a balanced account on this controversial topic. The text presents major developments of the last couple of decades, together with a unified, meta-analytic framework within which surrogates can be evaluated from several angles. Methodological development is coupled with perspectives on various therapeutic areas.

2005. 416 p. (Statistics for Biology and Health) Hardcover ISBN 0-387-20277-3

Easy Ways to Order ▶ Call: Toll-Free 1-800-SPRINGER • E-mail: orders-ny@springer.sbm.com • Write: Springer, Dept. S8113, PO Box 2485, Secaucus, NJ 07096-2485 • Visit: Your local scientific bookstore or urge your librarian to order.